Practical Biochemistry

With Clinical Correlation According to New Competency-Based Curriculum

Clinical cases, viva voce, AETCOM, SDL, ECE, Horizontal and vertical integration, log activity, interpretation of laboratory results, spotters, OSCE, OSPE, lesson plans

Practical Biochemistry

With Clinical Correlation According to New Competency-Based Curriculum

As per the Revised Competency-Based Medical Education Curriculum (NMC)

Second Edition

Nita Sahi
MSc (Medicine) Biochemistry PhD (Medicine) Biochemistry
Professor and Head
Department of Biochemistry
Dean Academics (UG, PG)
Pacific Medical College and Hospital
Udaipur, Rajasthan, India

Disha Sahi
MBBS
Pacific Medical College and Hospital
Udaipur, Rajasthan, India

JAYPEE

JAYPEE BROTHERS MEDICAL PUBLISHERS
The Health Sciences Publisher
New Delhi | London

Jaypee Brothers Medical Publishers (P) Ltd

Headquarters
EMCA House
23/23-B, Ansari Road, Daryaganj
New Delhi 110 002, India
Landline: +91-11-23272143, +91-11-23272703
+91-11-23282021, +91-11-23245672
E-mail: jaypee@jaypeebrothers.com

Corporate Office
4838/24, Ansari Road, Daryaganj
New Delhi 110 002, India
Phone: +91-11-43574357
Fax: +91-11-43574314
E-mail: jaypee@jaypeebrothers.com

Overseas Office
J.P. Medical Ltd
83 Victoria Street, London
SW1H 0HW (UK)
Phone: +44 20 3170 8910
E-mail: info@jpmedpub.com

EU GPSR Authorised Representative
Logos Europe, 9 rue Nicolas Poussin
17000, La Rochelle, France
Phone: +33 (0) 6 67 93 73 78
E-mail: contact@logoseurope.eu

Website: www.jaypeebrothers.com
Website: www.jaypeedigital.com

Inquiries for bulk sales may be solicited at: jaypee@jaypeebrothers.com

Practical Biochemistry with Clinical Correlation According to New Competency-Based Curriculum

First Edition: 2022
Second Edition: **2026**

ISBN: 978-93-5696-074-9

Dedicated to

My Husband

Dr Mukesh Sahi

and

Daughter

Dr Disha Sahi (MBBS)

Reviewers List

Ajay Jain
Assistant Professor
Department of Biochemistry
Jawaharlal Nehru Medical College
Ajmer, Rajasthan, India

Ashish Sharma
Professor and Head
Department of Biochemistry
Geetanjali Medical College
Udaipur, Rajasthan, India

Boinapalli Sudhakar
Professor
Department of Biochemistry
Surabhi Institute of Medical Sciences
Siddipet, Mundrai, Telangana, India

Deepa Thadani
Senior Professor
Department of Biochemistry
Jawaharlal Nehru Medical College
Ajmer, Rajasthan, India

Deepak Parchwani
Additional Professor and Head
Department of Biochemistry
All India Institute of Medical Sciences
Rajkot, Gujarat, India

Dharmveer Yadav
Associate Professor
Department of Biochemistry
All India Institute of Medical Sciences
Jodhpur, Rajasthan, India

Harish Kumawat
Professor
Tirupati College of Nursing
Udaipur, Rajasthan, India

Jairam Rawtani
Ex Senior Professor and Head
Department of Biochemistry
Dr SN Medical College
Jodhpur, Rajasthan, India

Kamlesh Kumar Swami
Professor and Head
Department of Biochemistry
CU Shah Medical College
Surendranagar, Gujarat, India

Ketan Mangukia
Associate Professor
Department of Biochemistry
Parul Institute of Medical Sciences and Research
Parul University
Vadodara, Gujarat, India

Neha Sharma
Professor
Department of Biochemistry
Geetanjali Medical College and Hospital
Udaipur, Rajasthan, India

Neeraj Mahajan
Associate Professor
Department of Physiology
Smt NHL Municipal Medical College
Ahmedabad, Gujarat, India

Nitin Sharma
Professor
Department of Biochemistry
Jawaharlal Nehru Medical College
Ajmer, Rajasthan, India

Rajul Lodha
Professor
Department of Biochemistry
Ravindra Nath Tagore Medical College
Udaipur, Rajasthan, India

Ravi Bhatia
Professor
Department of Pediatrics
Pacific Medical College and Hospital
Udaipur, Rajasthan, India

Ravi
Principal
Pacific Dental College and Research Center
Udaipur, Rajasthan, India

Renuka Z Lal
Professor
Department of Biochemistry
Ravindra Nath Tagore Medical College
Udaipur, Rajasthan, India

Richa K Lath
Professor and Head
Department of Biochemistry
Shri Shankaracharya Institute of Medical Sciences
Bhilai, Chhattisgarh, India

Ritu Bhatnagar
Professor and Head
Department of Microbiology
Pacific Medical College and Hospital
Udaipur, Rajasthan, India

SK Mehta
Professor
Department of Psychiatry
Pacific Medical College and Hospital
Udaipur, Rajasthan, India

Sarla Mahawar
Professor
Department of Biochemistry
Jawaharlal Nehru Medical College
Ajmer, Rajasthan, India

Shallu Gupta
Assistant Professor
Department of Biochemistry
SMS Medical College
Jaipur, Rajasthan, India

Shweta Biyani
Professor
Ravindra Nath Tagore Medical College
Udaipur, Rajasthan, India

Vandana Verma
Associate Professor
Department of Biochemistry
Mahatma Gandhi Memorial Medical College
Indore, Madhya Pradesh, India

Yogita Soni
Senior Professor and Head
Department of Biochemistry
Sardar Patel Medical College
Bikaner, Rajasthan, India

Advisory Committee

Preface to the Second Edition

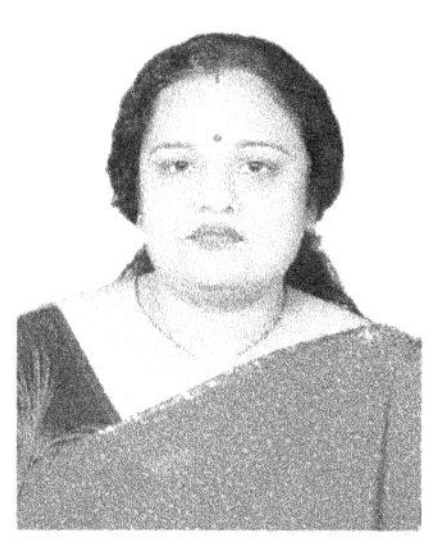

Biochemistry, as the molecular language of life, provides the essential framework for understanding the structure, function, and regulation of biomolecules within the human body. The practical component of biochemistry is not merely a laboratory extension of theory; it is a discipline in itself—training the mind in observation, interpretation, and scientific reasoning.

This book is conceived with the aim of introducing students to the fundamental principles and applied aspects of biochemistry through a structured and clinically conscious practical manual. Emphasis has been laid on accuracy in technique, clarity in documentation, and logical interpretation of biochemical findings.

Each exercise is methodically organized to include objectives, principles, procedures, observations, inferences, relevant viva voce questions, MCQs, Structured Clinical Case Scenarios, Spotters, OSCE, and OSPE. The intent is not merely to train students in laboratory techniques, but to foster a deeper conceptual understanding of biochemical processes and their interpretative relevance.

The content aligns with current medical education standards and seeks to cultivate critical thinking, scientific integrity, and a disciplined approach to experimental biochemistry. Clinical correlations are included selectively, only where they reinforce the core biochemical concept, thereby maintaining the academic purity of the subject.

It is hoped that this book will serve as a dependable and intellectually stimulating companion for undergraduate as well as postgraduate students, and also as a reference point for educators, clinicians, and examiners.

I express my sincere gratitude to all those who have contributed, directly or indirectly, to the development of this work. I welcome suggestions and constructive feedback for future editions.

The second edition of this book is based on competency-based medical education (CBME) curriculum implemented by the National Medical Council (NMC) in the year 2024. It focuses on the development of all the latest and updated required competencies for a successful Indian medical graduate. Care has been taken to provide horizontal and vertical integrations to develop the conceptual, clinical, correlated, and applied knowledge.

The book will be helpful for clinicians, MBBS (undergraduates) and MD Biochemistry (postgraduates), BDS, MDS, BSc Nursing, Post basic nursing, MSc Nursing, MSc Medicine Biochemistry, BPT, paramedical courses and most importantly for PG entrance examinations (NEXT/NEET-PG).

I sincerely hope and pray that the book will be appreciated by the medical, paramedical, and nonmedical students and faculties of both undergraduates and postgraduates.

The Medical Council of India has revised the undergraduate medical education curriculum so that an Indian Medical Graduate (IMG) is able to recognize "health for all" as a national goal. He/she should also be able to fulfill his/her societal obligations. The revised curriculum has specified the competencies that a student must attain and clearly defined teaching learning strategies for the same. With this goal in mind, early clinical exposure, integrated teaching—both horizontal and vertical, skill development, AETCOM and self-directed learning have been introduced in my book. There would be emphasis on communication skills, basic clinical skills, and professionalism. There is a paradigm shift from the traditional didactic classroom-based teaching to learning environments where there is emphasis on learning by exploring, questioning, applying, discussing, analyzing, reflecting, collaborating, and doing. The recognition of this need is enshrined by a greatly enhanced allocation of time to these methods and also the assessment techniques. With this view in mind, the book has been designed as per the guidelines of competency-based curriculum. The highlighted features of the book include skill-based competencies, clinical correlations of qualitative and quantitative experiments, group experiments and demonstrations, case histories, interpretations of laboratory results of all metabolisms, viva voce, integrated approach and early clinical exposure, and last but not the least clinical case spots.

Nita Sahi

Preface to the First Edition

This book is based on competency-based medical education (CBME) curriculum implemented by Medical Council of India (MCI). It focuses on development of all the required competencies for a successful Indian medical graduate. Care has been taken to provide horizontal and vertical integrations to develop the conceptual, clinical, correlated and applied knowledge.

The book will be helpful for MBBS, BDS, BSc nursing, Post basic nursing, MSc nursing, PG Biochemistry, paramedical courses and for PG entrance examinations.

I sincerely hope and pray that the book will be appreciated by the medical and paramedical students and faculties both undergraduates and postgraduates.

The Medical Council of India has revised the undergraduate medical education curriculum so that the Indian Medical Graduate (IMG) is able to recognize **"health for all"** as a national goal. He/she should also be able to fulfill his/her societal obligations. The revised curriculum has specified the competencies that a student must attain and clearly defined teaching learning strategies for the same. With this goal in mind, early clinical exposure, integrated teaching, skill development, AETCOM and self-directed learning have been introduced. There would be emphasis on communication skills, basic clinical skills and professionalism. There is a paradigm shift from the traditional didactic classroom-based teaching to learning environments where there is emphasis on learning by exploring, questioning, applying, discussing, analyzing, reflecting, collaborating and doing. The recognition of this need is enshrined by a greatly enhanced allocation of time to these methods and also the assessment techniques. With this view in mind, the book has been designed as per the guidelines of competency based curriculum.

Nita Sahi

Acknowledgments

First, I thank Almighty for giving me the courage to write the book and finally doing it with success.

My heartfelt thanks go to our management Mr Rahul Agarwal, Mrs Preeti Agarwal, and Mr Aman Agarwal.

I would like to thank respected Dr M M Mangal, President of PMU; Dr Ummed Parihar, Dean PMCH; Dr Apoorva Vohra, Professor, Department of Radiology; and Dr S K Verma, Professor Emeritus (General Medicine), for immense support and encouragement.

I will also like to acknowledge the whole team of M/s Jaypee Brothers Medical Publishers (P) Ltd, New Delhi, India, especially, Shri Jitendar P Vij (Group Chairman), Mr Ankit Vij (Managing Director), Mr MS Mani (Group President), Dr Madhu Choudhary (Director-Educational Publishing), Ms Pooja Bhandari [Director-Production (Books and Journals)], Mr Ajay Kumar Sharma [Deputy General Manager (Books and Journals)], Ms Sunita Katla (Executive Assistant to Group Chairman and Publishing Manager), Ms Samina Khan (Executive Assistant to Director-Educational Publishing), Dr Megha Jain (Editorial Manager), Mr Vijay Kumar Bhatia (Manager-Production), Bishan Singh (Production Manager), Ms Seema Dogra (Cover Visualizer), Ms Neha Verma (Graphic Designer-Cover), Mr Manoj Kushwaha (Proofreader), Mr Dinesh Bhardwaj (Typesetter), Mr Rajesh Ghurkundi (Graphic Designer) and the whole team members.

Motivation of my dear students is the driving force behind this accomplishment. Encouragement by my friends, seniors, and colleagues has helped me throughout this journey.

Words cannot express the gratitude I feel toward my husband Dr Mukesh Sahi and my daughter Dr Disha Sahi.

Nita Sahi

Department of Biochemistry

Student's Profile

ROLL NO: ______________________________

PASSPORT SIZE
PHOTO

DATE OF JOINING: ______________________________

NAME : ______________________________

FATHER'S NAME: ______________________________

DATE OF BIRTH: ______________________________

Email ID: ______________________________

MOBILE NO: ______________________________

ADDRESS (PRESENT): ______________________________

Student's Signature

Certificate

Department of Biochemistry

This is to certify that the candidate Mr/Ms ____

Roll no. ____________________ Course __________________________ admitted in the year ____________ has satisfactorily completed all assignments/requirements as per the Competency Based Curriculum in the subject of Biochemistry during the period from ________________ to ________________.

Date: ______/______/

Place: ____

Head of Department
Department of Biochemistry
(Signature & Seal)

Distribution of Subject Wise Teaching Hours for Phase-1 MBBS

Subject	Large group teaching	SGT/ Practical/Tutorials/ Seminars	SDL	Total
Foundation course				80
Anatomy	180	430	10	620
Physiology	130	305	10	445
Biochemistry*	82	157	10	249
Early clinical exposure (ECE)**	—	27	—	27
Community Medicine	20	20	—	40
Family adoption program (FAP)	—	24	—	24
(AETCOM)***	—	26	—	26
Sports and extra-curricular activities	—	—	—	10
Total	412	989	30	1521

SGT: Small group teaching; SDL: Self-directed learning
*Including molecular biology
**Minimum ECE hours. These hours are to be divided equally by anatomy, physiology and biochemistry.
***AETCOM module is a longitudinal program

Phase of course	Theory	Practicals	Passing criteria
Phase-I MBBS			
Biochemistry—2 papers	Paper 1-100 Paper 2-100	100	Mandatory to get 40% marks Theory and in practicals; and totally 50% for theory plus practicals

Suggested format for a theory paper—Universities and colleges may design their unique question paper blueprint as per the principles given in the format

Duration: 3 hours **100 marks**

	Type of question/ Number of questions	Marks per question
Q. No. 1	Scenario based MCQ/10–20	1–2
Q. No. 2	Long essay question/ONE	10–12
Q. No. 3	Reasoning Questions/FIVE	3
Q. No. 4	Short notes (applied aspects)/FOUR: All four subparts related to six integrated topics if subject is part of integrated modules. However, if a subject has less competencies in integrated module than at least 2 sub-parts from integrated modules	4–5
Q. No. 5	Short notes/THREE	5–6
Q. No. 6	Short notes/FOUR (one sub part of 5 marks from AETCOM)	4–5

SAMPLE OF INTEGRATED LECTURES OR SGT

Suggested Phase-I Alignment Table (Anatomy, Physiology and Biochemistry)
(Topics written here are indicative and can be adjusted if required)

Month	Anatomy	Physiology	Biochemistry
1	• General anatomy • Lower limb (LL)	General physiology, blood	Cell membrane and organelles, extracellular matrix, chemistry of carbohydrates, amino-acid and proteins, lab safety and biomedical waste management and chromatography (Demo)
2	• LL/UL • General embryology and histology	Blood, N-M	Plasma protein, immunoglobulins, enzymes, hemoglobin structure and hemoglobinopathies, electrophoresis (Demo), heme synthesis, porphyria's, hemecatabolism, iron metabolism (mineral) bilirubin formation, jaundice, colorimetry (Demo)
3	• UL • General embryology and histology	ANS, CVS	Clinical enzymology, chemistry of lipids, and lipoprotein metabolism, carbohydrate metabolism, vitamins, estimation of protein and albumin
4	• Abdomen • Related systemic embryology and histology	GIT, renal	Vitamins, nutrition, liver function tests, renal function tests, acid-base balance and its disorders, water and electrolyte normal and abnormal analysis of urine (DOAP), estimation of urea, creatinine
5	• Abdomen, Pelvis • Related systemic embryology and histology	GIT (contd.), Repro.	Metabolism of proteins and their metabolic disorders, metabolism of carbohydrates and their metabolic disorders, diabetes mellitus, electron transport chain and oxidative phosphorylation, xenobiotics, estimation of glucose
6	• Thorax • Related systemic embryology and histology	Repro (contd.), RS	Metabolism of lipids (remaining) and disorders, metabolism of proteins, minerals, vitamins, reproductive hormones, prenatal screening, new born screening
7	• H and N-I • Related systemic embryology and histology, genetics	Endocrine (Neck region), CNS	Hormone biochemistry; tumor markers, thyroid function tests, adrenal function tests, free radicals, and antioxidants
8	• H and N-II • Related systemic embryology and histology, genetics	CNS (contd.), special senses	Purine and pyrimidines metabolism, gout, purine salvage pathway, replication, DNA damage and repair mechanism, transcription, translation, posttranslational modifications, protein synthesis inhibitors, genetic code, and mutations, estimation of uric acid
9	• Neuroanatomy • Related systemic embryology and histology	CNS (contd.), integrated physiology	Molecular biology techniques and miscellaneous

Topic: Clinical enzymology: Integration of the topic in the department of biochemistry with department of internal medicine.

SLOs:

1. To know about the clinical application of various enzymes as biomarkers in diagnosis of diseases.
2. To know about the therapeutic use of enzymes in various diseased states.

Methodology:

1. Role play by an individual as a patient of myocardial infarction. Explain about the patients clinical symptoms and process of diagnosis with various lab reports and ECG reports.
2. Discuss cases of obstructive jaundice and viral hepatitis with various lab and radiological findings.
3. Knowledge about diagnostic approaches by clinical enzymology and further management.

Student's feedback for teaching—learning activity and reflection writing in log book as integrated SGT (vertical integration of biochemistry with department of internal medicine):

Certificate for Skill-based Competencies: (11)

This is to certify that Mr/Ms ____________________ Roll no. ____________________ Enrollment no. ____________

Batch ____________________ Course ____________________ has completed the following skill competencies in the department of Biochemistry and has achieved the required level of the given procedures and skill based competencies.

No.	Competency	Activity/ TL/No. Required to certify/ level	Full date of completion	Activity attempt F: (first) R: (repeat) Re: (remedial)	Rating B: (below) M: (meets) E: (exceeds expectation/ numerical score)	Faculty decision C: (completed) R: (repeat) Re: (remedial)	Signature of faculty with date	Received feedback/ signature of learner
BC14.3	Describe the physical properties chemical constituents of normal urine and abnormal constituents of urine and perform urine analysis to determine normal and abnormal constituents including dipsticks method demonstrations	LGT, SGD/ DOAP/1/P						
BC14.4 integrated with general medicine (vertical) integrated with physiology (horizontal)	Identify abnormal constituents of urine interpret the findings and correlate this with pathological states and prepare a urine report	LGT, SGD/ DOAP/1/P						
BC14.7	Perform estimation of glucose by manual or semi-automated analyzer method and demonstrate glucometer usage and interpretation of results with clinical scenarios	DOAPs/1/P						

Contd...

Contd...

No.	Competency	Activity/ TL/No. Required to certify/ level	Full date of completion	Activity attempt F: (first) R: (repeat) Re: (remedial)	Rating B: (below) M: (meets) E: (exceeds expectation/ numerical score)	Faculty decision C: (completed) R: (repeat) Re: (remedial)	Signature of faculty with date	Received feedback/ signature of learner
BC14.8	Perform estimation of urea and calculate BUN and interpretation of results in clinical scenarios	DOAPs/1/P						
BC14.9	Perform the estimation of serum creatinine and calculate creatinine clearance	DOAPs/1/P						
BC14.10	Perform the estimation of uric acid in serum and interpretation of results in clinical scenarios	DOAPs/1/P						
BC14.11	Perform estimation of serum proteins albumin and A: G ratio	DOAPs/1/P						
BC14.12	Perform the estimation of serum total cholesterol	DOAPs/1/P						
BC14.13	Perform the estimation of serum Bilirubin by manual or semi-automated analyzer	DOAPs/1/P						
BC14.21	Describe quality control and identify basic LJ charts in clinical Biochemistry lab.	DOAPs/1/P						

Head of Department

CERTIFICATE for ECE/Humanities

(75% Attendance/Assignments Certification)

This is to certify that Mr/Ms ______________________ Roll no. ____________ Enrollment no. ____________ Admission Year ____________ at ______________________ Medical college has completed the required 75% attendance during ECE. He/she has satisfactorily completed all assignments of ECE/Humanities.

Signature of student with date

Head of Department
Department of Biochemistry

CERTIFICATE for Integration

(75% Attendance/Assignments Certification)

This is to certify that Mr/Ms ______________________ Roll no. ____________ Enrollment no. ____________ Admission Year ____________ at ______________________ Medical college has completed the required 75% attendance during integration classes. He/she has satisfactorily completed all assignments of integration.

Signature of student with date

Head of Department
Department of Biochemistry
Signature with
Seal & Date

Record of Early Clinical Exposure

This is to certify that Mr/Ms ____________________ Roll no. ____________ Enrollment no. ____________

Batch ________ Course ________________ has completed the following modules and is recommended for appearing in the final university examinations.

No.	Competency	Activity Setting	Correlation	Full date of completion	Activity attempt F: (first) R: (repeat) Re: (remedial)	Rating B: (below) M: (meets) E: (exceeds expectation/ Numerical score)	Faculty decision C: (completed) R: (repeat) Re: (remedial)	Signature of faculty with date	Received feedback/ signature of learner
		Classroom/ hospital/ community	Basic science/ clinical skills						

Head of Department

Record of Self Directed Learning Sessions: (10)

This is to certify that Mr/Ms __________________________ Roll no. ___________________ Enrollment no. ___________

Batch ________________ Course ______________________ has completed the following modules and is recommended for appearing in the final university examinations.

No.	Competency/ seminars, tutorials, projects, quizzes, library assignments, other activities	Activity	Full date of completion	Activity attempt F: (first) R: (repeat) Re: (remedial)	Rating B: (below) M: (meets) E: (exceeds expectation/ Numerical score)	Faculty decision C: (completed) R: (repeat) Re: (remedial)	Signature of faculty with date	Received feedback/ signature of learner

Head of Department

Record of AETCOM (Attitude, Ethics and Communication: (Module 1.1/what does it mean to be a doctor?)

This is to certify that Mr/Ms ____________________ Roll no. ______________ Enrollment no. __________

Batch ____________ Course ________________ has completed the following modules and is recommended for appearing in the final university examinations.

Competency no.	Name of activity	Date	Attempt at activity	Rating	Decision	Signature of faculty and date	Feedback received/ Signature of learner
Module 1.1:	**What does it mean to be a doctor?**						
1.1.1	Enumerate and describe professional qualities and role of a physician		F/R/Re	B/M/E	C/Inc		
1.1.2	Describe and discuss commitment to lifelong learning as an important part of physician's growth		F/R/Re	B/M/E	C/Inc		
1.1.3	Describe and discuss the role of a physician in health care system		F/R/Re	B/M/E	C/Inc		
1.1.4	Identify and discuss physician's role and responsibility to society and the community that he/she serves		F/R/Re	B/M/E	C/Inc		

Remark: F: Attempt first; R: Repeat; Re: Remedial; B: Rating below; M: Meets; E: Exceed; C: Complete; Inc: Incomplete

PRACTICAL SESSIONS

Competency no.	Name of activity	Date	Attempt at activity	Rating	Decision	Signature of faculty and date	Feedback received/ signature of learner
BC14.1	Commonly used laboratory apparatus and equipments, good safe laboratory practice and waste disposal		F/R/Re	B/M/E	C/InC		
BC14.3	Urine analysis—physical properties, chemical constituents of normal urine and perform urine analysis to determine normal constituents (Dipsticks method demonstration)		F/R/Re	B/M/E	C/InC		
BC14.3	Urine analysis—physical properties, chemical constituents of abnormal urine and perform urine analysis to determine abnormal constituents (Dipsticks method demonstration)		F/R/Re	B/M/E	C/InC		
BC14.4	Identify abnormal constituents in urine, interpret the findings and correlate these with pathological states and prepare urine report		F/R/Re	B/M/E	C/InC		
BC14.6	Describe colorimeter and spectrophotometer		F/R/Re	B/M/E	C/InC		
BC14.7	Estimation of glucose, use of glucometer, interpretation of results with clinical scenarios		F/R/Re	B/M/E	C/InC		
BC14.8	Estimation of blood urea and calculate bun, interpretation of result with clinical scenarios		F/R/Re	B/M/E	C/InC		
BC14.9	Estimation of serum creatinine and calculate creatinine clearance		F/R/Re	B/M/E	C/InC		

Remark: F: Attempt first; R: Repeat; Re: Remedial; B: Rating below; M: Meets; E: Exceed; C: Complete; Inc: Incomplete

Contd...

Contd...

Competency no.	Name of activity	Date	Attempt at activity	Rating	Decision	Signature of faculty and date	Feedback received/ signature of learner
BC14.10	Estimation of uric acid, interpretation of results with clinical scenarios		F/R/Re	B/M/E	C/InC		
BC14.14	Describe the estimation of serum calcium, phosphorous (inorganic), interpretation of results		F/R/Re	B/M/E	C/InC		
BC14.12	Estimation of serum total cholesterol		F/R/Re	B/M/E	C/InC		
BC14.15	Describe the estimation of serum hdl-cholesterol and triglycerides, LDL calculation interpretation with clinical scenarios		F/R/Re	B/M/E	C/InC		
BC14.11	Estimation of serum total protein, albumin and A/G ratio		F/R/Re	B/M/E	C/InC		
BC14.13	Estimation of Serum Bilirubin		F/R/Re	B/M/E	C/InC		
BC14.16	Describe the estimation of serum SGOT, SGPT and ALP, interpretation with clinical scenarios		F/R/Re	B/M/E	C/InC		
BC14.17	Describe briefly various body fluids and discuss the composition of CSF		F/R/Re	B/M/E	C/InC		
BC14.18	Protein electrophoresis, PAGE and immunodiffusion		F/R/Re	B/M/E	C/InC		
BC14.18 BC14.5	Paper chromatography of amino acids, TLC and screening of urine for inborn errors		F/R/Re	B/M/E	C/InC		
BC14.18 BC14.2	pH meter, estimation of pH by pH meter and interpretation with paper case scenarios		F/R/Re	B/M/E	C/InC		

Remark: F: Attempt first; R: Repeat; Re: Remedial; B: Rating below; M: Meets; E: Exceed; C: Complete; Inc: Incomplete

Contd...

Competency no.	Name of activity	Date	Attempt at activity	Rating	Decision	Signature of faculty and date	Feedback received/ signature of learner
BC14.18	ELISA		F/R/Re	B/M/E	C/InC		
BC14.18	Auto analyzer		F/R/Re	B/M/E	C/InC		
BC14.18	Electrolyte analysis by ISE		F/R/Re	B/M/E	C/InC		
BC14.18 BC14.2	ABG analyzer, estimation of pH with ABG analyzer interpretation with paper case scenarios		F/R/Re	B/M/E	C/InC		
BC14.18	DNA isolation		F/R/Re	B/M/E	C/InC		
BC14.20	Describe and Identify Preanalytical (Order of draw, tourniquet technique), analytical and Postanalytical errors		F/R/Re	B/M/E	C/InC		
BC14.21	Describe quality control and identify basic L J charts in clinical biochemistry lab		F/R/Re	B/M/E	C/InC		
BC14.22	Describe performance of oral glucose tolerance test (OGTT), glucose challenge test (GCT), DIPsy and HbA1c and interpretation of results with clinical scenarios		F/R/Re	B/M/E	C/InC		
BC14.23	Calculate energy content of different food items, identify food Items with high and low glycemic index with its importance in diet		F/R/Re	B/M/E	C/InC		
BC14.24	SOP of clinical biochemistry, diagnostic, prognostic and discharge investigations		F/R/Re	B/M/E	C/InC		
BC14.24	Clinical lab visit		F/R/Re	B/M/E	C/InC		

Contd...

Remark: F: Attempt first; R: Repeat; Re: Remedial; B: Rating below; M: Meets; E: Exceed; C: Complete; Inc: Incomplete

Record of Qualitative Experiments and their Clinical Interpretations

This is to certify that Mr/Ms _________________________ Roll no. _______________ Enrollment no. ________________

Batch ____________ Course ______________________ has completed the following modules and is recommended for appearing in the final university examinations.

S. No.	Description	Dates From	Dates To	Percentage of attendance	Status Complete/incomplete	Signature of teacher	Signature of learner

Head of Department

Record of Quantitative Experiments and their Clinical Interpretations

This is to certify that Mr/Ms ______________________ Roll no. ________________ Enrollment no. ______________

Batch ___________ Course ____________________ has completed the following modules and is recommended for appearing in the final university examinations.

S. No.	Description	Dates From	To	Percentage of attendance	Status Complete/incomplete	Signature of teacher	Signature of learner

Head of Department

Record of Group Experiments and Demonstrations

This is to certify that Mr/Ms ______________________ Roll no. ________________ Enrollment no. ______________

Batch ___________ Course _____________________ has completed the following modules and is recommended for appearing in the final university examinations.

S. No.	Description	Dates		Percentage of attendance	Status Complete/incomplete	Signature of teacher	Signature of learner
		From	To				

Head of Department

Record of Humanities

This is to certify that Mr/Ms ________________________ Roll no. ________________ Enrollment no. _______________

Batch ____________ Course ______________________ has completed the following modules and is recommended for appearing in the final university examinations.

S. No.	Description	Dates		Percentage of attendance	Status Complete/incomplete	Signature of teacher	Signature of learner
		From	To				

Head of Department

Record of Integrated (Horizontal and Vertical) Biochemistry

This is to certify that Mr/Ms ____________________ Roll no. ____________ Enrollment no. ____________

Batch ________ course ______________ has completed the following modules and is recommended for appearing in the final university examinations.

S. No.	Description	Dates From	To	Percentage of attendance	Status Complete/incomplete	Signature of teacher	Signature of learner

Head of Department

Details of Attending Remedial Classes
(For Poor Attendance and poor internal assessment)

S. No	Date	Topic	Signature of student	Signature of teacher
1.				
2.				
3.				
4.				
5.				
6.				
7.				
8.				
9.				
10.				
11.				
12.				
13.				
14.				
15.				
16.				
17.				
18.				
19.				
20.				
21.				

Head of Department

Records of Internal Assessment/Part Completion Examinations

INTERNAL ASSESSMENT SCHEME

	I internal assessment	II internal assessment	III internal assessment
Theory I			
Theory II			
Practicals/OSCE/OSPE/viva			
Assignments			
Seminars, clinical case presentations, discussions projects, quiz, SDL, PBL exercises			
Log Book			
Grand Total			

Topics	I PCT	II PCT	III PCT	IV PCT	V PCT	VI PCT
Log Book status						
Other activities						
Grand Total						

Note: Above information is for the benefit of students and parents. In case of any discrepancy, departmental record will be treated as final.

Head of the Department
Biochemistry

Log Activities

REFLECTION PORTFOLIO OF EARLY CLINICAL EXPOSURE INCLUDING HORIZONTAL AND VERTICAL INTEGRATION

Session details	What happened?	What did the learner learn?
Session 1: Horizontal integration • Name of the topic • Faculty members • Date • Time • Duration		
Session 2: Vertical integration • Name of the topic • Faculty members • Date • Time • Duration		

REFLECTION PORTFOLIO OF EARLY CLINICAL EXPOSURE INCLUDING HORIZONTAL AND VERTICAL INTEGRATION

Session details	What happened?	What did the learner learn?
Session 1: Horizontal integration • Name of the topic • Faculty members • Date • Time • Duration		
Session 2: Vertical integration • Name of the topic • Faculty members • Date • Time • Duration		

REFLECTION PORTFOLIO OF EARLY CLINICAL EXPOSURE INCLUDING HORIZONTAL AND VERTICAL INTEGRATION

Session details	What happened?	What did the learner learn?
Session 1: Horizontal integration • Name of the topic • Faculty members • Date • Time • Duration		
Session 2: Vertical integration • Name of the topic • Faculty members • Date • Time • Duration		

REFLECTION PORTFOLIO OF EARLY CLINICAL EXPOSURE INCLUDING HORIZONTAL AND VERTICAL INTEGRATION

Session details	What happened?	What did the learner learn?
Session 1: Horizontal integration • Name of the topic • Faculty members • Date • Time • Duration		
Session 2: Vertical integration • Name of the topic • Faculty members • Date • Time • Duration		

REFLECTION PORTFOLIO OF EARLY CLINICAL EXPOSURE INCLUDING HORIZONTAL AND VERTICAL INTEGRATION

Session details	What happened?	What did the learner learn?
Session 1: Horizontal integration • Name of the topic • Faculty members • Date • Time • Duration		
Session 2: Vertical integration • Name of the topic • Faculty members • Date • Time • Duration		

REFLECTION PORTFOLIO OF EARLY CLINICAL EXPOSURE INCLUDING HORIZONTAL AND VERTICAL INTEGRATION

Session details	What happened?	What did the learner learn?
Session 1: Horizontal integration • Name of the topic • Faculty members • Date • Time • Duration		
Session 2: Vertical integration • Name of the topic • Faculty members • Date • Time • Duration		

REFLECTION PORTFOLIO OF EARLY CLINICAL EXPOSURE INCLUDING HORIZONTAL AND VERTICAL INTEGRATION

Session details	What happened?	What did the learner learn?
Session 1: Horizontal integration • Name of the topic • Faculty members • Date • Time • Duration		
Session 2: Vertical integration • Name of the topic • Faculty members • Date • Time • Duration		

REFLECTION PORTFOLIO OF EARLY CLINICAL EXPOSURE INCLUDING HORIZONTAL AND VERTICAL INTEGRATION

Session details	What happened?	What did the learner learn?
Session 1: Horizontal integration • Name of the topic • Faculty members • Date • Time • Duration		
Session 2: Vertical integration • Name of the topic • Faculty members • Date • Time • Duration		

Contents

SOME MORE INTEGRATED SKILL COMPETENCIES

Number	COMPETENCY The student should be able to	Suggested teaching learning method	Suggested assessment method	Integration
PE13.3	Identify the clinical features of dietary deficiency of Iron and make a diagnosis	Bedside clinics, skill lab	Documentin log book	Pathology, biochemistry
PE13.4	Interprethemogram and Iron Panel	Bedside clinic, small group discussion	Skill assessment	Pathology, biochemistry
PE21.11	Perform and interpret the common analytes in a Urine examination	Bedside clinic Labs, Skilll ab	Skill assessment	Biochemistry, pathology
PE29.16	Discuss the Indications for Hemoglobin electrophores is and interpret report	Small group discussion	Viva voce	Biochemistry
PE33.6	Perform and interpret Urine Dip Stick for Sugar	DOAP session	Skill assessment	Biochemistry
SU9.1	Chooseappropriate biochemical, microbiological, pathological, imaging investigations and interpret theinvestigative data in a surgical patient.	Lecture, small group discussion.	Written/Viva voce	Biochemistry, Microbiology, pathology
IM11.12	Perform and interpret a capillary blood glucose test	Bedside clinic, DOAP session	Skill assessment	Pathology, biochemistry
IM11.13	Perform and interpreta urinary ketone estimationwith a dip stick	Bedside clinic, DOAP session	Skill assessment	Pathology, biochemistry

CHAPTER 1

Laboratory Apparatus and Equipments, Good Safe Lab Practice and Waste Management

COMPETENCY

BC14.1: Describe commonly used laboratory apparatus and equipments, good/safe laboratory practice, biomedical hazards and waste management.

LEARNING OBJECTIVES

After reading this chapter, the readers should be able to:
- Identify and describe commonly used laboratory apparatus and equipment.
- Understand principles of good safe laboratory practice.
- Explain proper waste disposal procedures in the laboratory.
- Identify and write the applications of commonly used apparatus and equipment in the biochemistry laboratory.
- Describe the safe laboratory practices adopted in the laboratory while working.
- Mention the nature and method of disposal of waste generated in the laboratory.

BLUE PRINT

Lesson Plan

Objectives

By the end of the lecture, students should be able to:
1. Identify and describe commonly used laboratory apparatus and equipment.
2. Understand principles of good safe laboratory practice.
3. Explain proper waste disposal procedures in the laboratory.
4. Identify and write the applications of commonly used apparatus and equipment in the biochemistry laboratory.
5. Describe the safe laboratory practices adopted in the laboratory while working.
6. Mention the nature and method of disposal of waste generated in the laboratory.

Duration: *70 minutes*

Materials Needed

1. Presentation slides illustrating different laboratory apparatus and equipment.
2. Demonstration models or samples of laboratory apparatus for hands-on learning.
3. Safety guidelines and protocols for laboratory practice.
4. Visual aids such as posters or diagrams showing waste disposal procedures.
5. Handouts summarizing key points and safety protocols for students to reference.

Outline

Lecture, small group discussion

1. **Introduction** **(5 minutes)**
   - Welcome students and introduce the topic of laboratory apparatus, safety practices, and waste disposal.
   - Emphasize the importance of understanding and following safety protocols in the laboratory.

II. **Commonly used laboratory apparatus and equipment** **(20 minutes)**
- Present a comprehensive list of laboratory apparatus and equipment commonly used in scientific experiments, including:
  - *Glassware*: Beakers, flasks, test tubes, pipettes, graduated cylinders.
  - *Instruments*: Microscopes, spectrophotometers, centrifuges, pH meters.
  - *Safety equipment*: Goggles, gloves, lab coats, fire extinguishers.
- Describe the purpose and function of each piece of equipment, as well as proper handling and care.

III. **Principles of good safe laboratory practice** **(20 minutes)**
- Discuss fundamental principles of laboratory safety and good practice, including:
  - *Personal protective equipment (PPE)*: Wearing appropriate attire such as lab coats, gloves, and goggles.
  - *Chemical handling*: Proper storage, handling, and labeling of chemicals to prevent accidents and contamination.
  - *Equipment operation*: Following operating instructions, conducting equipment checks, and reporting malfunctions.
  - *Emergency procedures*: Familiarity with emergency exits, eyewash stations, and first aid kits.
  - *Hygiene and cleanliness*: Maintaining a clean and organized workspace to minimize hazards and contamination.
- Provide examples and scenarios to illustrate the application of safety principles in the laboratory.

IV. **Waste disposal procedures** **(10 minutes)**
- Explain the importance of proper waste disposal in maintaining a safe laboratory environment and protecting the environment.
- Describe different categories of laboratory waste (e.g., chemical, biological, sharps) and their respective disposal methods.
- Discuss segregation of waste, labeling requirements, and local regulations governing waste disposal.
- Provide guidelines for handling and disposing of hazardous materials safely.

V. **Demonstration and hands-on practice** **(5 minutes)**
- Conduct a demonstration of proper laboratory techniques and safety procedures using selected laboratory apparatus and equipment.
- Allow students to practice using equipment under supervision and guidance.

VI. **Review and summary** **(5 minutes)**
- Summarize key points covered in the lecture, emphasizing the importance of safety and proper waste disposal in the laboratory.
- Encourage students to ask questions and seek clarification on any topics discussed.

VII. **Conclusion** **(5 minutes)**
- Conclude the lecture by reiterating the significance of adhering to safety protocols and responsible laboratory practices.
- Remind students to apply the knowledge and skills learned in the lecture to their future laboratory work.

Assessment: Written/viva voce, direct observation.

INTRODUCTION TO CLINICAL LABORATORY OF BIOCHEMISTRY

Clinical biochemistry is an applied form of biochemistry in which there is analysis of body fluids that are required for the diagnosis of specific diseases and also for therapeutic purposes, also involving clinical research for development of various drugs.

Various specialties of clinical biochemistry are listed as: Carbohydrate clinical biochemistry, protein clinical biochemistry, lipid clinical biochemistry, renal clinical biochemistry, clinical endocrinology, electrophoresis, liver clinical chemistry and clotology, immunochemistry, cardio-chemistry, gastrointestinal clinical chemistry, fluid and electrolyte chemistry, tumor or cancer chemistry, microbial chemistry, serochemistry, vitaminology, toxicology and therapeutic drug monitoring, biotechnology, public health chemistry, epidemiology, forensic biochemistry, nucleic acid clinical biochemistry, nuclear clinical chemistry.

Various clinical diagnostic test lists: *Liver function tests*—total protein, albumin, globulin, A/G ratio, electrophoresis, urinary protein, total, direct, indirect bilirubin, aspartate transaminase (AST), alanine transaminase (ALT), gamma-glutamyl transpeptidase (GGT), alkaline phosphatase (ALP). *Cardiac profile*—heart-type fatty acid-binding protein (H-FABP), Troponin, Myoglobin, creatine kinase-MB (CK-MB), B type natriuretic peptide. *Electrolytes*—sodium, potassium, chloride, bicarbonates. *Renal function tests*—creatinine, urea, blood urea nitrogen. *Minerals*—calcium, magnesium, phosphate, potassium. *Disorders of blood*—iron, transferrin, TIBC, B12, vitamin D, folic acid. *Others*—CRP, HbA1C, glucose, uric acid, arterial blood gases, toxicological screening, forensic toxicology, neuron specific enolase, fecal occult blood test.

List of instruments and equipments present in undergraduate biochemistry laboratory and diagnostic clinical laboratory: Electronic balance, analytical balance, double pan balance, centigram balance, triple beam balance, fume cupboards, centrifuge, boiling water bath, constant temperature water bath, autoclave, vortex mixer, urinometer, incubator, hot air oven, magnetic stirrer, pump vacuum, flame photometer, primitive chromatographic chamber, water distillation plant, desiccators, homogenizer, ultraviolet lamp, refrigerator, electrophoresis—paper, polyacrylamide gel electrophoresis (PAGE), pH meter, colorimeter, spectrophotometer, semi-autoanalyzer, fully automated analyzer, wash bottle, reagent bottle, pipette, graduated cylinder, volumetric flask, erlenmeyer flask, beaker, thermometer, other glasswares.

BALANCES

Use: Balances are used to accurately weigh the chemicals in order to make good quality reagents and standard solutions. They can weigh very little amounts in milligrams or even less very accurately.

The two main types of balances are:
1. Physical/mechanical/double pan chemical balance
2. Single pan electric and electronic balance

Other Types of Balances

Triple Beam Balance

Mechanical balance used to determine the mass of the object, by moving sliders on three bars until the mass on the pan is balanced by the positions of the sliders.

Analytical Balance

This balance determines the mass of the object to high degree of precision.

Centigram Balance

It is used to precisely measure the mass of a substance more precise than the triple beam balance.

Centrifuge

Uses

- Centrifuge is used for separating serum or plasma from the whole blood.
- It separates urine sediments.
- It separates particulate matter from a liquid suspension.

Types

- Bench top/floor model/table top model (most convenient)
- Refrigerated (in built system for keeping low temperature) and without refrigeration
- Based on rotor (to hold the tubes), there are two types of centrifuge machines:
  1. Horizontal rotor type with a swing out head and has low speed
  2. Fixed angle rotor type with an angle head and has a high speed
- Based on speed there are two types of centrifuge machines:
  1. Normal centrifuge
  2. *Ultra centrifuge*: They are used for minute cell organelles and can generate very high speeds, even ranging between lacs of rotations per minutes (rpm).

Principle of Centrifuge

The factors which govern the speed of centrifugation are:
- The revolution per minute
- Length of radius
- Shape and size of the particles
- Viscosity and specific gravity of the fluid under centrifugation
- Gravitational force acting on the particles

It is based on the principle of relative centrifugal force (RCF)

$$RCF = R \times (RPM)^2 \times 118 \times 10^{-7}$$

R = rotating radius of the rotor

RPM: Revolutions per minute, that is, the number of rotor revolutions in one minute. We can preprogram RPM in any centrifuge machine.

There is an electric motor whose speed can be regulated, and it can rotate the sample container at different speeds as a result of which a centrifugal force is generated.

The centrifugal force depends on three factors:
1. Mass of the particles (kept constant)
2. Radius of their rotational path from the central axis (kept constant)
3. Speed (rpm)

'G' is the centrifugal force needed for proper separation and is measured in relation to gravitational force of the earth $(980\ cm/s)^2$.

The two types of centrifugal separations are:
1. Differential centrifugation type
2. Density gradient centrifugation type

Magnetic Stirrer

Use

This is used to make homogenous mixtures by vigorously mixing the solutes in the solution so that the mixture formed is homogenous in temperature as well as consistency. Bars or inductive agitators may be used for the thorough mixing of the solutes in the solution.

Hot Air Oven

- It was invented by Pasteur. It is widely used method of sterilization by dry heat.
- The holding period is 160°C for 1 hour.

Uses

- By the use of hot air oven we are able to dry various glasswares, syringes, forceps, etc.
- Many chemicals can be dried using hot air oven.
- Dry sterilization in various experiments especially in microbiology laboratory is done with the help of hot air oven.

Operation

There is an internal chamber, and there is production of dry heat, which is prevented from escaping out in the environment by a well-developed insulation technique in the instrument.

Incubator

It is an electrical device in which the incubation process is performed which conditions an enclosure to a predetermined temperature since it provides and maintains all artificial optimal conditions for growth of microbial culture as well as cell and tissue culture.

Uses

- This instrument can maintain optimum needed temperature and required humidity (temperature never crosses 100°C).
- Oxygen and carbon dioxide can also be accordingly maintained.
- In microbiology, it is used for various culture experiments.
- In biochemistry, the reaction mixture needs to be incubated at a particular temperature for a fixed period of time.

WATER BATH

Operation

There is water filled in water bath which can be electrically heated. It has a thermostatic temperature regulator by which temperature range can be set from room temperature to 100°C. For serological purpose, the temperature is maintained between 25–40°C and for boiling the temperature can be adjusted at 100°C.

Principle

Water baths are made of steel and are generally covered with electrostatic paint with high adherence and resistance to environmental laboratory conditions. It has an external panel on which a control can be found. They also have a tank made of rust-proof material with a collection of electrical resistors mounted on their lower parts. By the means of these, the heat is transferred to the medium until reaching the temperature selected with a controlled device.

Precautions

- De-ionized water should be used to avoid salt deposition.
- Bactericidal agents should be used to prevent bacterial growth.

Desiccators

They are air tight chambers having a lid and lubricated seal.

Uses

They are used to dry the chemicals before using them for analysis, they are kept with some drying agents called desiccants which are hygroscopic substances and can absorb water of the hydrated chemicals.

pH Meter

It can measure difference in the electric potential between a pH electrode and a reference electrode.

Parts of a pH Meter

- Glass electrode
- Calomel electrode
- Combined electrode

Thermometers

Use

It is a device for monitoring the temperature required for analytical reactions and enzymatic reactions.

Types

- Digital
- Thermistor (electronic)—required for swift and accurate measurements
- Liquid glass thermometer

Autoclave

They are electric device for killing microbes using steam heat by undergoing a full sterilization cycle.

Vortex Mixers

Use

They are required for mixing laboratory samples in test tubes flasks or well plates which use a simple mechanism to agitate samples and encourage reactions or homogenization at high degree of precision.

Operation

Motorized drive shafts beneath the sample platform oscillate rapidly, thereby transferring orbital motion to sample containers loaded into the mixer. This results in sample fluids circulating and undergoing turbulent flow, in other words, it creates a vortex.

Urinometer

Parts of a Urinometer

- Stem—has calibrations with numbers marked to measure the specific gravity
- Weight—lower end of the urinometer
- Float—air containing part

Operation and Principle

It is based on the principle of buoyancy. Urine is denser as compared to water so urinometer floats higher in urine than in water. Weighted float displaces the volume of the urine that is equal to its weight. The weight of the weighted float is designed in such a way that the urinometer sinks to the level of 1.000 in the distilled water.

Pump Vacuum

This instrument is required to remove the gas molecules from a sealed volume so that partial vacuum remains.

Water Distillation Plant (Metallic)

- Water distiller is used to purify water using distillation process, which is related to first boiling impure water after that collecting condensed water in a separate container.
- It is used for obtaining distilled water to be used in laboratory, organic chemistry labs, clinic, fermentation and medical industry.

All Glass Distillation Apparatus

Distillation is a widely used method for separating mixtures based on differences in the conditions required to change the phase of components of the mixture. To separate a mixture of liquids, the liquid can be heated to force components, which have different boiling points, into the gas phase. The gas is then condensed back into liquid form and collected. The reverse process can be used to separate gases by liquefying components using changes in temperature and/or pressure.

Primitive Chromatographic Chambers

They are used for separation and identification of the components of a mixture and for purification of proteins.

Homogenizer

They have prefilled micro tubes with ceramic beads to help in disruption and mixing of cells and are used for blending biological samples by disruption/mixing of the cells.

Ultraviolet Lamp

They are disinfectants.

Refrigerators

- Refrigerator is one of the most important equipment in laboratories. They maintain a temperature controlled environment for various fluids and substances. In laboratory different kinds of refrigerators are used. They can be grouped by temperature ranges.
- They maintain a temperature controlled environment for various fluids and substances.
- The temperature ranges between 2–8°C (conservation refrigeration), –15 to –30°C (low temperature freezer), and –60 to –86°C (ultralow temperature freezer). They are used to store the samples from 3 days to 3 months.

Fume Cupboards

They are very important in PCR laboratories. They are of two types:

1. Fume cupboard with a duct
2. Fume cupboard without a duct

The principle is the same for both types, air is drawn in from the front open side of the cabinet and either expelled outside the building or made safe through filtration and fed back into the room.

Uses

- They give protection to the user against toxic gases (fume hoods, biosafety cabinets and glove boxes).
- Protect the product or the experiment (biosafety cabinets and glove boxes).
- Protect the environment (recirculating fume hoods, certain biosafety cabinets, and any other type when fitted with appropriate filters in the exhaust airstream).

Flame Photometer

Flame photometry or flame atomic absorption spectrometry is a branch of spectroscopy in which the species examined in the spectrometer are in the form of atoms and flame photometer is used in inorganic chemical analysis to determine the concentration of certain metal ions.

They are used to know the concentration of metal ions, such as sodium, potassium, calcium, and lithium.

Principle

The principle is based on atomic spectroscopy for determining the composition of elements with the use of electromagnetic or mass spectrum.

Operation

Once a metal is introduced in the flame, light is emitted, and the intensity of this light emitted is measured. Wavelength of the color indicates the element (qualitative), and the intensity of the color indicates the concentration of the element (semiquantitative). Every metal emits a particular light, each atom of the element has different intensity of light emitted.

Semi-auto Analyzer

These are automated version of colorimeters and spectrophotometers, the pipetting of reagents and specimen mixing and incubation is done by technician, rest all procedure is carried out by analyzer.

Uses

- They are required for all types of routine investigations in clinical laboratories.
- They are required for the assays based on measurements of rate of reaction (kinetic assays).
- They are needed for hormonal assays.
- They can measure the concentration of electrolytes, therapeutic drugs, and drug enzyme assays.

Advantages

- They involve one or two step procedures and also require very small amounts of sample volumes (around 200–500 μL of reagent per test).
- There is facility of digital display and printing device.
- Very less calculations are required, as direct reports are produced, it displays and print the results.

Fully Automated Analyzers

Principle and Operation

The working of fully automated analyzer is based on the principle of colorimetry. They use mechanized operating procedures, such as automated pipetting, mixing and dispensing, etc.

Advantage

They efficiently provide best output rates for large loads of samples.

Glasswares

- **Composition:** Silicate with boron dioxide
- **Advantage:** They are resistant of acids, alkalis, temperature, radiations with low expansion coefficient.

Two types of glasswares are present which are used to transfer the liquids.

1. To contain (TC)
2. To deliver (TD)

Glasswares	Uses
Beakers (Griffin)	• They are used to hold liquids and sometimes solids • They are required for measuring approximate amounts
Erlenmeyer flask/conical flask	• They are used to hold liquids • They are splashing resistant • They are used for titrations • They are used for boiling (allows minimum evaporation)

Contd...

Contd...

Glasswares	**Uses**
Volumetric flask	• They are used for measuring exact amounts of liquids up to two decimal places, such as 200.00 µL • They are used for making specific concentrations of solutions
Graduated cylinder	They are used for accurate determination of volume of any liquid to accurately determine the volume of the liquid
Reagent dispensers	They are used to measure and transfer toxic chemicals which are otherwise harmful to the body
Test tubes and serum centrifuge tubes	They are used to perform experiments both in biochemistry and clinical laboratories
Burettes	• They are used to perform titrations • They put the exact amount/volume of liquid drop wise
Other instruments:	
Fluorometer	They are used to measure fluorescence used in detection of cancer cells, cell counting and estimation of catecholamines
Radioimmunology assay (RIA) instrument	This technique is used to measure concentration of antigens and hormones by using antibody in endocrinology, pharmacology, epidemiology, and oncology
Luminometry instrument	They are used for checking pollutants of atmosphere and DNA fingerprints
Atomic absorption spectrometry instrument: Atomic spectroscopy is of three types: 1. Absorption 2. Emission 3. Luminescence Absorption spectroscopy is further divided into three types: 1. Flame photometry/flame atomic emission spectrometry 2. Atomic absorption spectrometry (AAS) 3. Inductively coupled plasma-atomic emission spectrometry (ICP-AES)	They are used for estimation of calcium, magnesium and sodium in serum, (the determination of elemental composition by its electromagnetic or mass spectrum is one of the oldest method for determination of elements)
Mass spectroscopy instrument	They are used for detecting impurities
Arterial blood gas analyzer	They are used for cases of cyanosis, CPR and sudden dyspnea
Thermal cycler	They are used for amplifying DNA segments via PCR
HbA1c analyzer	They are used to estimate mean sugar over last 12 weeks
HPLC: High pressure liquid chromatography	They are used to separate proteins, vitamins, cortisol in blood and saliva
Micropipettes/Air displacement micropipette/ positive displacement pipette/macro-pipettes/ auto-pipettes	• They are comfortable to use, adjustable • They have high precision and accuracy • They save time when large number of samples need to be run in clinical laboratories • Positive displacement pipette are used to avoid contamination and for volatile and viscous substances at small volumes, such as DNA
Glass pipettes	• They may be TC (to contain) or TD (to deliver) type • The use of measuring or graduated type of pipettes is to dispense different volumes • Transfer pipettes are used to deliver a specific volume only

LABORATORY SAFETY

Safe laboratory practice includes recognition of different hazards, such as electrical shock, radioactive material hazard, gaseous hazard, corrosive substance hazard, infectious material hazard, and risk of handling potentially infectious materials, followed by taking appropriate safety measures both from the employer and the employee which includes biological safety, chemical safety, fire safety, radiation safety, disposal of hazardous material, handling of accidental exposure to acids and alkalis, etc.

Safety awareness includes: Effective implementation of safety rules, formulation of laboratory work methods, time to time trainings, providing personal protective equipment to the workers, employees should be following all the standard operating procedures with a positive attitude, signage and labeling for identification of critical hazards, guidelines for precaution and safety display.

Types of safety	Operation
Biological safety dealing with blood and biological samples	• Care should be taken in collection, transportation, processing and analyzing of potentially infectious biological samples • Use of gloves, gowns face shields • Spilling sites of samples should be treated with 10% bleach and rinsing with water
Chemical safety	Preparation of material safety data sheets for every hazardous chemicals along with proper trainings for their safe use
Fire safety	Proper training of using fire extinguisher by all workers
Radiation safety	• Cautious signage and labeling should be done • Restricted entry should be allowed
Disposal of hazardous material safety including chemical and radioactive disposal	• Water soluble chemicals can be drained out by water • Neutralization of strong acids and alkalis and then draining by water • Dilution of foul smelling chemicals followed by dumping in the drain • Solid chemical waste to be buried in landfill • Radioactive material to be handed over to licensed companies for safe disposal
Exposure to acid safety (hydrochloric acid, nitric acid, sulfuric acid, acetic acid, etc.)	• Skin exposure: – Wash with water – Treat with 5% sodium carbonate with the help of cotton • Eye exposure: – Spray water – Add two drops of 2% sodium carbonate • Acid swallow: – Ask the person to drink soap water – Gargle with the soap water – Drink half liter normal water – For mouth burn apply 2% sodium bicarbonate
Exposure to alkali safety (sodium hydroxide, ammonium hydroxide potassium hydroxide)	• Skin exposure: – Wash with water – Treat with 5% acetic acid with the help of cotton • Eye exposure: – Spray water – Add two drops of saturated boric acid • Acid swallow: – Ask the person to drink lemon water – Gargle with the lemon water – Drink half liter normal water – For mouth burn apply 5% acetic acid

Biomedical waste management: Major steps for managing biomedical waste are—generation, segregation, collection, storage, treatment, transport, and disposal.

Hospital waste	Biomedical waste
Discarded biological or nonbiological which is not to be used (discarded)	Any solid, fluid and liquid or liquid waste plus its container, and also any intermediate product formed during the diagnosis, treatment, immunization of living beings
According to WHO, it is approximately 80% of all the waste	According to WHO, it is approximately 15% of all the waste categorized as: • 10% infectious waste • 5% noninfectious waste, such as radioactive/chemical waste

BMW Segregation Categories and Processing

Category	Waste type	Type of container/ bag used	Treatment/disposal
Yellow	• Human anatomical waste • Animal anatomical waste • Chemical liquid waste: – Discarded/used disinfectants – Silver X-ray film developing liquid – Formalin – Infected secretions – Aspirated body fluids • Soiled waste: – Items contaminated with blood – Dressings – Plaster casts – Cotton swabs – Bags having discarded blood/blood components	Nonchlorinated plastic bags	• Incineration • Plasma pyrolysis • Deep burial If above facilities are not possible then: Autoclaving/ microwaving/ hydroclaving followed by shredding/ mutilation/sterilization + shredding
	• Expired/discarded medicines: – Antibiotics – Cytotoxic drugs – Glass/plastic ampoules – Vials		Return to manufacturer/supplier for incineration at temperature >1200°C
	Discarded linen, mattresses, contaminated beddings		• Nonchlorinated chemical disinfection + incineration/plasma pyrolysis/ energy recovery • In absence of above: Shredding/ mutilation/sterilization + shredding
	• Wastes from microbiology/ biotechnology: – Blood bags – Laboratory cultures – Specimens of microorganisms – Live/attenuated vaccines – Human/animal cell cultures – Industrial wastes	Autoclave plastic bags/ containers	Sterilize with nonchlorinated chemicals on site according to National AIDS Control Organization/WHO and finally incineration
Red	Recyclable contaminated waste: • Tubing • Bottles • Intravenous tubes and sets • Catheters • Urine bags • Syringes without needles and fixed needle syringes • Vacutainers • Gloves	Nonchlorinated containers/plastic bags	• Autoclaving/microwaving/ hydroclaving • Shredding/mutilation/sterilization + shredding • Treated material can be recycled
White translucent	Waste sharps and metals: • Needles • Syringes with fixed needles • Needles from needle tip cutter/burner • Scalpels • Blades • Any contaminated sharp object which can cause cuts	• Puncture-proof containers • Leak-proof containers • Tamper-proof containers	• Autoclaving/dry heat sterilization • Shredding/mutilation/encapsulation in a metal container • Shredding + autoclaving • Sent finally to be disposed to iron foundries
Blue	Glassware: • Broken/discarded/contaminated glass + medicine vials and ampoules except those contaminated with cytotoxic wastes • Metallic body implants	Cardboard boxes with blue color markings	• Disinfection by soaking in sodium hypochlorite/autoclaving/ microwaving/hydroclaving • Finally sent for recycling

OSPE—LABORATORY APPARATUS AND EQUIPMENTS

Q1. Define spectrophotometer? What is the working?

Ans: A spectrophotometer is used to measure the intensity of light absorbed by a solution at a particular and specific wavelength. The working is based on passing a beam of light through a solution, the instrument measures the absorbance/transmittance based on amount of light absorbed by the solution.

Q2. Explain the principle of a colorimeter?

Ans: The principle of a colorimeter is based on Beer-Lambert's law, and this law states that the absorbance of light is directly proportional to the concentration of the solution and the length of the path of the cuvette.

Q3. Differentiate between a colorimeter and a spectrophotometer?

Ans: A colorimeter makes use of a filter to isolate particular wavelengths and secondly it is suitable for visible light.

A spectrophotometer makes use of a monochromator for selecting wavelengths and can measure absorbance across a wider spectrum that is including UV and visible ranges.

Q4. Name important components of a spectrophotometer?

Ans:
1. Light source (usually tungsten or deuterium lamp)
2. Monochromator (for selecting specific wavelength)
3. Sample holder/cuvette
4. Detector (photodiode/photomultiplier)
5. Digital display or output system

Q5. Explain role of a centrifuge?

Ans: A centrifuge is made use of for separating components of a mixture based on their density by spinning the sample at high speeds, mainly for separating plasma, serum, or other cellular components in biochemistry labs

Q6. How do you ensure accuracy when you use a pH meter?

Ans:
1. Calibrate the pH meter with standard buffer solutions (like pH 4, 7, and 10) before the use.
2. Ensure the electrode is clean and immersed in the solution and is not having bubbles.
3. Rinse electrode with distilled water between the samples.

Q7. What is the use of electrophoresis apparatus?

Ans: It is used for separating charged biomolecules like DNA, RNA, or proteins based on their size/charges under an electric field, mainly using agarose/Polyacrylamide gels.

Q8. What precautions we must take when using a flame photometer?

Ans:
1. Use standard solution for calibrating
2. Ensure a stable gas supply like propane or acetylene.
3. Clean the burner plus avoid contamination of sample
4. Handle with care in order to avoid fire hazards.

Q9. What is chromatography and its types.

Ans: Chromatography is a technique that is used for to separating components of a mixture based on their affinity towards a stationary phase and a mobile phase.

Types:

Paper chromatography
Thin-layer chromatography (TLC)
Gas chromatography (GC)
High-performance liquid chromatography (HPLC)

Q10. What is an Autoanalyzer and its function in biochemistry?

Ans: An Autoanalyzer automates biochemical tests, like glucose/cholesterol measurement, by analyzing multiple samples simultaneously with minimum manual interventions.

OSPE—GOOD SAFE LAB PRACTICE

1. **Define good laboratory practices and also state their significance.**

   Good laboratory practices (GLP) are a set of principles laid down for ensuring the quality and integrity of nonclinical laboratory studies, like in the fields of chemical, biochemical, and toxicological researches. They are important as:

   They ensure safety towards laboratory personnels.

They maintain accuracy and reliability of the results of the experiments.
They prevent contamination/errors/and any kind of accidents.

2. **Name the essential components of a safe lab environment?**
Personal protective equipment (PPE): They include lab coats, gloves, safety goggles, masks.
Proper ventilation: Fume hoods for avoiding inhalation of poisonous fumes.
Chemical storage: Proper labeling/segregation of chemicals (acids, bases, flammable substances).
Disposal systems: Following biomedical waste disposal protocols for health hazardous materials.
Emergency equipment: Availability of fire extinguishers/eyewash stations/first aid kits.
Training: Regular safety trainings for all laboratory personnels.

3. **Explain the rules for handling hazardous chemicals in biochemistry labs?**
Always go through material safety data sheets (MSDS) for chemicals before using the labs.
Label all containers properly like chemical names, hazard classes, and dates mentioned.
Use proper PPE.
Never mix chemicals without proper knowledge of reactions.
Handle volatile/corrosive chemicals under a fume hood.
Store chemicals in designated proper cabinets according to compatibility

4. **Explain steps for spill management.**
Alert other people/evacuate if needed.
Wear proper PPE before handling the spill.
Contain the spill using absorbent material (e.g., spill kit).
Neutralize acids/bases by using proper neutralizers.
Dispose off the waste material in hazardous waste bins.
Report the spill to the lab supervisor and also document the same incident.

5. **Describe the important principles of waste disposal.**
Segregate waste into categories like biohazardous, chemical, glass, etc.
Dispose off the sharps in designated puncture-resistant containers.
Treat biohazardous waste like autoclaving before disposing.
Use labeled containers for liquid chemicals and waste.
Follow institutional along with government regulations for disposal.

6. **Explain role of standard operating procedures (SOPs).**
SOPs are the detailed, written instructions for achieving uniformity of performance for all specific procedures.
They ensure that the experiments are consistent and reproducible.
They help for training new personnel.
They decrease errors and enhance safety.
They comply with regulatory and accurate institutional guidelines.

7. **How can we avoid contamination in a biochemistry lab?**
Work in a clean and organized way.
Use sterile techniques while handling samples and reagents.
Avoid touching sterile surfaces with bare hands and without gloves.
Label all equipment and reagents properly.
Clean work stations with disinfectants before as well as after experiments.
Properly seal all the containers after the use.

8. **What are do's and don'ts in a biochemistry lab?**
Do's:
Wear PPE.
Follow protocols in a strict manner.
Dispose off the waste properly.
Report accidents urgently
Keep emergency contact information ready.

Don'ts:
Do not eat or drink or apply cosmetics.
Do not work alone without any supervision.
Do not use damaged glass wares.
Do not store food in lab refrigerators.
Do not pipette samples by mouth.

OSPE—WASTE MANAGEMENT

1. **Why is waste management a key in a biochemistry lab?**
   Waste management is important in a biochemistry lab to:
   Avoid contamination of the environment.
   Ensure the safety of lab personnels.
   Comply with legal and institutional rules and regulations.
   Minimize the exposure to hazardous substances.
   Promote sustainable practices.
2. **What are the different categories of waste generated in a biochemistry lab?**
   1. Biological waste like samples of blood, tissues, microorganisms, etc.
   2. Chemical waste like hazardous chemicals like acids, bases, solvents.
   3. Sharps: examples needles, syringes, broken glassware.
   4. General Waste such as Nonhazardous items like paper, gloves.
   5. E-waste like discarded electronic equipment such as pipette controllers.
3. **How is biological waste managed in a biochemistry lab?**
   Always collect waste in biohazard bags/containers.
   Treat waste autoclaving to sterilize pathogens.
   Dispose of the treated waste according to local biomedical waste disposal rules and regulations.
   Maintain a proper log of biological waste disposal.
4. **What are the different procedures for handling chemical wastes?**
   Segregate the waste based on chemical properties (like acids, bases, solvents).
   Store in leak-proof and properly labeled containers.
   Never mix incompatible chemicals randomly.
   Use appropriate neutralization techniques like neutralizing acids and bases.
   Follow institutional protocols for disposal through authorized vendors.
5. **How should sharps be disposed?**
   Collect all sharps like needles, broken glass in a puncture-resistant and proper labeled container.
   Ensure you do not overfill any container.
   Dispose of sharps containers by authorized biomedical waste handlers.
   Never throw sharps in general waste bins for avoiding various injuries.
6. **What are the steps for segregating waste in a lab?**
   1. *Color-coded bins*: Use different bins for every category of waste like use yellow for biomedical, red for sharps, and blue for recyclables.
   2. *Labeling*: Properly label clearly all the containers with the type of waste as well as date of collection.
   3. *Separation at source*: Ensure that waste is segregated quickly after generation of it.
   4. *Proper containers*: Use spill-proof/compatible containers for liquid and solid wastes.
7. **How do you ensure compliance with waste management rules and regulations?**
   Stay tuned and updated with local, national, and institutional guidelines for the disposal of wastes.
   Maintain adequate records for waste generation and disposal.
   Train lab personnels on waste management protocols.
   Collaborate with certified waste disposal vendors.
   Conduct periodic audits and inspections for adhering to standards.
8. **Give examples of waste treatment methods in a biochemistry lab?**
   1. Autoclaving—sterilization of biological waste.
   2. Neutralization—acidic or basic chemical wastes.
   3. Incineration—disposing of hazardous biomedical waste.
   4. Recycling—noncontaminated glass, plastic, and paper.
   5. Evaporation—small amounts of volatile solvents under a fume hood.
9. **What are the do's and don'ts of waste management in a biochemistry lab?**
   Do's:
   Wear PPE while handling all kinds of wastes.
   Segregate waste at the source itself.
   Use proper containers and labels every time.
   Report the spills/improper disposal urgently.

Don'ts:
Do not dispose of hazardous waste in general dustbins.
Do not mix waste types in a one single container.
Do not overfill waste container.
Do not ignore institutional protocols and regulations.

10. **What is the importance of material safety data sheets (MSDS) in waste management?**
MSDS give the detailed information regarding chemical properties, hazards, handling, and disposal methods for substances that are used in the lab. They also guide proper waste segregation methods along with ensuring safe disposal practices.

CLINICAL MCQS

1. **A 46-year-old patient with suspected diabetes mellitus needs a glucose estimation. Which equipment may be taken use of in a point-of-care setting?**
   a. Spectrophotometer
   b. Glucometer
   c. pH meter
   d. Autoanalyzer

   Answer: b. Glucometer
2. **A patient presents with jaundice, and liver function tests are advised. Which lab equipment is required for measuring serum bilirubin levels?**
   a. Centrifuge
   b. Spectrophotometer
   c. Electrophoresis apparatus
   d. Colorimeter

   Answer: b. Spectrophotometer
3. **During a clinical investigation of a patient with anemia, hemoglobin electrophoresis is advised. Which apparatus is needed for this test?**
   a. pH meter
   b. Electrophoresis chamber
   c. Photometer
   d. Water bath

   Answer: b. Electrophoresis chamber
4. **A patient's serum is sent for protein assay. Which method needs the use of a spectrophotometer?**
   a. Biuret method
   b. Western blotting
   c. Chromatography
   d. ELISA

   Answer: a. Biuret method
5. **A child with recurrent infections was investigated for immunoglobulin concentration. Which of the following equipment is important for doing ELISA?**
   a. Microplate reader
   b. Centrifuge
   c. PCR
   d. Gas chamber

   Answer: a. Microplate reader
6. **A blood sample is collected from a patient for arterial blood gas analysis. Which equipment is important for this test?**
   a. ABG analyzer
   b. Spectrophotometer
   c. Centrifuge
   d. Water bath

   Answer: a. ABG analyzer
7. **A patient with hyperlipidemia was going for a lipid profile assay. Which of the following steps involves the use of centrifuge?**
   a. Lipoprotein electrophoresis
   b. Separation of serum from blood

c. Determination of cholesterol
d. Measurement of HDL using precipitation methods

Answer: b. Separation of serum from blood

8. A neonate presents with suspected inborn errors of metabolism. Which equipment is important for tandem mass spectrometry?
a. Gas chromatography
b. pH meter
c. Mass spectrometer
d. Micropipette

Answer: c. Mass spectrometer

9. A patient presents with dehydration/serum electrolyte levels are to be measured. Which instrument is used for this analysis?
a. Flame photometer
b. Spectrophotometer
c. Electrophoresis apparatus
d. pH meter

Answer: a. Flame photometer

10. During an outbreak of viral infection, reverse transcriptase PCR was used for diagnosis. Which equipment is essential for this molecular diagnostic investigation?
a. Thermocycler
b. Photometer
c. Microplate reader
d. Electrophoresis apparatus

Answer: a. Thermocycler

11. A laboratory technician spills reagent on the work platform. What is the first step now to be taken?
a. Wipe it immediately
b. Inform the lab supervisor and follow material safety data sheet guidelines
c. Continue working/clean it after completing
d. Dilute the spill with water

Answer: b. Inform the lab supervisor and follow the material safety data sheet (MSDS) guidelines

12. While pipetting serum the technician accidentally aspirates the liquid. What should be done:
a. Dispose of the contaminated bulb and use a new one
b. Wash the bulb and reuse it
c. Continue using the same bulb after wiping
d. Ignore

Answer: a. Dispose of the contaminated bulb and use a new one

13. A lab technician handling blood samples develops a small cut on finger. What action must be taken?
a. Continue working with gloves
b. Wash the cut with soap and water, apply antiseptic, and report to the supervisor
c. Cover the cut with a tissue
d. Ignore it

Answer: b. Wash the cut with soap and water, apply antiseptic, and report to the supervisor

14. What is the correct method to dispose off used syringes in a clinical biochemistry lab?
a. Place them in a regular trash bin
b. Dispose of them in a puncture-resistant sharps container
c. Recap the needle and throw it in the biohazard bag
d. Disassemble the syringe and dispose of its parts separately

Answer: b. Dispose of them in a puncture-resistant sharps container

15. A chemical reagent splashes into a technician's eye. What is the appropriate action?
a. Rub the eye
b. Rinse the eye with water for at least 15 minutes and seek medical help
c. Use an antiseptic solution
d. Ignore the incident

Answer: b. Rinse the eye with water for at least 15 minutes and seek medical help

16. A worker processes patient samples for infectious disease testing. What is the safest way?
 a. Work in a biosafety cabinet/wear personal protective equipment
 b. Process the samples quickly
 c. Handle samples in an open area
 d. Rely on routine handwashing

Answer: a. Work in a biosafety cabinet (BSC) and wear personal protective equipment (PPE)

17. How should one transport biohazardous samples within the hospital?
 a. Carry in a plastic bag
 b. Place them in a sealed, labelled secondary container
 c. Transport them in tray
 d. Use a paper envelope

Answer: b. Place them in a sealed, labelled secondary container

18. Why is it important to sterilize lab equipment every time after processing samples?
 a. To ensure equipment functions
 b. To prevent contamination and cross-infection
 c. To meet regulatory requirements
 d. To increase speed of diagnostic tests

Answer: b. To prevent contamination and cross-infection

19. Which of the following describes the use of fume hoods?
 a. To store reagents
 b. To protect personnel from hazardous chemical fumes and vapors
 c. To incubate samples
 d. To maintain sterility

Answer: b. To protect personnel from hazardous chemical fumes and vapors

20. A technician drops a test tube having patient blood. What is the correct protocol?
 a. Pick up the broken pieces, wipe the blood with tissue
 b. Use gloves, disinfect the area with a suitable chemical, and dispose of materials in biohazard waste
 c. Allow the blood to dry
 d. Sweep the broken glass and dispose

Answer: b. Use gloves, disinfect the area with a suitable chemical, and dispose of materials in biohazard waste

21. Which color-coded bag is utilized to dispose human anatomical waste, in a clinical laboratory?
 a. Yellow
 b. Red
 c. Blue
 d. Black

Answer: a. Yellow

22. A technician is disposing of sharps. In which container can they be disposed of?
 a. Yellow bag
 b. Puncture-resistant sharps container
 c. Black bag
 d. Blue bag

Answer: b. Puncture-resistant sharps container

23. Which of the following waste is considered biomedical waste?
 a. Used gloves
 b. Patient blood samples and contaminated glassware
 c. Reagent bottles
 d. Broken furniture

Answer: b. Patient blood samples and contaminated glassware

24. What is the primary method to treat infectious biomedical waste to make it safe for disposal?
 a. Incineration
 b. Autoclaving
 c. Chemical disinfection
 d. Deep burial

Answer: b. Autoclaving

25. A technician drops a centrifuge tube having blood sample. What should be the first step?
a. Wear gloves and clean up the spill with disinfectant
b. Sweep the area and dispose of waste in a black bag
c. Leave the spill unattended and inform the supervisor
d. Pour water over the spill to dilute it

Answer: a. Wear gloves and clean up the spill with disinfectant

26. What type of waste is disposed of in the red-colored bag in biomedical waste management?
a. Expired medicines
b. Contaminated plastic items like syringes and tubing
c. General waste
d. Sharps

Answer: b. Contaminated plastic items like syringes and tubing

27. Why is it significant to segregate biomedical waste at the point of generation?
a. To decrease the cost of waste disposal
b. To ensure the safety of lab personnel and waste handlers
c. To comply with hospital rules
d. To prevent cross-contamination

Answer: b. To ensure the safety of lab personnel and waste handlers

28. What should be done with expired chemical reagents?
a. Dispose them in the black bag
b. Neutralize and discard them according to their hazard classification
c. Pour them down the sink
d. Store them indefinitely

Answer: b. Neutralize and discard them according to their hazard classification

29. Biomedical waste management rules recommend that waste bags should be replaced at what time:
a. They are completely full
b. They are three-fourths full
c. At the end of the day
d. Only when waste spills are there

Answer: b. They are three-fourths full

30. Which of the following is considered a chemical hazard?
a. Blood samples from a hepatitis patient
b. Unneutralized acids or alkali reagents
c. Broken glassware
d. Expired medicines

Answer: b. Unneutralized acids or alkali reagents

VIVA VOCE

Q1. What are the important principles of good laboratory practice/how do they ensure the safety/accuracy of laboratory?
Next question/Follow-up: Address the key risks of contamination/cross-contamination in a lab setting?

Q2. Explain the significance of proper waste management in a laboratory. What are the different kinds of laboratory waste, and how should they be disposed of properly?
Next question/Follow-up: How to ensure that chemical/biological/sharps waste is segregated/disposed of according to safety guidelines and regulations?

Q3. What is the role of a burette in volumetric analysis/how will you ensure accurate measurements while using burette?
Next question/Follow-up: What are the important differences between a burette/a pipette in terms of their applications and precision?

Q4. Discuss the principle of a centrifuge, and how will you choose appropriate speed/time settings for different types of samples?
Next question/Follow-up: Which precautions must be taken in operating a centrifuge for ensuring safety and avoid damage?

SPOTTERS

Q1. Show a laboratory setup with a volumetric flask/it is filled to the mark with a liquid. What is the procedure of using this apparatus/ what is the importance of the meniscus in getting accurate measurements?

Hints: The volumetric flask is utilized for preparing solutions of known volume. The meniscus must be read at eye level, and the liquid must be precisely at the calibration mark.

Q2. A lab centrifuge is shown with samples in the rotor. Which steps should be taken for ensuring that samples are properly balanced/ why is this important in centrifugation?

Hints: The samples must be balanced by placing equal volumes in opposite tubes which avoids the centrifuge from malfunctioning/plus ensures uniform separation of the components.

Q3. Show laboratory setup with an open chemical container/a spill on the work surface. What safety precautions the technicians are advised in such situation?

Hints: Wear personal protective equipment/cleaning spill according to the chemical's safety guidelines, informing authorities for waste disposal.

Q4. Show a waste bin in a lab that has chemical waste, glassware, and paper towels with biological residue. Ask to classify and manage this waste according to safety protocols?

Hints: Chemical waste must be segregated in designated containers with proper labeling/glassware must be disposed of in a sharps container if broken. Biological waste must be treated as biohazardous waste, disposed of in accordance with local protocols.

REFLECTION

Visit to the Diagnostic laboratory and narrate your experience about the instruments.

CHAPTER 2

Estimation of pH by pH Meter and ABG Analyzer

COMPETENCY

BC14.2: Describe the estimation of pH by pH meter or ABG analyzer and interpretation of results with paper case scenarios.

LEARNING OBJECTIVES

After reading this chapter, the readers should be able to:

- Understand the concepts of buffers along with their significance for maintaining pH stability.
- Describe the principles and methods for preparing buffer solutions.
- Demonstrate the estimation of pH using various techniques.
- Describe the applications and also the principle of ABG analyzer.
- Describe the interpretation of the results of case scenarios by ABG analysis.
- Observe and understand the arterial blood gas analysis.
- Discuss and interpret results of arterial blood gas analysis in various disorders.
- Describe the preparation of buffer and pH estimation.
- Explain the mechanisms of preparing buffer and its estimation of pH.
- Prepare phosphate buffer and its estimation of pH.

BLUE PRINT

Lesson Plan

Objectives

By the end of the lecture, students should be able to:

1. Understand the concepts of buffers along with their significance for maintaining pH stability.
2. Describe the principles and methods for preparing buffer solutions.
3. Demonstrate the estimation of pH using various techniques.
4. Describe the applications and also the principle of ABG analyzer.
5. Describe the interpretation of the results of case scenarios by ABG analysis.
6. Observe and understand the arterial blood gas analysis.
7. Discuss and interpret results of arterial blood gas analysis in various disorders.
8. Describe the preparation of buffer and pH estimation.
9. Explain the mechanisms of preparing buffer and its estimation of pH.
10. Prepare phosphate buffer and its estimation of pH.

Duration: ***70 minutes***

Materials Required

1. Presentation slides that outline the concepts of buffers and pH estimation methods.
2. Samples of common buffer solutions and pH indicators.
3. Laboratory glasswares and equipments needed to prepare buffer solutions.
4. pH meters, pH indicator strips, and other pH measuring devices.

5. Chemicals for buffer preparation, including acids, bases, and their conjugate salts.
6. Safety equipments like goggles, gloves and lab coats.

Outline

Lecture, small group discussion, case discussions

I. **Introduction to buffers** **(10 minutes)**
   - Define buffers and explain their roles for maintaining pH stability in biological and chemical systems.
   - Discuss the importance of buffers in different laboratory experiments and biochemical processes.

II. **Principles of buffer preparation** **(15 minutes)**
   - Explain the principles and mechanisms behind buffer solutions, and also the concept of buffering capacity along with Henderson-Hasselbalch equation.
   - Discuss the significance of selecting proper buffer components and their accurate concentrations.
   - Present common buffer systems and their pH ranges and values, like phosphate buffers, acetate buffers, and Tris buffers.
   - Describe the methodology to prepare buffer solutions, like:
     - Direct dissolution of buffer components.
     - Titration methodologies.
     - Combination of weak acids/bases along with their conjugate salts.

III. **Practical demonstration: Preparation of buffer solutions** **(15 minutes)**
   - Conduct a demonstration for preparing buffer by using selected buffer systems.
   - Guide student's step-by-step process for calculating buffer concentrations and mixing the components.
   - Focus on proper laboratory techniques, like accurate measurement and mixing techniques

IV. **Estimation of pH** **(15 minutes)**
   - Introduce various methods to estimate pH, including:
     - *pH meters*: principles of operation along with calibration techniques.
     - *pH indicator papers/strips*: selecting appropriate indicators and interpretation the different changes in colors.
     - *pH indicator solutions*: preparation and application in various titration and colorimetric assays.
   - Demonstrate the function of pH meters and pH indicator papers/strips for measuring pH in various solutions.
   - Discuss factors that affect pH measurement accuracy and troubleshooting common issues.

V. **Hands-on practice and application** **(5 minutes)**
   - Allow students to practice in preparing buffer solutions and estimating pH using laboratory equipment and techniques.
   - Encourage them to work in pairs or small groups and reinforce learning and collaboration.

VI. **Review and summary** **(5 minutes)**
   - Summarize key points taken in the lecture, like the principles of buffer preparation and pH estimation methods.
   - Highlight and emphasize on significance of accurate pH measurement in laboratory experiments and biological assays.

VII. **Conclusion** **(5 minutes)**
   - Conclude the small group discussion by emphasizing the practical applications of buffer solutions and pH estimation techniques in scientific research and clinical practice and in interpretation of results of clinical scenarios.
   - Encourage the students to apply their knowledge of buffers and pH measurement in future.

It is important to give enough hands-on practice opportunities to the students and guide during the practical demonstration for ensuring them to develop proficiency in this competency of buffer preparation and pH estimation additionally safety protocols must be strictly followed properly when handling the chemicals and laboratory equipments.

BLUE PRINT

BI6.8: Discuss and interpret results of arterial blood gas (ABG) analysis in various disorders.

Blueprint for small group teaching on BI6.8: Arterial blood gas (ABG) analysis Interpretation.

Objective

By the end of the lecture, students should be able to:

1. Understand the importance of arterial blood gas (ABG) analysis in assessing acid-base status along with respiratory functioning.

2. Interpret ABG results in different physiological as well as pathological states.
3. Discuss the clinical implications along with management strategies based on ABG findings.

Duration: ***60 minutes***

Materials Required

1. Presentation slides outlining the principles of ABG analysis along with interpretation.
2. Handouts that summarize important ABG parameters and common disorders.
3. Sample ABG reports as interactive interpretation exercises and activities.
4. Whiteboard/markers.

Outline

I. **Introduction to arterial blood gas (ABG) analysis** **(10 minutes)**
- Introduction to ABG analysis as a diagnostic tool for explaining acid-base balance and respiratory function.
- Overview/outline of objectives and structure of the lecture.

II. **Principles of ABG interpretation** **(15 minutes)**
- Explaining of the key parameters measured for ABG estimation: pH, partial pressure of oxygen (PaO_2), partial pressure of carbon dioxide ($PaCO_2$), bicarbonate (HCO_3^-), and oxygen saturation (SaO_2).
- Discussion of normal ranges and significance of ABG parameters.

III. **Interpretation of ABG parameters** **(20 minutes)**
- Detailed interpretation of ABG parameters in various acid-base disturbances:
  - Respiratory acidosis and alkalosis
  - Metabolic acidosis and alkalosis
  - Mixed acid-base disorders
- Explanation of compensatory mechanisms and various patterns seen for ABG results.

IV. **Clinical applications and case discussions** **(10 minutes)**
- Presentation of clinical scenarios and ABG reports for interactive interpretation activities.
- Discussion of the clinical applications and management strategies based on ABG findings.

V. **Advanced concepts and challenges** **(5 minutes)**
- Introduction to advanced updated concepts in ABG interpretation, like anion gap and delta gap.
- Discussion of challenges along with limitations in interpretations of ABG results, and factors affecting accuracy.

VI. **Review and summary** **(5 minutes)**
- Review of important points taken in the lecture.
- Summary of principles and guidelines needed for ABG interpretation.

VII. **Conclusion** **(5 minutes)**
- Concluding remarks on the significance of ABG analysis in clinical scenarios.
- Encouragement for further study and practice in ABG interpretation in projects.

Assessment: Written/viva voce, direct observation, OSPE.

Describe the estimation of pH with buffer preparation:

Objective
1. Prepare phosphate buffer solutions of pH 5.8 and 7.2
2. Measure the pH of a buffer by pH paper and indicators and verify by Henderson-Hasselbalch equation
3. Demonstrate that buffer resist the change in pH after adding an acid

Acid, base and buffer	
Acids	Proton donors
Bases	Proton acceptors
Strong acid	pK value is low
	Ionizes >a weak acid and forms more H^+ ions
Buffer	Mixture of a weak acid and its salt with a strong base/mixture of weak base and its salt with a strong acid
pH of a buffer	Depends on the pK value of its acids (remains constant) and the ratio of salt to acid concentration
	pH = pK + log [salt]/[acid]
Different pH buffers are made by	Varying the salt to acid ratios

Phosphate buffer with varying pH values		
pH	**mL of 1/15 M KH_2PO_4 (acid)**	**mL of 1/15 M Na_2HPO_4 (conjugate base)**
5.8	92	8.0
6.2	81.4	18.6
6.5	68.2	31.8
7.0	38.9	61.1
7.4	19.2	80.8
7.9	6.8	98.2

Buffer capacity	• Magnitude of resistance offered by the buffer to change in pH on addition of an acid or alkali • Defined as gram equivalent of acid or alkali required by 1 liter of a buffer to undergo a change of pH by 1
Buffer capacity depends on	Molar concentration of the buffer, and is maximum when salt to acid ratio is 1, that is they are present in equal concentrations
Indicators	• They change their color with change in the pH of the solution in which they are present • They are normally weak acids bases having various colors in ionized/unionized states
Acid color	An indicator that is a weak acid, is practically not dissociated in 'acid solutions' and forms the acid color
Alkaline color	In presence of a dilute alkali, the above will form a salt that will dissociate freely and will give 'alkaline color'
Mixture of an 'acid' or an 'alkaline' color	Will be obtained at an intermediate pH
Henderson-Hasselbalch equation	$H \rightarrow [H^+] + [I^-]$ (pH of a solution to which indicator HI is added) $K = [H^+] + [I^-]/[HI]$ $[H^+] = K \times [HI]/[I^-]$
Take negative log on both sides	$-\text{Log}\,[H^+] = -\log K - \log [I^-]/[HI]$
pH	$= pK + \log [\text{salt}]/[\text{acid}]$ (Henderson-Hasselbalch equation)
pH is dependent on	1. pK value of the indicator 2. Concentration of the 'salt' and 'acid' forms of the indicator represented by its 'dissociated' and 'undissociated' forms respectively There is an effective range of pH for every indicator over which it gives a detectable change in color Normally, this range is 1 pH unit around its pK value that is pK ± 1

Indicators with various colors at different pH			
Indicator	**pH undissociated acid form**	**pK**	**pH dissociated alkaline form**
Methyl orange	3 red	3.7 orange	4.4 yellow
Bromocresol green	3.8 yellow	4.7 green	5.4 blue
Methyl red	4.4 red	5.1 orange	5.8 yellow
Bromothymol blue	6 yellow	6.8 green	7.6 blue
Phenol red	6.8 yellow	7.6 orange	8.4 red
Phenolphthalein	8.3 colorless	9.0 pink	10 red

Acid base disorder	
Normal systemic pH	7.35–7.45
What are the organ systems and their role in maintaining the normal pH?	1. Respiratory system (controls the partial pressure of CO_2) 2. Renal system (controls the plasma bicarbonate/HCO_3^-)
Importance of Henderson-Hasselbalch equation $pH = 6.1 + \log HCO_3/PCO_2 \times 0.03001$	Provides the inter relation of partial pressure of CO_2 ($PaCO_2$) and plasma bicarbonate (HCO_3^-) on the plasma pH
What happens in acid base disorders?	Change in plasma bicarbonate (HCO_3^-) and partial pressure of CO_2 ($PaCO_2$) go hand in hand, that is in simple sense, if the plasma bicarbonate (HCO_3^-) decreases, such as in case of metabolic acidosis, then partial pressure of CO_2 ($PaCO_2$) also decreases by hyperventilation as a compensatory mechanism and vice versa
Degree of respiratory compensation in metabolic acidosis is given by the equation	$PaCO_2 = [HCO_3^-] + 15$
Clinical interpretation of the above	If a patient has metabolic acidosis having plasma bicarbonate (HCO_3^-) value of 15 mmol/L, then his $PaCO_2$ is expected to be 30 mm Hg, if there is variation in the level of $PaCO_2$ from the expected value, it will denote mixed disturbance If the change in $PaCO_2$ and plasma bicarbonate is in opposite direction, it denotes mixed acid base disorder

Normal serum levels	
pH	7.35–7.45
Plasma bicarbonate (HCO_3^-)	22–26 mmol/L
$PaCO_2$ (Partial pressure of CO_2)	35–45 mm Hg
H_2CO_3	1.2 mEq/L
PaO_2 (Partial pressure of oxygen)	85–105 mm Hg
O_2 saturation	95–100%

AIMS

Prepare a phosphate buffer solution of pH 5.8
Prepare a phosphate buffer solution of pH 7.2
Measurement of the pH along with verification by Henderson-Hasselbalch equation
Students should now that the there is no change in pH in buffer after we add acid so demonstrate to them

Notes

Acids: They are proton donors

Bases: They are proton acceptors
Indication of strength of acid by: pK value
pK is low for a strong acid
Strong acid ionizes more than a weak acid and forms more H^+ ions

Buffers

Mixture of a weak acid and its salt with a strong base or a mixture of weak base and its salt with a strong acid
pH of a buffer depends on: pK value of its acid and ratio of salt to acid concentration
$pH = pK + \log (salt)/(acid)$
For a given buffer there is constant pK of the acid so its pH depends on ratio of salt to acid
Preparation of buffers with different pH value is by varying the salt to acid ratio

Phosphate buffer having different pH values

pH	mL of 1 by 15 M KH_2PO_4	mL of 1 by 15 M Na_2HPO_4
5.8	92	8.0
6.2	81.4	18.6

Capacity of Buffer

Buffer can resist the alteration in pH when a small quantity of acid or base is mixed to it.
Buffer capacity is defined as gram equivalent of acid or alkali needed by one liter of a buffer to undergo change of pH by one, so we can say that a buffer that needs more acid or alkali is said to have more buffer value or buffer capacity.

Indicators

The substance that can change its color with variation in pH of solution in which it is present.
It is either weak acid or base having different colors in ionized state and unionized states.
A indicator that is a weak acid is actually undissociated in acid solutions and forms the acid color. In presence of a dilute base it will make salt that will dissociate and will form the alkaline color.
At an intermediate pH, the color will be a MIX of acid and alkaline color.
pH of a solution to which an indicator is added (HI) is given by the HH (Henderson-Hasselbalch) equation:

$$HI \leftrightarrow (H^+) + (I^-)$$
$$K = [H^+]\ [I^-]/[HI]$$
$$[H^+] = Ka\ [HI]/[I^-]$$
$$-\log [H^+] = -\log K - \log [I^-]/[HI]$$
$$pH = pK + \log [salt]/acid] \text{ (HH equation)}$$

OSPE—HENDERSON-HASSELBALCH EQUATION

Log Activity

Prepare buffers measure pH and verify by Henderson-Hasselbalch equation.

Reagents

1/15 M Na_2HPO_4
1/15 M KH_2PO_4
0.1 M acetic acid
0.1% sodium carbonate
pH papers
Universal indicator
Methyl red indicator
Phenol red indictor

Preparation of Buffers

Reagent	**Tube A of pH .8 (mL)**	**Tube B of pH 7.2 (mL)**
1/15 M Na_2HPO_4	2.0	14.4
1/15 M KH_2PO_4	23	5.6

Mix well

pH Measurement

By pH paper

Moisten pH paper having broad range of pH like 2 to 10 with buffer A

Use filter paper to wipe the excess solution

Find pH by comparing with color chart

Moisten pH paper having narrow range of pH with buffer A and find pH

Repeat process with buffer B

By universal indicator

Take 2 mL of buffer solution A and B in different tubes and mix few drops of universal indicator in both the tubes

Compare the color with the color chart

Verify the pH by HH Equation

We know the quantity of acid and salt to prepare the buffer
PK_2 value of H_2PO_4 of phosphate buffer is 7.2
Calculate the pH and see if it gets accurately determined by the indicator

Buffer resists a change in pH on addition of acid (buffer value):
Tae 5 mL of buffer A of pH 5.8 in tube A
Take 10 mL of buffer A of pH 5.8 in tube B
Add 5 mL distilled water in tube A and 2 drops of methyl red indicator to both the tubes and mix well
Since the pH values are greater than the pK value (5.1) both the tubes give yellow color
Now go on adding 0.1 N acetic acid drop wise to both tubes till you get red color
Note the volume of acid added in each tube and make a comment on the buffer capacity

Observation with Calculations

I. pH as got by pH paper
Buffer A:
Buffer B:
II. pH as got by universal indicator:
Buffer A:
Buffer B:
III. pH by HH equation:
Buffer A:
Concentration of salt (Na_2HPO_4):
Concentration of acid (KH_2PO_4):
pK of acid:
pH:

Buffer A:
Concentration of salt (Na_2HPO_4):
Concentration of acid (KH_2PO_4):
pK of acid:
pH:

IV. Buffer capacity:
Calculate the buffer capacity as gram equivalents of acetic acid needed by one liter of buffer:
Buffer A:

Buffer B:

Results, Interpretation and Comments

pH meter	Required for pH measurement
Principle	There is measurement of electromotive force generated between the 2 electrodes because of difference in $[H^+]$ concentration In pH meter, the electrode potential generated by H^+ concentration in any unknown solution is measured against a standard hydrogen electrode potential
Generation of emf between 2 electrodes	1. When a metal plate is kept in a solution of its own salt, e.g., Zn^{++} plate is kept in a solution of $ZnSO_4$, it loses ions into the solution and itself becomes negatively charged as compared to the solution 2. When this set up is made with 2 different metal electrodes connected, like Zn^{++} plate in $ZnSO_4$ solution connected to a Cu^{++} plate in $CuSO_4$ solution, the difference in their electrode potential is measured as emf/calculated as the net difference of the 2 electrode potentials 3. When one standard electrode of known potential is used, the electrode potential of the other can be easily measured by comparison 4. When there is a standard hydrogen electrode of known potential, the electrode potential of the unknown electrode, sensitive to the hydrogen ion concentration, can easily be measured
	pH measuring electrodes
1. Standard hydrogen electrode	1. The standard hydrogen electrode made of platinum plate coated with platinum black which absorbs hydrogen is dipped in a hydrogen ion solution of known concentration (0.1 M HCl) 2. For maintaining the H^+ concentration, we pass hydrogen gas constantly at 1 atmospheric pressure 3. The electrode potential of this is zero 4. When a same electrode is dipped in a solution of unknown H^+ concentration and connected by means of a bridge of potassium chloride solution, to allow the movement of ions and no cross mixing of the 2 solutions, the electrode potential of the unknown can easily be measured 5. This potential E has a relation with pH by the equation—$pH = E/0.0591$
2. Calomel electrode	1. There is mercury chloride electrode dipped in a solution of potassium chloride by a porous plug 2. There is a platinum wire whose potential varies with the concentration of potassium chloride (0.1 M–1.0 M/saturated KCl) 3. The Hg is in contact with the platinum wire 4. At 1.0 M KCl solution and at 25°C, its potential = 0.2444 volts 5. The potential at the temperature which is prevailing is given by: $V = 0.24444 - 0.0024(t-25)$ where t is the actual temperature in °C
3. Glass electrode	1. Used for $[H^+]$ measuring electrode 2. It has H^+ selective glass membrane that covers the tip of the glass electrode, made of 6% calcium oxide, 22% N_2O and 72% SiO_2 3. The membrane is delicate 4. There is a silver wire coated with silver chloride paste and dipped in 0.1 M HCl solution
4. Combined electrode	1. Consists of a reference electrode and measuring electrode 2. The pH of the unknown solution at 25°C is shown by the equation: - $pH = (E-K)/0.0591$ - E is the measured potential and K is a constant 3. The response of this electrode is linear with pH range 0–10
pH meter	Consists of combined electrode and electronic measuring and display device with a temperature correction also
	Reagents
Standard buffers	• pH = 4; pH = 7 • pH = 9; pH = 10

Contd...

Contd...

Unknown buffers/solutions	
Procedure	• Switch on • Give time to warm up the instrument • Note the room temperature • Adjust for temperature correction if needed • Take 250 mL beakers and fill all standards, sufficient enough that the electrode bulb dips in them • In the same way, take the unknown solution in other beaker • Calibrate the pH meter with standard buffer of pH 7 • Then calibrate the pH meter with the buffer of pH 4 if you feel that the pH of the unknown solution will fall in the acidic range • If you feel that the unknown solution will fall in the alkaline range, then calibrate the pH meter with the buffer of pH 9 or 10
Method of calibration with standard buffers	• Remove the excess DE from the electrode first by a soft tissue paper • Then lower the electrode carefully into the buffer solution of pH 7 taking care that the bulb dips properly in the solution • Adjust the instrument by coarse and fine adjustments to show the known pH value on the pH meter • Then lift the electrode and wash with DW, wipe with tissue paper • Now you can calibrate with other buffers (pH 4/9/10)
Wash the electrode and dip it into unknown solution, read the pH values and when the reading gets stable, note it	
Precautions: Handle the glass electrode with care as it is delicate The glass electrode should not be left dry Focus on temperature correction before the calibration Calibration should be done with the buffer of pH 7 first and if needed with other buffers of pH 4/9/10 After every change, wash and wipe	

Objective	Study of blood gas analyzer along with clinical advantages
Sample	Arterial blood sample
Method of collection	Tourniquet is not used Arterial blood pressure must be there to push the plunger and fill the syringe with blood otherwise of plunger is allowed to withdraw the blood, there will be mixing of air in the syringe with the blood sample, which will give false result for assessing O_2 transport
Amount of sample	50–100 µL
Precautions	Should be assessed immediately or if stored, the temperature should be 0–4°C only for 1 hour

Principle of parameters which are directly measured	
1. pH	• A glass electrode (Ag/AgCl) • A reference electrode (calomel) • Between the 2 electrodes, there is a liquid junction • There is a variation in the potential of the glass electrode because of variations in the H^+ of blood samples, which is measured in form of emf and calibrated to give the final result of pH
2. PCO_2	• A glass electrode is kept in a weak bicarbonate buffer that is separated from the sample by a membrane • The membrane is permeable to CO_2 present in the sample • The pH of the bicarbonate buffer changes with the diffusion of CO_2 from the blood sample to the bicarbonate buffer as: $CO_2 + H_2O \leftrightarrow H_2CO_3 \leftrightarrow H^+ + HCO_3^-$ • There is an alteration in the H^+ ion concentration in the buffer which is then measured

Contd...

Contd...

3. PO_2	• There is a Clark electrode made of silver anode and a platinum cathode kept in an electrolyte buffer • The buffer is made of potassium chloride and phosphate buffer • PO_2 is measured by electrochemical measurement of O_2 that diffuses across a gas permeable membrane into the electrolyte buffer, where it gets reduced by the platinum cathode: $2O_2 + 4H^+ + 4e^- \rightarrow H_2O_2 + 2e^- \rightarrow 2OH^-$ • Cathode electric potential is kept constant • When the O_2 gets reduced at the cathode, there is a current flow between the cathode and the anode • The amount of current is assessed which is related to the amount of CO_2 in the blood specimen
Precaution	Regular calibration of electrodes should be done against gases of known O_2 and CO_2 composition and used as standards
4. Electrolytes like Na^+, K^+, Cl^-, Li^+, Ca^{++}	Assessed by ion selective electrode-based measurements
5. Pressure of air (used during calibration)	There is an integrated air pressure sensor, PCO_2 and PO_2 values are affected by the air pressure
6. Hemoglobin	Assessed for percentage saturation
Principle of calculated parameters	
1. Actual HCO_3^-	Calculated by Henderson-Hasselbalch equation $pH = pK + \log [HCO_3^-]/alpha \cdot PCO_2$ where alpha is the solubility coefficient for CO_2 and in plasma its value at 37°C is 0.0306 mmol/L/mm Hg
Clinical significance	It is needed for diagnosing acid base misbalance (metabolic) and is affected by lung functions also
2. Standard HCO_3^-	Bicarbonate concentration in plasma at PCO_2 of 40 mm Hg, temperature –37°C and complete oxygen saturation of hemoglobin
3. Base excess (BE)	Concentration of titrable base in plasma We titrate the plasma with a strong acid at pH 7.4, at PCO_2 of 40 mm Hg and temperature of 37°C
4. Total carbon dioxide (tCO_2)	Dissolved CO_2 + CO_2 released from bicarbonate in the plasma when blood is drawn anaerobically There is change in the color of the indicator in a bicarbonate buffer due to release of carbon dioxide on acidification of the sample
5. Buffer bases (BB)	Sum of concentrations of all buffers, such as Hb, proteins, phosphates and bicarbonate
6. Oxygen saturation of hemoglobin	The binding sites of Hb are occupied with O_2 representing the% of Hb saturation, and is not affected by concentration of Hb
7. Total oxygen concentration	Physically dissolved + chemically bonded O_2 determined by PO_2 and oxyhemoglobin (oxyHb)
Alveolar arterial oxygen pressure difference	Difference of O_2 contact between alveolar air and arterial blood PO_2
Hematocrit	% of RBC to the total blood volume
Method of operation	• Injection of uncoagulated sample directly into the inlet from the syringe • Processing of the sample • Digital display/printout of the result • Rinse the instrument for next analysis
Precautions	• Sample must not come in contact with the air • The needle must be properly sealed • Sample must not clot • For analysis of oxygen transport, arterial sample is always used
Clinical significance	
Respiratory acidosis	↑ PCO_2
Respiratory alkalosis	↓ PCO_2
Metabolic acidosis	↓ HCO_3^-
Metabolic alkalosis	↑ HCO_3^-
Relation between HCO_3^- and tCO_2	tCO_2 is >HCO_3^- by 2 mm/L

	Normal values
PCO_2	35–48 mm Hg
PO_2	83–108 mm Hg
tCO_2	22–28 mm/L
pH	7.35–7.45
HCO_3^-	22–26 mm/L
Hb saturation of Hb	95–98%
Anion gap	8–18 mEq/L

Disease	Cause	Blood variation	Compensation
Respiratory acidosis	Less ventilation (pneumonia)	Increased PCO_2 Decreased pH	Increased HCO_3^- Renal retention
Respiratory alkalosis	More ventilation (salicylate poisoning, Thyrotoxicosis, hysteria)	Decreased PCO_2 Increased pH	Increased HCO_3^- Renal excretion
Metabolic acidosis	Increased acid load (diabetic ketoacidosis)	Decreased HCO_3^- Increased pH	Increased CO_2 removal by lungs (hyperventilation)
Metabolic alkalosis	Increased acid loss (pyloric obstruction)/ alkali intake (gastritis, peptic ulcer)	Increased HCO_3^- Decreased pH	Increased HCO_3^- Renal excretion

LOG ACTIVITY

Reagents

1. 1/15 M Na_2HPO_4
2. 1/15 M KH_2PO_4
3. 0.1 M acetic acid
4. 0.1% sodium carbonate
5. pH papers
6. Universal indicators
7. Methyl red indicator
8. Phenol red indicator

Procedure

Buffer preparation

Reagents	Tube A pH = 5.8	Tube B pH = 7.2
M/15 Na_2HPO_4	2 Ml	14.4 mL
M/15 KH_2PO_4	23 Ml	5.6 mL

Measurement of pH

1. By pH paper	• Take a piece of pH paper of broad range (pH 2–10) • Moist it with buffer A • Wipe the excess by filter paper • Compare with the color chart to get the approximate value of pH of the solution • Repeat the process by a narrow range of pH paper • Repeat the process with buffer B also
2. By universal indicator	• It is a broad range indicator • Take 2 mL of the buffer solutions A and B in two test tubes separately, and add few drops of universal indicator to both the test tubes • Mix, compare the color with the color chart
3. Verify the pH by Henderson-Hasselbalch equation	• The amount of acid and salt added to prepare the buffer is known to us • pK_2 value of KH_2PO_4 of phosphate buffer = 7.2 • Calculate the pH and see that it is accurately determined by the indicator

Contd...

Contd...

4. Buffer value	• Buffer resists the change in pH by adding acid • Take 5 mL of buffer A (pH = 5.8) in tube A • Take 10 mL of buffer A (pH = 5.8) in tube B • Add 5 mL DW in tube A • Add 2 drops of methyl red indicator in both tubes and mix • Because the pH values are greater than the pK value (5.1), both the tubes form yellow color • Add 0.1 N acetic acid drop wise by pipette to both the test tubes till we get a red color • Note the volume of acid added to each tube and see the buffer capacity of each

Calculations

1. pH as obtained by pH paper	Buffer A......
	Buffer B.......
2. pH as obtained by universal indicators	Buffer A........
	Buffer B.........

pH by H-H equation

Buffer A	
Concentration of salt (Na_2HPO_4)	....
Concentration of acid (KH_2PO_4)	....
pK of acid	....
pH	
Buffer B	
Concentration of salt (Na_2HPO_4)	....
Concentration of acid (KH_2PO_4)	....
pK of acid	....

pH

Buffer capacity	Calculate the buffer capacity as grams equivalents of acetic acid needed by 1 liter of buffer
Buffer A	
Buffer B	

Results

Method	Buffer A	Buffer B
1. pH paper		
2. Universal indicator		
3. H-H equation		
4. Capacity of buffer A, B		

Interpretation

OSPE—pH METER

1. **What is a pH meter, and what is its function in a biochemistry lab?**
   A pH meter is an electronic device required for measuring the hydrogen ion concentration (pH) of any solution. It gives accurate as well as reliable readings, significant for biochemical experiments where pH has an impact on enzyme activity, protein stability, as well as chemical reactions.
2. **What are the components of a pH meter?**
   Electrode (pH probe): A glass electrode to measures pH.
   Reference electrode: Provides a stable reference potential.

Digital display: exhibits the pH value.
Temperature probe (optional): Adjusts readings based on the temperature.

3. **What is the principle of pH measurement by pH meter?**
The pH meter is based on the mechanism of electrochemical measurement. It measures the potential difference between a glass electrode and reference electrode when immersed in any solution. This measured potential difference is proportional to the hydrogen ion concentration that is then converted to a pH value.

4. **Describe the procedure for estimating pH using a pH meter.**
   1. *Calibration*:
      Turn on the instrument.
      Use distilled water for rinsing the electrode.
      Immerse it in a standard buffer solution like pH 4.0, 7.0, or 10.0.
      Adjust the pH meter for displaying the buffer's pH.
   2. *Measurement*:
      Rinse the electrode with distilled water for avoiding contamination.
      Immerse it in the test solution.
      Wait for reading to stabilize, and then note the pH.
   3. *Post-use care*:
      Rinse the electrode.
      Store it in an appropriate storage solution.

5. **Why is calibration important before using pH meter?**
Calibration ensures the accuracy of pH readings by correcting any kind of drift or changes in the electrode's performance over time. It also adjusts the instrument to match the standard buffer solutions.

6. **What precautions should be taken while using pH meter?**
Always calibrate the pH meter.
Rinse the electrode with distilled water in between the measurements.
Avoid touching the glass electrode.
Use fresh buffer solutions for calibration purpose.
Do not try to immerse the electrode in solutions beyond the recommended depth.

7. **What are the common errors in pH measurement, and how can they be prevented?**
Contamination of the electrode: Rinse with distilled water before as well as after use.
Improper calibration: Use fresh buffers and follow all calibration steps.
Temperature variations: Preferably use a temperature-compensated pH meter.
Damaged electrode: Regularly inspect and replace the electrode if required.

8. **What is the role of temperature in pH measurement?**
Temperature affects the action of hydrogen ions, resulting in variations in pH readings. The modern pH meters have automatic temperature compensation (ATC) for correcting this. Always measure the pH at a consistent temperature for accuracy of results.

9. **What are standard buffer solutions, and why are they used?**
Standard buffer solutions are solutions with known and stable pH values like pH 4.0, 7.0, 10.0. They are required for calibrating the pH meter, ensuring its accuracy during all types of measurements.

10. **What are some applications of pH estimation?**
Monitoring pH during various enzymatic reactions
For preparing and maintaining buffer solutions
For studying protein stability along with folding
For determining the acidity or alkalinity of various biological samples

OSPE—ABG ANALYZER

1. **What is ABG analyzer?**
An ABG (arterial blood gas) analyzer is a medical device required for measuring the pH, partial pressures of oxygen (PaO_2), and also carbon dioxide ($PaCO_2$) in blood. It also gives other parameters like bicarbonates (HCO_3^-), oxygen saturation, base excess, that are significant to assess regulation of acids-bases, and respiratory functions.

2. What is the principle of pH estimation using an ABG analyzer?
The ABG analyzer measures pH by using an electrode system.
A glass electrode measures the hydrogen ion concentration of the test blood sample.
The potential difference between the reference electrode and the glass electrode corresponds to the pH value, calculation is based on the Nernst equation.

3. What is the normal pH range of arterial blood and its importance?
The normal arterial blood pH range: 7.35–7.45.
pH below 7.35 indicates acidosis /excess hydrogen ions.
pH above 7.45 indicates alkalosis /reduced hydrogen ions.
Maintaining this range is important for enzyme activity, cellular metabolism, and physiological stability overall.

4. Explain the procedure for pH estimation using an ABG analyzer.

1. *Sample collection*:
   Draw arterial blood by the use of a heparinized syringe for preventing clotting.
   Expel air bubbles if any, from the syringe, to avoid contamination.
2. *Sample handling*:
   Analyze the sample quickly for avoiding changes in pH due to continuous metabolism.
   If there is a delay, place the sample on ice.
3. *ABG analysis*:
   Insert the syringe into the ABG analyzer.
   The machine measures pH, PaO_2, and $PaCO_2$, and can also calculate bicarbonate levels.
4. *Interpretation*:
   Compare the pH values with normal ranges.
   Use associated parameters ($PaCO_2$, HCO_3^-) to assess the type of acid-base disturbance.

5. What precautions should be taken while using an ABG analyzer?
Ensure the syringe and blood sample do not have air bubbles.
Calibrate the ABG analyzer regularly and properly by using standard solutions.
Use heparin for avoiding clotting but at the same time avoid excess, because this can affect pH readings.
Analyze the sample within 15 minutes of collection for ensuring accuracy.

6. What are the errors in pH estimation using an ABG analyzer?
Air contamination: leads to falsely high pH and PaO_2 readings.
Delayed analysis: causes pH changes because of ongoing cellular metabolism.
Improper anticoagulant use: Excess heparin might dilute the samples thus affecting pH.
Calibration issues: Faulty calibration can provide improper results.

7. How do you interpret pH in acid-base disorders using ABG analysis?
Acidosis ($pH < 7.35$):
If $PaCO_2$ is high: Respiratory acidosis.
If HCO_3^- is low: Metabolic acidosis.

Alkalosis ($pH > 7.45$):
If $PaCO_2$ is low: Respiratory alkalosis.
If HCO_3^- is high: Metabolic alkalosis.

8. What is the function of ABG analysis in clinical practice?
To evaluate respiratory conditions like COPD and asthma
To diagnose and monitor acid-base disorders
To assess oxygenation in seriously sick patients
To guide ventilation settings in mechanically ventilated patients
To monitor electrolyte imbalances affecting the pH

9. How do we calibrate an ABG analyzer?
Use standard buffer solutions with known pH values like pH 7.0 and pH 4.0.
Perform a two-point calibration to set the range of measurements.
Regularly keep a check on the accuracy with quality control solutions.
Follow manufacturer guidelines for routine maintenance as well as calibration.

10. Compare ABG-based pH estimation with pH measurement using a standard pH meter.

Parameter	ABG analyzer	Standard pH meter
Sample	Arterial blood	Aqueous solutions
Application	Clinical diagnostics	Laboratory experiments
Speed	Rapid (immediate results)	Relatively slower
Portability	Compact, automated	Larger, semi-automated
Parameters measured	pH, PaO_2, $PaCO_2$, HCO_3^-, etc.	Only pH

OSCE

1. **What parameters are commonly given in an ABG report?**
   An ABG report typically includes:
   pH: for indicating acid-base balance; normal: 7.35–7.4.
   $PaCO_2$/partial pressure of carbon dioxide: for reflecting respiratory status; normal: 35–45 mm Hg.
   HCO_3^- (bicarbonate): for reflecting metabolic status; normal: 22–26 mmol/L.
   PaO_2 (partial pressure of oxygen): for indicating oxygenation status; normal: 80–100 mm Hg.
   SaO_2 (oxygen saturation): Percentage of hemoglobin saturated with oxygen; normal: >94%
   Base excess (BE): for indicating metabolic disturbance; normal: –2 to +2 mmol/L
2. **How do you interpret an ABG report?**
   1. *Check pH*:
      pH < 7.35 → Acidosis.
      pH > 7.45 → Alkalosis.
   2. *Analyze $PaCO_2$*:
      $PaCO_2$ > 45 mm Hg → Respiratory acidosis
      $PaCO_2$ < 35 mm Hg → Respiratory alkalosis
   3. *Evaluate HCO_3^-*:
      HCO_3^- < 22 mmol/L → Metabolic acidosis
      HCO_3^- > 26 mmol/L → Metabolic alkalosis
   4. *Assess compensation*: Is there any change in the parameter ($PaCO_2$ or HCO_3^-) not responsible for the primary disorder?
   5. *Check oxygenation (PaO_2 and SaO_2)*: PaO_2 < 80 mm Hg → Hypoxemia

CASE SCENARIOS

Case Scenario 1: pH 7.265, $PaCO_2$ 56 mmHg, HCO_3^- 25 mmol/L
Question: Interpret the ABG report.
Answer:
pH (7.26): Acidosis.
$PaCO_2$ (56 mmHg): High → Respiratory acidosis.
HCO_3^- (25 mmol/L): Normal → No metabolic compensation.
Conclusion: Uncompensated respiratory acidosis.

Case Scenario 2: pH 7.51, $PaCO_2$ 31 mmHg, HCO_3^- 21 mmol/L
Question: Interpret this ABG report?
Answer:
pH (7.51): Alkalosis.
$PaCO_2$ (31 mmHg): Low → Respiratory alkalosis.
HCO_3^- (21 mmol/L): Normal → No metabolic compensation.
Conclusion: Uncompensated respiratory alkalosis.

Case Scenario 3: pH 7.31, $PaCO_2$ 41 mmHg, HCO_3^- 19 mmol/L
Question: What is the likely diagnosis?

Answer:
pH (7.31): Acidosis.
$PaCO_2$ (41 mmHg): Normal → No respiratory involvement.
HCO_3^- (19 mmol/L): Low → metabolic acidosis.
Conclusion: Uncompensated metabolic acidosis.

Case Scenario 4: pH 7.39, $PaCO_2$ 51 mmHg, HCO_3^- 31 mmol/L
Question: Is there compensation?
Answer:
pH (7.39): Normal (on the acidic side).
$PaCO_2$ (51 mmHg): High → Respiratory acidosis.
HCO_3^- (31 mmol/L): High → metabolic compensation.
Conclusion: Fully compensated respiratory acidosis.

Case Scenario 5: pH 7.21, $PaCO_2$ 56 mmHg, HCO_3^- 19 mmol/L
Question: What does this ABG suggest?
Answer:
pH (7.21): Acidosis.
$PaCO_2$ (56 mmHg): Elevated → Respiratory acidosis.
HCO_3^- (19 mmol/L): Low → Metabolic acidosis.
Conclusion: Mixed acidosis (respiratory and metabolic).

Case Scenario 6: pH 7.47, $PaCO_2$ 41 mmHg, HCO_3^- 31 mmol/L
Question: Interpret the findings.
Answer:
pH (7.47): Alkalosis.
$PaCO_2$ (41 mmHg): Normal → No respiratory involvement.
HCO_3^- (31 mmol/L): Elevated → metabolic alkalosis.
Conclusion: Uncompensated metabolic alkalosis.

Case Scenario 7: pH 7.35, $PaCO_2$ 61 mmHg, HCO_3^- 35 mmol/L
Question: Is there compensation?
Answer:
pH (7.35): Normal (on the acidic side).
$PaCO_2$ (61 mmHg): High → Respiratory acidosis.
HCO_3^- (35 mmol/L): High → metabolic compensation.
Conclusion: Fully compensated respiratory acidosis.

Case Scenario 8: pH 7.55, $PaCO_2$ 20 mmHg, HCO_3^- 16 mmol/L
Question: What is the interpretation?
Answer:
pH (7.55): Alkalosis.
$PaCO_2$ (20 mmHg): Low → Respiratory alkalosis.
HCO_3^- (16 mmol/L): Low → metabolic compensation.
Conclusion: Partially compensated respiratory alkalosis.

VIVA VOCE

Q1. Discuss principle of a pH meter. How is it useful for measuring pH of a sample, and which factors affect the accuracy of its readings?
Next question/Follow-up: Which steps must be taken for calibrating pH meter before use, and why is calibration significant?

Q2. What is the principle behind the measurement of arterial blood gases by using an ABG analyzer? What parameters are measured/how do they aid in assessing a patient's respiratory and metabolic status?
Follow-up: Differentiate between metabolic and respiratory acidosis using an ABG analyzer?

SPOTTERS

Q1. Show a pH meter setup with a sample of blood/an electrode. How would you use this setup to get the pH of the sample/what precautions must be taken?

Hints: Focus on proper electrode placement/calibration with standard solutions/correct handling of the sample for preventing contamination.

Q2. Show an ABG report: pH 7.31, pCO_2 52 mmHg, HCO_3^- 22 mEq/L. Interpret findings/what condition do they indicate?

Hints: The decreased pH/elevated pCO_2 indicates respiratory acidosis. The bicarbonate level is in the normal range, suggesting that the kidneys have not yet compensated for the acidosis.

REFLECTION

Describe the applications and principle of ABG analyzer. Describe the interpretation of the results by ABG analysis. Describe the procedure, principle and applications of pH meter.

3 CHAPTER

Qualitative Assessments: Analysis of Normal Urine

COMPETENCY

BC14.3: Describe the physical properties chemical constituents of normal urine and abnormal constituents of urine and perform urine analysis to determine normal and abnormal constituents including dipsticks method demonstrations.

LEARNING OBJECTIVES

After reading this chapter, the readers should be able to:
- Describe the normal urine chemical composition.
- Perform analysis of urine for estimation of normal constituents of urine.
- Describe the chemical components of normal urine.
- Perform urine analysis to estimate and determine normal compounds in the urine.
- Perform and interpret the common constituent analyte in a urine examination.

BLUE PRINT

Lesson Plan: Chemical Components—Normal Urine

Objective

By the end of the lecture, students should be able to:
1. Understand the composition of normal urine and its chemical components.
2. Describe the physiological significance of each chemical component in urine.
3. Discuss the factors affecting the composition of urine.

Duration: *70 minutes*

Materials Required

1. Presentation slides outlining the chemical components of normal urine.
2. Samples of normal urine for demonstration and experiment.
3. Chemical reagents: (for urine testing) like dipsticks, reagent strips.
4. Laboratory glassware/equipment for urine analysis like test tubes, pipettes, etc.
5. Charts/diagrams illustrating the structure of urinary system.

Outline

Lecture, small group discussion, DOAP

I. **Introduction to urine composition** **(10 minutes)**
- Define urine, its significance in the excretory system.
- Explain the sources of urine formation along with role of the kidneys in regulation and its composition.
- Discuss the factors affecting urine composition, hydration status, diet, metabolic processes and reactions.

II. **Major chemical components of normal urine** **(30 minutes)**
- *Water*: Discuss the significance of water as the primary component of urine and its role in the solute transport/ waste excretion.

- *Electrolytes*: Describe the presence of electrolytes like sodium, potassium, chloride, and bicarbonate in urine along with their physiological importance.
- *Urea*: Explain the origin of urea in urine by protein metabolism and its role in nitrogen excretion.
- *Creatinine*: Discuss the formation of creatinine from muscle metabolism and its role as marker for renal function.
- *Uric acid*: Describe the synthesis of uric acid from purines metabolism and its excretion.
- *Other organic compounds*: Mention presence of other organic compounds in urine, including hormones, metabolites, and drugs.

III. **Physiological significance of urine components** **(10 minutes)**
- Explain the significance of maintaining electrolyte balance, osmolarity in urine for renal functions/body homeostasis.
- Discuss the importance of urea, creatinine, and uric acid in waste excretion and kidney function assessment.
- Highlight the diagnostic value of urine analysis in assessing the hydration status, renal functions and disorders.

IV. **Factors affecting urine composition** **(5 minutes)**
- Discuss how hydration status, dietary intake, physical activity, and hormonal factors have impact in the chemical composition of urine.
- Explain how certain medical conditions and medications may change the urine composition.

V. **Demonstration and hands-on activity** **(5 minutes)**
- Demonstrate use of urine test strips/reagents for analyzing the chemical composition of urine.
- Students to perform simple urine tests to identify like pH, protein, glucose, and ketones.

VI. **Review and summary** **(5 minutes)**
- Summarize the important points covered in the lecture.
- Emphasize the significance of urine analysis in clinical diagnosis and monitoring of renal and metabolic health in clinical scenarios.

VII. **Conclusion** **(5 minutes)**
- Conclude the lecture by encouraging students to focus on applying their knowledge in clinical practice and research settings.
- Invite questions from students and address any queries regarding interpretation.

Assessment: Written/viva voce, DOAP

INTRODUCTION

- ❖ Urine is the excretory waste product formed by the kidneys. It is the ultra filtrate of plasma which is formed when blood passes through both the glomeruli. Plasma is filtered by the glomerulus. The amount of glomerular filtrate for an adult is 180 liters per day.
- ❖ The final volume of urine in 24 hours is 1–2 liters because of reabsorption and secretion of water and solutes by kidney tubules. The normal glomerular filtration rate is 120 mL/minute. In this way, the kidneys excrete metabolic waste and retain important products and maintain acid-base balance.
- ❖ Routine urine examination is important to assess renal function tests and for the diagnosis and monitoring the severity of diseases, such as diabetes mellitus, nephrotic syndrome, jaundice, nephropathy, renal tuberculosis, nephrosclerosis and various aminoacidurias.

Urine Analysis

Bacteriological	Microscopic	Biochemical
For identification of infecting organism by doing culture	For detecting the presence of pus cells, RBCs casts, etc.	• Qualitative estimations • Quantitative estimations

Sample type	Sampling	Purpose
Random specimen	• No specific time • Very common • Taken anytime in the day	• Routine screening • Chemical and FEME
Morning sample	• First urine in the morning • Most concentrated	• Pregnancy test • Microscopic test

Contd....

Contd....

Sample type	Sampling	Purpose
Clean catch midstream	• Discard first few milliliters • Collect the rest of urine	Culture
24 hours	All the urine samples passed during the day, night and next day 1st sample is collected	• Qualitative analysis • Quantitative analysis
Postprandial	Two hours after meal	Determine glucose for monitoring of diabetes
Suprapubic aspired	Needle aspiration	Obtaining sterile urine

Specimen Collection

- For most of the urine investigations, fresh, midstream specimen of 10–20 mL urine is collected in a dry vial.
- In some cases, 24 hour urine sample is also collected.
- It should be done in clean sterile containers.
- The lid should be tight.
- It should be properly labeled.

Sample Preservation

- There is no single all-purpose preservative.
- Toluene is a very good and commonly used preservative for urine.

Type of urine investigation	Preservative used
Urea, ammonia, nitrogen, calcium	2N/concentrated HCl
Sodium, potassium, chloride, bicarbonate, calcium, phosphorus, urea, ammonia, amino acids, creatinine, proteins, reducing substances, ketone bodies	Thymol—5 mL of 100 g/L solution in iso-propanol (It is not used for 17-ketosteroids)
Ascorbic acid	Acetic acid

Organic Constituents of Urine

Sl. No.	Constituent	Concentration (G/day)
1.	Urea	25–30
2.	Uric acid	0.5–0.8
3.	Creatinine	1–1.8
4.	Hippuric acid	0.7–0.8

Inorganic Constituents of Urine

Sl. No.	Constituent	Concentration (G/day)
1.	Chlorides	10–15
2.	Sodium	3–5
3.	Potassium	2–2.5
4.	Calcium	0.1–0.3
5.	Phosphates	0.8–1.3
6.	Sulfates	1.0–1.2
7.	Ammonia	0.7–0.8

Characteristic	*Description*
Appearance	Clear, transparent, without turbidity and no sediments present
Amount	1–2 liters, depends on intake
Color	Straw/amber color (darker—more concentrated)

Contd....

Contd....

Characteristic	***Description***
Specific gravity	1.010–1.025, measure of dissolved material in urine, lower value = more diluted urine, depends on diet, fluid intake and renal functions, it is inversely related to urinary output except in diabetes mellitus where it is increased due to glucose excretion
pH	Diet has major effect on urine pH, varies between 4 to 8, usually 6.0
Odor	Slightly ammonical
Composition	95% water, 5% organic and inorganic solids
Nitrogenous wastes	• Urea—amino acid metabolism • Creatine—from muscle metabolism • Uric acid—from nucleic acid metabolism

PHYSICAL EXAMINATION OF URINE

Normal Color

It is mainly due to the presence of pigment urochrome, traces of uroerythrin, urobilin, uroporphyrin and coproporphyrin also contribute to the normal amber color of urine.

Physiological Variations in the Urine Color

S. No.	**Color**	**Interpretation**
1.	Dark yellow	• Concentrated urine • Mild dehydration • Vitamin B complex therapy specially riboflavin
2.	Orange	Drug induced
3.	Pinkish	Excess intake of beetroot, drug called pyridium
4.	Red	Intake of rifampicin
5.	Brownish yellow	Laxatives, such as rhubarb, senna

Pathological Variations in the Urine Color

S. No.	**Color**	**Interpretation**
1.	Deep yellow	Jaundice (presence of bile pigments in hepatic and obstructive cases)
2.	Reddish	Hematuria
3.	Brownish	Hemoglobinuria, myoglobinuria and porphyrias (porphyrins)
4.	Brown to black	Alkaptonuria—presence of homogentisic acid, (first inborn error of metabolism)
5.	Cloudy	Pus cells and bacteria in infected cells
6.	Smoky	Red blood cells
7.	Black	Iron therapy, melanotic sarcoma due to presence of melanin
8.	Pinkish brown	Presence of urobilin–hemolytic anemia
9.	Milky white	Chyluria (fat globules)

Normal Volume of Urine

- Around 800-2500 mL/day, average—1500 mL/day
- Around 500 mL/day is the minimum volume of urine needed in normal health to remove the waste products.

Factors Affecting Volume of Urine

- Fluid intake
- Fluid loss (output of urine may decrease due to heavy perspiration in summers and after exercise)
- Type of diet (salty, spicy foods, beverages, such as tea, coffee and alcohol increases the output of urine
- Cardiovascular status
- Renal functions

Variations in the Volume of Urine Excreted

Polyuria	Oliguria	Anuria
Increased volume of urine is excreted per day, exceeding 2500 mL/day	Volume of urine is less than 500 mL/day	Complete cessation of urine or volume of excreted urine is less than 100 mL/day
Conditions causing polyuria	Conditions causing oliguria	Conditions causing anuria
Diabetes mellitus	Fever	Acute tubular necrosis
Diabetes insipidus	Diarrhea (loss of fluid from extrarenal sites)	Blood transfusion reaction
Late stage of chronic glomerulonephritis	Severe edema	Severe shock/Surgical shock
Drug-induced diuretics	Acute nephritis	Bilateral renal stones
Alcohol	Early stage of acute glomerulonephritis	Sulfonamide therapy
Compulsive polydipsia	Cardiac failure and hypertension (decreased circulatory volume)	

Normal Specific Gravity of Urine

- The specific gravity indicates the concentrating ability of the kidneys; it is the crude measure of total solutes excreted in the urine.
- In normal health, the urinary specific gravity ranges between 1.016–1.025, the average being 1.020.

Factors Affecting Specific Gravity

- Volume of urine excreted
- The amount of solids present in the urine

Variations in the Specific Gravity of Urine

Low SG—1.016 or less	High SG—1.025 or more	Fixed SG (Isosthenuria): SG of urine is based on tubular function
Conditions causing decreased specific gravity	Conditions causing increased specific gravity	Conditions causing fixed specific gravity
Diabetes insipidus	Diabetes mellitus (due to glycosuria)	Fixed SG is seen in chronic renal failure, in the later stages of chronic renal failure, the kidneys fail to concentrate or dilute the urine which has a constant SG, ranging between 1.008–1.012, average–1.010, same as that of plasma
Polyuria	Severe dehydration	
Compulsive polydipsia	Nephrotic syndrome (due to proteinuria)	
Diuretics	Adrenal insufficiency (excess of sodium in urine)	
Glomerulonephritis	Congestive heart failure	
Pyelonephritis	Hepatic diseases	
	Extrarenal water loss (fever, vomiting, diarrhea)	
	Less water intake (passing concentrated urine)	

Measurement of Specific Gravity of Urine

Instrument—Urinometer

1. It is made of glass.
2. It has a bulb and a stem.
3. Bulb is filled with mercury and the stem has marks ranging from 1.000–1.060.
4. Because of the mercury weight, it dips into the urine to an extent depending on the SG of the urine sample.
5. The level of urine corresponding to the markings on the neck gives us the specific gravity measurement.
6. The instrument is calibrated at 15°C so the temperature correction is made based on at what RT you are doing the measurement.
7. For every 3°C of temperature more than 15°C, 0.001 is added in the measured value and for every 3°C temperature below 15°C, 0.001 is deducted from the measured value.

Operation:
- Fill 3/4th of a 100 mL cylinder with urine sample and gently dip the urinometer in the cylinder.
- Note the reading corresponding to the level of urine and calculate the SG.
- *Precaution*: The urinometer should not touch the walls of the cylinder.

8. **Examples:**
   - RT = 24°C
     - Calibration temperature = 15°C
     - Difference is plus 9°C
     - For every 3°C increase of temperature, correction factor is 0.001 therefore for 9°C increase, the correction factor will be +0.003
   - RT = 12°C
     - Calibration temperature = 15°C
     - Difference is minus 3°C
     - For every 3° decrease in temperature below 15°C, the correction factor to be deducted is 0.001.

Normal Odor of the Urine

Fresh Urine–Aromatic

Variations in the Odor of Urine

Odor	Characteristic
Ammonical	On keeping sample for long time due to decomposition of urea
Acetone	Ketonuria, such as diabetic ketoacidosis or starvation
Foul smell	Bacterial infections
Mousy/musty	Phenylketonuria
Cheesy	Isovaleric aciduria
Burnt sugar	Branched chain ketonuria (MSUD)
Cabbage	Tyrosinosis (tyrosinemia type 1)

Normal pH of Urine

Normal urine is acidic; pH range between 4.5–8.0 with a mean of 6.0 in 24 hours.

Variations in the pH of Urine

Acidic urine	Alkaline pH
Physiological factors: • Large intake of proteins in diet • Presence of sulfates, phosphates and chlorides in the diet	**Physiological factors:** • Fruits and vegetables/citrus fruits (alkaline tide is seen soon after meals) • Excess intake of milk and antacids • Ingestion of alkali, such as sodium bicarbonate • On standing it becomes alkaline due to decomposition of urea which forms ammonia
Pathological factors: • Acidosis • Diabetes mellitus • Starvation • Diarrhea	**Pathological factors:** • Severe vomiting • Infections of the urinary tract • Conditions of alkalosis

Measurement of Urinary pH

- pH papers
- Litmus papers

Normal Appearance of Urine

Fresh void urine is clear and transparent.

Variations in the Appearance of Urine

Appearance	Characteristic
Turbidity on standing	• Due to precipitation of mucoproteins and nucleoproteins • Ammonium urate precipitates in alkaline urine • Other urates precipitate in acidic urine
Fresh urine turbidity	Presence of cells, casts, crystals, chyle and pus

Chemical Composition of Normal Urine

Organic Constituents

Urea

- Exogenous and endogenous proteins catabolize to form waste product called urea.
- More than 75% of nonprotein nitrogen is excreted from our body in form of urea (blood urea is called BUN that is blood urea nitrogen).
- More than 90% of urea is excreted by the kidneys and the rest is excreted by skin and gastrointestinal tract.
- Urea is freely filtered by the glomerulus, and is not secreted by the renal tubules.
- Approximately 50–70% of filtered urea passively diffuses through the renal tubules and re-enters plasma.
- If the rate of urine flow is slow, this passive diffusion increases.
- Normally excretion of urea in urine is 25–30 g/day.
- Amount of protein intake influences the amount of urea in urine
- In renal disorders, the plasma urea becomes high than normal and urine urea is low than normal
- If the concentration power of the kidney is decreased, the urinary urea is higher than normal
- **General overview:** Tissue/diet → amino acids → transamination → amino nitrogen glutamate → deamination → toxic ammonia to less toxic urea

Creatinine (End Product of Creatine Metabolism)

- Nonenzymatic irreversible dehydration of creatine in muscles results in the formation of creatinine which is the waste end product of tissue proteins that is excreted by the kidneys.
- Creatine made in liver and kidneys with the help of three amino acids—glycine, arginine and methionine go to the muscles where creatine gets converted to creatine phosphate which acts as stored form of energy in skeletal muscles.
- Since creatine is involved in all processes that need energy, muscles, brain and nerve cell receive correspondingly larger amounts.
- Per day conversion of creatine to creatinine is around 2%.
- The amount of creatinine formation depends on the total muscle mass.
- Serum creatinine level is a very sensitive test for assessing renal functions as it depends on mass of the muscles and renal excretion.
- Its level does not change much with intake of dietary proteins.
- Normally excretion of creatinine in urine is 1–1.5 g in 24 hours.
- Its estimation in urine is preferred over urea estimation as it is constant on a day-to-day basis since the muscle mass does not change.
- Urinary creatinine is used as earliest test of glomerular dysfunctions.
- Creatinine excretion can be used to measure glomerular filtration rate.

Uric Acid (2, 6, 8 Trihydroxy Purine)

- It is the end product of catabolism of purine bases present in nucleoproteins, thus tissue nucleoprotein catabolism results in formation of most of the uric acid.
- It can act like a dibasic acid and can form mono sodium salts as well as disodium salts depending on the pH, which get deposited in the joints in our body to cause arthritis or gout.
- pKa of uric acid = 5.75, at pH >5.75 it act as monosodium urate ion whose solubility in water is 10 times more than uric acid, and at pH <5.75, it exists as uric acid.
- The four steps of renal picture of uric acid:
  1. Glomerular filtration of most of the plasma uric acid
  2. About 98% of filtered uric acid gets reabsorbed in the proximal convoluted tubules

3. Secretion of half of the reabsorbed uric acid into the lumen in the distal part of the proximal tubule
4. Reabsorption of 40% in the distal tubule

- Thus, the final excretion of uric acid in urine is about 12% of the amount filtered.
- The uric acid/urate pool in our body is around 1-2 g in men and 600 mg in women.
- Normally uric acid excretion in urine is 0.5–0.8 g in 24 hours.
- Its excretion is increased in basic urine (at pH more than 5.75, uric acid is soluble so taking base forming foods which increase the pH of urine, prevent calculi formation by increasing solubility of uric acid).
- **General overview:** Exogenous by diet, endogenous by tissue breakdown forms adenosine and guanosine which form hypoxanthine and xanthine, which finally forms uric acid.

Urobilinogen

- **General overview:** Reticuloendothelial cells: → RBC's lysis after 120 days → Hemoglobin released and splits to form heme and globin, globin gets degraded and heme in presence of heme oxygenase system forms bilirubin.
- **Blood:** Bilirubin is insoluble in blood so transported to liver by binding with albumin.
- **Liver:** Conjugation of bilirubin takes place by glucuronyl transferase enzyme to form bilirubin diglucuronide (conjugated bilirubin) which goes through bile duct to intestine.
- **Intestine:** Conjugated bilirubin gets reduced by intestinal bacteria to form urobilinogen.
- Most part of UBG is excreted in feces and the rest is reabsorbed, greater part of which is excreted in bile and small part goes to systemic circulation, filtered at glomerulus and excreted in urine.

Tests for Organic Constituents of Normal Urine

Tests for Urea

Experiment	Observation	Principle	Conclusion/Interpretation
Sodium hypobromite test: Urine sample = 2 mL + sodium hypobromite = 4 drops = see the effervescence of nitrogen	Brisk effervescence is observed	When urea is treated with alkaline hypobromite urea breaks to form nitrogen which is observed as brisk effervescence • $NH_2CONH_2 + 3NaOBr \rightarrow 3NaBr + N_2 + CO_2 + 2H$ • $CO_2 + 2NaOH \rightarrow Na_2CO_3 + 2H_2O$	• Urea is present in the urine • *BUN in blood*: 5–17 mg/dL • Normal urea in urine: 7–16 gm/day • *Increased urinary urea is seen in*: - Fever - Diabetes mellitus - Hyper functioning of adrenal cortical activity • *Decreased urinary urea is seen in*: - Liver disorders - Respiratory acidosis - Nephritis
Specific urease test: Urine sample = 2 mL + Phenol red = 2 drops → Phenol red turns red in basic medium + Drop wise add 2% acetic acid till the pink color disappears + Urease enzyme (soybean powder) = 1 mL	Solution turns pink	• Soybean powder has enzyme urease • This enzyme urease can break urea at pH 7–8 and temperature of 55°C to form ammonia and carbon dioxide $CO(NH_2)_2 + H_2O \rightarrow CO_2 + 2NH_3$ The evolution of ammonia is detected by indicator—phenol red • The above substrates join together to form alkaline ammonium carbonate which changes the slightly acidic reaction (yellow) to basic (pink)	
Biuret test: Urine sample = 2 mL + 10% sodium hydroxide = 2 mL, mix, heat + 0.5% solution of copper sulfate = 2 mL drop wise	Presence of purplish violet color indicate the presence of urea	• Urea decomposes to form ammonia and Biuret after heating $2CO(NH_2) \rightarrow NH_3 + \text{Biuret}$ • Biuret forms a violet color complex with alkaline copper sulfate solution	

Test for Creatinine

Experiment	Observation	Principle	Conclusion/Interpretation
Jaffe's test: Saturated picric acid = 5 mL + 5% sodium hydroxide = 5 mL Total solution = 10 mL Divide the solution in two equal halves in 2 test tubes **In test tube 1:** *Control tube* Add distilled water = 5 mL **In test tube 2:** *Test* Add urine solution = 5 mL	No change in color is seen Orange red color is seen	Creatinine reacts with alkaline picrate to form creatinine picrate which forms orange red color	• Creatinine is present in urine • *Normal creatinine level in blood*: – In males: 0.6–1.2 mg/dL – In females: 0.5–1.1 mg/dL • *Normal urinary creatinine is*: 1–2 gm/day • *Increased urinary creatinine is seen in*: – Muscular disorders – Myopathies – Muscle trauma and injury – Fever • *Decreased urinary creatinine is seen in*: Renal failure • *Creatinuria is generally seen in*: – Uncontrolled diabetes mellitus – Thyrotoxicosis – Myasthenia gravis – Starvation – Infancy – Pregnancy – Growing phase

Test for Uric Acid

Experiment	Observation	Principle	Conclusion/Interpretation
Shiff's test: A strip of filter paper is moistened with 3% ammonical silver nitrate + Urine drops	Filter paper turns black	This happens because of reduction of silver nitrate to free silver in basic medium in presence of uric acid	• Uric acid is present in the urine • *Uric acid in blood*: In males—3.6–7.8 mg% and in females—2.5–6.8 mg% • *Uric acid in urine*: 300–800 mg/day • *Increased urinary uric acid is seen in*: – Cancers – Leukemia – ACTH administration – Wilson's disease – High protein diet • *Decreased urinary uric acid id seen in*: – Purine free diet – Gout
Benedict's uric acid test: Urine = 5 mL + Anhydrous sodium carbonate = 2 gm + Benedict's uric acid reagent = 5 drops	Intense blue color is obtained	• Benedict's uric acid reagent contains arseno-phosphotungstate • Sodium carbonates provides alkaline medium • Arseno-phosphotungstate gets reduced to Arseno-phosphotungstite by uric acid in basic medium • Arseno-phosphotungstite is blue in color	
Murexide test for uric acid (generally done for stone analysis/solid uric acid) Pinch of uric acid in a petri dish + Concentrated nitric acid = 3 drops + Heat it on water bath till it becomes dry + Add a drop of ammonia	Purplish red color is seen	• Concentrated nitric acid oxidizes uric acid to produce dialuric acid and alloxan • These two condense to form alloxanthine • Alloxanthine reacts with dilute ammonia to form ammonium purpurate/murexide which forms a purplish red color	

Test for Urobilinogen (UBG)

Experiment	Observation	Principle	Conclusion/Interpretation
Ehrlich's test: Urine = 5 mL + Ehrlich reagent = 1 mL Let it stand for 5 minutes at room temperature Observe the change in color and compare with negative test	• Red color is seen for a positive UBG test • Fresh urine gives this test positive as urobilinogen is oxidized to urobilin in stored urine	• It confirms the presence of urobilinogen in urine • UBG reacts with para dimethylaminobenz-aldehyde and strong acid medium of Ehrlich's reagent to form a red color complex	• *Increase in urine urobilinogen is seen in*: – Viral hepatitis – Cirrhosis of liver – Obstruction of the gallbladder by gallstones (liver disorders that disturb normal passage of urobilinogen through the liver and gall bladder) – Hemolytic anemia – Pernicious anemia (destruction of many RBC's) • *Decreased levels of urine UBG is seen in*: – Obstructive jaundice – Broad spectrum antibiotics which destroy the bacterial flora (obstruction of bilirubin passage in the gut or failure of urobilinogen formation in the gut)

Tests for Inorganic Constituents of Normal Urine

Test for Urinary Chlorides

Experiment	Observation	Principle	Conclusion/Interpretation
Silver nitrate test: Urine = 2 mL + Concentrated nitric acid = 2 drops + 3% silver nitrate = 1–2 mL	White precipitate of silver chloride is seen	• Chlorides in urine react with silver nitrate to produce a white precipitate of silver chloride • Nitric acid prevents the precipitation of salts other than chlorides	• Chlorides are present in the urine sample • Dietary salts are sources of chlorides • Normal excretion of chlorides per day is 10–15 g • When reabsorption of sodium and chloride is impaired, the excretion of chloride is increased • *Increased chlorides in urine*: – Polydipsia – Use of diuretics – Addison's disease (aldosterone deficiency) • *Decreased chlorides in urine*: – Excess sweating – Fasting – Diarrhea – Excessive vomiting – Edema – Diabetes insipidus – Infections – Adrenocortical hyper functions (Cushing's syndrome)

Test for Urinary Sulfates

Experiment	Observation	Principle	Conclusion/Interpretation
Barium chloride test: Urine sample = 3 mL + Concentrated hydrochloric acid = 1 mL + 10% barium chloride = 2 mL	White precipitate of barium sulfate is seen	Urinary sulfate is precipitated as barium sulfate after reaction with barium chloride solution	• Sulphates are present in the urine • Dietary sulfur-containing amino acids are source of urinary sulfates • Normal excretion of sulfates per day is 0.8–1.0 g • *Increased urinary sulfates are seen in*: – Cystinuria – Homocystinuria – Melanuria – Obstructive jaundice – Hepatocellular jaundice – Cyanide poisoning – High protein diet intake • *Decreased urinary sulfates are seen in*: Renal function disorders

Test for Urinary Phosphates

Experiment	Observation	Principle	Conclusion/Interpretation
Ammonium Molybdate test: Urine sample = 3 mL + Concentrated nitric acid = few drops + Ammonium Molybdate = pinch Heat	Canary yellow precipitate is seen	After heating with ammonium molybdate in presence of nitric acid, inorganic phosphates get precipitated as canary yellow colored ammonium-phosphomolybdate precipitate	• Phosphates are present in the urine • Normal excretion of phosphates per day is 1 g • *Increased urinary phosphates are seen in*: – Rickets – Osteomalacia – Hyperparathyroidism – Acidosis • *Decreased urinary phosphates are seen in*: – Diarrhea – Nephritis – Parathyroid hypofunction – Pregnancy – Hereditary fructose intolerance – Galactosemia

Test for Urinary Calcium

Experiment	Observation	Principle	Conclusion/Interpretation
Potassium oxalate test: Urine sample = 2 mL + 1% acetic acid = 5 drops + Potassium oxalate = 5 mL	White precipitate of calcium oxalate is seen	In acidic medium and in presence of potassium oxalate, calcium gets precipitated as calcium oxalate	• Calcium is resent in the urine • Normal excretion of calcium is 0.1–0.3 g per day • *Increased urinary calcium is seen in*: – Hyperparathyroidism – Hyperthyroidism – Hypervitaminosis D – Multiple myeloma – Renal stones – Renal tubular acidosis – Steroid therapy – Diuretic therapy • *Decreased urinary calcium is seen in*: – Hypoparathyroidism – Pseudohypoparathyroidism (decreased response of PTH and not its decreased secretion) – Steatorrhea – Nephrosis

Test for Urinary Ammonia

Experiment	Observation	Principle	Conclusion/Interpretation
Phenolphthalein test: Urine sample = 8 mL + Phenolphthalein = 1 drop + 0.1 N NaOH = few drops + Hold a glass rod dipped in phenolphthalein at the mouth of the test tube + Heat all the contents	Phenolphthalein of glass rod changes pink	• pH range of phenolphthalein is 8.3–10.0 (colorless to pink) • Ammonium salts of urine, in basic medium, release ammonia vapors • Ammonia emerging out from the test tube turns the indicator to pink color as ammonia is basic	• Ammonium salts are present in the urine • Excretion of ammonia as ammonium salts is important in maintaining acid base balance of the body • Urinary ammonia is derived from glutamine and other amino acids • Normal excretion of ammonia in urine per day is 0.6–0.8 g • *Increased urinary ammonia is seen in*: – Diabetic ketoacidosis – Intake of foods which can form acids – Excess water intake – Infections of urinary tract • *Decreased urinary ammonia is seen in*: – Alkalosis – Nephritis

OSCE

1. **What are normal physical characteristics of urine?**
Color: Pale yellow to amber (due to urochrome pigment)
Clarity: Clear to slightly cloudy
Odor: Mildly aromatic
Volume: 800–2000 mL per day indicates normal hydration
Specific gravity: 1.005–1.030 shows urine concentration

2. **Case scenario 1:**
A healthy person gives a urine sample with these findings: pale yellow color, clear, specific gravity 1.015, no glucose, protein, or blood on dipstick. What is your interpretation?
Findings: Pale yellow, clear, specific gravity 1.015, no abnormal dipstick results
Interpretation: The sample is normal indicating adequate hydration without any pathological findings.

3. **Case scenario 2:**
A patient drinks 3 liters of water daily. Urine is colorless, specific gravity is 1.005. Assess this?
Findings: Colorless urine, specific gravity 1.005.
Interpretation: Normal dilute urine because of high water intake.
Explanation: High water intake results in increased urine output with less specific gravity, that is physiologically normal.

4. **Case scenario 3:**
Urine sample exhibits a mild ammonical odor after standing for some hours. Is it normal?
Findings: Mild ammonia odor after standing for few hours.
Interpretation: Normal.
Explanation: Urea of hydrolyzes down into ammonia as time passes due to bacterial action, leading to characteristic odor in stored urine.

5. **Case scenario 4:**
A healthy athlete gives a urine sample after a marathon. Sample is dark yellow, specific gravity is 1.030. What does it indicate?
Findings: Dark yellow urine, specific gravity 1.030.
Interpretation: Urine is concentrated, normal after excessive physical activity/dehydration.
Explanation: Exercise and dehydration results in reduced water excretion, leading to concentrated urine that is a normal physiological response.

6. **Case scenario 5:**
A pregnant woman's urine sample exhibits pale yellow color, clear, pH of 6.5, no protein, and no glucose. What does it indicate?
Findings: Pale yellow, pH 6.5, no protein or glucose.
Interpretation: Normal urine sample.
Explanation: Pregnancy results in high rate of glomerular filtration, but since there is absence of protein and/or glucose, this indicates towards normal renal function.

7. **Case scenario 6:**
Urine sample from a person on a high-protein diet exhibits pH of 5.5 with no other pathological findings. Is this normal?
Findings: pH 5.5, no other abnormalities.
Interpretation: Normal acidic urine because of high-protein intake.
Explanation: High-protein diets increase formation of acid and lowering the urine pH. This is normal physiological adaptation state.

8. **Case scenario 7:**
Urine is pale yellow and gives a negative result for ketones, glucose, protein, and blood. Patient has no complaints. How would you interpret this?
Findings: Pale yellow urine, no abnormal dipstick findings.
Interpretation: Normal urine sample exhibiting healthy renal and metabolic functions.

9. **Case scenario 8:**
A patient's urine has specific gravity: 1.020, pH: 7.0. No glucose, protein, or blood present. Give your interpretation.
Findings: Specific gravity 1.020, pH 7.0, no abnormalities found.
Interpretation: Normal urine sample with optimal hydration and no metabolic or renal issues in the patient.

10. **Case scenario 9:**
A urine sample from a fasting person is pale yellow with no abnormalities on dipstick testing. What does it indicate?
Findings: Pale yellow urine, no dipstick abnormalities.
Interpretation: Normal urine despite fasting.
Explanation: The body conserves glucose/ketone levels during fasting state, leading to normal urine composition unless prolonged fasting result in ketosis.

11. **Case scenario 10:**
Urine pH: 6.8, specific gravity: 1.010. The patient takes balanced diet with no complaints. Interpret this.
Findings: pH 6.8, specific gravity 1.010, no complaints.
Interpretation: Normal urine reflecting balanced diet/healthy hydration.

12. **What are the factors that influence normal urine composition?**
Diet: High protein/acidic urine), vegetarian/alkaline urine.
Hydration: More fluids dilute the urine; dehydration concentrates the urine.
Physical activity: Strenuous exercises increase urine concentration.
Circadian rhythm: Urine output/composition vary in between day and night.

CLINICAL MCQS

1. **What is the normal range for urine pH under physiological conditions?**
   a. 4.5–8.0
   b. 3.2–5.0
   c. 7.4–9.0
   d. 6.2–10.0

   Answer: a. 4.5–8.0

2. **A patient's urine sample turns red after standing. Which condition is associated with this finding?**
   a. Hematuria
   b. Porphyria
   c. APKU
   d. Glycosuria

   Answer: b. Porphyria

3. **Which test is done for detecting the presence of reducing sugars in urine?**
   a. Benedict's test
   b. Biuret assay
   c. Rothera's test
   d. Sulkowitch method

   Answer: a. Benedict's test

4. **In urine analysis, the presence of ketone bodies is suggestive of which clinical condition?**
   a. UTI
   b. Diabetic ketoacidosis
   c. Nephrosclerosis
   d. Glomerulonephritis

   Answer: b. Diabetic ketoacidosis

5. **Which parameter in a routine urine dipstick test is used to screen for UTI?**
   a. Plasma
   b. Leukocyte esterase
   c. Acetone
   d. Ketones

   Answer: b. Leukocyte esterase

6. **A urine sample exhibits frothy appearance with positive proteins. Which condition is most likely?**
   a. Nephrotic syndrome
   b. Diabetes insipidus
   c. Pyelonephritis
   d. Hematuria

   Answer: a. Nephrotic syndrome

7. **What does the presence of bilirubin in urine suggest?**
   a. Liver dysfunction or biliary obstruction
   b. Renal damage
   c. Hematuria
   d. Normal state

   Answer: a. Liver dysfunction or biliary obstruction

8. The presence of nitrites in a urine dipstick test is suggestive of which of the following?
   a. Albuminuria
   b. Bacterial infection, particularly by gram-negative bacteria
   c. Dehydration
   d. Heart failure

   Answer: b. Bacterial infection, particularly by gram-negative bacteria

9. A patient's urine sample is positive for glucose and negative for ketone bodies. What is the most likely cause?
   a. Diabetes insipidus
   b. Renal glycosuria
   c. Fasting
   d. Alcohol

   Answer: b. Renal glycosuria

10. Rothera's test is done to detect which substance in urine?
   a. Protein
   b. Ketone bodies
   c. Biliverdin
   d. Urea

   Answer: b. Ketone bodies

REFLECTION

Analysis of Physiological Urine Sample

Test	Observation	Inference

Result and Clinical Interpretation

....

....

....

....

....

....

....

....

....

....

....

....

....

....

Teacher's Signature with Date

REFLECTION

Analysis of Physiological Urine Sample

Test	Observation	Inference

Result and Clinical Interpretation

....

....

....

....

....

....

....

....

....

....

....

....

....

....

Teacher's Signature with Date

VIVA VOCE

Q1. Discuss normal constituents of urine/what is the significance of every constituent for maintaining body homeostasis?
Next question/Follow-up: How the factors like hydration status/diet influence the composition of normal urine?

Q2. Discuss about normal volume of urine produced in a 24-hour period/what factors can result in variations in urine output?
Next question/Follow-up: How do the renal system regulate urine concentration/volume in response to hydration levels?

SPOTTERS

Q1. Show a sample of normal urine having pale yellow color/no visible abnormal constituents. Interpret/what does this suggest about the patient's hydration status?

Hints: Pale yellow color suggests normal hydration. A clear sample with no visible abnormalities indicates the absence of infections/disease/other pathological conditions.

Q2. A urine sample shows specific gravity of 1.015, pH of 6.0/no protein/no glucose/no blood. Interpret/what does it suggest about the patient's renal function/health?

Hints: The results are typical for a healthy individual with normal renal functions. Specific gravity and pH are normal and indicative of proper kidney function in regulating water/electrolyte balance.

CHAPTER 4

Analysis of Abnormal Constituents in the Urine and their Clinical Correlation

COMPETENCY

BC14.4: Identify abnormal constituents in urine, interpret the findings and correlate this with pathological states and prepare a urine report.

LEARNING OBJECTIVES

After reading this chapter, the readers should be able to:
- Understand the principles of urine analysis.
- Perform urine analysis to estimate normal and abnormal constituents.
- Interpret urine analysis results and correlate them with clinical conditions.
- Perform urine analysis to estimate and determine normal compounds in the urine.
- **IM11.13:** Vertical integration—Perform and interpret urinary ketone estimation with a dipstick.
- **PE33.6:** Vertical integration—Perform and interpret urine dipstick for sugar.

BLUE PRINT

Lesson Plan: Blueprint for Lecture—Urine Analysis

Objective

By the end of the lecture, students should be able to:
1. Understand the principles of urine analysis.
2. Perform urine analysis to estimate normal and abnormal constituents.
3. Interpret urine analysis results and correlate them with clinical conditions.

Duration: ***105 minutes***

Materials Needed

1. Presentation slides outlining urine analysis, various principles/techniques.
2. Samples of normal and abnormal urine for demonstration and experiments.
3. Urine analysis kits with reagent strips for testing urine parameters like pH, protein, glucose, ketone, bilirubin, urobilinogen, nitrites, and leukocytes.
4. Laboratory glassware/equipment for urine testing.
5. **Microscopes:** Urine sediment analysis.
6. Charts/diagrams showing normal and abnormal urine constituents.

Outline

DOAP session

I. **Introduction to urine analysis** **(15 minutes)**
- Define urine, analysis of urine, importance in clinical interpretation.
- Explain the principles/mechanisms of urine analysis, including physical and visual inspection, chemical and microscopic examinations.
- Discuss the parameters that are routinely assessed with their clinical significance.

II. **Preparation and handling of urine samples** **(10 minutes)**
- Provide guidelines to collect, store, and transport urine samples for analysis.
- Discuss the significance of sample integrity, proper labeling for ensuring accurate results.
- Highlight safety precautions in handling infectious urine samples.

III. **Chemical analysis of urine** **(30 minutes)**
- *pH*: Explain the importance of urine pH/demonstrate pH testing with reagent strips.
- *Protein*: Discuss the presence of protein in urine that is proteinuria; perform protein testing with dipstick/chemical methods.
- *Glucose*: Explain detection of glucose in urine that is glycosuria/demonstrate glucose test with reagent strips.
- *Ketone*: Discuss the importance of ketone in urine that is ketonuria and perform ketone test with reagent strips.
- *Bilirubin and urobilinogen*: Explain detection of bilirubin, urobilinogen and perform testing with reagent strips.
- *Nitrites and leukocytes*: Discuss the presence of nitrites, leukocytes in urine in (UTIs) and perform testing using reagent strips.

IV. **Microscopic examination of urine sediment** **(20 minutes)**
- Explain the mechanisms of urine sediment analysis, importance of different cellular and noncellular elements.
- Demonstrate preparation of urine sediment slides.
- Identify and discuss normal and abnormal constituents like red blood cells, white blood cells, epithelial cells, casts, crystals, and microorganisms.

V. **Interpretation of urine analysis results** **(10 minutes)**
- Interpret the findings of urine analysis based on all aspects like visual inspection, chemical tests, along with microscopic examination.
- Correlate abnormal urine constituents with clinical states.
- Discuss limitations, potential sources of error in the analysis of urine.

VI. **Case studies and clinical correlations** **(10 minutes)**
- Present case studies/clinical scenarios that show abnormal urine analysis findings.
- Encourage students to analyze the data and make diagnostic clinical interpretations.

VII. **Review and summary** **(5 minutes)**
- Summarize the important points covered in the lecture.
- Emphasize the significance of urine analysis in clinical diagnosing, monitoring medical conditions.

VIII. **Conclusion** **(5 minutes)**
- Conclude by reinforcing the importance of urine analysis in clinical practice as well as research.
- Encourage students to apply their knowledge in their future medical research endeavors.

Identify abnormal constituents in urine, interpret the findings and correlate these with pathological states.

Lesson plan: Blueprint—Abnormal Constituents in Urine and Pathological Correlations

Objective

By the end of the lecture, students should be able to:
1. Identify common abnormal constituents in urine samples.
2. Interpret the importance of abnormal findings and correlate with different pathological conditions.
3. Understand the diagnostic value of urine analysis in detecting and monitoring diseases.

Duration: ***70 minutes***

Materials Needed

1. **Presentation slides:** For illustrating abnormal constituents in urine and their pathological correlations.
2. Examples of urine analysis reports exhibiting abnormal findings.
3. Case studies/clinical scenarios highlighting the diagnostic utility of urine analysis.

Outline

I. **Introduction to urine analysis** **(10 minutes)**
- Overview of the significance of urine analysis in diagnoses and monitoring of diseases.
- Discussion of the components that are generally assessed in urine analysis.

II. **Common abnormal constituents in urine** **(20 minutes)**
- Identification, description of abnormal constituents:
  - *Proteinuria*: Albumin, globulins, Bence Jones proteins

- *Hematuria*: RBC's, Hb, Mb
- *Glycosuria*: Glucose
- *Ketosis*: Ketone
- *Bilirubinuria*: Bilirubin
- *Pyuria*: WBC's
- *Crystalluria*: Crystals like calcium oxalate, uric acid

- Explanation of the pathological importance of each abnormal constituent

III. **Pathological correlations** **(20 minutes)**
- Correlation of abnormal urine constituents with specific disorders:
  - *Proteinuria*: Renal diseases like glomerulonephritis, nephrotic syndrome, systemic diseases like diabetes mellitus, hypertension.
  - *Hematuria*: Urinary tract infections, kidney stones, trauma, malignancies like bladder cancer.
  - *Glycosuria*: Diabetes mellitus, renal glycosuria.
  - *Ketosis*: Diabetic ketoacidosis, starvation, ketogenic diets.
  - *Bilirubinuria*: Liver diseases like hepatitis, cirrhosis, biliary tract obstruction.
  - *Pyuria*: Urinary tract infections, kidney inflammations.
  - *Crystalluria*: Kidney stones, metabolic disorders like gout.

IV. **Interpretation of urinalysis reports** **(5 minutes)**
- Demonstration of interpreting urinalysis reports and also recognize abnormal findings.
- Discussion of the significance of correlating urine analysis results with clinical symptoms and other diagnostic tests.

V. **Clinical case studies** **(5 minutes)**
- Presentation of clinical cases/scenarios and abnormal urine constituents.
- Group discussion on the differential diagnosis and management.

VI. **Conclusion and recap** **(5 minutes)**
- Summary of important points covered in the lecture
- Focus on the diagnostic value of urine analysis in identification/monitoring diseases.

VII. **Question and answer session** **(5 minutes)**
- Encourage the readers to ask questions and get clarifications.
- Discuss real-life examples/challenging cases.

Assessment: Skill assessment, OSCE

INTRODUCTION

Abnormal Constituents

Abnormal urinary constituents are reducing sugars, proteins, bile salts, bile pigments, ketone bodies and blood. In various pathological disorders, the glomerular filtration of plasma is defective, resulting in leakage of substances in the lumen of the tubules, from where they may/may not be absorbed. These substances are finally excreted in the urine, in which these are normally not present.

Physical Examinations as Discussed in Normal Urine Variations

Biochemical Examination

Reducing Sugars

Disorders in which reducing sugars appear in urine:

Disease	Type of reducing sugar and enzyme responsible
1. Diabetes mellitus	Glucose (renal threshold for glucose = 180 mg%, above which glucose start appearing in the urine)
2. Congenital galactosemia (recessive, inherited disorder of galactose metabolism). - Galactose of diet is not converted to glucose - Galactose gets accumulated in the blood and excreted in urine because it does not get reabsorbed by the renal tubules - Main symptom of galactosemia is mental retardation	• Galactose • The enzyme galactose-1-phosphate uridyl transferase is congenially absent

Contd....

Contd....

Disease	Type of reducing sugar and enzyme responsible
3. Essential Fructosuria	• Fructose • Inherited absence of enzyme fructokinase (harmless condition)
4. *Hereditary fructose intolerance*: It should be treated as it can cause liver damage and hypoglycemia	• Fructose • Inherited absence of enzyme aldolase B
5. Essential pentosuria (disorder of uronic acid pathway, harmless condition)	• L-Xylulose • Absence of xylitol dehydrogenase enzyme
6. Pregnancy	Lactose

Glycosuria

The presence of detectable amounts of reducing sugars in urine is called glycosuria.

Types and Causes of Glycosuria

Type of glycosuria	Characteristic
Alimentary glycosuria	Glucose appears in urine transiently after excess intake of carbohydrate diet, due to increased absorption, it is a benign or harmless condition
Renal glycosuria	The capacity of renal tubules of kidneys is subnormal, that is the renal threshold for glucose which is normally 180 mg/dL in normal people, is decreased in renal glycosuria
Emotional/stress glycosuria	It can be due to hyper-secretion of epinephrine because of emotional stress
Endocrine disorders	Diabetes mellitus, hyperpituitarism, hyperthyroidism, Cushing's syndrome, pheochromocytoma
During late pregnancy and lactation	Lactose appear in urine, it is a harmless condition

Test for reducing sugars:

Benedict's test: This test is also positive for some noncarbohydrate substances which are reducing, such as vitamin C, salicylates, creatinine, uric acid, homogentisic acid, drugs, such as salicylates, isoniazid

Significance	Reagents/method	Observation	Conclusion	Principle
• This test is positive for all reducing sugars with free aldehyde or ketone groups • It is a semi-quantitative test that is the color of the precipitate provide the concentration of the sugar • This test is done for the screening of diabetes mellitus and monitoring the effect of treatment	Benedict's reagent (copper sulfate, sodium carbonate, for providing basic medium as reduction occurs best in alkaline medium and sodium citrate to prevent the precipitation of cupric hydroxide) = 5 mL + Urine sample = 8 drops + Mix and boil for 2 minutes	• Blue color precipitate—no sugar • Green precipitate (+) 0.1–0.5% sugar • Yellow precipitate (++) 0.5–1.0% sugar • Orange precipitate (+++) 1.0–2.0% sugar • Red precipitate (++++) Above 2% sugar	• Reducing sugars are present • The reducing sugars can reduce solutions of metallic ions • It is also a test for detecting reducing sugars in urine: – Lactose in lactosuria – Fructose in fructosuria – Glucose in glucosuria – Galactose in galactosuria	• Reducing sugar in presence of hot alkaline medium forms enediol which are strong reducing agents • Cupric hydroxide $[2Cu(OH)_2]$ is formed by hydrolysis of copper sulfate • $(2Cu(OH)_2)$ is reduced by reducing sugars to cuprous oxide (Cu_2O) (red), the sugar is oxidized to corresponding aldonic acid

Dipstick method for detection of glucose

Significance	Method	Observation	Conclusion	Principle
It is a very specific and sensitive test as it can detect even traces of glucose in the urine sample (<0.1 g%)	Take 5 mL of urine in a test tube and dip one end of the strip in it and read the color after thirty seconds	The color changes to purple	Glucose is present in urine	• It is based on the principle of GOD-POD (glucose oxidase-peroxidase) • Stiff cellulose strips are coated with glucose oxidase Glucose → GOD Gluconic acid + H_2O_2 • $H_2O_2 \rightarrow$ POD $H_2O + [O]$ • Ortho-toluidine + [O] → colored complex

Proteins

Proteinuria

Presence of proteins in urine is called proteinuria. As albumin is smaller in size, it gets filtered and the major protein to be appearing in urine is albumin. Other proteins may be globulin and fibrinogen.

The main cause of proteinuria is any disorder leading to damage of basement membrane that is nephropathy.

Types of Proteinuria

	Prerenal	Renal	Postrenal
1. **Organic proteinuria:** It is due to some definite organic disorder, it may be divided into three types	The cause is outside the excretory system	The cause is in the kidneys	The cause lies in the urinary tract distal to the kidneys that is the urine passing out of kidneys is normal and the proteins enter the urine during its passage through pelvis, ureter, urinary bladder, prostate or urethra
	• Fever • Convulsions • Heart failure • Liver disorders • Collagen disorders • Toxemia of pregnancy	• Acute glomerulonephritis • Chronic glomerulonephritis • Nephrosclerosis • Nephrotic syndrome • Renal tuberculosis • Kidney cancer	Inflammatory or malignant lesions in the path/passage of urine

Bence-Jones proteins: They are gamma globulin proteins which appear in urine in multiple myeloma and leukemia, it consists of immunoglobin light chains, identified in urine by electrophoresis detected as M band (myeloma band), and it has a characteristic property of precipitating between 40–60°C on heating the urine and dissolves on further heating to 100°C. The precipitate reappear again on cooling between 40–60°C

2. **Functional proteinuria:** It is a temporary and benign condition and is not associated with any organic disorder, can be due to severe exertion or in pregnancy
3. **Postural proteinuria:** Proteinuria is in upright position but not in recumbent posture
4. **Microalbuminuria:** Excretion of albumin approximately 20–300 mg/day is called microalbuminuria, generally seen in patients with hypertension and diabetes mellitus as complication of clinical renal disorder

Methods based on precipitation of proteins:

The three criterion of protein solubility are:

1. Intact tertiary structure of protein
2. Net charge on the particles
3. Shell of hydration around protein particles

Name of the method	*Characteristic feature*
Heat coagulation test	Based on denaturation of protein where protein loses its quaternary, secondary and tertiary structures but the primary structure is intact
Heller's test	Concentrated nitric acid is a strong denaturing agent
Sulfosalicylic acid test	After centrifuging the urine 2.5 mL of supernatant is added to 7.5 mL of 3% sulfosalicylic acid, and the degree of turbidity is quantified
Salting out	The shell of hydration is disrupted by ammonium sulfate which is very soluble in polar medium, such as urine so precipitation of protein take place
Precipitation by acetone/alcohol	They are volatile solvents so they evaporate the shell of hydration around the protein, so precipitation of protein takes place
Isoelectric pH (pI)	It is the pH at which the protein exists in zwitter ion form so when the pH of the solution which contains the protein is brought to isoelectric point (pI), the protein will precipitate

Heat coagulation test: It involves dissociation of the protein subunits that is disruption of the quaternary structure, uncoiling of the polypeptide chains that is disruption of tertiary and secondary structure and matting together of the uncoiled polypeptide chains that is coagulation (irreversible denaturation)

Contd....

Contd....

Method	Observation	Inference
Take three fourth of the test tube of urine sample and heat the upper one-third of it for one minute, the lower portion of sample serves as control	1. White turbidity is seen on heating which is dissolved after adding 1% acetic acid 2. White turbidity is seen on heating which is intensified after adding 1% acetic acid	The white precipitate is because of phosphates/carbonates which were dissolved by acetic acid 1. The white precipitate is because of protein–albumin 2. Adding 1% acetic acid brought the pH of urine nearer to pI of albumin (5.4) and thus intensified the precipitate
	Heller's test	
Take 5 mL of urine in a test tube and add 1 mL of conc. Nitric acid in the urine drop-by-drop from the side walls of the test tube	A white ring is seen at the junction of two liquids which denotes denatured protein	Concentrated mineral acids cause intra-molecular changes in the protein molecules by changing the native proteins to insoluble acid metaproteins
	Sulfosalicylic acid test	
Take 5 mL of urine in a test tube and add sulfosalicylic acid (alkaloidal reagent) drop wise mixing after each addition	A white turbidity is seen Protein (mg%) — Degree of turbidity 0 mg% — Clear 1–10 — Opalescent 15–30 — Can read print through tube 40–100 — Can read only black line 150–400 — No visible black lines >500 — Flocculent	• Because of the amphoteric nature of proteins, they act as acids in basic medium and act as bases in acid medium • In presence of sulfosalicylic acid, they act as bases and react with the acid to form an insoluble salt, protein sulfosalicylate
	Precipitation of protein by alcohol/acetone	
Take 3 mL of urine in a test tube and mix 1 mL of alcohol/acetone vigorously shaking the test tube	White precipitate is seen	The volatile solvents have a tendency to precipitate the proteins by evaporating the shell of hydration from around the protein
	Bringing the pH to isoelectric pH (pI)	
Take 3 mL urine in a test tube and add conc. Nitric acid drop wise	White precipitate is seen	• The pI of albumin is 4.7 and the pH of urine is 6.5, so by adding acid drop wise in the urine, we bring the pH of urine nearer to isoelectric point of albumin (4.7) • The solubility of the proteins is minimum at their isoelectric pH because the protein molecules are electrically neutral at this pH, and exists as zwitter ion
	Salting out test	
Half saturation precipitation test: Make a saturated solution of ammonium sulfate in water and add 5 mL of this saturated solution in 5 mL of urine sample shake and let it stand for some time	Globulin present in urine gets precipitated in form of white precipitate	Proteins are colloidal so they are prevented from getting precipitated by 2 factors: • Electric charges—similar charged particles repel each other so prevents their coalescence • Shell of hydration—a thin film of water around each protein particle preventing their coalescence • We remove these 2 factors by adding a neutral salt—ammonium sulfate which neutralizes the electric charges and remove the shell of hydration as its affinity for water is more than the colloid

Contd....

Contd....

Full saturation precipitation test: Saturate 5 mL of urine sample with solid ammonium sulfate, shake and let it stand for some time	Albumin of urine gets precipitated in form of white precipitate	• The amount of ammonium sulfate needed to precipitate depends on surface area of the particles • The larger the surface area, the more is the number of electric charges and more is the shell of hydration, so the smaller molecules with a large surface area, such as albumin is precipitated with only full saturation test

Albustix test

Principle	Observation/Inference
• The proteins change the color of acid-base indicator, such as tetrabromophenol blue • When the dye is buffered at pH 3, it is yellow • The protein changes this yellow color to green to blue depending on the concentration of protein	We compare the developed color with color chart which aids in grading the protein concentration from traces (1–10 mg%) to +4 (>500 mg %)

BILE SALTS

They are salts of taurocholic acid and glycocholic acids; their functions are to help in digestion and absorption of fats by decreasing the surface tension and are excreted in urine in obstructive jaundice. They are made in liver and excreted in bile; about 1% is excreted in feces daily (400 mg/day) and the remaining 99% is reabsorbed from the intestine and return to liver by enterohepatic circulation.

They get regurgitated into systemic circulation in hepatic and posthepatic jaundice because of intra-/extra-hepatic biliary obstruction, as they are water soluble; they get excreted out in urine. They are absent in urine, in hemolytic jaundice, in hepatic jaundice, they are present in urine and in obstructive jaundice; they are present in urine in excess.

Hay's sulfur test

Procedure	Observation	Conclusion
• Take 2 test tubes • One test is marked T for sample and other test tube is marked C for control • Fill 5 mL water in C test tube and 5 mL of urine sample in T test tube • Sprinkle a pinch of sulfur powder in both the test tubes	Sulfur powder sinks at the bottom of the test tube containing urine and floats on surface in test tube containing water	Bile salt is present in the urine which decreases the surface tension so sulfur powder sinks at the bottom of the test tube

Precautions:
1. Do not shake the test tubes, let them stand for few minutes otherwise false results are produced
2. Do not excess of sulfur otherwise it will settle due to its mass
3. Use fresh sulfur so that it is moisture free

BILE PIGMENTS

Bilirubin is the main pigment in humans, formed from heme degradation in reticuloendothelial cells and is released in the circulation. This is called unconjugated bilirubin and is not soluble in plasma. It requires binding with albumin for its transportation so does not get filtered out in urine because of its large mass when combined with albumin. It is taken up by the hepatocytes, gets conjugated with glucuronic acid, forming bilirubin diglucuronide and is then excreted in bile. In the intestine, it gets changed to urobilinogen (red), most of which is reabsorbed and recirculated. Negligible amount of UBG is excreted in urine. The oxidized form of UBG is called urobilin (colorless). Some part of it is excreted in the feces which is responsible for the normal color of feces and is known as stercobilin.

Conjugated bilirubin regurgitates into systemic circulation in hepatic and posthepatic jaundice due to intra-hepatic and extra-hepatic obstructions respectively. As it is water soluble, it gets excreted out in urine. In prehepatic jaundice, unconjugated bilirubin is increased in the blood which cannot be excreted out in urine as it is water insoluble.

Test for bile pigment: Fouchet's test

Method	Observation and inference	Principle
Urine = 10 mL + $MgSO_4$ = 1 mL + Boil + 10% $BaCl_2$ is added drop wise to form a precipitate Filter the urine on a filter paper Discard the filtrate and dry the filter paper by keeping in hot air oven at 50°C for at least 5 minutes + Fresh Fouchet's reagent on the precipitate = 2 drops Keep the filter paper in hot air oven at 50°C for at least 2 minutes again Rosenbach's test is also done for bilirubin	• Bluish green color of precipitate is observed • Bilirubin diglucuronide (conjugated bilirubin) is excreted in urine in hepatic (+) and obstructive jaundice (++) and absent in urine in hemolytic jaundice	• Bilirubin is present in the urine which is oxidized to biliverdin by adding Fouchet's reagent which has $FeCl_3$ • Magnesium sulfate and barium chloride interact to form a precipitate of barium sulfate • Barium sulfate adsorbs bilirubin • After filtration, when we dry the precipitate and add Fouchet's reagent (10 mg of 10% ferric chloride and 100 mL of 25% trichloroacetic acid), the bilirubin gets oxidized to biliverdin which forms bluish-green color

KETONE BODIES

There are three ketone bodies:

1. Acetoacetate
2. Beta-hydroxybutyrate
3. Acetone

They are formed in liver from acetyl CoA in small amount. They are oxidized in extrahepatic tissues to release energy.

Ketonemia

Saturation of extra-hepatic machinery due to overproduction of ketone bodies leads to increased blood level of ketonebodies.

Causes of Ketonemia

- Improper carbohydrate metabolism
- Increased fatty acid oxidation
  (Excess acetyl CoA formed from increased fatty acid oxidation, is not able to get oxidized by TCA cycle because of impaired carbohydrate metabolism; and as intermediates of TCA are not available, this acetyl CoA is diverted to form ketone bodies).
- Intake of high fat and low carbohydrate diet

Ketonuria

The excretion of ketone bodies due to ketonemia is called ketonuria.

Ketosis

The excess formation of ketone bodies resulting in ketonemia and ketonuria cause ketosis which is seen in severe diabetes mellitus, starvation and toxemia of pregnancy.

Test for ketone bodies: Rothera's test

Method	Observation	Inference
Urine sample = 5 mL + Saturate with ammonium sulfate to precipitate the proteins in urine + Fresh 2% sodium nitroprusside solution + Liquor ammonia = 1 mL from the sides of the test tube	Purple color ring is seen at the junction of both the liquids	• Presence of acetone or acetoacetate in urine (keto group containing ketone body) • Beta-hydroxybutyrate (lacks keto group) is testes by modified Rothera's test in which it is first modified to acetoacetic acid by H_2O_2 and then tested • Sodium nitroprusside reacts with ketones to form a purple color complex in alkaline medium provided by ammonia

Blood

The presence of blood in urine includes hematuria and hemoglobinuria.

Hematuria	Hemoglobinuria
The presence of blood in urine is called hematuria	The presence of free hemoglobin in urine is called hemoglobinuria, occurring due to increased hemolysis
Acute glomerulonephritis	Hemolytic anemia
Bleeding disorders, such as hemophilia, purpura and leukemia	Typhoid fever
Injury/trauma to urinary tract	Black water fever
Urinary tract cancer	Burns
Stones in urinary tract	Mismatch blood transfusion
Tuberculosis	• Malignant hypertension • Sickle cell anemia • Clotting disorders • Polycystic kidney disorder

Benzidine test for detection of blood in urine

Method	Observation	Principle/Inference
Urine sample = 3 mL Boil for 3 minutes and cooled In other test tube: Benzidine solution = 3 mL + H_2O_2 = 3 mL Boiled and cooled urine is added to second test tube having benzidine and H_2O_2 **Precaution:** Benzidine is carcinogenic so handle with care	Transient blue color is observed	• Blood is present in the urine sample • The peroxidase activity of heme changes H_2O_2 to H_2O and nascent oxygen • Nascent oxygen act on benzidine to form blue color complex

Urobilinogen

UBG is colorless and is formed by bacterial oxidation of bilirubin in intestine, and is reabsorbed by the enterohepatic circulation and excreted in urine.

Test for urobilinogen in urine: Ehrlich's test

Method	Observation	Inference
Urine = 5 mL + Ehrich's reagent para-dimethyl-amino-benzal-dehyde in HCl) = 5 mL Wait for 10 minutes Saturated sodium acetate = 10 mL	A pinkish red color is observed	Urobilinogen is present in the urine
Hemolytic jaundice	Hepatocellular/hepatic	Obstructive jaundice
UBG = ++	UBG = +/absent	UBG = absent

OSCE

1. **What are abnormalities assessed in a urine sample?**
   Physical: Color, clarity, odor, volume
   Chemical: pH, protein, glucose, ketones, bilirubin, blood, urobilinogen, nitrites
   Microscopic: Red blood cells (RBCs), white blood cells (WBCs), casts, crystals, bacteria
2. **Case scenario 1:**
   A patient comes with symptoms of dark brown urine and yellow sclera. Urine dipstick exhibits positive bilirubin and negative urobilinogen. What is the diagnosis?

Abnormal findings: Dark brown urine, positive bilirubin, negative urobilinogen.
Interpretation: Suggest obstructive jaundice (e.g., bile duct obstruction).
Explanation: Conjugated bilirubin is water-soluble and also excreted out in urine, and urobilinogen is absent because of impaired bile flow in the intestine.

3. **Case scenario 2:**
   A patient's urine: Frothy, dip stick: +3 protein and microscopy: fatty casts. What is the diagnosis?
   Abnormal findings: Frothy urine, proteinuria, fatty casts.
   Interpretation: Suggests nephrotic syndrome.
   Explanation: Excess protein in urine and fatty casts are highlighting features of nephrotic syndrome due to glomerular damage.
4. **Case scenario 3:**
   Urine sample: reddish-brown. Dipstick: positive for blood, no RBCs are present on microscopy. What does this indicate?
   Abnormal findings: Positive blood on dipstick, no RBCs in microscopy.
   Interpretation: Myoglobinuria/rhabdomyolysis/hemoglobinuria/hemolysis.
   Explanation: The dipstick shows heme pigments that might indicate free hemoglobin/myoglobin in urine with no RBCs.
5. **Case scenario 4:**
   A patient comes with complains of frequent urination, burning micturition, with cloudy urine. Dipstick: positive nitrites + leukocytes. What is the likely diagnosis?
   Abnormal findings: Cloudy urine, positive nitrites and positive leukocytes.
   Interpretation: indicates a urinary tract infection.
   Explanation: Nitrites suggests bacterial conversion of nitrates, leukocytes indicate inflammation/infection.
6. **Case scenario 5:**
   Urine sample: fruity odor. Dipstick: positive for glucose, ketones. What does it indicate?
   Abnormal findings: Fruity odor, glycosuria, ketonuria.
   Interpretation: diabetic ketoacidosis
   Explanation: Glucose and ketones in urine are present because of uncontrolled diabetes, the body uses lipids for energy, forming ketones.
7. **Case scenario 6:**
   A patient comes with cola-colored urine and sore throat. Dipstick: blood + protein. Microscopy: RBC casts. What is the diagnosis?
   Abnormal findings: Cola-colored urine, blood, protein, RBC casts.
   Interpretation: indicative of acute glomerulonephritis/post-streptococcal glomerulonephritis
   Explanation: RBC casts show glomerular origin of hematuria, proteinuria shows glomerular damage.
8. **Case scenario 7:**
   Urine: pale yellow specific gravity is <1.005, no abnormal findings of dipstick. The patient complains of polyuria. What does this indicate?
   Abnormal findings: Low specific gravity, polyuria.
   Interpretation: suggests diabetes insipidus/dilute urine because of excessive water intake.
   Explanation: Low specific gravity plus dilute urine with polyuria suggests inability to concentrate urine, frequently observed in diabetes insipidus.
9. **Case scenario 8:**
   Urine: positive cystine crystals under polarized light. What is the condition?
   Abnormal findings: Cystine crystals.
   Interpretation: Suggest cystinuria.
   Explanation: Cystinuria is a genetic disease resulting in poor reabsorption of cystine in the kidneys, leading to its precipitation in urine.
10. **Case scenario 9:**
    Urine: dark plus turns black on standing. Dipstick: negative for blood. What is the diagnosis?
    Abnormal findings: Dark urine turning black after standing.
    Interpretation: Indicate Alkaptonuria
    Explanation: Alkaptonuria is a metabolic disorder due to by homogentisic acid buildup that oxidizes and darkens upon standing.
11. **Case scenario 10:**
    A dehydrated patient shows with concentrated urine. Dipstick: positive for ketones, no glucose. What does this indicate?
    Abnormal findings: Concentrated urine, positive ketones, no glucose.
    Interpretation: indicates starvation ketosis.
    Explanation: Ketones in the absence of glucose point towards fat metabolism because of prolonged fasting/starvation.

CLINICAL MCQS

1. **A 55-year-old male presents with frothy urine and edema. His urine analysis: 4+ proteinuria plus fatty casts. What is the diagnosis?**
   a. Nephropathy
   b. Nephrotic syndrome
   c. Glomerulonephritis
   d. Urinary tract infection

   Answer: b. Nephrotic syndrome

2. **A urine dipstick test: positive nitrites plus leukocyte esterase. The patient complains of dysuria plus fever. What is diagnosis?**
   a. Nephrosclerosis
   b. Acute pyelonephritis
   c. Glomerulonephritis
   d. Renal acidosis

   Answer: b. Acute pyelonephritis

3. **A patient comes with dark-colored urine and jaundice. Urinalysis: positive bilirubin and urobilinogen. What is the cause?**
   a. Acute liver failure
   b. Hemolysis
   c. Obstructive jaundice
   d. Hepatitis

   Answer: d. Hepatitis

4. **A urine sample appears red-brown, microscopic analysis: dysmorphic red blood cells and RBC casts. What is the diagnosis?**
   a. Acute glomerulonephritis
   b. Nephrosclerosis
   c. Hematuria
   d. Urinary tract infection

   Answer: a. Acute glomerulonephritis

5. **A child with vomiting, altered sensorium, urine is positive for ketones negative for glucose. What is the most likely reason?**
   a. Ketoacidosis
   b. Starvation ketosis
   c. UTI
   d. Alkaptonuria

   Answer: b. Starvation ketosis

6. **A 67-year-old male presents with hematuria. Urine microscopy: many red blood cells, no casts. What is the diagnosis?**
   a. Bladder carcinoma
   b. Glomerulonephritis
   c. Nephrosclerosis
   d. Chronic pyelonephritis

   Answer: a. Bladder carcinoma

7. **A urine sample has a sweet smell, positive for glucose plus ketones. What condition can be suspected?**
   a. Starvation ketosis
   b. DKA
   c. Glycosuria
   d. Fanconi syndrome

   Answer: b. DKA

8. **A patient has tea-colored urine and has muscle pain. The urine dipstick is positive for blood, microscopy shows no RBCs. What is the most probable reason?**
   a. Hematuria
   b. Rhabdomyolysis
   c. Nephrotic syndrome
   d. Chronic sclerosis

   Answer: b. Rhabdomyolysis

9. A neonate presents with dark urine which turns black after standing. Urine analysis shows presence of homogentisic acid. What is the likely diagnosis?
   a. MSUD
   b. PKU
   c. Alkaptonuria
   d. Homocystinuria

   Answer: c. Alkaptonuria

10. A 45-year-old diabetic patient has persistent glucosuria but normal blood glucose levels. What diagnosis is most likely?
   a. Diabetes insipidus
   b. Renal glycosuria
   c. Cushing syndrome
   d. Addisons disease

   Answer: b. Renal glycosuria

REFLECTION

Analysis of Pathological Urine Sample

Test	Observation	Inference

Result and Clinical Interpretation

....
....
....
....
....
....
....
....
....
....
....
....
....
....

Teacher's Signature with Date

REFLECTION

Analysis of Pathological Urine Sample

Test	Observation	Inference

Result and Clinical Interpretation

....

....

....

....

....

....

....

....

....

....

....

....

....

....

Teacher's Signature with Date

VIVA VOCE

Q1. Discuss common abnormal constituents of urine/what do they indicate about any patient's overall health?
Next question/Follow-up: Differentiate between physiological/pathological reasons for the presence of abnormal constituents like protein/glucose/blood in the urine?

Q2. Explain the importance of detecting protein in urine. What are the reasons behind proteinuria/how to further investigate a patient with proteinuria?
Next question/Follow-up: Differentiate between transient/persistent proteinuria?

SPOTTERS

Q1. Show urine sample with a positive dipstick test for blood, no red blood cells observed under the microscope. Interpret, and mention causes of this finding?

Hints: Suggests of presence of Hb/Mb in the urine that is hematuria vs. hemoglobinuria/myoglobinuria).
Reasons may be hemolysis/rhabdomyolysis/muscle injury.

Q2. Show sample of urine that has elevated levels of glucose but no ketones. Interpret/what further investigations are recommended?

Hints: Suggests hyperglycemia, mainly because of diabetes mellitus. Further investigations: FBG, HbA1c, proper clinical examination for confirming the diagnosis.

5

CHAPTER

Screening of Urine for Inborn Errors of Metabolism and Paper Chromatography

COMPETENCY

BC14.5: Describe screening of urine for inborn errors and describe the use of paper chromatography (Chapters 5 and 6).

LEARNING OBJECTIVES

After reading this chapter, the readers should be able to:

- Describe the important features of inborn errors of metabolism.
- Describe the biochemical basis of different tests performed in laboratory in urine for screening of IEM.
- Understand the concept of inborn errors of metabolism and their screening in urine.
- Describe the principles and techniques of paper chromatography.
- Perform paper chromatography for the detection of metabolic disorders in urine samples.

BLUE PRINT

Describe screening of urine for inborn errors and describe the use of paper chromatography.
Observe use of commonly used equipments and techniques in biochemistry laboratory, including paper chromatography of amino acid.

Lesson Plan: Screening of Urine for Inborn Errors and Paper Chromatography (Chapters 5, 6)

Objective

By the end of the lecture, students should be able to:

1. Understand the concept of inborn errors of metabolism and their screening in urine.
2. Describe the principles and techniques of paper chromatography.
3. Perform paper chromatography for the detection of metabolic disorders in urine samples.

Duration: ***120 minutes***

Materials Needed

1. Presentation slides outlining inborn errors of metabolism and principles of paper chromatography.
2. Samples of urine with known inborn errors for demonstration for the students.
3. Paper chromatography equipment like filter paper, solvent like isopropanol, pipettes, developing chamber, and drying rack.
4. Standard solutions of metabolites to compare.
5. Laboratory glassware, equipments for paper chromatography.
6. Charts/diagrams illustrating the mechanisms and principles of paper chromatography.

Outline

Lecture, small group discussion

I. **Introduction to inborn errors of metabolism** **(15 minutes)**
   - Define inborn errors of metabolism, along with genetic basis.
   - Discuss the importance of screening in newborns.
   - Provide examples of common IEMs along with clinical manifestations.

II. **Screening of urine for inborn errors** **(30 minutes)**
- Explain the principles of urine screening emphasizing on the detection of abnormal metabolites.
- Describe the methodology for urine sample collection and storage.
- Discuss the techniques used for urine analysis, chemical tests, enzymatic assays, and chromatography.
- Focus the significance of early detection along with intervention in management for avoiding diverse outcomes.

III. **Principles of paper chromatography** **(15 minutes)**
- Define paper chromatography, importance in separating, and analyzing mixtures of substances.
- Explain the principles of chromatography, concepts of stationary, mobile phase, adsorption, as well as partitioning.
- Discuss the causes influencing the chromatography, like polarity, size, solubility, etc.

IV. **Setup and procedure for paper chromatography** **(20 minutes)**
- Demonstrate the setup of paper chromatography, preparation of the chromatography chamber.
- Explain the process of spotting urine samples and standard solutions.
- Discuss the choice of solvents in the system along with chromatogram development.
- Highlight safety precautions and good laboratory practices.

V. **Interpretation of paper chromatography results** **(10 minutes)**
- Analyze chromatograms taken from urine samples and standard solutions.
- Identify and compare the migration patterns of metabolites.
- Interpret the results as presence or absence of abnormal metabolites.

VI. **Clinical applications and case studies** **(10 minutes)**
- Present case studies or clinical scenarios involving the screening of urine for IEMs using paper chromatography.
- Discuss the diagnostic implications in identifying and managing metabolic disorders.

VII. **Review and summary** **(5 minutes)**
- Summarize the important points regarding urine screening for IEMs and paper chromatography procedure.
- Focus the significance of early detection and intervention in management of metabolic disorders

VIII. **Conclusion** **(5 minutes)**
- Conclude by highlighting the role of urine screening and paper chromatography in the diagnosis plus management of inborn errors of metabolism.
- Encourage the readers for further exploring applications of chromatography in clinical practice.

IX. **Paper chromatography of amino acids** **(10 minutes)**
- Explanation of paper chromatography procedure for separating amino acids.
- Practical demonstration of sample preparation along with chromatography setup, and also visualization of amino acids.

Assessment: Written/viva voce, direct observation, OSPE

INTRODUCTION

Screening

It is a process of identifying apparently healthy people who may be at increased risk of a disease or a condition.

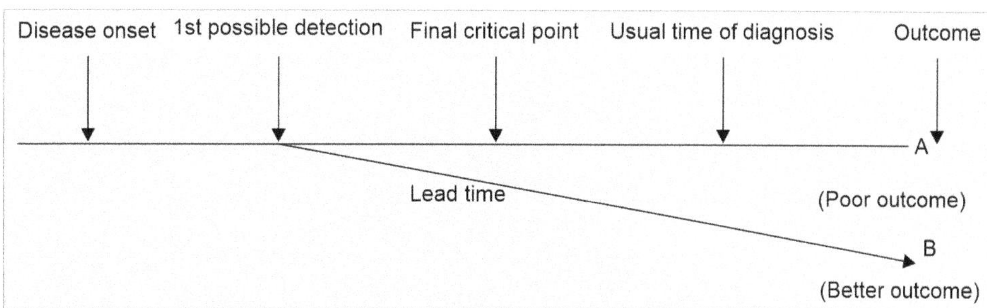

Screening	Diagnostic test
Done for apparently healthy	Done for sick with overt indications
More sensitive but less specific	More specific
Results are suggestive and give hints	Results are definitive
Positive result is not a basis of treatment	Positive result is not a basis of treatment
Economical	Comparatively costly

Inborn Errors of Metabolism

Inborn errors of metabolism (IEM): They are metabolic disorders, rare, detected most frequently at infancy, some IEM are fatal at early age.

IEM classes	
Disorders of carbohydrate metabolism	• Galactosemia • G6PD deficiency
Aminoacidopathies	Phenylketonuria
Urea cycle defects	• Hyperammonemia • Citrullinemia
Organic acidurias	Alkaptonuria
IEM causes	• Deficiency of enzyme • Absence of enzyme
IEM characteristics	• Substrate accumulation • Less formation/absence of products • The substrates get diverted to alternate pathways to form undesirable products • High morbidity and mortality • Commonly diagnosed in infancy • They can lead to fatal complications, such as brain damage
Suspected manifestations	• Poor growth • Delayed milestones • Damaged brain • High fatality rate • Children with seizures • Recurrent vomiting • History of consanguinity • Enlarged organs
Metabolic screening	• Complete blood cell count • ABG and electrolytes • Liver function tests and renal function tests • Blood glucose • Blood lactate • Serum uric acid • Urine all abnormal constituents, such as ketone bodies, reducing sugars, etc. • Specific screening tests according to clinical presentations • Lastly, confirmation of the diagnosis by special tests depending on the results of screening tests

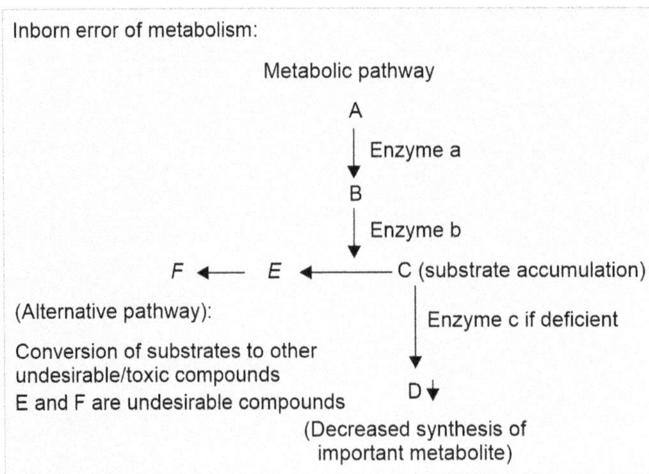

Phenylketonuria (PKU): Prevalence

- Very common IEM
- Seen in 1:10,000 live births
- Autosomal recessive

PKU: Cause

Deficiency of enzyme phenylalanine hydroxylase which converts phenylalanine to tyrosine

PKU: Biochemical effect

- Phenylalanine accumulates
- Tyrosine is not synthesized so it becomes essential amino acid/supplemented in diet in the treatment

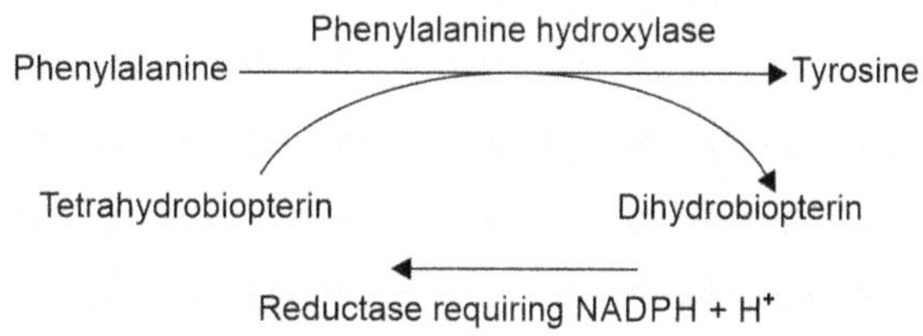

PKU: Alternate pathway

Forms phenylpyruvate, phenyllactate, and phenylacetate (neurotoxic metabolites)

PKU: Complications

- Excess phenylalanine inhibits tyrosinase enzyme which results in decreased formation of melanin leading to hypopigmentation and defect in protein synthesis
- Normal at birth but delayed milestones
- Irreversible damage to brain, cerebral disorders, such as convulsions, blank expressions, mental retardation (decreased formation of myelin, epinephrine, norepinephrine, serotonin and neurotransmitters)

Classical phenylketonuria (type 1 PKU): Cause

- Absence of phenylalanine hydroxylase
- Very severe

Malignant phenylketonuria: Cause

Defective tetrahydrobiopterin formation due to deficiency of phenylalanine hydroxylase

Malignant phenylketonuria: Effect

Neurotoxicity due to defect in the synthesis of other neurotransmitters, such as dopamine, serotonin, noradrenalin, etc.

Malignant phenylketonuria: Clinical features

- Seizures
- Mental retardation
- Eczema
- Mousy odor of urine and sweat (phenyl lactate)
- Hypopigmentation

Type II PKU

Deficiency of dihydrobiopterin reductase enzyme

Type III PKU

Deficiency of synthesis of tetrahydrobiopterin

Ferric chloride test: General test for phenol group (nonspecific test, so if positive, should be confirmed by a diagnostic test)

Method	**Observation**
Urine = 5 mL + 10 g% ferric chloride = 4 drops	Phenylpyruvate forms a green/blue color stable up to 2 minutes

Dinitrophenylhydrazine test (DNPH) (nonspecific)

Method	**Observation**
Urine = 2 mL + DNPH reagent = 2 mL	After 10 minutes, there is appearance of a yellow precipitate due to keto acid phenylpyruvate
Principle	DNPH + phenylpyruvate → Hydrazone (yellow precipitate)

Guthrie's bacterial inhibition test: Screening test done in blood

Bacillus subtilis

It is used in the test and it requires phenylalanine for growth in culture

Observation

If blood from normal infant is added, there is no growth of bacteria, but if blood from PKU patient is added, bacteria proliferate since phenylalanine is not metabolized, and is present in high amounts

Contd....

Contd....

Principle	• *Bacillus subtilis* needs phenylalanine in order to grow in culture • In presence of an phenylalanine antagonist that is beta-2-Thienylalanine in culture media the bacteria stops growing • So, if the serum has enough phenylalanine then growth of this *Bacillus* will be seen, but if the serum has deficient/normal phenylalanine, the growth of this *Bacillus* will not be seen
Diagnostic confirmatory tests	• Blood phenylalanine level (>4 mg/dL is indicative of phenylketonuria) • Activity of liver phenylalanine hydroxylase

Fructose intolerance

Cause	**Deficiency of enzyme aldolase B**
Clinical abnormality	Hypoglycemia
	Fructose $\xrightarrow{\text{Fructokinase + ATP}}$ Fructose1 phosphate $\xrightarrow{\text{Aldolase B}}$ Glyceraldehyde + dihydroxyacetone phosphate
Metabolic defects	Accumulation of fructose 1 phosphate in liver (hepatomegaly) Depletion of phosphate as it is continuously making fructose 1 phosphate Decreased ATP synthesis Phosphorylation of glucose does not take place Fructose 1 phosphate inhibits liver glycogen phosphorylase thus inhibiting glycogenolysis which is required to maintain blood sugar levels between the meals (high fructose in diet can cause hypoglycemia)
Confirmatory test	Fructose tolerance test: • A fructose load is given (3 g/sqm) as intravenous infusion • Periodical examination of samples is done • Within 45 minutes, hypoglycemia is observed which reaches peak by 1 hour • Blood fructose activity increases till 60 mg/dL within 15 minutes from zero base level • Fructose is present in urine, no presence of glucose in urine

Alkaptonuria

Alkaptonuria (definition)	• First disease to be identified as IEM • Autosomal recessive disorder of tyrosine metabolism
Cause	*Deficiency of enzyme homogentisic oxidase* Phenylalanine $\longrightarrow$ Tyrosine $\longrightarrow$ Homogentisic acid $\xrightarrow{\text{Homogentisic acid oxidase}}$ Malealyl-aceto-acetic acid
Biochemical effect	• Accumulation of homogentisic acid in blood along with its excretion • Homogentisic acid may convert to benzo-quinone acetate (black) on oxidation
Pathological effect/ Striking feature	• Polymerization of homogentisic acid of urine when exposed to atmospheric oxygen leading to formation of brownish-black colored pigment changing the color of urine to black • This pigment gets accumulated in eyes, sclera, ears, bones and even heart called ochronosis and bluish darkening of outer ears, nose and whites of eyes • Arthritis

Screening tests (done on basis of symptoms/complaints by the patient)

Method	**Observation**
Benedict's test	Reducing nature of homogentisic acid gives a positive test in form of brown color
Ferric chloride test	Phenol ring is present in homogentisic acid so this test is positive in form of immediate purple black color
Ammonical silver nitrate test: 3 g% silver nitrate = 5 mL + Urine = 0.5 mL + 10% Ammonia solution = few drops	A black precipitate is seen

Contd....

Contd....

X-ray of lumbar spine	• Bamboo-like appearance • Calcification seen • Arthritis changes seen
Diagnostic confirmation tests: They should be done in blood as well as urine, as homogentisic acid has a tendency to excrete rapidly in urine	• Chromatographic detection of homogentisic acid oxidase • Enzymatic estimation of homogentisic acid oxidase

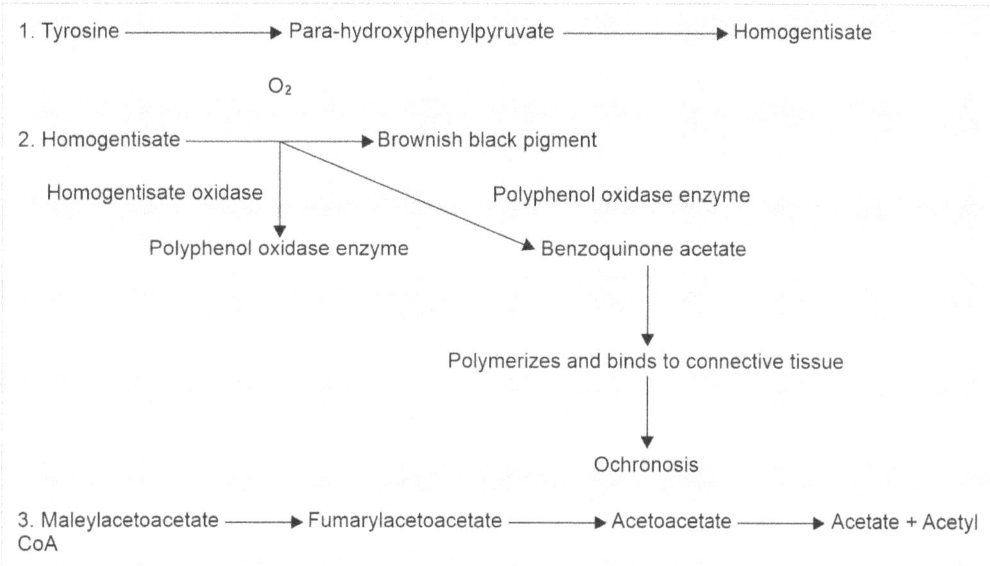

Maple Syrup Urine Disease

Maple syrup urine disease definition	• Autosomal recessive • Disorder of branched chain amino acid metabolism that is valine, leucine and isoleucine
Cause/metabolic defect: Branched chain amino acids in presence of transaminase enzyme converts to corresponding alpha-keto acids which in presence of alpha-keto acid dehydrogenase which is deficient in maple syrup urine disease, converts to corresponding CoA derivatives	• Deficiency of enzyme alpha-keto acid dehydrogenase • Plasma and urinary levels of leucine/isoleucine/valine and alpha-keto acids are raised
Symptoms	• Baby is normal at birth • At later stage may develop convulsions, spasticity, vomiting, tiredness • Smell of burnt sugar in urine due to keto acids
Screening test: • Ferric chloride test • Dinitrophenylhydrazine test	 • Positive (greenish gray color seen) • Positive
Guthrie's bacterial inhibition test: Diagnostic confirmatory test	Azaleucine antagonist of L leucine is used: • Plasma levels of branched chain amino acids • Activity of branched-chain alpha-ketoacid dehydrogenase enzyme in lymphocytes/ cultured fibroblasts

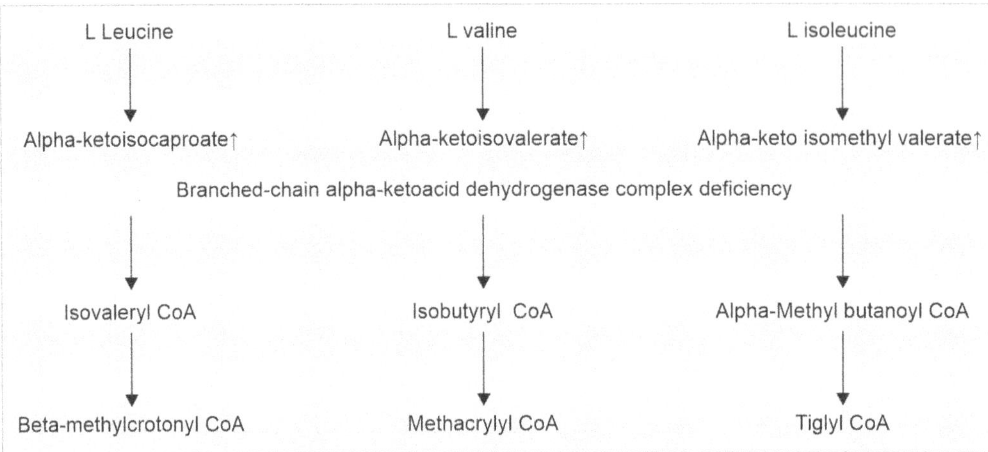

Glucose-6-phosphate Dehydrogenase Deficiency

Glucose-6-phosphate dehydrogenase deficiency: (definition)	X-linked disorder, most common deficiency and cause of hemolytic anemia
Glucose-6-phosphate dehydrogenase: (function)	Enzyme of HMP shunt an a very important source of NADPH + H^+ 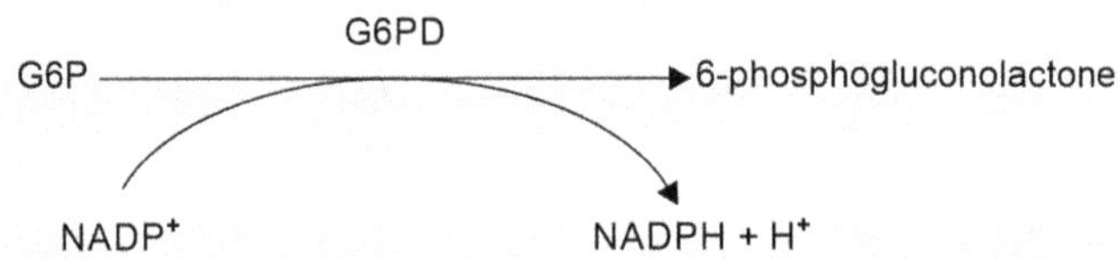
Importance of NADPH + H^+	• Keeps glutathione in reduced form In absence of NADPH oxidized glutathione will accumulate (GSSG), so oxidants will keep on accumulating (ROO) which can destroy lipid membrane, Hb, RBC membrane so lysis of red blood cells can occur) • Provides reducing equivalents for synthetic pathways • Reduced glutathione reduces H_2O_2 to H_2O otherwise H_2O_2 can form methemoglobin
Pathological effects	• Oxidative damage to red blood cells • Hemolytic anemia (decreased life span of RBC's)
Effect of drugs on G6PD deficiency	It is precipitated by drugs, such as: • Sulfonamides • Chloroquine/primaquine • Phenacetin • Nalidixic acid

Screening tests

Method	**Observation**	**Principle**
Sodium nitrite and methylene blue reduction test: (In blood) • Use citrated blood. • If G6PD deficiency is there then 1st reaction will occur but 2nd reaction does not occur due to deficient NADPH which is needed for conversion of chocolate brown color (Hb^{+++}) to dark red (Hb^{++}) • Thus, chocolate brown color is formed in all tests but it will not be persistent in normal G6PD samples as it will be converted to Hb^{++} in presence of methylene blue so persistence of chocolate brown color screens G6PD deficiency	Positive test is indicated by persistence of brown color Reaction: 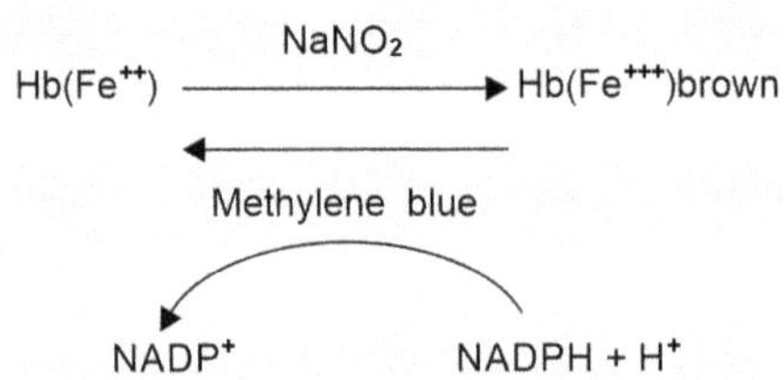	**State 1:** G6PD deficiency leading to NADPH deficiency—Hemoglobin is oxidized to methemoglobin by sodium nitrite, forming brown color **State 2:** If there is no G6PD deficiency—Methemoglobin (Fe^{+++}) is reduced back to normal hemoglobin (Fe^{++}) by methylene blue

Confirmatory test: Estimate G6PD activity in red blood cells

Galactosemia

Galactosemia: (Definition)	Galactose metabolism is defective
Cause	Deficiency of enzymes, such as: • Uridyltransferase (very common) • Galactokinase • UDP Galactose 4-epimerase
Biochemical effect	Accumulation of galactose in blood, excretion of galactose in urine (galactosuria)
Clinical manifestations	• Mental retardation (brain damage) • Hepatomegaly (due to deposition of galactose and other intermediates in the liver cells) • Jaundice (deposition of galactose and other intermediates leads to intrahepatic cholestasis) • Renal damage • Cataract (due to conversion of excess galactose to excess sorbitol and sorbitol accumulates in eyes to form cataract) Galactose —Aldose reductase→ dulcitol Effect of dulcitol: • Hygroscopic • Impermeable It has a tendency to draw in water so it is responsible for the opaque lens in cataract
Principle of treatment	Galactose free diet is given to the patient so as to prevent severe damage of brain

Screening Tests

Galactosuria

Method	**Observation**
Benedict's test: In addition to Benedict's test, to rule out the possibilities of reducing natured glucose	Positive test due to reducing nature of galactose in urine
Oxidase strip method	Negative (reducing sugar in Benedict's test is not glucose)
Seliwanoff's test	Negative (reducing sugar in Benedict's test is not fructose)
Beutler enzyme spot test: All the dots where light blue color is there, that shows normal galactose-1-phosphate uridylyltransferase, if no color develops, that shows galactose-1-phosphate uridylyltransferase deficiency	• Galactose-1-phosphate uridylyltransferase activity is monitored on blood dried on filter disc, followed by measurement of absorbance of reduced $NADP^+$ under UV light • NADPH is chromogenic substance so it absorbs light, so whenever NADPH is able to absorb light, it means galactose-1-phosphate uridylyltransferase enzyme is normal, and when light is not present, that means deficiency of enzyme is there
Confirmatory test	• Galactose in urine can be detected by chromatography • Enzyme deficiency that is galactokinase can be estimated in red blood cells

Homocystinuria

Homocystinuria: (Definition)	Metabolic disorder of amino acid Methionine
Cause	Deficiency of enzyme cystathionine synthase
Biochemical effect	• Excretion of homocystine in urine • Accumulation of homocystine, homocysteine and methionine in blood

Other types of homocystinuria:
1. Homocystinuria type II: Deficiency of reductase enzyme
2. Homocystinuria type III: Defective formation of methylcobalamin
3. Homocystinuria type IV: Defective B12 absorption

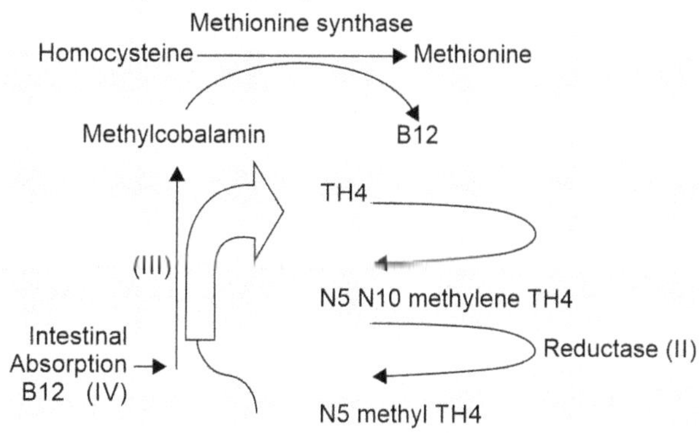

Contd....

Contd....

Role of coenzymes in homocystinuria	B6, B12, folic acid deficiencies, which are used as coenzymes in homocysteine metabolism
Types according to B6 responsiveness	• Vitamin B6 responsive (B6 act as coenzyme for the enzyme cystathionine synthase) • Vitamin B6 resistant
Metabolic defect in type I/classical homocystinuria	Methionine → S-Adenosine methionine (SAM) → S-Synthase, B6, Serine Adenosyl homocysteine → L homocysteine → Cystathionine —(Cystathioninase, B6)→ Homoserine + cysteine → Propionyl-CoA → Succinyl CoA → TCA cycle
Complications	• Thromboembolic vascular disorders (altered vascular endothelial cell adherence) • Delayed milestones—mental retardation (cerebrovascular thrombosis in early age) • Osteoporosis (lysyl semialdehyde is needed for cross linking of collagen fibers, but homocysteine and homocystine both react with lysyl semialdehyde and also interfere with lysyl oxidase action by binding with copper ions which are needed for collagen formation) • Dislocation of lens (immature collagen and improper connective tissue proteins) • Homocysteinemia can lead to atherosclerosis, MI and cerebral stroke
Basis of treatment	Avoid methionine in diet and take proper vitamins for proper metabolism

Screening test

Cyanide nitroprusside test	SH group of homocysteine is tested by nitroprusside test

In cystinuria, cysteine is excreted in urine, so silver nitroprusside test is done, which is positive for cystinuria, but this test does not reduce the disulfide bond, so we can differentiate between homocystinuria and cystinuria

Diagnostic test	• Estimation of level of homocysteine in blood • Estimation of level of methionine in blood • Activity of enzyme cystathionine synthase in tissue extract
Normal homocysteine level in plasma	4–12 mmol/liter
Homocysteine level in plasma in homocystinuria	>100 mmol/liter

Mucopolysaccharidosis

Type	Eponym	Deficient enzyme	Clinical picture	
I	Hurler's	L-iduronidase	Mental retardation, skeletal deformity, corneal opacity	Dermatan sulfate and heparin sulfate in urine
II	Hunter's	Iduronate sulfatase	Deafness, mental retardation, no corneal clouding, skeletal deformity	Dermatan sulfate and heparin sulfate in urine
III	Sanfili-ppo's	N-acetyl glucosaminidase, heparin sulfatase	Mental retardation, corneal clouding, skeletal deformity	• Heparin sulfate in urine • Three types reported
IV	Morquio's	Galactosamine sulfatase, beta D galactosidase	Mental retardation, skeletal deformity, epiphyseal dysplasia, corneal opacity	• Keratan sulfate and chondroitin sulfate in urine • Two types reported

Screening test

Alcian blue spot test

Alcian blue	It is a copper phthalocyanine dye and contains positively charged groups, capable of making salt linkages with certain poly anions (sulfate and carboxyl radicals of acid mucin)
Method	10 mL urine is dried on filter paper and Alcian blue is added
Observation	Urine appears as a blue spot on a white background
Principle	Mucopolysaccharides/GAG accumulate in blood and come out in urine, where they react with Alcian blue

Case study 1: Galactosemia

Baby presenting with jaundice, cataract, vomiting and convulsions, enlarged liver, urine showed positive reducing sugar. His condition improved by stopping milk feed

1. What is the diagnosis?
2. What is the cause of cataract?
3. What is the reason behind enlarged liver?
4. Write the main symptoms of the disease?
5. What is the line of treatment?
6. What may be the cause of jaundice?

1. Diagnosis	Galactosemia
Deficient enzymes	• Galactokinase • Galactosyl uridyl transferase • Uridyl galactose phosphate epimerase
2. Cataract	• Aldose reductase • Galactose ⟶ Dulcitol
Properties of dulcitol	• Hygroscopic • Unable to come out of the cell
Effect of dulcitol on the eye lens	Attracts water inside the lens making it opaque
3. Enlarged liver	Impaired metabolism of galactose leads to deposition of galactose in the liver, making it enlarged
4. Important symptoms	• Cataract of the lens of eye • Neurological defect resulting in brain damage
5. Line of treatment	• Diet should be devoid of galactose for prevention of more brain damage • Cataract can be treated by surgery
6. Jaundice in galactosemia	Galactose deposits causing intra hepatic cholestasis

Case study 2: Phenylketonuria

A 5-month-old baby presenting with blank expressions, small head, delayed milestones, not holding his neck, could not sit without support, mother complained about the mousy odor of urine no weight gain as his age, with no history of abnormal child in the family

1. What is the diagnosis? Justify your statement.
2. What is the cause and types of phenylketonuria?
3. What is the reason behind mousy smell of urine?
4. Write the main causes of mental retardation and convulsions?
5. What is the line of treatment and what is the right age of starting the treatment?
6. What may be the confirmation test?
7. What is the screening test and what is the principle of the same?
8. What is the reason behind supplementing the diet with tyrosine?

1. Diagnosis	• Phenylketonuria • Improper growth • Mental retardation • Mousy odor in urine
2. Cause and types	• Deficient enzyme—phenylalanine hydroxylase due to which phenylalanine is not further metabolized and tyrosine is not formed • Classical phenylketonuria/Type 1 • Type II–deficient enzyme is dihydrobiopterin reductase • Type III–deficient formation of tetrahydrobiopterin • Malignant phenylketonuria
3. Mousy smell in urine	• There is opening of an alternate pathway where phenylpyruvate and phenyllactate are formed from accumulated phenylalanine • Phenyllactate gives mousy odor to urine
4. Main causes of mental retardation	• Decreased myelin • Decreased epinephrine • Low level of nor epinephrine • Reduced serotonin

Contd....

Contd....

5. Line of treatment	• Normal level of phenylalanine in blood is up to 6 mg% • Prescribe a diet having very less phenylalanine, but tyrosine supplements must be given along with it
6. Confirmation test	• Phenylalanine level in blood (should not be more than 6 mg%) • Estimation of enzyme phenylalanine hydroxylase
7. Screening tests	• Ferric chloride test Urine + $FeCl_3$ forms permanent dark blue color (phenylpyruvate) • In alkaptonuria, a temporary light blue color is obtained due to homogentisic acid • Confirm the above diagnosis by estimating phenylalanine level in blood • DNPH test • Guthrie's test
8. Tyrosine supplementation	Although tyrosine is nonessential as it can be made in our body by phenylalanine, but in phenylketonuria, tyrosine synthesis does not take place, hence its supplementation is important part of treatment

Case study 3: Homocystinuria

A 5-year-old baby presenting with lens dislocation in left eye, delayed milestones, delayed speech and osteoporosis

1. What is the diagnosis? Justify your statement.
2. What is the biochemical cause and types of homocystinuria?
3. What is the reason behind osteoporosis?
4. Write the main causes of mental retardation and convulsions.
5. What is the line of treatment?
6. What is the fate of homocysteine in homocystinuria type I?
7. What are the functions of vitamins in homocystinuria?
8. What is the screening test done?

1. Diagnosis	Homocystinuria type I, disease progresses to thrombovascular defects in future
2. Biochemical cause and other types of homocystinuria	Deficient enzyme–cystathionine synthase, requiring coenzyme pyridoxine 1. Homocystinuria type II: Deficiency of reductase enzyme 2. Homocystinuria type III: Defective formation of methylcobalamine 3. Homocystinuria type IV: Defective B12 absorption
3. Osteoporosis	Osteoporosis (lysyl semialdehyde is needed for cross linking of collagen fibers, but homocysteine and homocystine both react with lysyl semialdehyde and also interfere with lysyl oxidase action by binding with copper ions which are needed for collagen formation)
4. Mental retardation and convulsions	Cerebrovascular thrombosis in early age
5. Line of treatment	Avoid methionine in diet and take proper vitamins for proper metabolism
6. Fate of homocysteine in homocystinuria type I	With the support of methylcobalamine, it changes to Methionine
7. Functions of vitamins	Folate, B12 (supplementation decreases homocysteine and methyl malonic acid levels), B6 (causing homocysteine breakdown), riboflavin, choline are involved in homocysteine metabolism
8. Screening test	Urine screening test called cyanide nitroprusside test and neonatal screening test called Guthrie test detects methionine in heel stick blood

Case study 4: Fructose intolerance

A child presented with dizziness, weakness, limbs trembling, sweating, felt ill after taking fruit juices. After examination, he had symptoms of hypoglycemia and low blood pressure, blood sugar was 60 mg/dL and urine tested positive Benedict's test

1. What is the diagnosis? Justify your statement.
2. What is the confirmatory test?
3. Why it causes hypoglycemia?
4. What are the metabolic defects?

1. Diagnosis	Fructose intolerance
2. Confirmatory test	Fructose tolerance test
3. Hypoglycemia	Fructose 1 phosphate inhibits liver glycogen phosphorylase thus inhibiting glycogenolysis which is required to maintain blood sugar levels between the meals (high fructose in diet can cause hypoglycemia)
4. Metabolic defects	• Accumulation of fructose 1 phosphate in liver (hepatomegaly) • Depletion of phosphate as it is continuously making fructose 1phophate • Decreased ATP synthesis • Phosphorylation of glucose does not take place

OSPE

Paper Chromatography

Aim

Separation of amino acids from a mixture of amino acids.

Mechanism/Principle

1. It is a physical mechanism of separating the components of a mixture when they are passed by a media that is porous by virtue of their differential distribution along with rate of migration in 2 phases that are immiscible—mobile phase and stationary phase.
2. Distribution coefficient/partition coefficient is defined as concentration of the substance in solvent A divided by the concentration of the substance in solvent B.
3. $Kd = \dfrac{\text{Concentration of the substance in solvent A}}{\text{Concentration of the substance in solvent B}}$
4. $\text{Retention factor (Rf)} = \dfrac{\text{Distance covered by the substance}}{\text{Distance covered by the solvent}}$
5. Different amino acids possess different Rf values in a biphasic system like water (stationary phase) and butanol (mobile phase) solvent system.
6. Role of acids or bases: To increase their ionization, migration, and better separation.

Kinds of Chromatography

1. **Planar chromatography:**
   Vertical plane—paper/glass/plastic.
   It is saturated with stationary phase solvent or is coated with silica gel which then carry stationary phase (thin layer chromatography).
   The mobile phase solvent moves over the stationary phase.
2. **Column chromatography:**
   The inert particles coated with stationary phase are packed in a column.
   Mobile phase is passed through this column.
   If the mobile phase is gas, it is known as gas chromatography.
   If the mobile phase is liquid, it is known as liquid chromatography.

The factors which affect the differential distribution of the mixture components:

1. Adsorption of solute in both phases—adsorption chromatography
2. Affinity of the solute in both phases—affinity chromatography
3. Ionic bond (ion exchange chromatography
4. Partition between both phases—partition chromatography

Applications of chromatography:

1. Separation of carbohydrates, fats, amino acids, hormones, growth factors
2. Identification of inborn errors of metabolism (paper chromatography)
3. Estimation of glycosylated hemoglobin (HPLC)
4. Detection of thalassemia (HPLC)

Experiment

Aim

Use paper chromatography for separation of amino acids.

Materials Required

1. Whatman number 1 filter paper strips (in cm - 1.5 × 15)
2. Lead pencil
3. Test tube with cork that is split in center
4. *Mixture of amino acid*: N/10 glycine, N/10 leucine (ratio—2:1 in H_2O)

5. Mixture of solvent—n-butanol, acetic acid, distilled H_2O (ratio—12:3:5)
6. Auto pipettes (1-5 micro L)
7. Solution of ninhydrin (0.1%)

Methodology/Steps

1. Wear gloves and make strips of Whatman filter paper (1.5 cm × 15 cm).
2. Using lead pencil make a line 2.5 cm above one end of all the filter paper strips, mark these strips as 1, 2, 3 below the line.
3. Take 3 test tubes and add 2 mL solvent in all test tubes in test tube stand.
4. Apply 1 to 2 µL of the amino acid mixture at a spot in the middle on marked line on strip 3.
5. Apply pure glycine on strip 1, pure leucine solution on strip 2.
6. Put the other end of the strip in the cork slit gently in a way that it holds the strip in a tight manner.
7. Lower the cork carrying the strip in its slit in the test tube containing the solvent in a way that the low end on which the sample was applied dips into the solvent.
8. Precaution is that the strip must not touch any side of the test tube, level of the solvent in the tube must touch the edge of the paper but at the same time it must remain below the amino acid mixture spot.
9. Leave the system to stand for 45 minutes.
10. The solvent migrates up to the upper end of the strip near the cork.
11. Remove the strip and mark the solvent front with lead pencil.
12. Dry in oven at 100 degree centigrade for 15 minutes.
13. Dip strips in ninhydrin, dry.
14. There is appearance of violet spots that show the positions of amino acids.
15. Compare the position of separated amino acid spots on strip 3 with position of glycine spot on strip 1 and leucine spot on strip 2.
16. Calculate and compare Rf values.

Observations and Calculations

1. Distance traveled by solvent in: (in cm)
   Tube 1 =
   Tube 2 =
   Tube 3 =
2. Distance traveled by amino acid in: (in cm)
   Tube 1 =
   Tube 2 =
   Tube 3 =
3. Rf value of glycine: (tube 1)
   Rf value of leucine: (tube 2)
4. Rf value of spot A: (tube 3)
   Rf value of spot B: (tube 3)

Take the center point of the spot in order to measure the distance.

Results

Following amino acids are present in the mixture:

Significance of Urine Paper Chromatography

1. For metabolic disorder of glycinuria the excretory product is glycine.
2. For metabolic disorder of phenylketonuria the excretory product is phenylpyruvate.
3. For metabolic disorder of maple syrup urine disease the excretory product are branched chain amino acids like valine, leucine, isoleucine.
4. For metabolic disorder of tyrosinemia the excretory product is tyrosine.
5. Detection of disorders such as galactosemia, lactosuria.

CLINICAL MCQS

1. **A neonate presents with musty body odor, urine screening: increased phenylpyruvic acid. What is the likely diagnosis?**
   a. Phenylketonuria
   b. Alkaptonuria
   c. MSUD
   d. Cystinuria

   Answer: a. Phenylketonuria
2. **A 6-month-old infant presents with dark urine that turns black on standing. Urine analysis reveals homogentisic acid. What is the most probable diagnosis?**
   a. PKU
   b. Alkaptonuria
   c. Tyrosinosis
   d. Cystinuria

   Answer: b. Alkaptonuria
3. **A newborn exhibits lethargy, poor feeding, and seizures. Urine analysis reveals a burnt sugar-like odor and the presence of branched-chain amino acids. What is the likely diagnosis?**
   a. MSUD
   b. PKU
   c. Tyrosinosis
   d. Hyperglycemia

   Answer: a. MSUD
4. **A 2-year-old child presents with recurrent kidney stones and sulfur-like urine odor. Urine screening detects elevated cystine levels. What is the most likely diagnosis?**
   a. Cystinuria
   b. Tyrosinosis
   c. Homocystinuria
   d. PKU

   Answer: a. Cystinuria
5. **An infant has jaundice, hepatomegaly, and cataracts. Urine analysis is positive for reducing substances but negative for glucose. What is the likely diagnosis?**
   a. Galactosemia
   b. GSD
   c. Glucosuria
   d. Alkaptonuria

   Answer: a. Galactosemia
6. **A 5-year-old presents with lens dislocation, thromboembolism, and developmental delay. Urine analysis reveals increased methionine and homocysteine. What is the likely diagnosis?**
   a. Homocystinuria
   b. Tyrosinosis
   c. Cystinuria
   d. PKU

   Answer: a. Homocystinuria

7. **A child with a history of seizures and vomiting has urine that smells of sweaty feet. Urine organic acid analysis reveals isovaleric acid. What is the most probable diagnosis?**
   a. Isovaleric acidemia
   b. PKU
   c. MSUD
   d. Alkaptonuria

   Answer: a. Isovaleric acidemia

8. **A neonate presents with jaundice, vomiting, and cabbage-like odor of urine. Urine analysis shows succinylacetone. What is the likely diagnosis?**
   a. Tyrosinemia type 1
   b. MUD
   c. Alkaptonuria
   d. Galactosuria

   Answer: a. Tyrosinemia type 1

9. **A child presents with vomiting, lethargy, and hypoglycemia after fruit consumption. Urine analysis is positive for reducing substances. What is the most probable diagnosis?**
   a. Hereditary fructose intolerance
   b. Galactosuria
   c. Tyrosinosis
   d. GSD

   Answer: a. Hereditary fructose intolerance

10. **A patient presents with neurological symptoms and blue diaper syndrome. Urine analysis reveals elevated tryptophan metabolites. What is the likely diagnosis?**
    a. Hartnup disease
    b. PKU
    c. Tyrosinosis
    d. Alkaptonuria

    Answer: a. Hartnup disease

VIVA VOCE

Q1. Explain inborn errors of metabolism/how can urine screening aid in their diagnosis?
Next question/Follow-up: Which metabolites are usually tested in urine for the screening of these disorders/why?

Q2. Discuss principle behind the use of urine tests, like ferric chloride test, in diagnosing inborn errors of metabolism as phenylketonuria/alkaptonuria.
Next question/Follow-up: How will you interpret a positive result in these tests, and what follow-up investigations are required for confirmation?

SPOTTERS

Q1. Show a urine sample with positive ferric chloride test, as finding of green color. What inborn error of metabolism does this indicate, and how will you proceed for further tests?

Hints: This is characteristic of phenylketonuria. Further testing-quantitative analysis for phenylalanine levels/genetic testing.

Q2. Show a sample of urine that darkens on standing and a positive test for homogentisic acid. Interpret/discuss condition that might be indicated?

Hints: Suggestive of alkaptonuria that is disorder characterized by the accumulation of homogentisic acid. Further confirmation by urine organic acid analysis.

REFLECTION

Visit to Central diagnostic laboratory and try to correlate the clinical findings with lab results about the important features of inborn errors of metabolism and describe the biochemical basis of different tests performed in laboratory in urine for screening of IEM.

6

CHAPTER

Paper Chromatography

COMPETENCY

BC14.5: Describe screening of urine for inborn errors and describe the use of paper chromatography.

LEARNING OBJECTIVES

After reading this chapter, the readers should be able to:

- Describe the principle, types, applications of chromatography.
- Describe the separation of amino acids by this application.
- Understand use of commonly used equipment/techniques in biochemistry laboratory including paper chromatography of amino acid.

Objective	Separation of individual amino acids from a mixture of amino acids by paper chromatography
Definition	Physical method of separation of the components of a mixture when they are passed through a porous media on the basis of their differential distribution and migration rates in 2 immiscible phases—stationary and mobile phase
Principle	• Distribution of a substance in a given biphasic solvent system at a given temperature is constant • When the mixture reacts with 2 immiscible phases, the components of the mixture distribute themselves differentially according to their Kd value resulting in their different migrations and Rf value
Distribution coefficient/ partition coefficient (Kd)	Concentration of the substance in solvent A/Concentration of the substance in solvent B Kd values of different components of the mixture varies, so their mobility in the 2 phases differ, measurement of this mobility is known as retention factor
Retention factor (Rf)	Distance covered by the substance/distance covered by the solvent
When will the separation	• The substance that is more distributed in the mobile phase will definitely migrate faster than the one that is more distributed in the stationary phase • Various amino acids have different Rf values in a given biphasic system, such as of water (stationary phase) and butanol (mobile phase) solvent system
What is the need to add acids/alkalies	They may be added to increase the ionization/migration/separation like acetic acid in this experiment
Advantages/uses	• Separation of carbohydrates, amino acids, lipids hormones growth factors, etc. • Paper chromatography is used for assessing inborn errors of metabolism • Estimation of HbA1c is detected by high pressure liquid chromatography • Detection of thalassemia by HPLC
Types of chromatography	• Planar • Column
Planar chromatography	• There is a vertical or horizontal plane • The plane may be in form a paper/glass/plastic as support • It has to be saturated with the stationary phase solvent directly or coated with thin layer of silica gel which then carries the stationary phase • The mobile phase solvent moves over the stationary phase

Column chromatography	• There is a glass tube or column in which we pack the inert particles coated/chemically bonded with the stationary phase • The mobile phase is then passed through the column • If the mobile phase is liquid, it is called liquid chromatography or if the mobile phase is gas, it is called gas chromatography
Physical/chemical basis of differential distribution of the components of mixture in 2 phases depends on:	• Adsorption of the solute in 2 phases (adsorption chromatography) • Affinity of the solute in 2 phases (affinity chromatography) • Ionic bonding (ion exchange chromatography) • Partition between the 2 phases (partition chromatography)

LOG ACTIVITY

Aim	Separation of amino acids by paper chromatography
Materials required	• Whatman No. 1 filter paper strips sized 1.5 cm × 15 cm • Lead pencil • Test tube with rubber stopper, split in the center • Mixture of amino acid made of N/10 glycine and N/10 leucine in the ratio of 2:1 in water • Solvent mixture containing n-butanol, acetic acid and DW in the ratio of 12:3:5 respectively • 1–5 μL auto pipettes • Ninhydrin solution 0.1%
Method	• Cut a sheet of Whatman's filter paper no. 1 into strips of 1.5 cm × 15 cm • Mark a line with a pencil 2.5 cm above one end of all the strips • Mark these strips as 1, 2, 3 with the pencil below the line • Take 2 mL of the solvent in each of the 3 test tubes and keep in test tube stands • Put 1–2 μL of amino acid mixture at a spot in the center on the marked line on strip no 3 • In the same way put pure glycine and leucine solution only on strips 1 and 2 respectively • Gently put the other end of the strip into the slit made in the rubber cork so that it holds the strip tightly • Then lower the cork carrying the paper strip in its slit into the test tube containing the solvent • The lower end of the strip, on which the sample has been applied must dip in the solvent • Then cork the tube • Be sure that the paper strip hangs vertically and does not touch any side of the test tube • In the beginning, the solvent level in the tube should touch the edge of the paper strip but should remain below the amino acid mixture spot • Let the tube untouched in the stand for 45 minutes so that the solvent migrates up to the upper end of the strip near the cork/to about 10 cm • Remove the strip and mark the solvent front • Dry it in oven at around 100°C for 15 minutes • Dip the strips in ninhydrin solution and again dry • Purple spots show the amino acid positions • Compare the position of the separated amino acid spots in the strip C with the position of glycine spot and leucine spot in strip A and B respectively • Calculate the Rf values and compare
Urine paper chromatography	The technique is used for metabolic diseases and galactosemia, lactosuria, etc.
Glycinuria	Glycine is the excretory product
Phenylketonuria	Phenylpyruvate is the excretory product
Maple syrup urine disease	Valine, leucine, isoleucine are the excretory products
Tyrosinemia	Tyrosine Is the excretory product

Observations

Distance covered by the solvent in

Tube 1 ....cm

Tube 2 ....cm

Tube 3 ....cm

Distance covered by the amino acid in

Tube 1 ....cm

Tube 2 ....cm

Tube 3 ....cm

Rf value of glycine (tube1)

Rf value of leucine (tube 2)

Rf value of spot A (tube 3)

Rf value of spot B (tube 3)

RESULTS AND CLINICAL INTERPRETATION

....

....

....

....

....

....

....

....

....

....

....

....

....

....

....

....

....

....

....

....

....

....

....

....

....

OSPE

1. **Explain the technique of paper chromatography?**
Paper chromatography is a simple as well as cost-effective procedure required for separating and analyzing mixtures of chemical substances, based on their differential partitioning between a stationary phase that is filter paper and a mobile phase that is solvent.

2. **What is the principle of paper chromatography?**
The principle is based on partition chromatography, in which the substances are separated because of their different and varied solubilities in the mobile phase that is solvent and their different affinities for the stationary phase that is paper. The compounds move at variable rates, producing distinct spots on the paper.

3. **What are the applications of paper chromatography?**
   1. *Separation of amino acids*:
   This is taken to identify amino acids in biological fluids like in urine and plasma.
   Applied in diagnosing aminoacidurias like phenylketonuria/maple syrup urine disease/cystinuria.
   2. *Detection of sugars*:
   Separation and identification of reducing and nonreducing sugars.
   Used in disorders such as galactosemia/fructosuria.
   3. *Separation of nucleic acids*: Identification of purines/pyrimidines/nucleotides in the samples.
   4. *Analysis of organic acids*: Detection of metabolic products in states such as methylmalonic acidemia.
   5. *Drug and metabolite analysis*: Identification of drug metabolites/toxic compounds in various biological fluids.

4. **How is paper chromatography useful for diagnosing inborn errors of metabolism?**
   1. *Phenylketonuria (PKU)*: Detects high levels of phenylalanine in the urine.
   2. *Maple syrup urine disease (MSUD)*: Separates branched-chain amino acids that are leucine, isoleucine, and valine in urine.
   3. *Cystinuria*: Identifies cystine in the urine samples.
   4. *Galactosemia*: Differentiates galactose from other sugars in the sample of urine.

5. **What are the applications of paper chromatography?**
Simple, not costly
Need minimal equipments
Suits for small sample volumes
Able to separate a wide range of substances like amino acids along with sugars, and also drugs

6. **What are the limitations of technique of paper chromatography?**
Limited sensitivity in comparison to advanced techniques like HPLC/GC.
Takes a lot of time
Difficulty faced in quantification
Inability to separate extremely similar compounds properly and effectively

7. **What are the steps in paper chromatography?**
   1. *Sample application*: A small drop of the sample is applied on base of the paper.
   2. *Development*: The paper is placed in a solvent, and we allow the mobile phase to move up the paper.
   3. *Separation*: Components of the sample separate as the solvent moves up, and spots are formed.
   4. *Detection*: The separated spots are visualized by using proper and appropriate reagents such as ninhydrin for amino acids/ $AgNO_3$ for sugars.

8. **How are the results analyzed in paper chromatography?**
The retardation factor is calculated:
Rf = Distance traveled by the substance/Distance traveled by the solvent front.
Every compound has a specific and unique Rf value under particular conditions, thus allowing identification.

9. **Which stains are used in paper chromatography?**
   1. *Ninhydrin*: For detecting amino acids; forms a purple/yellow color
   2. *Aniline phthalate*: For staining the sugars for analysis of carbohydrate
   3. *Silver nitrate*: For detecting the presence of reducing sugars
   4. *Iodine vapors*: For Visualizing lipids/nonpolar compounds

10. **Give an example of how paper chromatography is utilized in clinical biochemistry.**
For diagnosis of phenylketonuria (PKU):
Urine/blood sample is applied on the filter paper.
Paper is developed in solvent for separation of amino acids.
Ninhydrin spray is utilized for visualizing the spots.
An increased intensity of the phenylalanine spot compared to controls confirms the diagnosis of PKU.

CLINICAL MCQS

1. **Paper chromatography is used in clinical biochemistry to separate which type of molecules?**
   a. Fats
   b. Proteins
   c. Amino acids and sugars
   d. Nucleotides

   Answer: c. Amino acids and sugars

2. **Paper chromatography is used to analyze amino acid composition in a patient's urine. What condition may be diagnosed by detecting high phenylalanine?**
   a. MSUD
   b. Phenylketonuria
   c. Alkaptonuria
   d. Tyrosinosis

   Answer: b. Phenylketonuria

3. **What is the stationary phase?**
   a. Solvent
   b. Filter paper
   c. Glass tube
   d. Silica gel

   Answer: b. Filter paper

4. **Which of the solvents is commonly used as mobile phase in paper chromatography for separating amino acids?**
   a. H_2O
   b. Acetoacetate
   c. Aqueous ethanol with buffer
   d. Ether

   Answer: c. Aqueous ethanol with buffer

5. **Paper chromatography is used to separate sugars in urine. The presence of high galactose shows which condition?**
   a. GSD
   b. Fructosuria
   c. Galactosemia
   d. Diabetes insipidus

   Answer: c. Galactosemia

6. **In paper chromatography, what determines the separation of components on the paper?**
   a. Molecular weight
   b. Polarity/solubility in the solvent
   c. Charge
   d. Concentration in the sample

   Answer: b. Their polarity/solubility in the solvent

7. **After paper chromatography, how are amino acids visualized?**
   a. Using iodine
   b. By exposing to sunlight
   c. Spraying with ninhydrin reagent
   d. Spraying with sulfuric acid

   Answer: c. Spraying with ninhydrin reagent

8. **A urine sample is analyzed to detect organic acids. If high homogentisic acid is observed what is the diagnosis?**
   a. PKU
   b. Alkaptonuria
   c. Tyrosinosis
   d. Cystinuria

   Answer: b. Alkaptonuria

9. A important application of paper chromatography in a clinical setting is:
a. It needs expensive equipment
b. It is rapid, inexpensive, and simple
c. It analyses all biomolecules
d. It gives quantitative analysis

Answer: b. It is rapid, inexpensive, and simple

10. The retention factor is calculated by?
a. Distance traveled by the solute ÷ Distance traveled by the solute
b. Distance traveled by the solute ÷ Distance traveled by the solvent
c. Distance traveled by the solvent × Distance traveled by the solvent
d. Distance traveled by the solution – Distance traveled by the solvent

Answer: b. Distance traveled by the solute ÷ Distance traveled by the solvent

VIVA VOCE

Q1. Explain principle of paper chromatography/how is it useful?
Next question/Follow-up: Discuss how the stationary phase/mobile phase work in these technique/how different substances are separated on the basis of their polarity.

Q2. What are the types of paper chromatography/differentiate them according to their applications?
Next question/Follow-up: Discuss importance of the Rf value/how it is calculated.

SPOTTERS

Q1. Show paper chromatography setup with a mixture of colored substances that is separated into different spots. Interpret result/ what does the number of spots suggest about the mixture?

Hints: Number of distinct spots–the number of components in the mixture. Every spot corresponds to a different substance based on its interaction with the stationary phase.

Q2. Show a chromatogram with many separated spots on the paper. Calculate the Rf value/what are the factors that affect its accuracy?

Hints: Rf: Distance traveled by the compound divided by the distance traveled by the solvent front. Focus on factors such as solvent polarity/temperature/type of paper used.

REFLECTION

Enumerate principle, types and applications of chromatography and also explain the separation of amino acids by this technique.

CHAPTER 7

Principles of Colorimetry and Spectrophotometry

COMPETENCY

BC14.6: Describe the principles of colorimetry and spectrophotometry.

LEARNING OBJECTIVES

After reading this chapter, the readers should be able to:

- Explain the principles and working of the colorimeter and spectrophotometer.
- Mention the advantages of spectrophotometer over colorimeter.
- Observe the working of colorimeter.
- Describe the components of a colorimeter and their functions.
- Explain the applications of Colorimetry in biochemical analysis.

BLUE PRINT

Principles of Colorimetry

Objective

By the end of the lecture, students should be able to:

1. Understand the principles of colorimetry.
2. Describe the components of a colorimeter and their functions.
3. Explain the applications of colorimetry in biochemical analysis.

Duration: *70 minutes*

Materials Needed

1. Presentation slides for explaining principles of colorimetry.
2. Examples of colorimetric assays with their results.
3. Colorimeter/spectrophotometer for demonstration purpose.
4. Samples of standard solutions with known concentrations.
5. Charts/diagrams for illustration of principles of colorimetry.

Outline

I. **Introduction to colorimetry** **(10 minutes)**
- Define colorimetry, its importance in biochemical assays.
- Explain the concept of absorbance, its relationship with concentration.
- Discuss the principles of Beer–Lambert Law, its use in different colorimetric assays.

II. **Components of a colorimeter** **(10 minutes)**
- Describe the components of a colorimeter, including the light source, filters, sample holder, and detector.
- Explain the function of every component in the measurement of absorbance/transmittance of light.
- Discuss the significance of calibration, quality control in different colorimetric measurements.

III. **Measurement of absorbance** **(15 minutes)**
- Demonstrate preparation of samples and setting up the instruments.
- Explain the methodology to measure the absorbance by using standard solutions and unknown samples.
- Discuss the causes and factors that affect absorbance measurements, like path length, wavelength, and turbidity in sample.

IV. **Calibration and standardization** **(10 minutes)**
- Discuss the significance of calibration curves in different colorimetric assays.
- Explain the methodology for preparing standard solutions of known concentrations.
- Demonstrate construction of a calibration curve and application for determining the concentration of unknown samples.

V. **Applications of colorimetry** **(10 minutes)**
- Provide different examples of colorimetric assays used in biochemical analysis, like enzyme assays, protein quantification/detecting specific analytes.
- Discuss the advantages and limitations of colorimetry in comparison to other analytical techniques.
- Highlight the applications of colorimetry in the diagnosis, monitoring, and pharmaceutical assays

VI. **Hands-on activity** **(5 minutes)**
- Conduct a hands-on activity for the students to perform a simple colorimetric assay by using a colorimeter/spectrophotometer.
- Provides guidance/assistance as students' themselves measure the absorbance and calculate concentrations of standard solutions.

VII. **Interpretation of results** **(5 minutes)**
- Analyze the absorbance readings taken by colorimetric assay.
- Interpretation of results by reading the concentration.
- Discuss any potential sources of error/strategy for getting accuracy and precision in the measurements.

VIII. **Review and summary** **(5 minutes)**
- Summarize the important points covered in the lecture.
- Reinforce the significant colorimetric techniques.

IX. **Conclusion** **(5 minutes)**
- Conclude the lecture by emphasizing the significance of colorimetry as a quantitative analytical tool.
- Encourage students to explore further applications in scientific research and technology.

Discuss the Principles of Spectrophotometry

Blueprint: Principles of spectrophotometry.

Objective

By the end of the lecture, students should be able to:
1. Understand the basic principles of spectrophotometry.
2. Explain how spectrophotometry is used to quantify the concentration of substances in a sample.
3. Describe the components of a spectrophotometer and their functions.
4. Apply the Beer-Lambert law to calculate concentration from absorbance measurements.

Duration: *60 minutes*

Materials Needed

1. Presentation slides explaining principles/applications of spectrophotometry.
2. Examples of spectra and absorbance curves.
3. Spectrophotometer for demonstration purposes
4. Handouts for summarizing important concepts and formulas.

Outline

I. **Introduction to spectrophotometry** **(10 minutes)**
- Definition/importance of spectrophotometry in analytical chemistry/biochemistry.
- Brief history/development of spectrophotometric procedures.

II. **Basic principles of spectrophotometry** **(15 minutes)**
- Explanation of absorption spectroscopy.
- Beer–Lambert law/its significance for quantifying concentration based on absorbance measurements.
- Factor impact on absorbance like path length/concentration/molar absorptivity.

III. **Components of a spectrophotometer** **(10 minutes)**
- Description of light source/monochromator/sample holder/cuvette/detector.
- Functions of components in the spectrophotometric measurement techniques.

IV. **Operation of a spectrophotometer** **(10 minutes)**
- Overview of the spectrophotometric workflow like calibration/blank correction/sample measurement.
- Demonstration of preparing samples, setting wavelength, and measuring absorbance by a spectrophotometer.

V. **Applications of spectrophotometry** **(10 minutes)**
- Discussion of different applications in fields like biochemistry, pharmaceuticals, environmental analysis, and clinical diagnostics.
- Examples of substances mainly analyzed by using spectrophotometry like nucleic acids/proteins/pharmaceuticals.

VI. **Calculations and data analysis** **(5 minutes)**
- Practice problems like use of Beer–Lambert law for calculating concentration from absorbance measurements.
- Explanation of plotting standard curves and interpreting results.

VII. **Conclusion and recap** **(5 minutes)**
- Summary of important points regarding principles/applications of spectrophotometry.
- Emphasize the significance of spectrophotometry in quantitative analysis/research.

VIII. **Question and answer session** **(5 minutes)**
- Encourage students to ask questions and clarify
- Discuss potential challenges/troubleshooting for spectrophotometric measurements.

INTRODUCTION

Photometry

Importance: Analytical technique used in laboratories based on measurement of absorbance of light.

Principle: When we pass white light through a solution which is colored, the colored substance that is chromogen absorbs a part of this light and the remaining light is transmitted. This transmitted light depends on following factors:
- Nature of chromogen
- Concentration of substance in the colored solution
- Wavelength of incident light
- Path length of the solution through which the light passes

Transmittance: Ratio of intensity of transmitted light (Ie) that is how much light comes out of the solution, to the intensity of incident light (I_0) that is how much light was given to the solution, across a solution.
- The photometric instruments measure the emerging light from the solution in form of transmittance (T).
- T = that proportion of total incident light that is transmitted by the solution.
- If total incident light = I_0 and the light which is transmitted by the solution after absorption = Ie then the formula becomes:
  $T = Ie/I_0$
  Percent T (% T) = $Ie/I_0 \times 100$
  The transmittance is measured in the range of 0–100%.
- % T is inversely proportional to absorption (If more light is absorbed, % T is less).
- 100% T reflects no absorption of light at all.
- 0% T reflects all light has been absorbed and no light is transmitted.
- When we keep all other factors constant and just increase the concentration of light absorbing substance, then we will see that T will become less and gradually decrease.
- In the same way if we increase the light path length, then also T will decrease.
- Thus, we see that T varies inversely with concentration change and path length of the light (T varies exponentially) therefore, there is one more term called absorbance (A), which gives a direct relation with the concentration of the substance in the solution at a constant path length.

- A = – log T or log 1/T
- If percentage transmittance is used, then:
  - % T = Ie/I_0 × 100
  - A = $\log_{10}$ 1/T
  - A = $\log_{10}$ 100/% T
  - A = 2–log % T
  - T is inversely and logarithmically proportional to concentration that is:
    - T α log 1/C
    - Absorbance was amount of light absorbed by the solution and transmittance is amount of light transmitted by the solution.
  - We have 2 solutions:
    1. A = 100 mg/dL glucose (less glucose)
    2. B = 200 mg/dL glucose (more glucose)
       - 'A' compared to 'B' will have less absorbance but its T will be more (if it has not absorbed much light that means it has transmitted more light).
       - For B, if the absorbed amount is very high, then transmitted light will be low.
- Absorbance is also known as optical density (OD) which is the amount of light absorbed by any colored compound; it is logarithmic ratio of incident light to that of transmitted light.
- **Photometry is based on 2 laws:** When a monochromatic light is passed through any colored solution, the solution will absorb certain wavelength of light. The amount of absorbed light or amount of transmitted light by any colored solution falls in accordance with two laws:
  1. *Beer's law*: When a parallel beam of monochromatic light is passed through a solution, then the absorbance (A) of the solution is directly proportional to the concentration (C) of the substance in the solution or in other words, when monochromatic light passes through a light absorbing medium, the intensity of the transmitted light decreases exponentially as the concentration of the light absorbing material increases:
     A α C, where A = light absorbed, and C = concentration of the solution that is the absorbance (A) or optical density (OD) is directly proportional to the concentration of the solution: A = K C.
     To understand this more, we take an example: We select a particular wavelength of light, and then we allow this particular wavelength of light to pass through a colored solution, then, the absorbance that is the amount of light absorbed will be directly proportional to the concentration of the solution, suppose we have 2 solutions with 2 different concentrations of glucose:
     Solution A = 100 mg/dL (less glucose)
     Solution B = 150 mg/l (more glucose)
     The color developed will be more for solution B (more glucose means more reaction means more intensity of color). Since in solution B, the color developed is more, there will be more absorbance also, so once monochromatic light is passed through cuvette having solution, the amount of light absorbed will depend upon the concentration of the unknown solution.
  2. *Lambert's law*: states that when monochromatic light is passed through a colored solution, the amount of light absorbed, increases with the increase in thickness of the layer of solution through which the light passes
     The absorbance (A) is directly proportional to the path length of light or the thickness of the solution (I) A α I (length of the light path)
     A = K I
     We have 2 cuvettes:
     A = 1 cm diameter
     B = 5 cm diameter
     Absorbance will be more for B (path length is more, the more the path length is to be covered, the more will be the light absorbed).

On Combining Beer–Lambert Law

- A = KCI
- Where K = proportionality constant/extinction coefficient/absorption coefficient and is constant/fixed at particular concentration and wavelength for a given substance.
- Molecular extinction coefficient/absorption coefficient is the absorbance of one molar solution of a substance at a path length of 1 cm, it is used to calculate the concentration of an unknown sample.
- Beer's law is obeyed only by dilute solutions.

- In laboratories, the concentration of the test sample is calculated by comparing its absorbance with the absorbance of a solution of known concentration that is standard.
- If Ct = concentration of urea in the test sample and Cs is the concentration of urea in standard sample, then:
  - Absorbance of test sample (At) = KCt I
  - Absorbance of standard sample (As) = KCs I
- For the same substance and at constant path length under the same conditions, K and I are constant (we are adding the standard and test samples in the same cuvette so length will be same).

  At = Ct
  As = Cs
  At/As = Ct/Cs
  Ct = At/As × Cs

$$\text{Concentration of test/100 mL} = \frac{\text{Absorbance of test}}{\text{Absorbance of standard}} \times \frac{\text{Concentration of standard}}{\text{X mL}} \times 100$$

Standard solution/calibrator: Solution of the same substance as of the test but of known concentration. Both OD and concentration is known to us.

A series of standards of known concentrations are taken and their absorption is plotted against concentration, this gives us a standard curve/calibration curve so that we know the concentration over which Beer's law is obeyed.

Blank: It has all the solvents and the reagents except the test substance, and is used to exclude the absorbance contributed by the solvents and reagents.

Standard Calibration Curve

Standard curve is constructed by plotting a vertical axis (y-axis, ordinate) for optical density/absorbance and a horizontal axis (x-axis, abscissa) for the concentration of standard solution.

The concentration of unknown can be measured from the standard curve

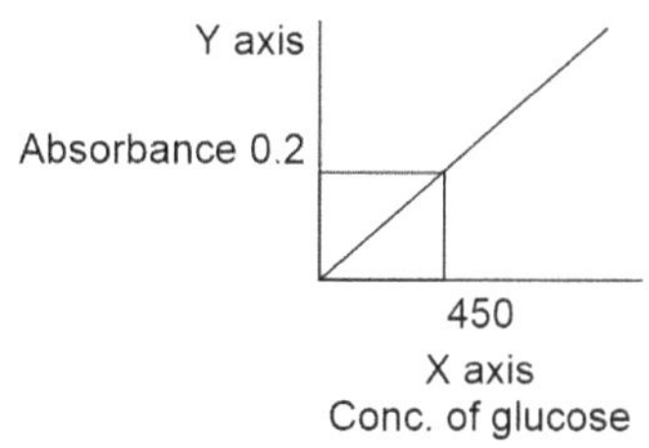

We give 5 glucose samples: (1) having glucose 10 mg/dL, (2) having glucose 100 mg/dL, (3) having glucose 350 mg/dL, (4) Having glucose 500 mg/dL, (5) having glucose 750 mg/dL. You are asked to find their optical densities. Whatever OD's are found, plot the graph, accuracy of pipetting is required. We get a straight curve.

Significance of Standard Curve

Suppose we have an unknown solution, X, and you find its OD, which came out to be 0.2, now extrapolate it on graph and from there, allow a perpendicular to fall on the X axis, and suppose this value on X axis is 450 mg/dL, then this will be the concentration of X sample given to you.

Thus, if we have a standard curve, we just need to find the OD of the unknown solution so every time, blank and standard are not required.

Blank has reagents without the sample and standard. It is to compensate any nonspecific color and to set the instrument at 100% transmittance and 0% OD (no absorbance means everything got transmitted). The use of distilled water in blank is to equal the ultimate volume as that of standard and test.

If we set the instrument at zero after keeping blank in cuvette, then we need not subtract the OD of blank, it will automatically subtract it for us, so that the reagent color does not interfere in actual reading. To omit the reagents color and false high values of our test samples, we set the colorimeter after putting blank in it to zero so practically for examination of test and standard, the reagent has no color, since it has allowed 100% T and 0% a (no absorbance means everything got transmitted).

Test sample = Reagent + unknown solution whose OD is to be measured

Colorimetry

Definition and Principle

This refers to the measurement of intensity of color in a solution. So, we can calculate the concentration of any colorless compound or metabolite which can be changed into colored compound by various chemical reactions under specific conditions by measurement of intensity of the color that is proportional to the concentration of the compound.

Photo Colorimeter

They are the instruments to measure the intensity of transmitted light through a colored solution.

Design

Light source	• Tungsten filament lamp which can emit light in visible range • High power tungsten halogen (quartz–iodine) lamp
Filters type	Colored glass filters
Filters function	They absorb most of the light and allows light of corresponding color only with a specific wavelength
Filters operation	A particular wavelength of light is selected for every estimation, by using a particular filter of known wavelength given in the instrument
Factor on which use of filter depends	It depends on the color of the resultant solution, we use filters of complementary colors as the absorbance is maximum of the corresponding light

Color filters and wavelength of light transmitted by them

Color wheel (ROYGBIV): The complementary colors fall across the diameter of color wheel and combine to produce white light. So, the color of the solution which we see by our eyes is compliment to the color of light absorbed by that colored compound. Absorption of blue color is maximum with yellow color filter and as the absorption is maximum, we use the complementary color. Thus, if we are given a blue-colored solution, we will use yellow color filter because absorption is maximum at this particular wavelength

Color of the solution	Filter color	Wavelength range (nm)
Bluish green	Red	650–700
Green blue	Orange	600–650
Blue	Yellow	575–600
Violet	Yellow green	55–575
Purple	Green	505–555
Red	Blue green	495–505
Orange	Green blue	475–495
Yellow	Blue	430–475
Yellowish blue	Violet	350–430

Wavelength <350–UV region (not visible), wavelength >750–IR (not visible)

Cuvettes	1. Glass tubes of 1 cm diameter and uniform thickness—used in visible range colorimetry 2. Quartz or fuse silica cuvettes are used for measurements in ultra violet range
Cuvette function	To hold the solutions
Cuvette types	1. Square 2. Rectangular 3. Circular
Precautions taken for cuvettes	1. It should be optically transparent 2. Clean and dry 3. No scratches/contamination should be present 4. One side is from where the light will cross called as clear side and the other side should be frosted to avoid dispersion 5. Flat surface is generally preferred 6. Optical path is always 1 cm

Contd....

Contd....

Photosensitive detectors	They may have a photocell or a phototube			
Photosensitive detectors function	Conversion of transmitted light to electrical energy			
Types of photo detectors	Barrier layer cells	Photoemissive tubes	Photomultiplier tubes	Photoconductor cells
Design of photocell	1. Metal plate is coated with thin layered photosensitive element called selenium 2. This in turn is coated with transparent layer of gold/copper			
Mechanism of photocell	When light strikes selenium, electrons are generated which go to the metal layer and there is generation of emf			
Design of phototube	1. It has a cathode made of metal plate coated with photosensitive element 2. An anode is present made of metal wire			
Mechanism of photocell	When light strikes the photosensitive element, electrons move from cathode towards anode thus generating a potential difference			
Measuring device: Read out devices—the signal may be transmitted to a computer system	Galvanometer	Ammeter	Recorder	Digital read out

Advantages of colorimeter

1. Not costly
2. It is used for quantitative analysis of colored substances
3. Easy transport

Disadvantages of colorimeter

1. Cannot be used for uncolored compounds
2. Does not work in UV and IR regions
3. Cannot set a particular wavelength as we have to set a range
4. Similar colors from interfering substances can give errors

Applications of colorimeter

- It can be used for samples, such as plasma, serum, CSF and urine
- Quantitative estimations of various parameters can be done
- Can be used in food industry, paint industry or textile industry

Spectrophotometer	It measures the ratio or a function of the two, of the radiant power of two electromagnetic beams over a large wavelength range and uses dispersing elements (prisms/gratings) instead of filters to scan a large wavelength region					
Components	Source of radiant energy	Collimating system	Monochromator system	Sample container	Detector for collecting transmitted radiations	Suitable amplifier or read out device
Source of radiant energy	For visible radiation—tungsten halogen lamp			For UV radiation—hydrogen discharge lamp		
Collimating system	The radiation emitted by the source is made parallel by lens/mirrors/slits so that each ray can be diffracted into colors and UV radiations					
Monochromator system	It is required to isolate radiation of specific wavelength from wavelength of continuous spectra					
	Prisms			Gratings		
Sample container	For UV region study, we use quartz/fused silica cuvettes			For visible region study, we use color corrected fused glass		
Precautions	They should be clean without any finger marks					
Detector for collecting transmitted radiations	Device to change light energy into electrical energy					
	Photovoltaic cells		Phototubes		Photo multiplier tube	
Suitable amplifier	The finally obtained mechanical energy is seen on read out device					

Characteristic	Colorimeter	Spectrophotometer
Monochromator	Filter	Prism/gratings
Spectrum band width	Broad band	Narrow band
Spectrum purity	Less	More
Spectral isolation	Change the filter	Specific wavelength can be adjusted
Stray light	Maximum	Minimum
Accuracy	Less	More
Sample	More	Less
Cost	Cheap	Costly
Light source	Visible range of light	Beyond visible range
Sensitivity	Less	More
Advantage	The compound to be estimated needs to form a color	The compound to be estimated need not form a color

End Point and Kinetic Estimations

End point	Kinetic
Reaction is carried out for specific period of time	Monitoring of reaction takes place regularly
We measure the absorbance in the last	Absorbance is read at serial intervals
Standard is used	Standard is not used
Slow, less sensitive, less accurate	• Fast, sensitive, more accurate • Mainly used for enzyme estimations • Use NAD, NADP as co substrates and NADH, NADPH absorb light at 340 nm

Semi-auto Analyzers

Semi-auto analyzers	Automated photometers
Operation for end point methods	End point methods are programmed by entering volume of reagent, volume of sample, standard concentration and wavelength
Use for end point methods	Instrument measures the absorbance, concentration is calculated and print out is given
Operation for kinetic methods	Kinetic methods are programmed by entering volume of reagents, volume of sample, temperature, number of readings, molar absorption, and gap between readings
Use for kinetic methods	Absorbance is read by the instrument at specific intervals of time, concentration is calculated and display of results is given

	Fully automated analyzers
Advantage	They offer enhanced efficiency, convenience and superior accuracy
	They efficiently provide best output rates for large loads of samples
Principle and operation	The working of fully automated analyzer is based on the principle of colorimetry. They use mechanized operating procedures, such as automated pipetting, mixing and dispensing, etc.
Parts/components of the instrument	Dilution turn table, dilution pipettes, dilution mixer, dilution cleansing mechanism sampling pipettes, reaction cleansing mechanism cell, rotation reactor, mixer 1 and 2, reagent pipettes 1 and 2, reagent bar code reader, reagent turn table 1 and 2, multiwavelength photometer, thermostatic oven, bar code reader

EXPERIMENT

Aim

To verify Beer's Lambert's law.

Requirements

Test tubes, standard of albumin (1 mg/mL), distilled water, Biuret reagent, colorimeter.

Procedure/Steps

1. Take one blank test tube, take 2.5 mL distilled water and 5 mL Biuret reagent in it
2. Take 5 test tubes and label them as tests—T1, T2, T3, T4, T5
3. In T1, take 0.5 mL albumin standard, 2 mL DW and 5 mL Biuret reagent
4. In T2, take 1.0 mL albumin standard, 1.5 mL DW and 5 mL Biuret reagent
5. In T3, take 1.5 mL albumin standard, 1.0 mL DW and 5 mL Biuret reagent
6. In T4, take 2.0 mL albumin standard, 0.5 mL DW and 5 mL Biuret reagent
7. In T5, take 2.5 mL albumin standard, no DW and 5 mL Biuret reagent
8. After mixing well, measure absorbance of all the solutions after 10 minutes
9. Take albumin concentration on X axis and optical density on Y axis, plot the graph, linear curve should be obtained

Observation

Tubes	Optical density
T1	
T2	
T3	
T4	
T5	

GRAPH

RESULTS AND INTERPRETATION

OSPE

1. **What is colorimetry?**
Colorimetry is a technique used to determine the concentration of colored substances in a solution by measuring the absorption of light at a specific wavelength.

2. **What is the principle of colorimetry?**
The principle of colorimetry is based on Beer–Lambert's law, which states that the absorption of light is directly proportional to the concentration of the absorbing substance and the path length of the light through the solution.

Formula:
$A = \varepsilon \times c \times l$

Where:
A = Absorbance
ε = Molar absorptivity
c = Concentration of the solution
l = Path length (usually 1 cm).

3. **What are the main components of a colorimeter?**
   1. *Light source*: Provides a beam of light (often a tungsten lamp).
   2. *Filter*: Selects the desired wavelength of light.
   3. *Cuvette*: Holds the sample solution.
   4. *Photoelectric detector*: Measures the light intensity passing through the solution.
   5. *Display unit*: Shows the absorbance or transmittance reading.

4. **What is the difference between absorbance and transmittance?**
Absorbance (A): The amount of light absorbed by a solution. It has no units.
Transmittance (T): The fraction of light that passes through the solution.
$T = I/I_0$, where I_0 is the incident light intensity and I is the transmitted light intensity.
$A = -\log(T)$

5. **What are the applications of colorimetry in biochemistry?**
   1. *Estimation of hemoglobin*: Cyanmethemoglobin method.
   2. *Quantification of glucose*: Glucose oxidase-peroxidase method.
   3. *Protein estimation*: Lowry's or Biuret method.
   4. *Enzyme activity assays*: Measuring product formation or substrate consumption.
   5. *Analysis of drug concentration*: For therapeutic drug monitoring.

6. **What are the limitations of colorimetry?**
   1. Can only be used for colored substances.
   2. Requires a suitable filter to select the appropriate wavelength.
   3. Less sensitive compared to spectrophotometry.

7. **What is spectrophotometry?**
Spectrophotometry is a technique used to measure the intensity of light absorbed by a solution over a range of wavelengths.

8. **What is the principle of spectrophotometry?**
Spectrophotometry also follows Beer–Lambert's law, where the absorbance is directly proportional to the concentration of the solute and the path length.
Unlike colorimetry, spectrophotometry measures absorbance over a broad range of wavelengths and can detect substances that are colorless or absorb in the UV range.

9. **What are the components of a spectrophotometer?**
   1. *Light source*: Usually a tungsten lamp for visible light and deuterium lamp for UV light.
   2. *Monochromator*: Separates light into its component wavelengths.
   3. *Cuvette*: Holds the sample.
   4. *Detector*: Measures the intensity of transmitted light.
   5. *Output display*: Shows the absorbance or transmittance.

10. **What are the applications of spectrophotometry in biochemistry?**
   1. *DNA/RNA quantification*: Using absorbance at 260 nm.
   2. *Protein concentration estimation*: Using absorbance at 280 nm or colorimetric assays (e.g., Bradford method).
   3. *Enzyme kinetics*: Monitoring reaction progress by measuring absorbance of substrates/products.
   4. *Drug analysis*: Determining purity and concentration.
   5. *Estimation of bilirubin*: In liver function tests.

11. Why is 260/280 ratio important in spectrophotometry?
The 260/280 ratio is used to assess the purity of nucleic acid samples.
DNA and RNA absorb at 260 nm, while proteins absorb at 280 nm.
A ratio of ~1.8 indicates pure DNA, while a ratio of ~2.0 indicates pure RNA.

12. What are some examples of spectrophotometric assays?
1. *Glucose estimation*: Hexokinase or glucose oxidase method
2. *Lipid analysis*: Cholesterol estimation using enzymatic assays
3. *Liver function tests*: Bilirubin estimation
4. *Kidney function tests*: Creatinine and urea quantification

13. What is the importance of calibration in colorimetry and spectrophotometry?
Calibration ensures accurate/reproducible results by setting a baseline with known standards. It involves:
Zeroing the instrument with a blank solution
Measuring standard solutions of known concentration to construct a calibration curve

14. What are the advantages of spectrophotometry over colorimetry?
1. Measures colored as well as colorless substances
2. High sensitivity/specificity
3. Analyze wide range of wavelengths
4. Gives precise quantitative results

15. What is the function of Beer-Lambert's law in spectrophotometry?
Beer-Lambert's law relates absorbance to concentration, enabling the quantification of substances in a sample. Deviations from the law might be seen at high concentrations because of scattering or chemical interactions.

16. What is the difference between UV-Vis spectrophotometry and IR spectrophotometry?
UV-Vis spectrophotometry: Measures absorption in the ultraviolet/200–400 nm/visible/400–700 nm regions. Used for analyzing nucleic acids/proteins.
IR spectrophotometry: Measures absorption in the infrared region (>700 nm). Used for studying molecular vibrations/functional groups.

17. What are some common light sources used in spectrophotometry?
1. *Tungsten lamp*: For visible light/400–700 nm
2. *Deuterium lamp*: For ultraviolet light/200–400 nm
3. *Xenon lamp*: Covers UV and visible ranges

CLINICAL MCQS

1. In spectrophotometry, absorbance of solution is directly proportional to:
a. The path length/concentration of the analyte
b. The molecular weight
c. The temperature
d. The refractive index

Answer: a. The path length and concentration of the analyte

2. Which law forms the basis of colorimetry and spectrophotometry?
a. Beer-Lambert law
b. Charles' rule
c. Henry's rule
d. Avogadro's rule

Answer: a. Beer-Lambert law

3. A spectrophotometric analysis of hemoglobin exhibits an abnormal absorbance peak at 630 nm. What could this suggest?
a. Carboxyhaemoglobin
b. Oxyhaemoglobin
c. Methaemoglobin
d. Deoxyhaemoglobin

Answer: c. Methaemoglobin

4. Presence of bilirubin is detected by measuring absorbance at what wavelength?
a. 280 nm
b. 548 nm

c. 450 nm
d. 628 nm

Answer: c. 450 nm

5. **Glucose estimation using spectrophotometry include GOD-POD technique. The final-colored product is measured at what wavelength?**
   a. 520 nm
   b. 350 nm
   c. 650 nm
   d. 456 nm

   Answer: a. 520 nm

6. **During spectrophotometric analysis of creatinine by Jaffe reaction, interference from ketones may result in:**
   a. A false increase in measured creatinine
   b. A decrease in creatinine
   c. No effect
   d. Complete inability

   Answer: a. A false increase in measured creatinine

7. **Which cuvette is needed for spectrophotometric measurements in UV range?**
   a. Glass
   b. Copper
   c. Quartz
   d. Plastic

   Answer: c. Quartz

8. **Total protein level is estimated using biuret reagent in a colorimetric assay. The intensity of the color is directly proportional to:**
   a. Albumin volume
   b. Protein concentration
   c. pH
   d. Temperature

   Answer: b. Protein concentration

9. **Spectrophotometric analysis of lactate dehydrogenase involves monitoring production of NADH. At what wavelength NADH is measured?**
   a. 270 nm
   b. 440 nm
   c. 340 nm
   d. 625 nm

   Answer: c. 340 nm

10. **A colorimetric assay measures alkaline phosphatase using para-nitrophenyl phosphate as substrate. The yellow compound is measured at what wavelength?**
    a. 405 nm
    b. 545 nm
    c. 345 nm
    d. 625 nm

    Answer: a. 405 nm

VIVA VOCE

Q1. Discuss principle of colorimetry/its clinical diagnostics?
Next question/Follow-up: How is Beer's Law relating with colorimetry/how is it applied to find concentration of a substance in a sample?

Q2. Discuss principle of spectrophotometry. Differentiate from colorimetry/what are its applications?
Next question/Follow-up: What are the factors that affect the accuracy of spectrophotometric measurements, and how can we correct these errors

SPOTTERS

Q1. Show a spectrophotometric setup with a sample in a cuvette. Ask about the purpose of using blank solution/how is it used in the calibration?

Hints: Focus on the role of the blank in setting the baseline/zero absorbance/ensuring that only the absorbance from the sample is measured.

Q2. A colorimeter is used for measuring the concentration of Hb a blood sample. The absorbance at a particular wavelength is measured. What does the absorbance reading suggest/how would you calculate the hemoglobin concentration?

Hints: Focus on Beer's Law ($A = \varepsilon lc$) is applied, where A is absorbance, ε is the molar absorption coefficient, l is the path length, and c is the concentration.

REFLECTION

Visit the hospital laboratory and learn the principles and working of the colorimeter and spectrophotometer, Mention the advantages of spectrophotometer over colorimeter and observe the working of colorimeter.

8

CHAPTER

Estimation of Glucose in Serum and Other Biological Fluids

COMPETENCIES

BC14.7: Perform estimation of glucose by manual or semi-automated analyzer method and demonstrates glucometer usage and interpretation of results with clinical scenarios.
BC14.22: Describe performance of OGTT, glucose challenge test and HbA1c and interpretation of results with clinical scenarios.

LEARNING OBJECTIVES

After reading this chapter, the readers should be able to:
- Describe the significance and principle of estimation of blood glucose level in clinical chemistry.
- Perform the estimation of blood sugar level and interpretation of the results with clinical correlation.

BLUE PRINT

Demonstration of Serum Biochemical Assays

Objective

By the end of the lecture, students should be able to:
1. Understand the principles and techniques involved in estimating glucose, creatinine, urea, and total protein levels in serum.
2. Perform the biochemical assays accurately and safely.
3. Interpret the results obtained from the assays.

Duration: ***90 minutes***

Materials Needed

1. Laboratory equipments, reagents to perform biochemical assay of glucose.
2. Serum samples for assay.
3. *Demonstration requirement*: Spectrophotometer/pipettes/test tubes/colorimetric reagents.
4. *Safety equipment*: Gloves/lab coats/goggles.
5. Worksheets/handouts for detailing the techniques/procedures/calculations of every assay.

Outline

I. **Introduction to serum biochemical assays** **(15 minutes)**
   - Overview of the significance of biochemical assays in clinical approaches.
   - Explanation of the principles mechanisms/required for estimation of glucose in serum and plasma.
   - Discussion of the relevance of every assay in assessing different physiological/pathological conditions.

II. **Demonstration of glucose estimation** **(20 minutes)**
   - Explanation of enzymatic methodology for assay of glucose.
   - Step-by-step demonstration of the techniques, procedure, sample preparation, reagent mixing, and spectrophotometric measurement.
   - Interpretation of the results received/discussion of the factors which have an impact on glucose levels in serum.

III. **Safety precautions and quality control** **(10 minutes)**
- Review of the different safety measures procedures for handling biohazardous substances/laboratory chemicals.
- Significance of maintaining quality control measures for ensuring accuracy/reliability of results.

IV. **Conclusion and recap** **(5 minutes)**
- Summary of key points.
- Emphasis on the significant techniques, proper sticking to protocols, along with interpretation of results in clinical practice.

V. **Question and answer session** **(10 minutes)**
- Encourage the students to ask questions and get clarification on every aspect.
- Discuss real-life case scenarios/challenging conditions in relation to serum biochemical analysis for further research work and proper understanding.

INTRODUCTION

Sample Collection

- Plasma is the preferred sample for estimation of glucose.
- Blood sample is taken from cubital vein.
- Gray-colored capped vacutainers containing sodium fluoride to inhibit enzyme of glycolysis at enolase step otherwise the glucose level may drop at a rate of 10 mg/dL/hour and potassium oxalate as anticoagulant are used (NaF and Potassium oxalate ratio is 1:3).
- In fed condition, capillary (arterialized) blood sugar may be higher by 35 mg% as compared to venous blood.

Conditions when Blood Glucose Estimation may be Indicated

- Symptoms of hyperglycemia
- Symptoms of hypoglycemia
- Obese people
- Hypertension
- Complications of diabetes mellitus
- All pregnant women especially with bad obstetric history
- Preoperative cases
- Monitoring the therapy for diabetes mellitus and effectiveness of the treatment

Clinical Classification of Blood Sugar

Fasting blood sugar	Blood sample collected after overnight fast of at least twelve hours
Postprandial blood sugar	Blood sample collected two hours after taking a normal diet
Postprandial blood sugar	Blood sample collected two hours after taking 75 g of glucose load
Random blood sugar	Blood is taken anytime in the day without preparation of the patient

Estimation of Blood Glucose Includes the Following Methods

Enzymatic methods	Reduction methods	Chemical tests	Other tests
Glucose oxidase	Ferricyanide Hoffman's method	Modified King and Asatoor	Clinistix test
Hexokinase	Copper sulfate method	Ortho-Toluidine	Diastix
	Aromatic amines method		Capillary blood glucose test

Enzymatic method: Glucose oxidase method

Reagents	Blank (B)	Standard (S)	Test (T)
Enzyme reagent	2 mL	2 mL	2 mL
Standard (100 mg%)		20 µL	
Plasma			20 µL
Distilled water	20 µL		

Reagents needed	• Enzyme reagent – Glucose oxidase – Peroxidase – 4-Aminoantipyrine dye – Phenol in phosphate buffer • Glucose standard: 100 mg%
Method/ procedure	• Take three test tubes, mark them as blank, standard and test, take 2 mL enzyme reagent in all the three test tubes • Add 20 μL of DW in 'B' test tube, 20 μL sample in the 'T' test tube and 20 μL standard in 'S' test tube • Mix well and incubate at 37°C for 15 minutes and take reading at 540 nm in colorimeter and record the OD
Principle	**Reaction 1:** Aldehyde group of beta D glucose gets oxidized by glucose oxidase enzyme to form gluconic acid and H_2O_2 is also released — $\text{Glucose} \xrightarrow{\text{GOD (enzyme)}} \text{Gluconic acid} + H_2O_2$ **Reaction 2:** H_2O_2 forms nascent oxygen in presence of enzyme peroxidase — $H_2O_2 \xrightarrow{\text{POD (enzyme)}} H_2O + \{O\}$ **Reaction 3:** Nascent oxygen reacts with 4-Aminoantipyrine dye to form pink-colored complex of quinoneimine — $4\ \text{AAP} + \{O\} \longrightarrow \text{Quinoneimine complex}$ **Reaction 4:** The pink color is read colorimetrically at 540 nm and the color absorbance that is OD is directly proportional to the amount of nascent oxygen which in turn is directly proportional to the amount of glucose in the sample
Calculations	Amount of glucose = OD (T)/OD (S) × amount of standard (mg)/volume of serum (mL) × 100 — OD (T)/OD (S) × 0.02/0.02 × 100 — OD (T)/OD (S) × 1 × 100
Disadvantage	Ascorbic acid, uric acid and glutathione interfere with GOD enzyme due to which this method is not done in urine glucose estimation
Hexokinase method	Reference method as it uses glucose-6-phosphate dehydrogenase enzyme acting specifically on glucose 6-phosphate moiety alone
Principle:	$\text{Glucose} + \text{ATP} \xrightarrow{\text{Hexokinase}} \text{Glucose-6-phosphate} + \text{ADP}$ $\text{Glucose-6-phosphate} + \text{NADP} \xrightarrow{\text{Glucose-6-phosphate dehydrogenase (G6PD)}} \text{6-phosphogluconate} + \text{NADPH}$ NADPH formed is directly proportional to the amount of glucose, NADPH absorbs wavelength at 340 nm and can be quantified by increase in absorbance at 340 nm

Advantages of enzymatic methods	Specific for glucose, accurate and precise	Minute amount of sample is required	Single step process, room temperature is needed so convenient	NaF does not interfere in estimations	Linearity is high around 700 mg/dL (a test is considered best which can give us wide range and even very abnormal high values can be obtained)

Chemical methods: Modified King and Asatoor method

Reagents	Isotonic copper sulfate solution 10% sodium tungstate Alkaline copper sulfate solution Phosphomolybdic acid reagent Glucose standard 10 mg%
Principle Cupric ions (alkaline cupric sulfate) ↓ Reducing blood glucose Cuprous ions ↓ Phosphomolybdic acid Blue-colored complex	Based on reducing property of glucose which occurs best in basic medium In basic medium, glucose is heated, which forms enediol form, which has the tendency to reduce cupric ions (Cu^{++}) to cuprous ions (Cu^{+}) which precipitates as insoluble cuprous oxide (Cu_2O) Cu_2O then reduces phosphomolybdate to molybdenum blue which is measured at 610 nm Amount of molybdenum blue is directly proportional to amount of Cu_2O, which in turn is directly proportional to amount of glucose in the sample

Contd....

Contd....

Calculations	Amount of glucose = OD of test/OD of standard × amount of standard/volume of serum × 100 OD of test/OD of standard × 0.05/0.05 × 100 OD of test/OD of standard × 1 × 100 (Amount of standard: 100 mL has 10 mg so 0.5 mL has 0.05 mg) and 8 mL of solution prepared in test tube A has 0.2 mL of blood, so 2 mL of protein free filtrate has 0.05 mL of serum)		

Modified King and Asatoor method

Reagents	**B (Blank) mL**	**S (Standard) mL**	**T (Test) mL**
Distilled water	2	1.5	-
Glucose standard (10 mg%)	–	0.5	-
Protein free filtrate: Take a centrifuge tube and add: $CuSO_4$ = 7.4 mL Whole blood = 0.2 mL Sodium tungstate = 0.4 mL (total 8 mL) Centrifuged and supernatant is used as protein free filtrate			2
Alkaline copper sulfate	2	2	2
Total	4	4	4

All the test tubes are boiled for 10 minutes, cooled, and then add 3 mL of Phosphomolybdic acid and 8 mL of distilled water in all the tree test tubes and then OD is read at 610 nm

Ortho-Toluidine method

Reagents	• 10% trichloroacetic acid • O-Toluidine reagent (5 g thiourea is dissolved in 90 mL of ortho-Toluidine and made up to 1 liter with glacial acetic acid and stored in brown bottle) • Glucose standard 10 mg%
Principle Glucose + Ortho-Toluidine Hot ↓ acid medium Green-colored complex (N-glycosylamine)	When glucose reacts with ortho-Toluidine at boiling temperature forms a blue-green colored derivative called N-glycosylamine, the intensity of which is directly proportional to the concentration of glucose in the solution and is read at 600 nm or 630 nm
Calculations	Amount of glucose = OD of test/OD of standard × amount of standard/volume of serum × 100 OD of test/OD of standard × 0.1/0.1 × 100 OD of test/OD of standard × 1 × 100 (Amount of standard: 100 mL has 10 mg so 1.0 mL has 0.1 mg) (5 mL of the filtrate has 0.5 mL of serum so 1 mL has 0.1 mL of serum)

Ortho-Toluidine method

Reagents	**B (Blank) mL**	**S (Standard) mL**	**T (Test) mL**
Distilled water	1		
Glucose standard (10 mg%)		1	
Filtrate: Take a test tube and add: Blood sample = 0.5 mL DW = 3 mL 10% Trichloroacetic acid = 1.5 mL (total 5 mL) Keep for 10 minutes Filter Keep the filtrate for adding in T test tube (5 mL of this solution has 0.5 mL of serum so 1 mL has 0.1 mL of serum)			1
Ortho-Toluidine reagent	5	5	5
Total	6	6	6

All the test tubes are boiled for 10 minutes, cooled, then OD is read at 600/630 nm

Reduction methods	
Ferricyanide Hoffman's test: Based on reducing property of glucose	It uses Ferricyanide which gets reduced by glucose (Fe^{+++} to Fe^{++}), and color changes from yellow to colorless
Copper sulfate method	• Folin-Wu method using alkaline copper sulfate and Phosphomolybdic acid forming • Nelson–Somogyi method using copper sulfate and arsenomolybdate • Fehling's test using copper sulfate, KOH and sodium potassium tartrate
Aromatic amines method	Ortho-Toluidine reacts with colorless glucose and on heating and acid pH, a colored complex called glucosamine is formed

Clinistix test	To confirm presence of glucose in urine
Kit	An area on the stick is coated with o-Toluidine, glucose oxidase and a pink background dye
Procedure	Take 5 mL urine in a test tube and dip the stick in it for 10 seconds
Observation	If the stick area turns shades of blue, it confirms the presence of glucose in urine (glucose concentration should be more than 1 g/L)
Principle	O-Toluidine gets oxidized to a blue substance forming different blue shades
Capillary blood glucose test	Based on enzymatic estimation of blood glucose
Kit of dry chemistry technique	• Instrument—glucometer • Test strips (has enzyme—glucose oxidase peroxidase, in dried form at one end) • Needle/lancet • Lancet device • Alcohol swab
Sample type	Whole blood (its glucose concentration is 15% low as compared to plasma/serum glucose concentration)
Sample requirement	Varies from 0.3 to 1.5 µL
Incubation time	Varies from 5 to 45 seconds
Range of values which can be measured	(0–600 mg/dL/30–500 mg/dL)
Operation	• Machine is switched on • Correct the placement of test strip in the socket • Use alcohol swab for cleaning the tip of the finger • Place the lancet in lancet holder • Prick the finger • Put a blood drop at correct spot and the drop of capillary arterial blood is made to react with the enzyme in the strip • Read the screen result after 5 to 45 seconds • Dispose the test strip
Advantages	• Accurate • Self-monitoring can be done and patient can modulate the dose of insulin accordingly • Portable • Bed side measurement done
Diastix test	To confirm presence of glucose in urine
Kit	An area on the stick is coated with potassium iodide, glucose oxidase and a blue background dye
Procedure	Take 5 mL urine in a test tube and dip the stick in it for 30 seconds
Observation	If the stick area turns shades of green to blue, it confirms the presence of glucose in urine

Observation and conclusion	**Normal ranges**
Fasting blood sugar	70–100 mg/dL (plasma)
	60–100 mg% (whole blood)
Post prandial (PP)	100–140 mg%
Impaired fasting glucose	110–126 mg%

Contd....

Contd....

Impaired fasting glycemia	Fasting plasma sugar is more than normal, but 2 hour post glucose value is in normal range, patient is at high risk of diabetes
Impaired post prandial sugar (impaired glucose tolerance)	140–200 mg%
Impaired glucose tolerance	Blood sugar values are more than normal but below diabetic levels, and proper diet and exercise is recommended
Random blood sugar	<126 mg/dL
Random blood sugar Pre diabetics	126–140 mg/dL
Hyperglycemia	Fasting >110 mg%
	Post prandial >140 mg%
Hypoglycemia	Less than 60 mg%
Children	60–110 mg/dL
Newborns	40–60 mg/dL

All hyperglycemic are not diabetics: (other causes may be present)

Hyperglycemia	**Hypoglycemia**
Due to over activity of thyroid/adrenal gland	Hypo activity of endocrinal glands
Due to excess formation of epinephrine/norepinephrine	Improper absorption of glucose
Pancreatic disorders	Pancreatic beta cell tumor
Mild exercise	Severe exercise
Postoperative anesthesia effect	Starvation

American Diabetes Association diagnostic criterion for diabetes: (results must be confirmed by repeated testing)

Test	**Threshold**	**Qualifier**
HbA1c	>6.5%	National GHb standardization program certified, standardized diabetes control and complications trial
Fasting glucose	>126 mg%/7mol/L	No calorie intake for eight hours
2 hour glucose	>200 mg%/11.1 mmol/L	After 75 g of anhydrous glucose
Random glucose	>200 mg%/11.1 mmol/L	Plus classic hyperglycemia symptoms/crisis

Gestational diabetes mellitus (GDM)
Complications: Mother should be examined again well after child birth

- Carbohydrate intolerance seen for the 1st time during pregnancy
- Fasting blood glucose is more than 126 mg%
- Increased risk of developing frank diabetes
- Increased risk of neonatal mortality
- Mother hyperglycemia leads to more secretion of insulin in the fetus, leading to more weight at birth

Glycosylated hemoglobin (HbA1c)	A hemoglobin which forms a non-enzymatic Schiff base with glucose Hb + glucose → Aldimine → Glycated hemoglobin
Importance	The measurement of HbA1c is not dependent on one day diet or medications (as of fasting/PP/random), and can give information about long-term control of diabetes mellitus (whether a long-term diabetic patient's sugar who is undergoing treatment is under control or not)
Formation	Nonenzymatic glycosylation of beta chain N-terminal valine amino acid with glucose, rate and extent of this reaction depends on average blood glucose concentration
Unit	Percentage
Measurement	Cation exchange chromatography

Contd....

Contd....

Principle of cation exchange chromatography	• Hemolyzed preparation of whole blood is mixed with weak binding cation exchange resin, in this period of five minutes, non-glycated Hb binds to the resin • A filter is present to separate the supernatant which has glycated Hb from the resin, which is the fast fraction, elutes first in column chromatography with cation exchange resin • The percentage of glycated Hb is estimated by measuring the absorbance at 415 nm of glyco-Hb fraction and total hemoglobin fraction
Applications	• We get to know about average blood sugar in preceding 8–12 weeks (life of red blood cells is 120 days, so it can tell that whether any glycation during last 120 days has taken place or not) • Only one value of 6.5% of random blood sample is enough for diagnosing diabetes mellitus • We get to know about the patient response to treatment • We get to know about that whether the therapy given to a diabetic patient is effective or not • We can calculate mean plasma glucose according to rule of 8 • Estimation of HbA1c throws light on blood sugar control between 2 successive investigations • Provides a reliable measure of degree of metabolic control in diabetics
Limitations	Since the interpretation of glycosylated Hb depend on red blood cells with a normal life span of 120 days we can get abnormal values of GHb in conditions, such as we can get falsely high value in iron deficiency anemia and falsely low values in hemolytic disorder and blood loss

Types of glycated hemoglobin: HbA forms 90% of total hemoglobin HbA1a, HbA1b, HbA1c are together called glycated Hb	HbA1a1	Binds with fructose 1,6-bisphosphate
	HbA1a2	Binds with glucose 6 phosphate
	HbA1b	Binds with pyruvate
	HbA1c (found in red blood cells of diabetic patient)	Binds with glucose

HbA1c and the status of diabetic person

HbA1c	**Status**
<5.7% (normal range = 4.5% to 6.3%)	Nondiabetic
5.7–6.4%	Good control
>6.5%	Diabetic (there is high amount of circulating HbA1c that is blood glucose is not under control)
7–8%	Fair control
>8%	Poor control/uncontrolled DM
Interpretation	1% decrease in HbA1c means decrease in risk of death due to diabetes by 21%, myocardial infarction by 14% and microvascular abnormalities by 37%
Rule of 8:	For HbA1c value of 8%, mean plasma glucose value is 180 mg%, and for every 1% increase/decrease of HbA1c, 35 mg% of glucose is added/subtracted respectively from 180 mg% value to get the mean plasma glucose value
HbA1c	Mean plasma glucose in mg%
5	75
6	75 + 35 = 110
7	110 + 35 = 145
8	145 + 35 = 180
9	180 + 35 = 215
For Type 1 DM (minimum treatment)	HbA1c should be done 4 times annually
For Type 1 DM (intensive treatment)	HbA1c should be done once in 2 months
For Type 2 DM	HbA1c should be done 2 times in one year

Fructosamine Assay

Measures average blood glucose over the past 2–3 weeks.

CASE STUDY

A 50-year-old man came with complaints of increased thirst and appetite and increased urine frequency for last 5 months.

Blood Report

- Fasting plasma glucose—150 mg%
- Postprandial glucose—215 mg%
- HbA1c—7%
- Urine is positive for sugar by dipstick
- What is the diagnosis?
- What is the reason of excess urination frequency?
- What other investigations are required?
- Comment on glycosylated value.
- What is the American Diabetes Association criterion for diabetes?
- What is the line of treatment?

Age	**50 years**
Complains	Weakness, frequency of passing urine increased from past few months
On examination	Blood pressure was slightly raised, eye balls were sunken
	Blood report
Fasting blood sugar	160 mg%
Postprandial blood sugar	250 mg%
HbA1c	15% (uncontrolled blood sugar from past 8–12 weeks)
Diagnosis	Type II diabetes mellitus–NIDDM (onset is 50 years)
Reason behind weakness	There is no transport of glucose inside the cells due to insulin deficiency which otherwise promotes the entry of glucose inside the cells, thus glycolysis is decreased which lowers ATP release
Reason behind increased frequency of urine	Glucosuria is associated with polyuria, because glucose present in the urine exerts osmotic effect, renal threshold for glucose is 180 mg%, resulting in glycosuria in the patient
Reason behind sunken eye balls	Polyuria results in dehydration causing polyphagia, so we need to test the serum electrolytes also
Normal range of serum sodium, potassium and chlorides (mEq/L)	136–143, 3.5–5.5, 95–105 respectively

Age	**13 years**
On hospitalization	Tachypnea, fruity smell, dehydrated
History	Weight loss
	Investigations
Random blood glucose	400 mg%
Urinary ketone bodies	++
Glycosuria	+++
	ABG analysis
pH	7.1
Serum potassium	6.2 mEq/L (deficiency of insulin decreases the entry of potassium in the cells, resulting in hyperkalemia, all the more, ketone bodies increases $H^+ - K^+$ antiport, so the exit of potassium out of the cells take place)
pCO_2	45 mm Hg
HCO_3	20 mEq/L

Contd....

Contd....

Serum chlorides	114 mEq/L
Serum sodium	150 mEq/L
Diagnosis	Type I DM and ketoacidosis (juvenile, presence of ketone bodies, extremely raised blood glucose)
Reason behind presence of ketone bodies	Insulin is deficient → transport of glucose inside the cells is deficient leading to deficient production of ATP → energy demands of the cells is met by excess oxidation of fatty acids resulting in production of excess ketone bodies → ketoacidosis
Immediate treatment	Insulin administration, IV fluids for electrolytes and water balance, IV bicarbonates administration for acidosis, monitor pulse, blood pressure and respiration
Line of treatment	Check for complications by doing lipid profile, renal profile urinary proteins, examination of cardiac functions and eye

VIVA VOCE

Q1. What is the preferred methods for blood glucose estimation and why?

Q2. What are the chemical methods for glucose estimation?

Q3. Explain the glucose oxidase method.

Q4. What is the hexokinase method for glucose estimation?

Q5. What is the function of anticoagulant and antiglycolytic agent in glucose estimation?

Q6. What is hypoglycemia, mention causes of the same?

Q7. What is the mechanism of action of insulin in blood glucose regulation?

Q8. What is impaired fasting glucose?

Q9. Define impaired glucose tolerance.

Q10. What is the difference between glycated and glycosylated Hb?

Q11. Which metabolic pathway is responsible for maintaining glucose levels in hypoglycemia?

Q12. Which sample is preferred for routine biochemical analysis?

Q13. What is the use of sodium fluoride in sample collection?

Q14. What are the fasting, PP, and random samples?

Q15. What are the probable causes of hyperglycemia?

Q16. What is gestational diabetes?

OSCE

Case 1: Fasting Blood Glucose Estimation

A 53-year-old male presents with: fatigue, frequent urination, fasting blood glucose: 153 mg/dL.

1. **Give the normal range of fasting blood glucose?**
   70–100 mg/dL
2. **What is the interpretation?**
   Normal: 70–100 mg/dL
   Impaired fasting glucose/prediabetes: 100–125 mg/dL
   Diabetes mellitus: ≥126 mg/dL
   In the clinical scenario fasting blood glucose of 153 mg/dL is indicating diabetes mellitus.
3. **Give the principle of the GOD-POD method?**
   It is based on the enzymatic oxidation of glucose:
   - Glucose oxidase oxidizes glucose forming gluconic acid + hydrogen peroxide.
   - Peroxidase + hydrogen peroxide + chromogen like o-dianisidine forms a colored compound.
   - The intensity of the color can be measured at 505 nm, which is proportional to the concentration of glucose.
4. **What is the clinical significance of fasting blood glucose estimation?**
   For diagnosing diabetes mellitus/prediabetes
   For monitoring the control of glucose control in diabetic patients
   For screening of metabolic disorders

Case 2: Postprandial Blood Glucose Estimation

A 61-year-old female has family history of diabetes. Her PPBG: 198 mg/dL.

1. **Give the normal reference range for PPBG?**
   PPBG is <140 mg/dL
2. **Interpret the findings.**
   Normal: <140 mg/dL
   Impaired glucose tolerance/prediabetes: 140–199 mg/dL
   Diabetes mellitus: ≥200 mg/dL
   198 mg/dL is indicating impaired glucose tolerance/prediabetes.
3. **What conditions can result in high PPBG levels?**
   Diabetes mellitus, Hyperglycemia that is induced by stress, Cushing's syndrome/other endocrinopathies.

Case 3: Random Blood Glucose (RBG) Estimation

A 61-year-old male presents with excessive thirst/frequent urination/lethargy, random blood glucose: 333 mg/dL.

1. **What is the diagnostic significance of RBG?**
   Random blood glucose levels assay is needed for diagnosing diabetes in symptomatic patients:
   Normal: <140 mg/dL.
   Diabetes mellitus: ≥200 mg/dL with associated classic symptoms of hyperglycemia.
2. **What is the interpretation?**
   Random blood glucose: 333 mg/dL, associated with the mentioned symptoms, confirms the disorder of diabetes mellitus.
3. **What are the complications of uncontrolled hyperglycemia?**
   Acute complications: Diabetic ketoacidosis/hyperosmolar hyperglycemic coma.
   Chronic complications: Retinopathy/nephropathy/neuropathy/CVD.

Case 4: Glycated Hemoglobin Investigation

A 39-year-old female with known diabetes investigated for HbA1c test. The result: 9.0%.

1. **What is the normal range for HbA1c?**
   Normal: <5.7%.
   Prediabetes: 5.7–6.4%.
   Diabetes: ≥6.5%.
2. **What does an HbA1c of 9.0% suggesting?**
   An HbA1c of 9.0% is suggestive of poor glycemic control, corresponding to an average blood glucose level of ~213 mg/dL.

3. **What are the applications of HbA1c assay over simple glucose estimation?**
   It reflects long-term glycemic control/average glucose levels over 2–3 months
   Does not require fasting of 12 hours
   It is less affected by daily glucose fluctuations by different factors

Case 5: Hypoglycemia

A 25-year-old male presents with confusion and palpitations, random blood glucose: 41 mg/dL.

1. **What is the diagnostic threshold for hypoglycemia?**
   Hypoglycemia: blood glucose level of <70 mg/dL, along with symptoms occurring less than 50–60 mg/dL.
2. **What can be the reasons of hypoglycemia?**
   - Overdose of Insulin in diabetic patients.
   - Fasting hypoglycemia because of prolonged starvation
   - Hypoglycemia that is induced by alcohol
   - Insulinoma that may be due to pancreatic β-cell tumor
3. **What can be management of hypoglycemia in this scenario?**
   Immediate administration of oral glucose/intravenous dextrose
   Identify/treat the underlying reason

Case 6: Oral Glucose Tolerance Test

A 30-year-old pregnant woman goes for OGTT for gestational diabetes screening.
Fasting: 98 mg/dL.
1-hour: 195 mg/dL.
2-hour: 165 mg/dL.

1. **What are the diagnostic criteria for gestational diabetes in OGT test?**
   Gestational diabetes is diagnosed if any one of the following thresholds is met that is:
   Fasting: ≥92 mg/dL.
   1-hour: ≥180 mg/dL.
   2-hour: ≥153 mg/dL.
2. **How should this patient's results be interpreted?**
   This patient meets the criteria for gestational diabetes that is based on high fasting, 1-hour, and 2-hour glucose concentration.
3. **What are the risks of gestational diabetes for the mother/fetus?**
   Mother: High risk of preeclampsia, facing cesarean delivery/type 2 diabetes in future
   Fetus: Macrosomia/neonatal hypoglycemia/and high risk of obesity/diabetes later in future

Case 7: Diagnosis of Diabetes

A 46-year-old male having family history of diabetes presents with HbA1c: 7.9%.

1. **What is the normal range for HbA1c?**
   HbA1c is <5.7%.
   Prediabetes/impaired glucose tolerance: 5.7–6.4%.
   Diabetes: ≥6.5%.
2. **How should this be interpreted?**
   An HbA1c of 7.9% is suggestive of diabetes mellitus. The threshold for diagnosing diabetes: (with HbA1c): ≥6.5%, and the result is more than threshold, it confirms a diagnosis of type 2 diabetes.
3. **What is the clinical importance of testing of HbA1c?**
   HbA1c testing shows long-term glycemic control, over a period of 2–3 months, and is utilized to:
   Diagnose diabetes/prediabetes.
   Monitor the effectiveness of therapy/treatment of diabetes control over time.
   Assess risk of diabetes-related complications.

Case 8: Monitoring of Diabetes Control

A 62-year-old female with known type 2 diabetes mellitus has been taking metformin for the past one year. On her follow-up investigation visit, HbA1c is 8.5%.

1. **What does this result indicate in a patient with known diabetes?**
   An HbA1c of 8.5% indicates suboptimal glycemic control. In patients with diabetes, the target HbA1c is generally <7% to decrease the risk of long-term side effects This result indicates that her blood glucose concentration has been increased over the past few months, despite taking treatment.

2. **What are the potential long-term complications associated with poorly controlled diabetes?**
   Microvascular side effects: Retinopathy, nephropathy, neuropathy.
   Macrovascular side effects: Cardiovascular disease, stroke, peripheral arterial disease.
   High risk of infections as well as wound healing disorders.
3. **What measures can be taken to improve this case HbA1c?**
   Review the diet, physical activities/medication therapy.
   Adjust for diabetes medication regimen if required that is adding an SGLT2 inhibitor/GLP-1 agonist.
   Encourage to go for changes in lifestyle doing regular exercise/physical activities/balanced diet with emphasis on control of carbohydrates in diet.

Case 9: Prediabetes Diagnosis

A 39-year-male comes for a routine check-up. His HbA1c: 6.3%. He is obese and has family history of diabetes.

1. **What does an HbA1c of 6.3% indicate in this patient?**
   An HbA1c of 6.3% falls in range for prediabetes/impaired glucose tolerance that can be defined as an HbA1c between 5.7% and 6.4%. This is suggestive of being at risk for the development of type 2 diabetes.
2. **What measures might be taken to avoid the progression to state of diabetes in this patient?**
   Lifestyle modifications
   Weight loss by taking balanced diet/regular physical activity/exercise
   Exercise minimum 180 minutes per week.
   Dietary alterations for decreasing refined carbohydrates and more of fiber advised
   Monitor blood glucose frequently for tracking any changes
3. **How frequent should HbA1c be tested in a patient having prediabetes?**
   For persons having prediabetes, HbA1c must be monitored every 6 months to assess progression to stage of diabetes. Regular screening can aid for making timely interventions.

Case 10: False Positive Result because of Hemoglobin Variants

A 51-year-old woman reports as HbA1c: 9.6%. Known history of sickle cell trait.

1. **How can sickle cell trait affect this result?**
   Some hemoglobin variants such as sickle cell trait, hemoglobin C/miscellaneous hemoglobinopathies, might lead to false low/false high HbA1c due to changed red blood cell lifespan/interference with the estimation methodology. In this case, the sickle cell trait may have affected the accuracy of the HbA1c test.
2. **What is another test for assessing long-term glycemic control in patients having hemoglobinopathies?**
   Fructosamine test that reflects glycemic control over the past 2–3 weeks can be done/the 2-hour postprandial glucose measurement can be done. The glycated albumin test can be done because it remains unaffected by hemoglobin variants.
3. **What can be done in this case for confirming diagnosis?**
   We can go for repeat HbA1c test/high-performance liquid chromatography which can identify hemoglobin variants.
   Or do fructosamine/glycated albumin for assessing long-term glucose control.
   Can perform random glucose/OGTT for coming to more definitive diagnosis.

Case 11: HbA1c for Monitoring Glucose Control in Pregnancy

A 29-year-old pregnant woman was diagnosed with gestational diabetes at 26 weeks of gestation. HbA1c at 24 weeks: 5.7%.

1. **What does this indicate during pregnancy?**
   This value of HbA1c is within the normal range, indicative of blood glucose levels are in good controlled in the months prior to her diagnosis of gestational diabetes. However, HbA1c is not the preferred method for monitoring glucose control during pregnancy because of the potential physiological alterations in pregnancy can affect red blood cell turnover.
2. **How glucose control be tested in pregnancy?**
   Self-monitoring of blood glucose: This generally involves pre-meal and postprandial blood sugar measurements.
   Frequent OGTT in the postpartum time can help assess persistent gestational diabetes.
3. **What are the complications of uncontrolled sugar in pregnancy?**
   Macrosomia has more chances of C-section delivery/birth injuries.
   Neonatal hypoglycemia post delivery
   High risk of preterm baby/preeclampsia

Case 12 : Monitoring Type 1 Diabetes

A 21-year-old male with type 1 diabetes presents for HbA1c: 9.3%, and increased thirst and frequent urination.

1. **What does this interpret?**
   Poor glycemic control. In type 1 diabetes, the target HbA1c is commonly <7% to decrease other complications.

2. **What steps can be taken for management?**
   Review of insulin regimen/adjust insulin doses/switch to an insulin pump.
   Improve diet as well as carbohydrate count.
   Encourage frequent blood glucose monitoring.
   Refer to endocrinologist/dietitian A.

CLINICAL MCQS

1. **Which method is commonly utilized for estimating plasma glucose?**
   a. Glucose oxidase-peroxidase method
   b. Folin-Wu
   c. Glucokinase method
   d. Ortho-toluidine

   Answer: a. Glucose oxidase-peroxidase method

2. **Fasting blood glucose is measured using the GOD-POD method. The intensity of the color formed is directly proportional to which of the following?**
   a. Glucose concentration
   b. Hb
   c. Oxygen
   d. Enzyme activity

   Answer: a. Glucose concentration

3. **In the GOD-POD method, what is the function of peroxidase?**
   a. Changes glucose to gluconic acid
   b. Catalyzes the oxidation
   c. Reduces hydrogen peroxide
   d. Catalyzes the reaction between hydrogen peroxide and chromogen

   Answer: d. Catalyzes the reaction between hydrogen peroxide and chromogen

4. **The hexokinase method for glucose estimation depends on the measurement of what coenzyme?**
   a. NADH
   b. NADPH
   c. FADH2
   d. ADP

   Answer: b. NADPH

5. **A diabetic patient for glucose estimation exhibits fasting plasma glucose: 130 mg/dL. According to ADA guidelines, this is classified as:**
   a. Normal
   b. Impaired
   c. Diabetes mellitus
   d. Hypoglycemia

   Answer: c. Diabetes mellitus

6. **A glucose assay which involves glucose oxidase cannot be used in which of the following scenarios?**
   a. Lipemic sample
   b. Presence of ascorbic acid
   c. Hemolyzed
   d. Icteric serum

   Answer: b. Presence of ascorbic acid

7. **A patient's random blood glucose level is: 255 mg/dL. What is the next step for diagnosing diabetes mellitus?**
   a. Repeat glucose measurement
   b. Perform a fasting plasma glucose test
   c. OGTT
   d. HbA1c levels

   Answer: b. Perform a fasting plasma glucose test

8. **Reference range for fasting plasma glucose is:**
   a. 50–88 mg/dL
   b. 70–99 mg/dL
   c. 100–127 mg/dL
   d. 126–142 mg/dL

   Answer: b. 70–99 mg/dL

9. **A glucose estimation is done blood sample taken in plain tube and left at room temperature for 3 hours. The glucose levels are likely to be:**
   a. Accurate
   b. Lower than the actual value
   c. Lower than the actual value
   d. Unaffected

   Answer: c. Lower than the actual value

10. **In a glucose tolerance test, blood glucose values are measured at fasting, 1 hour, and 2 hours after glucose intake. A 2-hour glucose level of 180 mg/dL shows:**
    a. Normal glucose tolerance
    b. Impaired glucose tolerance
    c. Diabetes insipidus
    d. Hypoglycemia

    Answer: b. Impaired glucose tolerance

VIVA VOCE

Q1. What is the physiological importance of glucose in the body/how is blood glucose controlled and regulated?
Next question/Follow-up: What is the role of insulin/glucagon in regulating blood glucose levels/discuss pathophysiology of diabetes mellitus?

Q2. A patient presents with high FBG. What are the key reasons of hyperglycemia/differentiate between type 1 and type 2 diabetes mellitus on the basis of clinical presentation/lab results?
Next question/Follow-up: Which investigations are advised for confirming diagnosis of diabetes?

SPOTTERS

Q1. A patient shows symptoms of excessive thirst/frequent urination/blurred vision. RBG: 350 mg/dL. Interpret/what is your next step in diagnosis/management?

Hints: Focus diagnosing diabetes, possibly type 1, and further investigations such as HbA1c/urinalysis/FBG.

Q2. A patient has hypoglycemia and symptoms of sweating/trembling/confusion. Mention causes of hypoglycemia/how to manage further?

Hints: Focus on causes like insulin overdose/adrenal insufficiency/hypoglycemic drugs/immediate administer glucose.

REFLECTION

Visit the central diagnostic laboratory to discuss and interpret laboratory results of analytes with metabolism of carbohydrates and try to interpret the results of blood glucose levels and other laboratory investigations related to disorders of carbohydrate metabolism along with estimation of glucose in serum.

CHAPTER 9

Estimation of Urea in Serum and Other Biological Fluids

COMPETENCY

BC14.8: Perform estimation of urea and calculate BUN and interpretation of results in clinical scenarios.

LEARNING OBJECTIVES

After reading this chapter, the readers should be able to:
- Describe the significance and principle of blood urea and urea clearance.
- Perform the estimation of blood urea and calculation of urea clearance along with the clinical interpretation.

BLUE PRINT

Demonstration of Serum Biochemical Assays

Objective

By the end of the lecture, students should be able to:
1. Understand the principles and techniques involved in estimating urea in serum.
2. Perform the biochemical assays accurately and safely.
3. Interpret the results obtained from the assays.

Duration: *50 minutes*

Materials Needed

1. Laboratory equipment and reagents for biochemical assays (glucose, creatinine, urea, and total protein).
2. Serum samples for analysis.
3. Demonstration apparatus, such as spectrophotometer, pipettes, test tubes, and colorimetric reagents.
4. Safety equipment including gloves, lab coats, and goggles.
5. Worksheets or handouts detailing the procedures and calculations involved in each assay.

Outline

I. **Introduction to serum biochemical assays** **(15 minutes)**
- Overview of the importance of biochemical assays in clinical diagnostics.
- Explanation of the principles underlying the estimation of urea in serum.
- Discussion of the relevance of each assay in assessing various physiological and pathological conditions.

II. **Demonstration of urea estimation** **(20 minutes)**
- Explanation of the enzymatic urease method for urea estimation.
- Demonstration of the procedure, including sample dilution, addition of reagents, and spectrophotometric analysis.
- Discussion of urea levels in serum and their implications in kidney function and protein metabolism.

III. **Conclusion and recap** **(5 minutes)**
- Summary of key points covered in the demonstration of serum biochemical assays.
- Emphasis on the importance of proper technique, adherence to protocols, and interpretation of results in clinical practice.

IV. **Question and answer session** **(10 minutes)**
- Encourage students to ask questions and seek clarification on any aspects of the assays demonstrated.
- Discuss real-life case scenarios or challenging situations related to serum biochemical analysis for further understanding.

INTRODUCTION

Urea is the end product of protein metabolism:
- *Ammonia formation*: Protein digestion → amino acids → deaminated to form ammonia (toxic)
- *Formation of CO_2*: It is ending product of fat/carbohydrate metabolism.
- Both waste products that are ammonia and CO_2 condense in liver forming urea (non-toxic) by urea cycle.
- It is the major non-protein nitrogenous (NPN) waste substance in urine constituting about 75% of it.
- Other NPN substances are ammonia, creatinine, and uric acid.
- It is freely filtered by glomeruli so whenever filtration is affected due to any disorder, urea accumulates in plasma and by measuring its concentration in plasma we get an idea about renal functions.

Berthelot's Method	
Principle	$\text{Urea} + H_2O \xrightarrow{\text{Urease}} NH_3 + CO_2$ $NH_3 + \text{phenol} + \text{hypochlorite} \xrightarrow{\text{Nitroprusside (alkaline medium)}}$ Indophenol (blue green-colored complex) intensity is measured at 580 nm $\text{Urea} + 2H_2O \xrightarrow{\text{Urease}} 2NH_4^+ + CO_2^{-}$-- $NH_4^+ + \text{2-oxoglutarate} \xrightarrow{\text{Glutamate dehydrogenase}} \text{Glutamate} + H_2O$ (NADH → NAD^+) Rate of disappearance of NADH is measured at 340 nm We can quantify the released NH_4^+ by • Color change associated with pH indicator • Glutamine synthetase • Pyruvate kinase • Pyruvate oxidase
Berthelot's method	DAM method
Requires less time	Requires more time
Requires less sample	Requires more sample
It is less accurate as atmospheric ammonia and that present in the reagent interferes	It is more better as it measures urea directly
Physiological variations	• Depends on dietary intake of proteins • Values are more in males as compared to females • Due to hemodilution the urea values are low in early pregnancy • High in old age
	Pathological Variations
Azotemia	**Uremia/end-age renal disease**
Increased blood urea and other nitrogenous substances only due to inability of renal mechanisms to filter these waste products properly	• Increased blood urea + clinical symptoms + multiorgan failure • Nausea, vomiting, anorexia, metallic taste in mouth, muscle pain, mental confusion, acid base disbalance

Contd....

Contd....

Decreased urea levels	• Severe liver disorders (loss of synthetic ability of liver like in cirrhosis) • Liver cancer			
Increased urea levels	Prerenal azotemia (due to decreased GFR)	Renal azotemia (Due to decreased GFR and non-functional nephrons)		Postrenal azotemia
	Hypovolemia (plasma volume/body fluids are reduced)	Renal/kidney disorder		Urine flow obstruction leads to urine retention which results in reduced effective filtration pressure at glomerulus
	Shock/hemorrhage	Acute glomerulonephritis		Prostate enlargement
	Salt/water decrease	Nephrotic syndrome		Urinary tract stones
	Dehydration (vomiting/ diarrhea)	Malignant nephrosclerosis		Urethral stricture
	Chloride loss like in ulcerative colitis	Chronic pyelonephritis		Tumor of bladder
	Pyloric stenosis	Renal TB		
	Obstruction of the intestine	Mercury poisoning	Ethylene glycol toxicity	Rupture of urinary outflow tracts
	Extensive burns			

Diacetyl monoxime method/DAM-TSC

Reagents required	Acid reagent: $FeCl_3$ in orthophosphoric acid Color reagent: Diacetyl monoxime and thiosemicarbazide in H_2SO_4 Urea standard 1 mg%
Method	Take 3 test tubes and mark them as blank (B), standard (S) and test (T)
Principle	• Urea reacts with DAM in strong acid medium and ferric ions • DAM gets hydrolyzed to form diacetyl + hydroxylamine • Urea + diacetyl = Diazine (pink-colored complex) which is read at 540 nm
Calculations	Urea concentration in serum = OD test/OD standard × amount of standard in mg/volume of serum in mL × 100

Plot a standard curve	It is plotted by treating the standard solution of different concentrations in the same way as standard Different standards are made by diluting the stock standard (100 mg%) with water				
Stand. Conc. (mg%)	0.25	0.5	1.0	2.0	3.0
Blood urea level (mg%)	25	50	100	200	300
Reagents	Blank (B) mL		Standard (S) mL	Test (T) mL	
Standard urea 1 mg%			1		
Serum (1 :100 dil)				1	
DW	2		1	1	
Coloring reagent	2		2	2	
Acid reagent	2		2	2	
Total	6		6	6	
All test tubes are boiled in water bath for 20 minutes, cooled and OD read at 520 nm					
Interpretation	Reference range		Urine	Blood urea nitrogen (BUN)	
	15–50 mg% Conversion factor for converting mg/dL to mmol/L is 0.357 15 mg/dL is 15 × 0.357 = ...mmol/L		23–30 g/day	7–25 mg/dL (1 mg of BUN = 2.14 mg of urea	
Bed side measurement of blood urea		Azostix			
Sample		Whole blood			
Principle		Strip has urease enzyme and bromothymol blue indicator Ammonia is released due to action of urease on urea and this ammonia changes the color of the indicator from yellow to green to blue			

UREA ESTIMATION IN URINE

- Daily excretion of urea in urine = 30 g/day, depends on intake of water and proteins along with the catabolism of proteins.
- Thus, we need to dilute the urine 1:20 with distilled water and results are expressed in mg/dL or g/dL.

Urea clearance: Actually, plasma is not cleared off urea, there is removal of only 10% urea 750 mL plasma pass through the kidney in one minute and only 10% urea is removed which is equivalent to completely clearing only 75 mL plasma in one minute	Volume of plasma that is cleared of that amount of urea which is excreted by the kidneys in one minute
Importance	It is the measure of GFR
Unit	Milliliters/minute
Formula: Urea clearance is expressed as percentage of normal maximum or normal standard urea clearance depending on the output of urine	$C = U \times V/P$ Where U = concentration of urea in urine (mg/dL) V = volume of urine excreted per minute (mL/min) P = concentration of urea in plasma (mg/dL)
Factors on which clearance depends	Directly proportional to body surface area
	Urinary flow rate
Maximum clearance	Urine volume = 2 mL/min or more Then the rate of urea eliminated is maximum and is directly proportional to blood urea concentration This is called maximum urea clearance Cm and the normal value is 75 mL/min $C = U \times V/P$
Standard clearance	Urine volume is <2 mL/min Then the rate of urea eliminated is decreased as more urea gets reabsorbed in the tubules and is directly proportional to square root of urinary volume. It is called standard clearance of urea Cs and the normal value is 54 mL/min $C = U \times V/P$
Two hour test	• The patient is given two glasses of water to drink and asked to completely empty the bladder, this urine sample is discarded • After 1 hour, urine sample is collected • Venous blood sample is also taken • He is given one more glass of water to drink • After 1 hour, collect another urine sample • Determine the urea concentration in plasma and urine samples and urine flow rate from the two urine samples • Calculate the standard or maximum urea clearance according to the flow rates • The 2 clearance values must not vary by more than 10% • The average of the 2 values is finally reported
Clinical interpretation	Maximum urea clearance = 75 mL/min
	Standard urea clearance = 54 mL/min
Deviations	• 40–70% shows mild impairment • 20–40% shows moderate impairment • Below 20% shows severe impairment • Below 5% shows uremic coma imminent
Why creatinine clearance is better index than urea	• Creatinine levels are more or less constant (renal excretion does not vary much with protein intake) • Creatinine clearance is not dependent on urine flow rate
Clearance study vs blood urea estimation	In early renal damage conditions, clearance is likely to indicate renal damage due to less GFR, at this stage, blood urea is likely to be normal. But in later stages of renal damage, clearance holds no value and blood urea levels are better indicators of renal damage

OSCE

Case 1: Acute Kidney Injury (AKI)

A 50-year-old male presents with low urine output/swelled legs, BUN: 41 mg/dL, creatinine: 2.6 mg/dL.

1. **What does this interpret?**
   Renal dysfunction is indicated. BUN is a product of protein metabolism which gets excreted by kidneys. High BUN is seen in acute and chronic kidney injury, conditions that impair renal perfusion, such as dehydration/heart failure.
2. **What is the normal range for BUN?**
   7–20 mg/dL is the reference range. Elevated BUN suggests renal dysfunction/dehydration. Decreased BUN is observed in malnutrition/liver disease/overhydration.
3. **What is the BUN-to-creatinine ratio?**
   It is diagnostic tool for distinguishing between prerenal/intrinsic renal reasons of renal dysfunction.
   A ratio of >20:1 is observed for prerenal reasons, such as dehydration/heart failure.
   A ratio of <10:1 indicates intrinsic renal damage, such as acute tubular necrosis.
   In this case, the scenario suggests prerenal azotemia.

Case 2: Chronic Kidney Disease (CKD)

A 68-year-old female having history of hypertension plus diabetes presents with BUN: 36 mg/dL, /creatinine: 3.1 mg/dL.

1. **What does this interpret?**
   Chronic kidney disease is indicated associated to her history of hypertension and diabetes, that are quite common reasons of CKD. Kidney function seem to be compromised over time, resulting in accumulation of nitrogenous waste products such as urea/creatinine in the blood.
2. **How kidney function is monitored?**
   Serum creatinine, glomerular filtration rate, BUN levels, urine albumin-to-creatinine ratio, keep a check on proteinuria which is key marker for CKD progression.
3. **What is the significance of high BUN?**
   Impaired kidney function, decreased ability of the kidneys to excrete nitrogenous waste products.

Case 3: Liver Disease

A 43-year-old male with a history of alcohol use disorder presents with ascites/jaundice, BUN: 23 mg/dL, creatinine: 0.8 mg/dL.

1. **What is the interpretation?**
   The normal creatinine level indicate that kidneys are functioning normally, despite the liver disease. In liver disorders, BUN can be affected impaired liver function, because liver is responsible for making urea.
2. **How liver disease affects BUN levels?**
   In liver disease, specifically cirrhosis, the liver's ability to form urea is compromised, resulting in lower BUN levels.

Case 4: High-protein Intake in a Healthy Individual

A 43-year-old male athlete presents serum urea: 53 mg/dL, serum creatinine: 1.1 mg/dL. He takes high-protein diet.

1. **What does this interpret?**
   The high urea of healthy individual taking high-protein diet is probably because of high protein metabolism. High protein diet results in more urea formation as the body metabolizes proteins for energy. The normal creatinine level indicate kidney function is normal and the high urea is not because of kidney dysfunction.
2. **Why is creatinine level normal despite the high urea?**
   The creatinine level remains normal as creatinine is a byproduct of muscle metabolism and is not usually affected by dietary protein intake. Urea is a byproduct of protein metabolism, so high-protein diet may increase urea formation resulting in high levels. The normal creatinine indicates unaffected kidney functions.
3. **What advice regarding high-protein diet can be given?**
   Encourage proper hydration to aid kidneys excrete the high urea.
   Monitor urea/creatinine frequently for ensuring kidney function is normal.
   If any underlying kidney disorder is present then advise that more protein intake might raise the burden on the kidneys.

CLINICAL MCQS

1. **The common method to assay for urea:**
   a. Urease
   b. Uricase method
   c. Creatine oxidase
   d. Oxidase

   Answer: a. Urease

2. **For urease method of urea estimation, what compound is measured spectrophotometrically?**
   a. Ammonia
   b. CO_2
   c. Urea
   d. NO

   Answer: a. Ammonia

3. **A 67-year-old patient having chronic kidney disease shows serum urea: 80 mg/dL. This shows:**
   a. Normal kidney function
   b. Azotemia
   c. Postrenal defect
   d. Uremia

   Answer: d. Uremia

4. **Reference range for serum urea in adults:**
   a. 10–25 mg/dL
   b. 20–40 mg/dL
   c. 40–65 mg/dL
   d. 50–82 mg/dL

   Answer: b. 20–40 mg/dL

5. **For urea estimation blood is taken/stored at room temperature for 4 hours. What effect can be there on the urea concentration?**
   a. Decrease due to hemolysis
   b. Decrease due to bacterial decomposition
   c. No change
   d. Increase because of enzymatic reactions

   Answer: b. Decrease due to bacterial decomposition

6. **In urea estimation by Berthelot's methodology, the blue-color complex formed is because of reaction between ammonia and:**
   a. Phenol and hypochlorite
   b. Nessler's dye
   c. Nitroprusside
   d. Ninhydrin solution

   Answer: a. Phenol and hypochlorite

7. **A 47-year-old male having dehydration shows elevated urea level but a normal creatinine level. This indicates:**
   a. Prerenal azotemia
   b. Renal disease
   c. Postrenal azotemia
   d. Abnormal renal function

   Answer: a. Prerenal azotemia

8. **A patient's blood urea nitrogen is: 28 mg/dL. What is the serum urea concentration?**
   a. 11 mg/dL
   b. 24 mg/dL
   c. 60 mg/dL
   d. 82 mg/dL

   Answer: c. 60 mg/dL
   (Serum urea = BUN × 2.14)

9. **A urea-creatinine ratio more than 20:1 is observed in:**
   a. Prerenal azotemia
   b. Intrinsic disease

   c. Postrenal azotemia
   d. Normal kidney function

   Answer: a. Prerenal azotemia

10. **Which of the conditions is least likely to result in high serum urea levels?**
    a. Dehydration state
    b. High-protein intake
    c. Liver failure
    d. Heart failure

    Answer: c. Liver failure

VIVA VOCE

Q1. What is urea/how is it formed in the body?

Next question/Follow-up: How urea formation in the liver associated with protein metabolism/why is it used as a marker for renal function?

Q2. A patient presents with high BUN levels. What are the important causes of high urea, and how can you approach the diagnostic evaluation?

Next question/Follow-up: Differentiate between prerenal/renal reasons of increased urea?

SPOTTERS

Q1. A patient presents with dehydration/high urea levels/normal creatinine. Interpret urea-creatinine ratio/what follow up steps for management are taken?

Hints: Focus on prerenal causes, such as dehydration/investigate for possible causes, such as gastrointestinal loss/bleeding.

Q2. A patient with CKD) presents with high urea levels/symptoms of fatigue/nausea. Interpret/how would you assess the severity of kidney dysfunction?

Hints: Focus on uremia, the progression of CKD, requirement to assess the GFR/perform a creatinine clearance test.

REFLECTION

Describe the significance and principle of blood urea and urea clearance. Perform the estimation of blood urea, urine urea and calculation of urea clearance along with the clinical correlation.

CHAPTER 10

Estimation of Creatinine in Serum and Other Biological Fluids

COMPETENCY

BC14.9: Perform the estimation of serum creatinine and calculate creatinine clearance.

LEARNING OBJECTIVES

After reading this chapter, the readers should be able to:

- Describe the significance and principle of blood creatinine and creatinine clearance.
- Perform the estimation of blood creatinine, urine creatinine and calculation of creatinine clearance along with the clinical interpretations.

BLUE PRINT

Estimation of Serum Creatinine and Creatinine Clearance

Objective

By the end of the lecture, students should be able to:

1. Understand the principles behind the estimation of serum creatinine and creatinine clearance.
2. Describe the methods used for the measurement of serum creatinine and calculation of creatinine clearance.
3. Explain the clinical significance of serum creatinine and creatinine clearance in assessing renal function.

Duration: ***60 minutes***

Materials Needed

1. Presentation slides explaining the principles of creatinine estimation and creatinine clearance calculation.
2. Charts or diagrams illustrating the renal clearance concept.
3. Examples of laboratory reports showing serum creatinine levels and creatinine clearance values.
4. Sample data for creatinine clearance calculation.
5. Calculators for students use during hands-on calculation exercises.

Outline

I. **Introduction to serum creatinine and creatinine clearance** **(10 minutes)**
- Define serum creatinine and creatinine clearance.
- Explain the significance of these parameters in assessing renal function.
- Discuss the relationship between creatinine production, filtration, and excretion by the kidneys.

II. **Principles of creatinine estimation** **(10 minutes)**
- Describe the chemical basis of the Jaffe reaction, the most common method for serum creatinine measurement.
- Explain how creatinine reacts with alkaline picrate to form a colored complex.
- Discuss factors that may interfere with the accuracy of creatinine measurements and methods to minimize these interferences.

III. **Methods for serum creatinine measurement** **(10 minutes)**
- Discuss laboratory techniques for measuring serum creatinine, including manual and automated methods.
- Explain the advantages and limitations of each method in terms of accuracy, precision, and turnaround time.
- Provide examples of instruments and reagents commonly used for creatinine analysis in clinical laboratories.

IV. **Creatinine clearance calculation** **(15 minutes)**
- Introduce the concept of renal clearance and its importance in assessing kidney function.
- Explain the formula for calculating creatinine clearance using serum creatinine concentration, urine creatinine concentration, and urine volume.
- Demonstrate step-by-step calculations for determining creatinine clearance in hypothetical patient scenarios.
- Discuss the interpretation of creatinine clearance values in different clinical contexts.

V. **Clinical applications of serum creatinine and creatinine clearance** **(10 minutes)**
- Describe how serum creatinine levels and creatinine clearance values are used to diagnose and monitor renal diseases, such as acute kidney injury and chronic kidney disease.
- Discuss the role of creatinine clearance in adjusting drug dosages in patients with impaired renal function.
- Highlight the importance of serial measurements of serum creatinine and creatinine clearance in evaluating treatment responses and disease progression.

VI. **Hands-on activity** **(5 minutes)**
- Provide sample data for serum creatinine and urine creatinine concentrations.
- Guide students through the calculation of creatinine clearance using the Cockcroft-Gault formula or other appropriate equations.
- Encourage students to work in pairs or small groups to enhance collaboration and problem- solving skills.

VII. **Interpretation of results** **(5 minutes)**
- Review the calculated creatinine clearance values obtained by students.
- Discuss the clinical implications of these results in terms of renal function and disease severity.
- Address any questions or concerns raised by students regarding the calculation process or interpretation of results.

VIII. **Review and summary** **(5 minutes)**
- Summarize the key points covered in the lecture regarding the estimation of serum creatinine and creatinine clearance.
- Reinforce the importance of these parameters in clinical practice and research.
- Provide additional resources for further reading and self-study on renal function assessment.

IX. **Conclusion** **(5 minutes)**
- Conclude the lecture by emphasizing the role of serum creatinine and creatinine clearance in evaluating kidney function and diagnosing renal disorders.
- Encourage students to apply the knowledge gained in the lecture to their clinical practice or future research endeavors.

INTRODUCTION

Serum creatinine assessment	For assessment of glomerular filtration rate
Formation of creatinine: 2% of total creatine is converted to creatinine daily	Creatine $\xrightarrow{H_2O}$ Creatinine (non-toxic excretory compound)
Creatine	Creatine is made in liver by glycine, arginine and methionine, goes to skeletal muscles, converts to creatine phosphate which serve as stored form of energy for skeletal muscles
Creatinine is a good marker for assessing the kidney functions	• Amount of creatine and thus creatinine is directly proportional to the muscle mass which remains constant • Its level does not vary with the dietary intake of proteins
Factors affecting the creatinine level	Muscle mass; Rate of creatine turnover; Renal functions

Estimation of serum creatinine	**Chemical method: Jaffe's reaction**
Reagents required	**For making protein free filtrate:** • 2/3 M H_2SO_4 • 10% sodium tungstate **For Jaffe's reaction:** • Saturated picric acid • 5% NaOH • Creatinine standard 1 mg%
Method: Whole blood is not preferred as red blood cells are rich in non-creatinine chromogen, such as glucose, vitamin C so serum is used generally	**Step 1:** Prepare protein free filtrate: 1 mL DW + 1 mL serum + 1 mL sodium tungstate + 1 mL H_2SO_4, (total 4 mL) and centrifuged for 3 minutes, the supernatant is used for creatinine estimation which is protein free
	Step 2: Three test tubes that are blank, standard and test are taken

Reagents	**Blank (B) mL**	**Standard (S) mL**	**Test (T) mL**
5% NaOH	1	1	1
Saturated picric acid	1	1	1
Creatinine standard 1 mg%		1	
DW	4	3	2
PFF			2
Total	6	6	6

Test tubes are shaken well and kept at 37°C for 10 minutes and OD taken at 520 nm

Calculations	• Creatinine concentration in serum = OD test/OD standard × amount of standard in mg/volume of serum in mL × 100 • OD test/OD standard × 0.01/0.5 × 100 • OD test/OD standard × 2

Standard = 1 mg% means in 100 mL creatinine is 1 mg so in 1 mL creatinine is .01, we are using 1 mL standard so amount of standard is .01 mg

For making PFF, we used 1.0 mL of serum and total volume was 4 mL, so in 4 mL sample is 1.0, so in 1 mL of this the sample will be 0.25, we are using 2 mL of PFF, so volume of serum becomes 0.5 mL

Principle	Creatinine + saturated picric acid $\xrightarrow{\text{Alkaline medium}}$ Creatinine picrate (red color complex) to be measured at 520 nm
Interpretation	• In healthy males, normal creatinine level is 0.9–1.3 mg/dL (more in males due to high muscle mass) • In healthy females, normal creatinine level is 0.6–1.1 mg/dL • Whole blood = 0.70–1.2 mg/dL • In muscles = 10 mg/dL • Creatinine urea ratio = 1:20
Which is better renal function test, blood urea or serum creatinine?	Serum creatinine is better as its level is dependent on glomerular filtration and not on diet, tubular reabsorption and secretion
Which is better, creatinine clearance or urea clearance?	Creatinine clearance is better as it is freely filtered by the glomeruli but not reabsorbed and secreted very little by renal tubules, it is not affected by dietary intake of proteins, so creatinine clearance is closely equal to GFR
Normal daily excretion of creatinine in urine	1–2 g/day
Linearity	Up to 20%
Variations	• Increased levels are observed for renal failure/renal disorders • Increased levels are observed for muscular dystrophies and poliomyelitis at early stages • High catabolic states, such as fever • Decreased levels are seen in muscle wasting disorders at late stages

Contd....

Contd....

Disadvantages	• Jaffe's reaction is nonspecific and pseudo-positive results are due to acetone, acetoacetic acid so high values can be obtained in diabetic ketoacidosis • Lack of specificity also means that only eighty percent of the developed color is because of creatinine and the rest 20% is due to substances, such as glucose, uric acid, urea, and proteins that can react with alkaline picrate to give false higher results • Jaffe's reaction is sensitive to change in atmospheric conditions, such as temperature and pH		
Can we overcome this disadvantage?	• Yes, we can get rid of nonspecific chromogen by using hydrated aluminum silicate called Lloyd's reagent that will adsorb creatinine in acid medium • After centrifugation, we can resuspend the pellet in basic medium to elude the creatinine that can be then estimated		
New methods which are more specific	**Kinetic Jaffe's method**	**Coupled enzymatic method (costly so not commonly used)**	**Isotope dilution mass spectroscopy (IDMS)**
	To find out the true creatinine levels and to minimize the effect of non-creatinine chromogen, rate of change of absorbance is measured after we add the serum with alkaline picrate	We take into consideration the reaction with combination of different enzymes, such as CPK, PK, LDH, and creatininase	Reference method for creatinine estimation
	Non-creatinine chromogen react differentially: Acetoacetate reacts in first 20 seconds to form color complex, proteins react with it after 90 seconds so we can measure the rate of reaction 20 to 80 seconds after the mixing of sample with picric Acid	Creatinine + H_2O →(Creatinine hydrolase) creatine Creatine + ATP →(CK) Creatine phosphate + ATP ADP + PEP →(Pyruvate kinase) ATP + pyruvate Pyruvate →(LDH) Lactate $NADH + H^+$ → NAD	

ESTIMATION OF CREATININE IN URINE

We need to dilute the urine 1:100 with distilled water due to following reasons:

1. Creatinine values to come within the range of Beer-Lambert law
2. To dilute the interfering substances

Jaffe's Method

Reagents	**Blank (B) mL**	**Standard (S) mL**	**Test (T) mL**
Dilute urine			3
DW	3		
Standard (0.01 mg/dL)		3	
5% NaOH	1	1	1
Saturated picric acid	1	1	1
Mix and keep the test tubes at room temperature for 15 minutes, measure the optical density at 520 nm			

Creatinine clearance	That volume of plasma which is cleared of that amount of creatinine which is excreted by the kidneys in one minute
Creatinine clearance is fair marker of GFR	1. After filtration, there is no reabsorption 2. Creatinine secretion from the tubules is very less 3. Endogenously formed in body 4. Rate of its release in body fluids is constant 5. Plasma levels are maintained within narrow limits
Method	• Advice for restriction of drugs and caffeine on the day of test • Ask to drink half liter water • He is asked to empty the bladder but discard this sample • Collect the rest of the samples of urine in next 24 hours • A blood sample is taken in between • Creatinine is estimated in urine as well as in serum
Formula for creatinine clearance	C = U V/P Where C = clearance (mL/min) U = urine creatinine (mg/dL) V = flow of urine (mL/min) P = serum creatinine (mg/dL)
Interpretation	Reference range: • In males: 95–140 mL/min • In females: 85–125 mL/min
Variation	Creatinine clearance is decreased in impaired renal function

Taking 125 mL/min = 100%, the cut off level for calculated creatinine clearance is 70%, any further decrease means renal abnormality

Up to 70%	Normal
70%–50%	Mild renal damage
49%–20%	Moderate
Below 20%	Severe damage

In early stages of glomerular damage, serum creatinine levels can be normal, but its clearance is affected

OSCE

Case 1: Acute Kidney Injury (AKI)

A 62-year male having history of hypertension presents with serum creatinine: 3.3 mg/dL, blood urea nitrogen: 46 mg/dL. Urine output is less than 400 mL per day.

1. **What does this interpret?**
   The high serum creatinine indicates acute kidney injury, where kidneys' ability to excrete creatinine is damaged that is a feature of AKI.
2. **What another test is recommended?**
   Serum creatinine/creatinine clearance
   A low creatinine clearance suggests decrease in renal function, further confirming the diagnosis of AKI.
3. **What is the management?**
   Fluid management/correction of dehydration/hypoperfusion/regular monitor creatinine/electrolytes/discontinuing nephrotoxic medications/treat infections depending on the reason behind AKI, dialysis.

Case 2: Chronic Kidney Disease (CKD)

A 46-year female with diabetes mellitus presents with pedal edema/hypertension, serum creatinine: 2.6 mg/dL, estimated glomerular filtration rate: 46 mL/min.

1. **What does this interpret?**
   The high serum creatinine indicates CKD. The rise in creatinine shows a decrease in kidney function, that is common in patients of long-standing diabetes, a known complication of CKD.

2. **How is the kidney function evaluated in CKD patients?**
   Serum creatinine, creatinine clearance eGFR are the assays for kidney functions. The formula for eGFR is Cockcroft-Gault/MDRD equation on the basis of serum creatinine/age/sex/race. An eGFR less than 60 mL/min suggests moderate to severe kidney dysfunction, in support of the diagnosis of CKD in the patient.
3. **What are the management strategies?**
   Blood sugar control to avoid any more renal damage.
   Target blood pressure <130/80 mmHg
   Diet control/weight control/stop smoking
   Regular testing of serum creatinine/eGFR/urine albumin to track for the progression

Case 3: Dehydration

A 37-year-old male presents with dry mouth/dizziness/decreased urine output after diarrhea for some days, serum creatinine: 1.9 mg/dL, BUN is high.

1. **What does this interpret?**
   Prerenal azotemia is indicated that may be because of dehydration due to prolonged diarrhea. Dehydration results in reduced renal perfusion, leading to high serum creatinine because of impaired clearance by the kidneys.
2. **Why dehydration affect creatinine?**
   Dehydration results in decreased renal blood flow, resulting in prerenal azotemia. In this state, the kidneys try to conserve water by reabsorption of solutes such as sodium/urea, but creatinine clearance gets impaired, resulting in increase in serum creatinine. The kidneys function properly but the reduced perfusion leads to decreased excretion of creatinine.
3. **What is the management?**
   Rehydrate with fluids for restoring hydration/improve kidney perfusion.
   Repeat creatinine/BUN after rehydration for assessing improvement in renal function.
   Treat diarrhea/prevent any more fluid loss.

Case 4: Acute Glomerulonephritis (AGN)

A 33-year-old male presents with edema/hematuria/high blood pressure, serum creatinine: 2.6 mg/dL. Urinalysis: red blood cell casts/proteinuria.

1. **What is the interpretation?**
   Acute glomerulonephritis is a kidney disease which results in inflammation of the glomeruli, leading to impaired filtration plus high creatinine. Hematuria along with presence of red blood cell casts/proteinuria is supporting the diagnosis.
2. **How to monitor renal functions?**
   Creatinine clearance: To assess the glomerular filtration rate/evaluating extent of kidney dysfunction. Decreased creatinine clearance suggests decreased kidney function.
   Monitor urine protein/urine output
3. **What is the management?**
   Control hypertension to protect kidneys, steroids for immune-mediated AGN, diuretics for treating edema, fluid management, monitor renal functions, electrolytes, and urine output.

CLINICAL MCQS

1. **The common method for creatinine estimation:**
   a. End point method
   b. Jaffe's reaction
   c. Glucokinase method
   d. Urease method
   Answer: b. Jaffe's reaction
2. **In the Jaffe method, creatinine + picric acid in a basic medium forms:**
   a. Red complex
   b. Yellow complex
   c. Orange complex
   d. Violet complex
   Answer: a. A red-colored complex

3. **A 59-year-old male presents with serum creatinine: 3.6 mg/dL. This report is consistent with:**
   a. Abnormal renal function
   b. Azotemia
   c. Chronic kidney disease
   d. Acute renal disease

   Answer: c. Chronic kidney disease

4. **Creatinine clearance is used for estimating:**
   a. Renal tubule function
   b. GFR
   c. Renal blood flow
   d. Protein metabolism

   Answer: b. GFR

5. **The normal range of serum creatinine in adults:**
   a. 0.2–0.8 mg/dL
   b. 0.6–1.2 mg/dL
   c. 1.5–2.8 mg/dL
   d. 2.5–3.8 mg/dL

   Answer: b. 0.6–1.2 mg/dL

6. **A 69-year-old patient has serum creatinine: 5.0 mg/dL, urine creatinine: 50 mg/dL, urine output: 1 Liter/day. What is the creatinine clearance?**
   a. 10 mL/min
   b. 25 mL/min
   c. 55 mL/min
   d. 105 mL/min

   Answer: a. 10 mL/min

7. **Which of the conditions is linked with falsely elevated creatinine values in the Jaffe method?**
   a. Hyperbilirubinemia
   b. Hypoglycemia
   c. Dyslipidemia
   d. Ketosis

   Answer: d. Ketosis

8. **A less serum creatinine value in a malnourished patient is because of:**
   a. Decreased muscle mass
   b. Decreased GFR
   c. Decreased tubular secretion
   d. Acute kidney disease

   Answer: a. Decreased muscle mass

9. **In enzymatic method of creatinine estimation, what enzyme is required?**
   a. Creatinase oxidase
   b. Creatinine oxidase
   c. Uricase
   d. Glucokinase

   Answer: b. Creatinine oxidase

10. **A 72-year-old diabetic patient presents with normal serum creatinine but low GFR. The condition is best explained by:**
    a. Early diabetic nephropathy
    b. Chronic renal disease
    c. Azotemia
    d. Renal hyperfiltration

    Answer: a. Early diabetic nephropathy

VIVA VOCE

Q1. What is creatinine/how is it made in the body?

Next question/Follow-up: Why is creatinine a key marker for assessing renal function? How does the GFR correlate with creatinine concentration?

Q2. A patient comes with high creatinine level. What are the main causes of this rise/how would you approach to diagnosis and management?

Next question/Follow-up: Differentiate between prerenal/renal/postrenal reasons of high creatinine?

SPOTTERS

Q1. A patient has a markedly high serum creatinine level, oliguria/edema. Interpret these findings/what is your next step in investigation?

Hints: Consider AKI, and causes like acute glomerulonephritis/dehydration/obstructive uropathy.

Q2. A patient with CKD presents with a gradual increase in creatinine, interpret/how will you monitor the progression of the disease?

Hints: Emphasize on the staging of CKD based on creatinine/GFR/consider any linked complications like electrolyte imbalances/ anemia.

REFLECTION

Describe the significance and principle of blood creatinine and creatinine clearance.
Perform the estimation of blood creatinine, urine creatinine and calculation of creatinine clearance along with clinical interpretations.

11

CHAPTER

Estimation of Uric Acid in Serum

COMPETENCY

BC14.10: Perform the estimation of uric acid in serum and interpretation of results in clinical scenarios.

LEARNING OBJECTIVES

After reading this chapter, the readers should be able to:
- Describe the significance and principle of serum uric acid.
- Perform the estimation of serum uric acid along with the clinical interpretations.

CLINICAL SIGNIFICANCE OF URIC ACID

Chemically	2,4,6-trihydroxy purine			
Uric acid	Catabolic end product of purine nucleotide metabolism			
Formation	• Originate from endogenous purine nucleotides • Also formed by catabolism of dietary nucleotides			
Excretion	Kidney eliminates 70% of the total uric acid and the remaining goes to GIT to be degraded by intestinal enzymes			
Properties	pKa = 5.7 (dissociation constant) • At pH more than this 5.7, that is at physiological pH of 7.4, it exists in ionized form (urate/monosodium urate) and is sparingly soluble, and definitely more soluble than uric acid • The characteristic feature of monosodium urate crystals in gout is they are negatively birefringent crystals • At low pH that is acidic condition, it is in form of uric acid that is insoluble and has a tendency to make uric acid crystals			
Clinical importance	When monosodium urate concentration exceeds 6.8 mg/dL, it gets precipitated in joints and tissues and results in swelling and pain in joints along with deposition of tophi which are crystalline deposits of uric acid and urates			
Estimation holds importance in	Diagnosing gout	Managing gout	Monitoring of chemotherapy	Assess RFT

	Chemical method/caraway method: Phosphotungstic method
Reagents required	• 10% sodium carbonate • Tungstic acid • Phosphotungstic acid • Uric acid standard 1 mg%
Method	Step 1: Make protein free filtrate: Take a centrifuge tube and add tungstic acid = 5.4 mL + whole blood = 0.6 mL (total 6 mL), keep at room temperature for 10 minutes and centrifuge at 3000 rpm for 5 minutes, use the supernatant as PFF for uric acid estimation Step 2: Take 3 test tubes and mark them as blank, standard and test

Contd....

Contd....

Reagents	**B (Blank) mL**	**S (Standard) mL**	**T (Test) mL**
Standard uric acid (1 mg%)		3	
PFF			3
DW	3		
Sodium carbonate	1	1	1
Phosphotungstic acid	1	1	1
Total	5	5	5

Calculations
- Uric acid concentration in serum = OD test/OD standard × amount of standard in mg/volume of serum in mL × 100
- OD test/OD standard × 0.03/0.3 × 100
- OD test/OD standard × 10

Standard = 1 mg% means in 100 mL uric acid is 1 mg so in 1 mL uric acid is .01, we are using 3 mL standard so amount of standard is .03 mg

For making PFF we used 0.6 mL of whole blood and total volume was 6 mL, so in 6 mL sample is 0.6, so in 1 mL of this the sample will be 0.1, we are using 3 mL of PFF, so volume of serum becomes 0.3 mL

Principle
- It is based on the reducing property of uric acid
- It reduces Phosphotungstic acid in alkaline medium and form tungsten blue
- The amount of tungsten blue formed is directly proportional to the amount of uric acid in the sample. The color formed is read at 650 nm

Coupled enzymatic method: Uricase peroxidase reaction

Principle

$$\text{Uric acid} + 2H_2O + O_2 \xrightarrow{\text{Uricase}} \text{Allantoin} + CO_2 + H_2O_2$$

$$2H_2O_2 + \text{4-Aminophenazone} + \text{2,4-Dichlorophenol sulfonate} \xrightarrow{\text{Peroxidase}} \text{Quinoneimine complex}$$

(red colored, stable for half hour) + $4H_2O$, intensity of red color is directly proportional to the concentration of uric acid

Interference
- Bilirubin >170 mmol/L (destroys H_2O_2)
- Vitamin C >570 mmol/L
- Hb >130 mg/dL

Method

Reagents	**Blank**	**Standard**	**Test**
Working reagent	1 mL	1 mL	1 mL
Standard		25 µL	
Sample			25 µL

Mix, incubate for 2 minutes at 37°C and read OD at 650 nm

Calculation: Uric acid (mg/dL) = OD test/OD standard × amount of standard used/volume of serum × 100

Clinical interpretation: **Reference range:** 2.5–7.0 mg/dL or 149–458 mmol/L
- In males = 3.6–7.2 mg/dL
- In females = 2.6–6.0 mg/dL

Conversion factor: mg/dL × 59.5 = mmol/L

Variations	Hyperuricemia		Hypouricemia
Causes	1. Excess formation of urates as in gout, Lesch–Nyhan syndrome	2. Decreased excretion of uric acid/normal formation	1. Liver diseases

Contd....

Contd....

Primary cause (defective enzymes)	1. Over activity/mutation of enzyme PRPP synthetase	1. Lactic acidosis	2. Fanconi syndrome (tubular reabsorption defect)
	2. Deficiency of enzyme HGPRTase	2. Alcoholism	3. Excess treatment with allopurinol
	3. Deficiency of enzyme G6PD (Von Gierke's disease)	3. Von Gierke's disease	
		4. Renal failure	
Secondary cause: Some other disorder is responsible for over production (too much production/destruction of cells resulting in uric acid excess production)	1. Cancer 2. Psoriasis		
Miscellaneous causes	Chemotherapy for leukemia/lymphoma, purine rich diet, fructose intolerance		
Use of alcohol precipitates gout	Alcohol metabolism → Increased NADH concentration → Increased formation of lactate from pyruvate (LDH) → Lactic acidosis → Impaired excretion of uric acid → Hyperuricemia and gout		
Primary gout	Secondary gout		
The reason behind hyperuricemia and gout is defects in purine nucleotide metabolism	The reason behind hyperuricemia and gout is other disorders, such as defects in carbohydrate metabolism, such as in Von Gierke's disease, fructose intolerance, galactosemia, or any other defect		

OSCE

Case 1: Gout Diagnosis

A 61-year-old male with a history of recurrent joint pain, high blood pressure, alcohol use, presents with severe pain and swelling in his big toe, serum uric acid: 9.3 mg/dL.

1. **What does this interpret?**
   Hyperuricemia/elevated uric acid in the blood and this results in deposition of urate crystals in joints, specifically in the big toe/podagra.
2. **What another diagnostic test is needed?**
   For confirming the diagnosis of gout, a joint aspiration performed for examining synovial fluid for the presence of monosodium urate crystals under polarized light microscopy. X-ray of the affected joint can exhibit presence of tophi/urate crystal deposits in chronic state of gout.
3. **What is the management?**
   NSAIDs for pain/inflammation control, Colchicine for its anti-inflammatory effects, corticosteroids if NSAIDs are ineffective, long-term control needs allopurinol or febuxostat to decrease uric acid levels/avoiding future attacks, lifestyle changes that include reducing alcohol, loss in weight, avoid purine-rich foods.

Case 2: Hyperuricemia and Cardiovascular Risk

A 59-year-old male with a history of high blood pressure, obesity presents with serum uric acid: 8.01 mg/dL, blood pressure: 148/90 mm Hg.

1. **What does this interpret?**
   The high serum uric acid level suggests hyperuricemia, that is a risk factor for both gout as well as cardiovascular disease. Chronic hyperuricemia is linked with a high risk of hypertension/atherosclerosis/ischemic heart disease. As the patient has the history of hypertension along with obesity the risk of CVD is more
2. **How does hyperuricemia associate with cardiovascular risk? through:**
   Endothelial dysfunctioning: Resulting in more vascular resistance.
   Inflammation: Uric acid increase inflammation in the blood vessels, contributing all the more to atherosclerosis.
   Oxidative stress: High levels of uric acid may increase oxidative stress, resulting in vascular endothelial cells damage along with plaque formation.

3. **What is the management?**
Weight loss/no alcohol/low purine diet, hypertension control for protecting the kidneys, uric acid-lowering therapy—allopurinol for hyperuricemia, regular monitoring for preventing complications.

Case 3: Uric Acid and Diabetes Management

A 51-year-old male with Type 2 Diabetes Mellitus presents with increased thirst/frequent urination, serum uric acid: 7.6 mg/dL, HbA1c: 8.6%.

1. **What does this interpret?**
The clinical scenario indicates hyperuricemia which is common in patients of Type 2 diabetes because of insulin resistance, that impairs renal excretion of uric acid. The high uric acid is linked with more risk for cardiovascular disease in diabetic patients.
2. **What is the link between hyperuricemia and Type 2 Diabetes?**
Hyperuricemia and insulin resistance in Type 2 diabetes are associated. Elevated uric acid may impair endothelial functions, raising risk of high blood pressure and atherosclerosis and these two are very common comorbidities in diabetes. Uric acid may worsen insulin resistance also leading to a cycle that exacerbates both conditions.
3. **What is the management?**
   - Control blood glucose
   - Address hyperuricemia
   - Cardiovascular protection

Case 4: Hyperuricemia in Pregnancy

A 29-year-old pregnant woman in her second trimester presents swelling in legs/hypertension, serum uric acid: 6.8 mg/dL.

1. **What is the interpretation?**
The serum uric acid is high pregnancy, because expected normal uric acid range is typically lower in pregnant woman because of more renal clearance. The high level of uric acid suggests preeclampsia which is pregnancy-related condition involving high blood pressure/proteinuria/edema
2. **What other signs assess the complication of preeclampsia?**
High blood pressure, proteinuria, edema, headaches, vision changes, upper abdominal pain.
3. **What is the management?**
Monitor uric acid levels, controlling hypertension, proper antenatal check-ups, early delivery might be considered if preeclampsia gets worse/when fetus is at risk.

Case 5: Hyperuricemia Due to Renal Disease

A 69-year-old male with chronic kidney disease and hypertension presents serum uric acid: 10.6 mg/dL.

1. **What is the interpretation?**
The high serum uric acid with chronic kidney disease is probably because of impaired renal excretion of uric acid. In the disorder of CKD, low glomerular filtration rate decreases kidneys' ability to excrete uric acid, that result in hyperuricemia.
2. **How is chronic kidney disease linked to hyperuricemia?**
In CKD, the kidneys' ability to filter/excrete uric acid diminishes because of decreased GFR. This results in more retention of uric acid in the circulation contributing to hyperuricemia and this finally leads to gout/nephropathy.
3. **What is the management?**
Optimize renal functions, control hypertension, allopurinol for lowering uric acid adjusting the dose according to the kidney function, low-purine diet, adequate hydration regular monitor serum uric acid/creatinine/GFR.

Case 6: Hyperuricemia and Obesity

A 36-year-old obese male presents for weight loss counseling, serum uric acid: 8.3 mg/dL, with no history of gout

1. **What is the interpretation?**
Obesity is a key risk factor for hyperuricemia, because it is linked with insulin resistance, that impairs renal clearance of uric acid. High uric acid may raise risk of gout/cardiovascular diseases
2. **How is obesity linked to hyperuricemia?**
   - Insulin resistance that decreases kidney's ability to excrete out uric acid
   - High production of uric acid because of high turnover of cells in adipose tissue
   - Obesity is frequently accompanied by more inflammation/oxidative stress, and these result in elevated uric acid
3. **What is the management?**
Weight loss: By dietary modifications/increased physical activity.
Monitor uric acid: For detecting whether hyperuricemia results to gout.

Adequate hydration: To increase uric acid excretion.
Low-purine diet, allopurinol to reduce uric acid.

Case 7: Uric Acid and Cancer Therapy

A 44-year-old male taking chemotherapy for leukemia presents with serum uric acid: 15.2 mg/dL.

1. **What does this interpret?**
   Tumor lysis syndrome which is complication of cancer treatment, in which chemotherapy result in quick cell destruction, resulting in release of purines, that are metabolized to uric acid. This finally results in hyperuricemia, that may lead to kidney injury.
2. **What other findings support the diagnosis?**
   Hyperkalemia because of cell breakdown, hyperphosphatemia, hypocalcemia because of phosphate binding with calcium, acute renal failure, metabolic acidosis, renal functions
3. **What is the management?**
   Proper hydration for avoiding renal failure, allopurinol/rasburicase for decreasing uric acid, correction of electrolyte imbalances, such as hyperkalemia/hypocalcemia, dialysis

CLINICAL MCQS

1. **Uric acid assay is commonly performed in labs using:**
   a. Enzymatic method using uricase
   b. Alkaline picrate method
   c. Hexokinase
   d. Folin-Wu
   Answer: a. Enzymatic method using uricase
2. **In uricase methodology, uric acid is hydrolysed into what products?**
   a. Allantoin and ammonia
   b. Urea
   c. Allantoin only
   d. Creatinine ammonia
   Answer: c. Allantoin and carbon dioxide
3. **A 53-year-old male presents with symptoms of swelling/pain in his big toe, serum uric acid: 9. 1 mg/dL. What is the diagnosis?**
   a. Osteoarthritis
   b. Arthritis
   c. Gout
   d. Hypoparathyroidism
   Answer: c. Gout
4. **The normal range of serum uric acid in adult males:**
   a. 2.0–5.4 mg/dL
   b. 3.5–7.2 mg/dL
   c. 4.5–8.2 mg/dL
   d. 6.0–9.8 mg/dL
   Answer: b. 3.5–7.2 mg/dL
5. **In the phosphotungstic acid method of uric acid assay, which compound is produced?**
   a. Blue-colored complex
   b. Yellow complex
   c. Red
   d. Orange
   Answer: a. Blue-colored complex
6. **A 68-year-old patient with CKD shows serum uric acid level: 12 mg/dL. This condition is because of:**
   a. Increased production of uric acid
   b. Decreased renal excretion of uric acid
   c. Increased tubular secretion of uric acid
   d. Increased intestinal excretion of uric acid
   Answer: b. Decreased renal excretion of uric acid

7. Which of the following drugs can artificially low-down serum uric acid levels during assay?
   a. Aspirin high dose
   b. Allopurinol
   c. Furosemide
   d. Thiazide

   Answer: b. Allopurinol

8. A pregnant woman is diagnosed with preeclampsia. Which findings is associated with high serum uric acid level?
   a. Decreased renal filtration of uric acid
   b. Decreased formation of uric acid
   c. Decreased tubular excretion of uric acid
   d. Decreased intestinal excretion of uric acid

   Answer: a. Decreased renal filtration of uric acid

9. Which condition is least likely to result into hyperuricemia?
   a. Lesch-Nyhan syndrome
   b. Proliferative disease
   c. Wilson's disease
   d. Tumor lysis

   Answer: c. Wilson's disease

10. A uric acid level: 2 mg/dL is most commonly associated with:
   a. Pseudogout
   b. Tumor lysis syndrome
   c. Deficient Xanthine oxidase
   d. Acute kidney disease

   Answer: c. Deficient Xanthine oxidase

VIVA VOCE

Q1. What is uric acid/how is it formed in the body?
Next question/Follow-up: What function does the enzyme xanthine oxidase has in the production of uric acid/how is this related to clinical conditions like gout?

Q2. A patient presents with high uric acid levels. Give causes of hyperuricemia/how to manage the condition?
Next question/Follow-up: Can hyperuricemia happen without symptoms? What is the importance of uric acid levels in asymptomatic patients?

SPOTTERS

Q1. A patient has an elevated uric acid level, symptoms of joint pain/swelling, mainly in the big toe. Interpret/what diagnostic tests will you advise?

Hints: Focus on gout/joint aspiration for crystal analysis.

Q2. The uric acid level is low in a patient having signs of malabsorption/fatigue/weakness. Interpret/what further investigations to be recommended?

Hints: Focus on Fanconi syndrome/other renal tubular disorders.

REFLECTION

Describe the significance and principle of serum uric acid. Perform the estimation of serum uric acid along with the clinical interpretations.

12

CHAPTER

Estimation of Total Protein in Serum and Other Biological Fluids

COMPETENCY

BC14.11: Perform estimation of serum proteins, albumin and A:G ratio.

LEARNING OBJECTIVES

After reading this chapter, the readers should be able to:

- Describe the significance and principle of serum total proteins, albumin and A:G ratio in clinical medicine.
- Perform the estimation of serum total proteins, albumin and A:G ratio along with the clinical interpretations.

BLUE PRINT

Estimation of Serum Proteins, Albumin, and A:G Ratio

Objective

By the end of the lecture, students should be able to:

1. Understand the significance of serum proteins, albumin, and the albumin-to-globulin (A:G) ratio in clinical diagnosis.
2. Describe the principles behind the estimation of serum proteins and albumin.
3. Demonstrate the calculation of the A:G ratio.
4. Interpret laboratory results of serum protein and albumin levels in various pathological conditions.

Duration: ***70 minutes***

Materials Needed

1. Presentation slides explaining the principles of serum protein and albumin estimation.
2. Charts or diagrams illustrating the structure and functions of serum proteins.
3. Examples of laboratory reports showing serum protein and albumin levels.
4. Sample data for A:G ratio calculation.
5. Calculators for students use during hands-on calculation exercises.

Outline

I. **Introduction to serum proteins and albumin** **(10 minutes)**
   - Define serum proteins and albumin.
   - Explain the physiological functions of serum proteins, including transport, immunity, and osmotic pressure regulation.
   - Discuss the clinical significance of serum albumin levels in assessing nutritional status and liver function.

II. **Principles of serum protein estimation** **(10 minutes)**
   - Describe the biuret method; the most commonly used technique for serum protein estimation.
   - Explain how protein reacts with copper ions in alkaline conditions to form a colored complex.
   - Discuss factors that may interfere with the accuracy of protein measurements and methods to minimize these interferences.

III. **Methods for albumin estimation** **(10 minutes)**
- Discuss laboratory techniques for measuring serum albumin, including colorimetric and immunological methods.
- Explain the advantages and limitations of each method in terms of sensitivity, specificity, and turnaround time.
- Provide examples of instruments and reagents commonly used for albumin analysis in clinical laboratories.

IV. **Calculation of A:G ratio** **(10 minutes)**
- Define the A:G ratio and its significance in assessing immune function and protein distribution.
- Explain how to calculate the A:G ratio using serum albumin and total protein concentrations.
- Demonstrate step-by-step calculations for determining the A:G ratio in hypothetical patient scenarios.
- Discuss the interpretation of A:G ratio values in different clinical contexts.

V. **Clinical applications of serum proteins and albumin** **(10 minutes)**
- Describe how serum protein and albumin levels are used to diagnose and monitor various medical conditions, such as liver disease, kidney disease, and inflammatory disorders.
- Discuss the prognostic value of serum albumin in predicting outcomes in critically ill patients.
- Highlight the importance of serial measurements of serum proteins and albumin in evaluating treatment responses and disease progression.

VI. **Hands-on activity** **(5 minutes)**
- Provide sample data for serum protein and albumin concentrations.
- Guide students through the calculation of the A:G ratio using the obtained values.
- Encourage students to work in pairs or small groups to enhance collaboration and problem-solving skills.

VII. **Interpretation of results** **(5 minutes)**
- Review the calculated A:G ratio values obtained by students.
- Discuss the clinical implications of these results in terms of immune function and protein metabolism.
- Address any questions or concerns raised by students regarding the calculation process or interpretation of results.

VIII. **Review and summary** **(5 minutes)**
- Summarize the key points covered in the lecture regarding the estimation of serum proteins, albumin, and the A:G ratio.
- Reinforce the importance of these parameters in clinical diagnosis and patient management.
- Provide additional resources for further reading and self-study on serum protein analysis and interpretation.

IX. **Conclusion** **(5 minutes)**
- Conclude the lecture by emphasizing the role of serum proteins and albumin in assessing nutritional status, liver function, and immune function.
- Encourage students to apply the knowledge gained in the lecture to their clinical practice or future research endeavors.

Plasma proteins	Complex mixture of albumin, globulin, fibrinogen, proteoglycans, metalloproteins, lipoproteins, transferrin, ceruloplasmin, alpha 1 antitrypsin, clotting factors, etc.
Functions of proteins	Act as enzymes, hormones, clotting factors, transport agents, protective agents, nutrient agents, immunity, etc.
Synthesis	Except enzymes, hormones and immunoglobulins, other proteins are mainly synthesized in liver
Serum proteins	Definite ratio of albumins and globulins, as fibrinogen is used up in clotting so it is not present in serum
Factors deciding the level of proteins/A:G ratio	• Proper dietary intake of essential amino acids • Liver synthesis • Normal renal functions so that there is no major urinary loss of proteins

	Estimation of total protein
Biuret method	Violet color chelate in presence of cupric ions is formed
Limitation	Minimum 2 peptide bonds are needed for getting a positive test, so dipeptides with only 1 peptide bond do not respond to this test
Principle	• Biuret reagent has copper sulfate, NaOH, sodium potassium tartrate and KI • Cupric ion (Cu^{++}) of $CuSO_4$ react with $NH^{-}CO$ group (peptide bond) in basic medium and violet color complex is formed, the absorbance of this is measured • Pink to different shades of purple are obtained, that depends on the number of copper coordinate complexes formed, which in turn depends on number of peptide bonds/(size of protein) present in the protein • Sodium potassium tartrate prevents the precipitation of copper in basic medium and KI is an antioxidant
Reagents	Biuret reagent, protein standard (280 mg/dL or 2.8 mg/mL)

Reagents	(B) Blank mL	(S) Standard mL	(T) Test mL
Serum			100 μL
Standard		2.5	
DW	2.5		
Biuret reagent	3.5	3.5	3.5
Total	6	6	6

Mix and incubate for 10 minutes at 37°C, read the absorbance at 540 nm

Precautions:
- Excess sugar in serum or lipemic serum decreases the intensity of the color
- Avoid hemolyzed samples as they increase the intensity of color

Calculations

Protein concentration in serum
- OD test/OD standard × amount of standard in mg/volume of serum in mL × 100
- OD test/OD standard × 7/0.1 × 100
  (Amount of standard = 1 mL contains 2.8 mg so 2.5 mL will have 2.8 × 2.5 = 7 mg)
- OD test/OD standard × 7000 mg/dL
- OD test/OD standard × 7 g/dL

Clinical Interpretation

Normal range
- Males: 6.5–8.0 g/dL
- Females: 5.5–7.5 g/dL
- Fibrinogen should be between the range of 2–4 g/dL

Hyperproteinemia is observed in:
- Multiple myeloma
- Vomiting/sweating/hemoconcentration as diarrhea
- Macroglobulinemia
- Autoimmune diseases like sarcoidosis and rheumatoid arthritis
- Chronic infections like kala-azar
- Excess infusion of albumin
- Collagen diseases
- Hemoconcentration means false hyperproteinemia due to decrease in plasma volume in conditions like diarrhea, vomiting, inadequate water intake, excess sweating and burns. Here A:G ratio remains same

Hypoproteinemia is observed in (common in India due to inadequate protein intake):
- Liver disorder (impaired synthesis)
- Hemodilution/overhydration
- Proteinuria (loss of albumin during nephropathy and nephrotic syndrome)
- Hyperthyroidism/wasting disorder/high fever (due to increased catabolism)
- Malnutrition/kwashiorkor/starvation (poor intake of essential amino acids resulting in impaired synthesis of proteins)
- Malabsorption (less intestinal absorption)
- Agammaglobulinemia (congenital disease)
- Uncontrolled diabetes mellitus
- Chronic infections
- Through skin loss (extensive burns)
- Trauma (increased blood loss)

Other causes of hypoproteinemia other than hypoalbuminemia: Hemodilution (does not change A:G ratio) because of overloading of water causing false hypoproteinemia, which can be due to excess steroids which cause water retention, diabetes insipidus, compulsive polydipsia, etc. In true hypoproteinemia, A:G ratio is decreased.

Some more methods of estimation of protein:
1. Kjeldahl's method
2. Lowry method (Phosphotungstic and Phosphomolybdic acid called as Folin–Ciocalteu reagent forming blue color with the protein depending on tyrosine or tryptophan content of the protein)
3. Direct photometric method (absorption assessed at 280 nm)
4. Dye binding method
5. Refractometry
6. Turbidimetric method [when protein level is low like in cerebrospinal fluid (CSF)]
7. Nephelometric method

Serum albumin	Present in highest concentration in plasma
Synthesis	In liver
Functions	• Act as carrier molecule for fatty acids, urates, bilirubin, calcium ions magnesium ions antibiotics, drugs like digoxin, thyroid hormone, salicylates • Maintains plasma colloidal osmotic pressure (80% contribution in maintaining the intravascular fluid colloidal OP) • It is a negative acute-phase reactant protein

Estimation of albumin	Bromocresol green (BCG) method and Bromocresol purple (BCP) method
Bromocresol green method (BCG)	Binding of protein to the indicator changes its color
Principle Albumin + BCG $\xrightarrow{\text{Acid pH}}$ Albumin-BCG complex	• The pI (pH at which the protein has no net charge) of albumin is 4.7 • BCG is yellow in undissociated form at pH <4.7, and blue in dissociated form at pH >4.7 • At pH below this pI, albumin act as cation and has binding affinity for ionized BCG • BCG (3′,3″,5′,5″-Tetrabromo-m-cresol-sulfonephthalein) is an anionic dye that specifically gets bound to albumin at acidic pH and forms yellow green to green blue color, the concentration of this complex is proportional to albumin in sample which is read at 620 nm
Reagents	• BCG dye solution in succinate buffer • Normal saline • Albumin standard (0.5 g/dL)

Reagents	**B (Blank) mL**	**S (Standard) mL**	**T (Test) mL**
Normal saline	0.2		
Albumin standard (5 mg/mL)		0.2	
Diluted serum: (Normal saline = 1.8 mL + Serum = 0.2 mL = total volume = 2 mL)			0.2
BCG dye	5	5	5
Total	5.2	5.2	5.2

Keep at room temperature for 10 minutes and read at 620 nm

Calculations

- OD test/OD standard × amount of standard in mg/volume of serum in mL × 100
- OD test/OD standard × 1/0.02 × 100
  (Amount of standard = 1 mL contains 5 mg so 0.2 mL will have 0.2 × 5 = 1 mg)
  (Volume of serum = in 2 mL total volume, the amount of serum is 0.2) so in 0.2 mL the amount will be 0.02
- OD test/OD standard × 5000 mg/dL
- OD test/OD standard × 5 g/dL

Clinical interpretation

Normal range of serum albumin	3.7–5.3 g%
Hyperalbuminaemia	• Tissue damage • Inflammation • Dehydration • Shock • Malignancy • Hemoconcentration
Hypoalbuminemia leading to edema around soft tissues like face and eyelids because of decreased plasma colloidal osmotic pressure that favors water retention in tissue spaces:	• Malnutrition • Liver disorders (synthesis of albumin is in liver) • Loss of albumin in urine in nephropathy (normally, negatively charged albumin is repelled by negatively charged basement membrane but any disruption in the intactness of basement membrane leads to loss of negative charge on it so now albumin is no more repulsed, also the size of albumin is smaller than globulin so easily filtered by glomerulus) • Hemorrhages, burns, trauma • Uncontrolled DM, hyperthyroidism, psoriasis (excess protein breakdown) • Neoplastic disease • Leukemia • Plasma dilution • Genetic disorders

	Serum globulin
Four types:	1. Alpha 1 globulins like alpha 1 antitrypsin, alpha 1 fetoprotein, alpha 1 glycoprotein 2. Alpha 2 globulins like ceruloplasmin, haptoglobin, alpha 2 macroglobulin 3. Beta globulin like transferrin, hemopexin, beta 2 microglobulin, C-reactive protein 4. Gamma globulin like immunoglobulins like IgG, IgA, IgM, IgD, IgE
Calculations	Total protein—serum albumin
Normal range of serum globulin	2.5–3.5 g/dL
	Clinical interpretation
Hyperglobulinemia	• Acute and chronic bacterial infections • Malaria • Leishmaniasis • Schistosomiasis • Infective hepatitis • Liver cirrhosis • Biliary cirrhosis • Hemochromatosis • Sarcoidosis • Multiple myeloma (malignancy of plasma cells that synthesize immunoglobulins, huge increase of gamma globulins occur, mainly of L chain type and being small in size and easily filtered by the glomeruli, they get excreted out in urine called Bence–Jones proteins) • Electrophoresis is the method by which presence of myeloma protein is detected in blood and urine. A sharp, intense and dark band known as M band is seen in the gamma globulin region near the origin. Scanning is done to estimate the concentration which is more than normal • Lymphoprolferative disorders
Hypoglobulinemia	• Malnutrition • Congenital agammaglobulinemia • Acquired hypogammaglobulinemia • Lymphatic leukemia
Albumin: Globulin ratio (A:G ratio)	Level of plasma albumin/level of plasma globulin
Clinical importance	For assessing the nutritive status of our body, liver function test (LFT) and renal function test (RFT) In false alterations of total protein levels, this ratio does not change, but in actual alterations of total protein levels, mainly due to renal or liver disorders, this ratio is also altered more commonly decreased
Normal ratio	1.5:1–2.5:1
The ratio is reversed in	• Multiple myeloma (excess formation of globulin) • Chronic liver disorder (less albumin formation) • Nephrotic syndrome (loss of albumin in urine)

Zone electrophoresis: Protein separation technique
There is migration of charged macromolecules in porous supporting medium like agarose gel, cellulose acetate strips
Electrophoretogram is formed that displays zones of proteins, each zone being sharply separated from the neighboring zone on electrophoretic medium

Age	1.5 years
Complains	Fever, diarrhea, cough, swelling on body, loss of appetite, weakness
History	Low socioeconomic status, eats mainly starchy foods, weight and height less as compared to the ideal for the age
On examination	Distended abdomen, enlarged liver

Contd....

Contd....

Investigations	
Hb	9.0 g/dL
DLC	P77 L17 E4 M1
TLC	9200/cu.mm
RBC's	43 million/cmm
Urine	Normal, pus cells 1–2 HPF
Serum total proteins	4.2 g/dL
Serum albumin	1.2 g/dL
Stool	Normal
X-ray chest	Normal
Diagnosis	Kwashiorkor (deficiency of protein, generalized edema, anemia, low weight, skin was flaky)
Reason behind edema	Hypoproteinemia → less plasma oncotic pressure → fluid moves into the interstitial compartment
Reason behind anemia	Globin deficiency due to essential amino acids deficiency, iron and vitamins deficiency
Reason behind hepatomegaly	Fatty liver due to impaired lipoprotein synthesis
Management of the disease	Balanced diet, groundnuts, Jaggery, pulses, etc.

Clinical picture	Marasmus	Kwashiorkor
Edema	–	+
Enlarged liver	–	+
Wasting of muscles	Severe	Not so severe
Body fats	–	Decreased
Serum proteins	Mild deficiency	Severe deficiency
Main deficiency	Carbohydrates, proteins	Proteins

OSCE

Case 1: Hypoalbuminemia in Liver Disease

A 45-year-old male presents with ascites/jaundice, serum albumin: 2.1 g/dL (normal range: 3.5–5.0 g/dL).

1. **What does this interpret?**
   Hypoalbuminemia that is commonly observed in liver disease like cirrhosis/chronic hepatitis. The liver is the main site of albumin formation therefore liver dysfunction ultimately impairs its formation. Other causes of hypoalbuminemia are nephrotic syndrome/malnutrition/protein-losing enteropathy.
2. **What additional tests confirms the diagnosis?**
   Liver function tests: AST, ALT, ALP, bilirubin/prothrombin time.
   Ultrasound: To check for signs of cirrhosis/ascites/liver lesions.
   Serum globulin levels: albumin-to-globulin ratio in distinguishing between liver disease and other causes of hypoalbuminemia
3. **What is the management?**
   Treating the underlying liver condition, managing complications, Albumin supplementation, Nutritional support to correct any deficiencies

Case 2: Increased Serum Globulin in Multiple Myeloma

A 61-year-old female presents with bone pain and anemia, serum total protein: 8.6 g/dL (normal range: 6.0–8.0 g/dL), serum albumin-to-globulin ratio: low. Serum electrophoresis shows a monoclonal spike.

1. **What does this interpret?**
   Monoclonal gammopathy, commonly observed in multiple myeloma. The M spike on serum electrophoresis is characteristic of monoclonal immunoglobulin formation that is feature of multiple myeloma. Malignant plasma cells form single type of immunoglobulin that results in high globulin levels.

2. **What additional tests confirm multiple myeloma?**
   Bone marrow biopsy: For assessing plasma cell infiltration.
   Serum free light chains assay: For detection of high light chains/Bence-Jones proteins.
   X-rays: To assess bone lesions/lytic lesions.
   24-hour urine collection: For detection of Bence-Jones proteins that are light chains excreted out in urine in multiple myeloma.
3. **What is the management?**
   Chemotherapy/immunotherapy, prevention of bone destruction/manage bone pain, Autologous stem cell transplant, pain management, treatment of anemia

Case 3: Proteinuria and Nephrotic Syndrome

A 41-year-old female presents with edema, especially around the eyes and legs, serum albumin: 1.7 g/dL, total serum protein: 4.1 g/dL, urine analysis: proteinuria (3+ protein).

1. **What does this interpret?**
   Nephrotic syndrome where there is high loss of proteins specially albumin in the urine, resulting in hypoalbuminemia and decreased total serum protein levels. This leads to edema, that is feature of nephrotic syndrome.
2. **What is the principle behind protein loss in nephrotic syndrome?**
   Glomerular basement membrane is damaged in this disease so large amounts of plasma proteins, especially albumin, leaks into the urine leading to hypoalbuminemia, ending up in fluid accumulation in tissues or edema. The proteinuria in nephrotic syndrome is typically more than 3.5 g/day.
3. **What other investigations are required?**
   Urine protein quantification: For measuring exact amount of protein in the urine.
   Serum cholesterol and triglycerides: These are generally high in nephrotic syndrome.
   Renal biopsy: For assessing underlying cause like minimal change disease/focal segmental glomerulosclerosis/membranous nephropathy.
   Serum creatinine/GFR: To assess for kidney functions.

CLINICAL MCQS

1. **The most common method for total protein assay:**
   a. Biuret method
   b. Lowry technique
   c. Bradford methodology
   d. Kjeldahl methodology

   Answer: a. Biuret method
2. **In the Biuret method, the purple color produced is because of the reaction between proteins and:**
   a. Copper ions in an alkaline medium
   b. Tungstic acid
   c. Ninhydrin
   d. Bromocresol green dye

   Answer: a. Copper ions in an alkaline medium
3. **A 62-year-old patient diagnosed with liver cirrhosis shows total serum protein level: 4.5 g/dL. This is suggestive of:**
   a. Normal protein
   b. Hypoproteinemia
   c. Hyperproteinemia
   d. Nephrosclerosis

   Answer: b. Hypoproteinemia
4. **The normal range for total serum protein in adults:**
   a. 3.0–5.2 g/dL
   b. 6.0–8.0 g/dL
   c. 8.0–10.5 g/dL
   d. 4.0–6.2 g/dL

   Answer: b. 6.0–8.0 g/dL

5. **In which of the conditions we expect to find high total protein levels?**
   a. Nephrosclerosis
   b. Malnutrition
   c. Chronic inflammatory conditions
   d. Glomerulonephritis

   Answer: c. Chronic inflammatory conditions

VIVA VOCE

Q1. Mention components measured in total protein/how they are clinically significant?
Next question/Follow-up: Differentiate between primary/secondary reasons of hypoalbuminemia in total protein interpretation?

Q2. What are the likely causes of high total protein level/how to approach the diagnosis based on other clinical findings?
Next question/Follow-up: Is it possible that increase in total protein occur without hyperglobulinemia? justify.

SPOTTERS

Q1. A patient presents with low total protein levels, low albumin level, but globulin levels are normal. Interpret/mention causes of this finding?

Hints: Look for signs of liver disease/malnutrition/nephrotic syndrome/gastrointestinal loss.

Q2. The total protein level is significantly high in a patient with symptoms of some chronic infection. The globulin fraction is significantly high. What is your interpretation/which further tests would you advise to confirm your diagnosis?

Hints: Consider states such as multiple myeloma/chronic inflammation/paraproteinemia.

REFLECTION

Describe the significance and principle of estimation of serum TP, albumin and A: G ratio and also perform the estimation and clinically correlate with lab reports and diagnosis

13

CHAPTER

Estimation of Total Cholesterol and HDL Cholesterol

COMPETENCY

BC14.12: Perform the estimation of serum total cholesterol.

LEARNING OBJECTIVES

After reading this chapter, the readers should be able to:

- Describe the significance and principle of estimation of serum total cholesterol and HDL cholesterol in clinical chemistry.
- Perform the estimation of serum total cholesterol and HDL cholesterol along with clinical interpretations.

BLUE PRINT

To Estimate Total Cholesterol and HDL Cholesterol

Objective

By the end of the lecture, students should be able to:

1. Understand the significance of serum cholesterol levels in cardiovascular health.
2. Describe the principles behind the estimation of serum total cholesterol and HDL-cholesterol.
3. Demonstrate the laboratory techniques used for the estimation of serum cholesterol levels.
4. Interpret laboratory results of serum cholesterol levels in the context of cardiovascular risk assessment.

Duration: ***60 minutes***

Materials Needed

1. Presentation slides explaining the principles of cholesterol metabolism and laboratory techniques for cholesterol estimation.
2. Charts or diagrams illustrating the structure and functions of cholesterol and lipoproteins.
3. Examples of laboratory reports showing serum cholesterol levels.
4. Laboratory equipment and reagents for cholesterol estimation demonstration.
5. Calculators for student use during hands-on calculation exercises.

Outline

I. **Introduction to cholesterol and lipoproteins** **(10 minutes)**
   - Define cholesterol and lipoproteins.
   - Explain the physiological functions of cholesterol, including membrane structure, hormone synthesis, and bile acid production.
   - Discuss the role of lipoproteins in cholesterol transport and metabolism.

II. **Significance of serum cholesterol levels** **(10 minutes)**
   - Describe the association between elevated serum cholesterol levels and cardiovascular risk.
   - Explain the concept of high-density lipoprotein (HDL) cholesterol as "good" cholesterol and its protective effect against cardiovascular disease.
   - Discuss the importance of monitoring serum cholesterol levels in cardiovascular risk assessment and disease prevention.

III. **Principles of serum cholesterol estimation** **(10 minutes)**
- Describe laboratory techniques for measuring serum total cholesterol and HDL-cholesterol, including enzymatic methods and precipitation methods.
- Explain how cholesterol reacts with specific enzymes or reagents to produce colorimetric or turbidimetric signals.
- Discuss factors that may affect the accuracy of cholesterol measurements and strategies for quality control.

IV. **Laboratory demonstration of cholesterol estimation** **(15 minutes)**
- Perform a step-by-step demonstration of the enzymatic method for measuring serum total cholesterol.
- Explain the procedure for isolating HDL-cholesterol using precipitation methods or ultracentrifugation.
- Involve students in the demonstration process by allowing them to observe and ask questions about the techniques used.

V. **Interpretation of results** **(10 minutes)**
- Review sample laboratory reports showing serum total cholesterol and HDL-cholesterol levels.
- Discuss the optimal ranges for serum cholesterol levels based on cardiovascular risk assessment guidelines.
- Interpret the significance of abnormal cholesterol levels in terms of cardiovascular risk and potential interventions.

VI. **Hands-on activity** **(5 minutes)**
- Provide sample data for serum total cholesterol and HDL-cholesterol concentrations.
- Guide students through the calculation of cholesterol ratios, such as the total cholesterol to HDL-cholesterol ratio.
- Encourage students to work in pairs or small groups to analyze and interpret the provided data.

VII. **Clinical applications of cholesterol estimation** **(5 minutes)**
- Describe how serum cholesterol levels are used in clinical practice to assess cardiovascular risk and guide treatment decisions.
- Highlight the role of lifestyle modifications, medications, and dietary interventions in managing dyslipidemia and reducing cardiovascular risk.

VIII. **Review and summary** **(5 minutes)**
- Summarize the key points covered in the lecture regarding the estimation of serum total cholesterol and HDL-cholesterol.
- Reinforce the importance of cholesterol monitoring in cardiovascular disease prevention and management.
- Provide additional resources for further reading and self-study on cholesterol metabolism and laboratory techniques.

IX. **Conclusion** **(5 minutes)**
- Conclude the lecture by emphasizing the significance of serum cholesterol levels in cardiovascular health and disease.
- Encourage students to apply the knowledge gained in the lecture to their clinical practice or research endeavors.

BLUE PRINT

Understanding Laboratory Results in Lipid Metabolism

Objective

By the end of the lecture, students should be able to:

1. Interpret laboratory results of analytes associated with lipid metabolism.
2. Understand the significance of lipid-related parameters in health and disease.
3. Apply knowledge of lipid metabolism to clinical scenarios.

Duration: *90 minutes*

Materials Needed

1. PowerPoint presentation or visual aids
2. Whiteboard and markers
3. Handouts with key lipid-related laboratory parameters and their interpretation
4. Clinical case studies related to lipid metabolism

Outline

I. **Introduction to lipid-related laboratory parameters** **(10 minutes)**
- Overview of the lecture's objectives and agenda.
- Explanation of the importance of lipid-related laboratory tests in clinical practice.

II. **Common lipid profile tests** **(20 minutes)**
- Description of common lipid profile tests, including:
  - Total cholesterol
  - LDL cholesterol
  - HDL cholesterol
  - Triglycerides
  - Lipoprotein(a) [Lp(a)]
- Explanation of reference ranges and interpretation of results for each parameter.

III. **Additional lipid-related tests** **(20 minutes)**
- Discussion on additional lipid-related tests, including:
  - Apolipoproteins (apoB, apoA1)
  - Lipoprotein particle size and density
  - Lipid ratios (e.g., LDL/HDL ratio)
- Interpretation of results and clinical significance of these tests.

IV. **Clinical correlation and case studies** **(30 minutes)**
- Present clinical case studies related to lipid metabolism disorders.
- Facilitate a discussion on how to interpret laboratory results in the context of specific clinical scenarios.

V. **Quality control and assurance** **(5 minutes)**
- Brief overview of quality control measures for lipid-related laboratory tests.
- Importance of accurate and reliable lipid testing for patient care.

VI. **Conclusion and recap** **(5 minutes)**
- Summary of key points covered in the lecture.
- Emphasis on the importance of interpreting lipid-related laboratory results in clinical practice.
- Encouragement for further study and research in lipid metabolism and laboratory medicine.

Cholesterol	• Abundant form of sterol in human tissues and body fluids, 27 carbon tetracyclic structure with cyclopentanoperhydrophenanthrene ring • In the extrahepatic cell, it is used for making cell membrane, steroids, bile acids and vitamin D
Types 2: Exogenous cholesterol is the dietary cholesterol and endogenous cholesterol is synthesized in tissue	• Free cholesterol (30% of the total cholesterol, and active, amphipathic form) • Esterified cholesterol (70% of total cholesterol, inert, nonpolar and stored form) • Cholesterol ester has a fatty acid chain esterified at 3rd OH group of cholesterol
Acyl-CoA cholesterol acyl-transferase	• Enzyme required for esterification of cholesterol in plasma • Exogenous cholesterol is absorbed from intestinal lumen with the help of chylomicrons
Diet sources	• Milk, butter, egg, meat • Polyunsaturated fatty acids (PUFA) decrease serum cholesterol
Excretion	It is excreted in bile through the intestines
Transport	Transported after it binds to lipoproteins mainly high-density lipoprotein (HDL) and low-density lipoprotein (LDL)
Clinical significance of assessment	Hypercholesterolemia is associated with atherosclerosis, myocardial infarction (MI), cerebral hemorrhage and thrombosis
	Methods of estimation
Two methods	1. Zak's method which is a chemical method 2. Cholesterol oxidase peroxidase method which is an enzymatic method
Liebermann Burchard reaction used in colorimetric assays/ manual method	Cholesterol + acetic anhydride + H_2SO_4 $\xrightarrow{\text{Dehydration/oxidation}}$ monosulfonic acid derivatives of Cholesta-3,5-diene (green)
Sample	Serum after overnight fasting of 12 hours as dietary cholesterol increases serum cholesterol, avoid taking alcohol, oral contraceptives, steroids, lipid lowering drugs, exercise and medications before 48 hours, it should not be hemolyzed
Interfering substances of blood:	Sterols, bilirubin, Hb

Contd....

Contd....

Zak's method: Serum is used for total cholesterol estimation, which estimates the value of cholesterol of all lipoproteins and also free cholesterol

Principle

Bischolesta-3,5-diene is red complex and is proportional to the cholesterol concentration, measured optically at 540 nm

For HDL cholesterol estimation: Precipitation method	We precipitate other lipoproteins other than HDL, such as chylomicrons, LDL, VLDL by Phosphotungstic acid and magnesium chloride
Principle	Plasma or serum is treated with phosphotungstic acid and magnesium chloride, LDL, VLDL and chylomicrons get precipitated, supernatant has HDL and then its cholesterol content is estimated
Reagents	Acetic acid ferric chloride reagent Cholesterol standard (200 mg%) Concentrated H_2SO_4 Phosphotungstic acid Magnesium chloride

Procedure

Reagents	**Test**	**Standard**
Serum	0.2 mL	
Cholesterol standard		0.2 mL
$FeCl_3$ acetic acid reagent	9.8 mL	9.8 mL
Total	10 mL	10 mL

Mix well for 15 minutes by a glass rod to extract cholesterol, centrifuge, use supernatant for total cholesterol estimation

Precipitation for HDL: Add the following:

Serum	0.5 mL
Phosphotungstic acid	0.05 mL
Magnesium chloride	0.02 mL

Mix and centrifuge, Take the clear supernatant, add 9.4 mL of $FeCl_3$ acetic acid reagent and again centrifuge, use supernatant for HDL cholesterol estimation

Reagents	**B (blank)**	**T (test)**	**S (standard)**	**HC (HDL cholesterol)**
Ferric chloride reagent	5 Ml			
Standard supernatant			5 mL	
Test supernatant		5 mL		5 mL
Concentrated H_2SO_4	3 mL	3 mL	3 mL	3 mL

Mix and keep in water bath for 10 minutes at 6°C, cool and read at 540 nm, do not rinse the cuvette with water, note the OD and calculate

Standard curve: Cholesterol standards of 50, 100, 200, 300 and 400 are treated as 'S' and OD values are plotted against the concentration

Precautions	Use clean and dry glasswares, no mouth pipetting should be done as the reagents are corrosive, due to high viscosity of reagents, proper mixing should be done

Observations and Calculations

Total cholesterol (mg/dL)	• OD test/OD standard × amount of standard/volume of sample × 100 • OD test/OD standard × 0.2/0.1 × 100 • OD test/OD standard × 2 × 100 • OD test/OD standard × 200 mg%
Amount of standard	• 10 mL supernatant has 0.2 mL of standard • So, 5 mL supernatant has 0.1 mL of standard • 100 mL of standard has 200 mg of cholesterol • So, 0.1 mL of standard will have 0.2 mg of cholesterol
Volume of serum	• 10 mL of supernatant has 0.2 mL of serum • So, 5 mL of supernatant will have 0.1 mL of serum
HDL-cholesterol (mg/dL)	OD test (HDL-C)/OD standard × amount of standard/volume of sample × 100

Reference range of HDL-cholesterol: HDL is cardioprotective (good cholesterol)

Adult males	35–60 mg%
Adult females	40–75 mg%
Low risk	>60 mg%
High risk for atherosclerosis	<35 mg%
For every 1 mg% decrease in HDL	Risk of chronic heart disease (CHD) increase by 3%
HDL is low in	Tangier disease

Enzymatic method: Cholesterol oxidase-peroxidase method (CHOD-POD method)

Principle: Cholesterol ester + H_2O forms Cholesterol + Fatty acid in presence of cholesterol esterase

$$\text{Cholesterol} + O_2 \xrightarrow{\text{Cholesterol oxidase}} \text{Cholestenone} + H_2O_2$$

$$H_2O_2 \xrightarrow{\text{Peroxidase}} H_2O + [O]$$

$$H_2O_2 + \text{4-Aminoantipyrine} \xrightarrow{\text{Peroxidase}} \text{Quinoneimine (pink) read at 540 nm}$$

Advantages of the enzymatic method:
- Sensitive and specific for cholesterol
- Linearity is up to 700 mg%
- Requires less sample
- Less time consumption
- Reagents are noncorrosive
- No deproteinization is required and because of low sample volume, no interference by icteric and hemolyzed serum

Procedure

Reagent	Blank	Standard	Test
Working enzymatic reagent	3 mL	3 mL	3 mL
Standard (200 mg%)		0.1 mL	
Serum			0.1 mL

Incubate all test tubes at 37°C for 5 minutes, read at 520 nm

Precautions: Cholesterol is stable in the sample for a week if stored at 2–8°C and if frozen can be stored for one month, If stored at room temperature, the proportion of free and esterified cholesterol may change due to serum lecithin cholesterol acyltransferase (LCAT) but the total cholesterol concentration is not changed

Clinical interpretation

Normal level in adults	<200 mg%
In high incidence of central obesity and high waist hip ratio and lipoprotein a	<180 mg%
Physiological variations: Vary with age, sex, diet, seasonal variations	• It rises with age; rise is more under 50 years in men than in women due to estrogen • May increase in pregnant women by 20–25% of the normal value
Hypercholesterolemia seen in/causes	• Diabetes mellitus (DM) • Nephrotic syndrome • Type II hyperlipoproteinemia (familial hypercholesterolemia) • Hypothyroidism • Hypopituitarism • Myxedema • Obstructive jaundice • Von Gierke's disease
Hypocholesterolemia	• Hyperthyroidism (80–100 mg%) • Pernicious anemia • Hemolytic jaundice • Malabsorption • Hepatic disorder • Wasting disorders • Abeta/hypobetalipoproteinemias

Contd....

Contd....

Lifestyle modifications to reduce serum cholesterol	Vegetarian diet, fiber diet, low fat diet, regular exercise, avoid stress, smoking and alcohol, maintain ideal weight
LDL-cholesterol assessment	**LDL-cholesterol can measured as well as can be calculated**
Measurement of LDL cholesterol	Beta quantification method and direct method
Beta quantification method	• Ultracentrifugation to float VLDL and chylomicrons • Precipitation by chemicals of LDL from infranate got by step 1 • Assessment of cholesterol in infranate from step 1 • This gives the value of sum total of LDL and HDL-cholesterol and assessment of cholesterol in supernatant from step 2 which gives the value of HDL-cholesterol only • LDL cholesterol is calculated by deducting the value of HDL-cholesterol from sum total of LDL and HDL-cholesterol
Direct method/immune separation	• Latex beads are used which are coated with anti-VLDL and anti-HDL antibodies • Anti-VLDL binds with VLDL and anti HDL binds with HDL • Centrifugation is done to remove this complex • In the remaining fluid, LDL-cholesterol is measured by using appropriate method to estimate cholesterol
Calculation of LDL-cholesterol by Friedewald formula	• When the level of triacylglycerols (TAG) is <400 mg%, this formula is used to calculate LDL-cholesterol • HDL-cholesterol is measured by direct or precipitation method • Total cholesterol (TC) and TAG are measured • VLDL is calculated as TAG/5
LDL-cholesterol	Total cholesterol (TC)–HDL cholesterol–TAG/5
VLDL	TAG/5
Reference range for VLDL	Up to 38 mg%
Reference range for LDL	<100 mg%
LDL increases the risk of CHD	It carries 70% of total cholesterol to the tissues, oxidized LDL is taken up by macrophages to form fatty streaks causing atheromatous plaques
LDL oxidation is more in smokers	Nicotine causes increased lipolysis of adipose tissue which results in increased free fatty acid (FFA) and serum cholesterol, DM and insulin resistance

Desired lipid profile		**Extended lipid profile**		
Cholesterol	<200 mg%	Apo A1	94–199 mg%	Rise means decreased CHD risk
TG	<150 mg%	Apo B	60–133 mg%	Rise means increased CHD risk
HDL-C	>35 mg%	Lipoprotein a	<20 mg%	–
LDL-C	<100 mg%			
VLDL-C	Up to 38 mg%			

OSCE

Case 1: Dyslipidemia in a Middle-aged Man

A 55-year-old male with a history of smoking/high blood pressure shows with total serum cholesterol: 258 mg/dL (normal range: 140–200 mg/dL), HDL: 36 mg/dL (normal range: >40 mg/dL), LDL: 168 mg/dL (normal range: <100 mg/dL), triglycerides: 210 mg/dL (normal range: <150 mg/dL).

1. **What is the interpretation?**
   Dyslipidemia characterized by high total cholesterol/LDL both of these are more than normal range for cardiovascular health, Low HDL that is a negative risk factor for CVD because HDL aids in removing excess cholesterol from the circulation, high triglycerides also contribute to the risk of CVD, so patient is at very high risk for atherosclerotic cardiovascular disease because of these lipid abnormalities.
2. **What are the underlying reasons?**
   Primary hyperlipidemia, such as genetic disorders of familial hypercholesterolemia/familial combined hyperlipidemia
   Secondary causes, such as uncontrolled hypertension, smoking that decreases HDL/increase LDL/triglycerides, sedentary lifestyle that leads to decreased HDL and high triglycerides, obesity mainly abdominal obesity that leads to excess LDL/triglycerides/low HDL, diet that is high in saturated fats and cholesterol can raise LDL, diabetes that is not controlled.

3. **What further investigations are needed?**
   Lipoprotein assay: For checking other lipid subfractions, such as VLDL and IDL and also to see pattern of lipid abnormalities.
   Liver function tests: To exclude liver disease as contributing reason.
   Thyroid function tests: Hypothyroidism can raise cholesterol.
   Renal function tests: Kidney disease can contribute more to dyslipidemia.
   HbA1c and fasting blood glucose: To evaluate undiagnosed diabetes/poor glycemic control.
   Apolipoprotein B: To assess risk linked with atherosclerosis.
4. **What is the management?**
   Diet low in saturated fats/cholesterol/more fiber/rich in fruits, vegetables, regular exercise to increase HDL and decrease LDL plus triglycerides, smoking cessation that improves HDL levels and cardiovascular health, obesity control that may improve lipid levels, pharmacologic therapies, such as statins to lower LDL cholesterol, fibrates to decrease triglycerides, niacin to increase HDL cholesterol, PCSK9 inhibitors for familial hypercholesterolemia

Case 2: Hypercholesterolemia in a Young Female

A 29-year-old woman presents with a total serum cholesterol: 310 mg/dL (normal range: 140–200 mg/dL), HDL: 61 mg/dL (normal range: >40 mg/dL), LDL: 248 mg/dL (normal range: <100 mg/dL). She has premature cardiovascular disease as family history.

1. **What is the likely diagnosis?**
   Cholesterol profile indicates familial hypercholesterolemia genetic disease characterized by significant high total cholesterol and LDL
   Normal HDL is usually preserved in familial hypercholesterolemia.
   A family history of premature cardiovascular disease indicative of genetic predisposition, FH is characterized by a defect in LDL receptors, resulting in decreased clearance of LDL from the bloodstream leading to high LDL cholesterol.
2. **What is the genetic cause of genetic disease?**
   Familial hypercholesterolemia is a result of mutations in the LDL receptor gene/LDLR resulting in defective/absent LDL receptors on hepatocytes. This impairs the capacity of hepatocytes to clear LDL cholesterol from the circulation leading to persistent hypercholesterolemia. FH can also be due to mutations in other genes, such as APOB (apolipoprotein B)/PCSK9.
3. **What is the complication of uncontrolled familial hypercholesterolemia?**
   It may lead to premature cardiovascular events, such as CAD/heart attacks, aortic stenosis because of high deposition of cholesterol in aortic valve, xanthomas that is cholesterol deposits in skin/tendons, higher risk for atherosclerotic cardiovascular disease at young stages.
4. **What further investigations confirms familial hypercholesterolemia?**
   Genetic testing: For mutations in the genes—LDLR/APOB/PCSK9.
   Apolipoprotein B levels: high in FH, because of increase in the number of atherogenic particles.
   LDL receptor activity.
   Family screening: (FH is an inherited condition).
5. **What is the treatment?**
   Statins to decrease LDL cholesterol levels.
   Ezetimibe: To inhibit absorption of cholesterol in the intestines and decrease LDL levels.
   PCSK9 inhibitors for very high cholesterol/not responding to statins.
   Lipid apheresis that is method for removing cholesterol from the blood.
   Dietary control: low-cholesterol/low-saturated-fat diet.

Case 3: Hypercholesterolemia in a Patient with Hypothyroidism

A 60-year-old female with a history of hypothyroidism presents with a total cholesterol level of 280 mg/dL (normal range: 140–200 mg/dL). Her LDL is 180 mg/dL, and her HDL is 45 mg/dL.

1. **How does hypothyroidism affect cholesterol metabolism in this patient?**
   In hypothyroidism, there is a decrease in the activity of the LDL receptor, leading to impaired clearance of LDL cholesterol from the blood. This results in elevated total cholesterol and LDL levels. Additionally, hypothyroidism can reduce the synthesis of thyroid hormone-dependent lipoprotein lipase, which may contribute to an increase in cholesterol levels.
2. **What other lab tests would be helpful in this patient?**
   The following tests would be helpful:
   Thyroid function tests (TSH, free T4) to assess the degree of hypothyroidism.
   Liver function tests: To rule out any liver involvement in lipid metabolism.
   Apolipoprotein B levels: To assess the number of atherogenic particles.
   C-reactive protein (CRP): To check for any underlying inflammation.

3. **What is the treatment plan for this patient?**
   Management includes:
   Thyroid hormone replacement (e.g., levothyroxine) to correct hypothyroidism, which can help normalize lipid levels.
   Statins to lower LDL cholesterol and reduce cardiovascular risk
   Dietary modifications to improve overall cholesterol levels, focusing on reducing saturated fat intake.

Case 4: Hypercholesterolemia in a Diabetic Patient

A 58-year-old male with a history of type 2 diabetes mellitus presents with a total serum cholesterol: 279 mg/dL (normal range: 140–200 mg/dL), HDL: 37 mg/dL (normal range: >40 mg/dL), LDL: 191 mg/dL (normal range: <100 mg/dL), HbA1c: 8.7% (normal range: <5.7%).

1. **What is the interpretation of the cholesterol profile?**
   Dyslipidemia is indicated that is complication of diabetes, High total cholesterol and LDL raises cardiovascular risk, low HDL is a major risk factor for cardiovascular disease, hyperglycemia as indicated by the high HbA1c contributes more to dyslipidemia, as high glucose levels result in more formation of VLDL and less clearance of LDL, further increasing cholesterol levels. This patient is at high risk for atherosclerotic cardiovascular disease because of a dyslipidemia as well as poor glycemic control.
2. **How diabetes can contribute to dyslipidemia?**
   More VLDL formation: Hyperglycemia stimulates liver to form more VLDL, that is rich in triglycerides. VLDL is changed into LDL, thereby increasing its concentration.
   Reduced HDL: High blood glucose may decrease formation of HDL, resulting in lower levels of good cholesterol. HDL has protective role in cardiovascular health by removing the cholesterol from arteries.
   Insulin resistance: It alters lipid metabolism leading to increased level of free fatty acids plus triglycerides in the blood.
3. **What further investigations are needed?**
   Lipid assay:
   Apolipoprotein B (apoB) assay: For evaluating number of atherogenic particles.
   Liver function tests: To exclude liver disease, that may exacerbate lipid abnormalities.
   Renal function tests: Diabetic nephropathy might contribute to lipid abnormalities.
   Thyroid function tests: Hypothyroidism might worsen lipid levels.
   HbA1c: for assessing long-term glycemic regulation.
4. **What is the management?**
   Optimal diabetes control: HbA1c <7% by lifestyle modification that is diet/exercise/medications
   Statins: To decrease LDL cholesterol/decreasing cardiovascular risk.
   Fibrates/niacin: To control high triglycerides.
   Ezetimibe: LDL-lowering effects if statins alone do not work.
   Lifestyle changes

Case 5: Hypercholesterolemia in a Post-menopausal Woman

A 62-year-old post-menopausal woman presents total serum cholesterol: 317 mg/dL (normal range: 140–200 mg/dL), HDL: 44 mg/dL (normal range: >40 mg/dL), LDL: 239 mg/dL (normal range: <100 mg/dL), blood pressure: 130/85 mm Hg.

1. **What are the risk factors contributing to high cholesterol?**
   Post-menopausal status: Decreased estrogen results in high LDL and low HDL (Estrogen has protective effect on lipid metabolism).
   High total cholesterol/LDL: this is a risk factor for CVD.
   Age: Age increases the risk of getting dyslipidemia, because lipid metabolism generally becomes less efficient with increasing age.
   Blood pressure: A sign of mild hypertension adds to cardiovascular risk.
2. **What is the clinical interpretation of the cholesterol profile?**
   High total cholesterol increases the complication of atherosclerosis/coronary artery disease.
   High LDL is primary atherogenic lipoprotein, significant contributor of plaque formation in arteries.
   Normal HDL is a protective factor against cardiovascular disease but not sufficient enough to offset the high LDL levels.
   The patient is at high risk for coronary artery disease/stroke.
3. **What additional investigations are required?**
   Lipid subfraction analysis, Apolipoprotein B, Carotid intima-media thickness/coronary artery calcium score: Non-invasive tests for assessing subclinical atherosclerosis, Thyroid function tests: To exclude hypothyroidism as a risk factor, Liver function tests: To exclude liver dysfunction, that may impact lipid metabolism
4. **What treatment options are present?**
   Statins to decrease LDL cholesterol/reducing cardiovascular risk.
   Ezetimibe: To decrease LDL cholesterol by inhibiting absorption of cholesterol, PCSK9 inhibitors for patients with statin resistance.
   Lifestyle modification, blood pressure control.

CLINICAL MCQS

1. **The common method of cholesterol estimation is:**
   a. Enzymatic method
   b. Liebermann-Burchard method
   c. Alkaline Picrate method
   d. GOD POD method

   Answer: a. Enzymatic method

2. **In the enzymatic methodology of cholesterol assay, the enzyme which catalyzes the breakdown of cholesterol esters is:**
   a. Cholesterol esterase
   b. Elastase
   c. Lipase
   d. Cholesterol oxidase

   Answer: a. Cholesterol esterase

3. **A patient's serum cholesterol level: 300 mg/dL. According to the National Cholesterol Education Program (NCEP) guidelines, this value indicates:**
   a. Desirable cholesterol level
   b. Borderline low cholesterol
   c. High cholesterol
   d. Very low cholesterol

   Answer: c. High cholesterol

4. **The normal reference range for total cholesterol in adults is:**
   a. 100–200 mg/dL
   b. 120–250 mg/dL
   c. 140–260 mg/dL
   d. 160–310 mg/dL

   Answer: a. 100–200 mg/dL

5. **A 48-year-old male with a cholesterol level: 220 mg/dL, a low HDL: 30 mg/dL, and a elevated LDL: 170 mg/dL is at high risk for:**
   a. Hypolipidemia
   b. Cardiovascular disease
   c. Gallbladder stones
   d. Chronic pancreatitis

   Answer: b. Cardiovascular disease

6. **The Liebermann-Burchard methodology of cholesterol assay includes reaction of cholesterol with:**
   a. Sulfuric acid and acetic anhydride
   b. Phosphoric acid
   c. Acetone
   d. Bromine

   Answer: a. Sulfuric acid and acetic anhydride

7. **Which of the conditions is likely to lead to a high total cholesterol level?**
   a. Hypothyroidism
   b. Chronic liver disease
   c. Diabetes insipidus
   d. Chronic pancreatitis

   Answer: b. Chronic liver disease

8. **In a patient having diagnosed with hyperlipidemia, a cholesterol level amore than 240 mg/dL is typically linked with a high risk of:**
   a. Coronary artery disorder
   b. Stroke
   c. Peripheral vascular disease
   d. All of the above

   Answer: d. All of the above

9. **A fasting cholesterol estimation is preferred because of:**
   a. It prevents interference from dietary fats
   b. It reduces variability of LDL
   c. It allows estimation of total cholesterol
   d. It provides a accurate reflection of liver functions

   Answer: a. It prevents interference from dietary fats

10. **A patient having cholesterol level: 400 mg/dL. The next best step to include is:**
    a. Initiate statins
    b. Reassess after doing exercise
    c. Perform an LDL cholesterol measurement
    d. Recommend a cholesterol free diet

    Answer: c. Perform an LDL cholesterol measurement

VIVA VOCE

Q1. What are the normal levels of total cholesterol/HDL cholesterol/why are they significant in cardiovascular risk assessment?

Total cholesterol:

Desirable: <200 mg/dL
Borderline high: 200–239 mg/dL
High: ≥240 mg/dL

HDL cholesterol:

Low (high risk): <40 mg/dL (men), <50 mg/dL (women)
Protective (low risk): ≥60 mg/dL
Importance: Elevated total cholesterol increases risk of atherosclerosis/cardiovascular disease, and HDL cholesterol is cardioprotective because it aids to remove excess cholesterol from blood vessels.

Q2. What are the reasons of high/low HDL cholesterol/how does it affect cardiovascular risk?

Low HDL (<40 mg/dL): Observed in obesity/smoking/sedentary lifestyle/diabetes mellitus/metabolic syndrome/high carbohydrate consumption.
High HDL (>60 mg/dL): Oftenly considered protective, but extremely more levels (>100 mg/dL) may sometimes be dysfunctional.

SPOTTERS

Q1. Show lipid profile report having elevated total cholesterol/low HDL cholesterol.

Increased cardiovascular risk, generally observed in dyslipidemia/metabolic syndrome/sedentary lifestyle. Lifestyle modifications/lipid-lowering therapy like statins are needed.

Q2. Show an image of a corneal arcus in a patient having hypercholesterolemia.

Corneal arcus/arcus senilis is a white or grayish ring around the cornea, generally observed in hypercholesterolemia. In young individuals that is less than forty years, it indicates familial hypercholesterolemia, needing aggressive lipid management.

REFLECTION

Describe the significance and principle of estimation of serum TC and HDL-C and also perform the estimation and clinically correlate with lab reports and diagnosis.

14

CHAPTER

Estimation of Triglycerides

COMPETENCY

BC14.15: Describe the estimation of triglycerides, HDL and calculation of LDL and interpretation of results in clinical scenarios.

LEARNING OBJECTIVES

After reading this chapter, the readers should be able to:

- Describe the significance and principle of estimation of triglyceride level in blood and its significance.
- Perform the estimation of triglyceride level in blood along with clinical interpretations.

BLUE PRINT

Estimation of Triglycerides

Objective

By the end of the lecture, students should be able to:

1. Understand the significance of triglyceride levels in health and disease.
2. Describe the principles behind the estimation of serum triglycerides.
3. Demonstrate the laboratory techniques used for the estimation of serum triglycerides.
4. Interpret laboratory results of serum triglyceride levels in the context of cardiovascular risk assessment.

Duration: ***60 minutes***

Materials Needed

1. Presentation slides explaining the principles of triglyceride metabolism and laboratory techniques for triglyceride estimation.
2. Charts or diagrams illustrating the structure and functions of triglycerides.
3. Examples of laboratory reports showing serum triglyceride levels.
4. Laboratory equipment and reagents for triglyceride estimation demonstration.
5. Calculators for students use during hands-on calculation exercises.

Outline

I. **Introduction to triglycerides** **(10 minutes)**
   - Define triglycerides and their role in lipid metabolism.
   - Discuss sources of triglycerides in the diet and endogenous triglyceride synthesis.
   - Explain the physiological functions of triglycerides and their relevance to health and disease.

II. **Significance of serum triglyceride levels** **(10 minutes)**
   - Describe the association between elevated serum triglyceride levels and cardiovascular risk.
   - Discuss the role of triglycerides in atherosclerosis, pancreatitis, and metabolic syndrome.
   - Highlight the importance of monitoring serum triglyceride levels in cardiovascular risk assessment and disease management.

III. **Principles of serum triglyceride estimation** **(10 minutes)**
- Describe laboratory techniques for measuring serum triglycerides, including enzymatic methods and colorimetric assays.
- Explain how triglycerides are hydrolyzed into glycerol and fatty acids for detection.
- Discuss factors that may affect the accuracy of triglyceride measurements and strategies for quality control.

IV. **Laboratory demonstration of triglyceride estimation** **(15 minutes)**
- Perform a step-by-step demonstration of the enzymatic method for measuring serum triglycerides.
- Explain the procedure for sample preparation, reagent mixing, and absorbance measurement.
- Involve students in the demonstration process by allowing them to observe and ask questions about the techniques used.

V. **Interpretation of results** **(10 minutes)**
- Review sample laboratory reports showing serum triglyceride levels.
- Discuss the optimal ranges for serum triglyceride levels based on cardiovascular risk assessment guidelines.
- Interpret the significance of abnormal triglyceride levels in terms of cardiovascular risk and potential interventions.

VI. **Hands-on activity** **(5 minutes)**
- Provide sample data for serum triglyceride concentrations.
- Guide students through the calculation of triglyceride concentrations and the determination of lipid profiles.
- Encourage students to work in pairs or small groups to analyze and interpret the provided data.

VII. **Clinical applications of triglyceride estimation** **(5 minutes)**
- Describe how serum triglyceride levels are used in clinical practice to assess cardiovascular risk and guide treatment decisions.
- Highlight the role of lifestyle modifications, medications, and dietary interventions in managing dyslipidemia and reducing cardiovascular risk.

VIII. **Review and summary** **(5 minutes)**
- Summarize the key points covered in the lecture regarding the estimation of serum triglycerides.
- Reinforce the importance of triglyceride monitoring in cardiovascular disease prevention and management.
- Provide additional resources for further reading and self-study on triglyceride metabolism and laboratory techniques.

IX. **Conclusion** **(5 minutes)**
- Conclude the lecture by emphasizing the significance of serum triglyceride levels in cardiovascular health and disease.
- Encourage students to apply the knowledge gained in the lecture to their clinical practice or research endeavors.

Triglycerides are of two types	Dietary/exogenous and hepatic/endogenous
Triacylglycerols (TAG) are present in	• Chylomicrons (dietary TAG are absorbed via chylomicrons which are made in intestinal mucosa) act as carrier of exogenous TAG in the plasma • Very low-density lipoprotein (VLDL) (hepatic/endogenous) act as a carrier of endogenous TAG in the plasma • Phospholipids are also derived from triglycerides (TG)
TAG estimation is a part of lipid profile done for	• Evaluating the risk of atherosclerosis • High TAG may lead to pancreatitis • High TAG may lead to insulin resistance/metabolic syndrome
Some reference methods of TAG estimation	• Alkaline hydrolysis, solvent extraction and color reaction with chromotropic acid • Colorimetric method using Zeolite
Estimation of TAG by enzymatic method	Enzymatic end point method/Trinder method
Sample	Collected after 10 hours of fasting in a plain vial or with ethylenediaminetetraacetic acid (EDTA) as anticoagulant
Kit	Readymade kit is available which contains: Two reagents: 1. R1 which is TG reagent 2. R2 which is TG standard of 200 mg%

Contd....

Contd....

Method	**Reagent**	**Blank**	**Standard**	**Test**
	TG reagent R1	1 mL	1 mL	1 mL
	TG standard R2		10 µL	
	Serum			10 µL
	DW	10 µL		

Mix, incubate at 37°C for 5 minutes, read at 505 nm

Principle

$$TG \xrightarrow{\text{Lipase}} \text{Glycerol} + 3 \text{ free fatty acids}$$

1. Either H_2O_2 formed is measured by the action of peroxidase enzyme which forms nascent oxygen [O] which acts on a dye Aminoantipyrene to convert it into quinoneimine dye
2. Or glycerophosphates can be measured by NADH formation in a reaction, and this NADH can be measured spectrophotometrically at 340 nm

$$\text{Glycerol} + ATP \xrightarrow{\text{Glycerokinase}} \text{Glycerol 3 phosphate} + ADP$$

$$\text{Glycerol 3 phosphate} + O_2 \xrightarrow{\text{Oxidase}} \text{Dihydroxyacetone phosphate} + H_2O_2$$

$$2H_2O_2 + 4\ AAP + \text{Phenol} \xrightarrow{\text{Peroxidase}} \text{Quinoneimine} + 4H_2O \text{ (pink colored)}$$

measured at 5050 nm (AAP is Aminoantipyrene)

Calculation

Concentration of serum TG (mg/dL) — OD of test/OD of standard × amount of standard/volume of sample used × 100

Interfering substance — Endogenous plasma glycerol which can be high in plasma because of IV fluids having glycerol, DM or contamination

Clinical interpretation

Normal level of TAG in adults	<200 mg% (50–150 mg/dL)
Borderline high	200–400 mg%
High	400–1,000 mg%
Very high	>1,000 mg%
Hypertriacylglyceridemia seen in	• DM • Nephrotic syndrome • Type I hyperlipoproteinemias (familial Hypertriacylglyceridemia) • Type III, IV, V hyperlipoproteinemias • Hypothyroidism • Obesity • Pregnancy • Alcoholism • Oral contraceptive pills • Coronary artery disease (CAD), ischemic heart disease and atherosclerosis
Lipemic serum	When TAG levels are very high, TAG settles at the top of the serum seen as an opaque yellow fatty layer

CLINICAL MCQS

1. **A very common method of triglyceride estimation:**
   a. Enzymatic method
   b. GOD method
   c. POD method
   d. Liebermann-Burchard reaction

   Answer: a. Enzymatic method

2. **In enzymatic methodology of triglyceride assay, triglycerides are first broken up/hydrolysed by the enzyme:**
   a. Lipase
   b. Phosphatase
   c. Esterase
   d. Creatine Kinase

   Answer: a. Lipase

3. **A 53-year-old patient with serum triglyceride level: 359 mg/dL. According to the American Heart Association guidelines, this level is classified as:**
   a. Normal
   b. On border
   c. High
   d. Very low

   Answer: c. High

4. **The normal reference of serum triglycerides in adults is:**
   a. 50–110 mg/dL
   b. 100–150 mg/dL
   c. 150–210 mg/dL
   d. 150–280 mg/dL

   Answer: b. 100–150 mg/dL

5. **Which of the conditions is likely to result in high triglyceride level?**
   a. Hyperparathyroidism
   b. Hypothyroidism
   c. Renal failure
   d. Acute kidney disease

   Answer: b. Hypothyroidism

6. **High serum triglyceride is commonly linked with which risk factors?**
   a. High alcohol
   b. Low carbohydrate
   c. Physical inactivity
   d. All of the above

   Answer: d. All of the above

7. **A 69-year-old male with diabetes mellitus and obesity has elevated triglycerides. Which of the following would be the most appropriate intervention to help reduce triglyceride levels?**
   a. High dietary fats
   b. Increase fiber intake and exercise
   c. Increase protein intake
   d. Decrease alcohol consumption

   Answer: b. Increase fiber intake and exercise

8. **In the Van Handel and Zilversmit method for triglyceride estimation, triglycerides are hydrolyzed to produce:**
   a. Glycerol/free fatty acids
   b. Glycerol only
   c. Phospholipids
   d. Free fatty acids

   Answer: a. Glycerol/free fatty acids

9. **A fasting serum triglyceride level: 519 mg/dL is linked with a high risk of:**
   a. Pancreatitis
   b. Heart attack
   c. Stroke
   d. CVD

   Answer: a. Pancreatitis

10. **The triglyceride level can be affected by factors:**
    a. Food intake before the test
    b. Physical activity
    c. Use of certain medications
    d. All of the above

    Answer: d. All of the above

VIVA VOCE

Q1. What are the normal TG levels/conditions causing hypertriglyceridemia/hypotriglyceridemia?

Normal triglyceride levels: <150 mg/dL

Hypertriglyceridemia (>200 mg/dL):

Primary/genetic causes: Familial hypertriglyceridemia/deficient lipoprotein lipase.

Secondary causes: Diabetes mellitus/metabolic syndrome/obesity/hypothyroidism/alcohol use/nephrotic syndrome/medications like corticosteroids, beta-blockers.

Hypotriglyceridemia (<50 mg/dL): In malabsorption syndromes/hyperthyroidism/chronic illness/severe malnutrition.

Q2. What are the clinical effects of severe hypertriglyceridemia (>500 mg/dL)?

Acute pancreatitis where Triglycerides >1000 mg/dL.

Eruptive xanthomas—yellowish papules on skin.

Hepatosplenomegaly like in familial hyperlipoproteinemia.

Increased CVD risk, when associated with low HDL and high LDL.

SPOTTERS

Q1. Show lipid profile report having triglyceride levels >1000 mg/dL.

Severe hypertriglyceridemia, that may be because of familial chylomicronemia syndrome/poorly controlled diabetes/excessive alcohol use. Advised low-fat diet/fibrates/omega-3 fatty acids/insulin if diabetic.

Q2. Show an image of eruptive xanthomas.

They are small/yellow-red papules which appear on buttocks, extensor surfaces, and back because of high triglycerides (>1000 mg/dL).

REFLECTION

Describe the significance and principle of estimation of serum TG and also perform the estimation and clinically correlate with lab reports and diagnosis.

15

Estimation of Bilirubin

CHAPTER

COMPETENCY

BC14.13: Perform the estimation of serum bilirubin by manual or semi-automated analyzer.

LEARNING OBJECTIVES

After reading this chapter, the readers should be able to:
- Describe the significance and principle of serum bilirubin estimation.
- Perform the estimation of serum bilirubin along with the clinical interpretations.

BLUE PRINT

Estimation of Serum Bilirubin

Objective

By the end of the lecture, students should be able to:
1. Understand the significance of serum bilirubin in clinical practice.
2. Describe the principles and laboratory methods for the estimation of serum bilirubin.
3. Demonstrate the laboratory techniques for the estimation of serum bilirubin levels.
4. Interpret laboratory results of serum bilirubin levels in health and disease.

Duration: *75 minutes*

Materials Needed

1. Presentation slides explaining the physiology of bilirubin metabolism, laboratory techniques, and interpretation of results.
2. Charts or diagrams illustrating the structure and metabolism of bilirubin.
3. Examples of laboratory reports showing serum bilirubin levels.
4. Laboratory equipment and reagents for bilirubin estimation demonstration.
5. Calculators for students use during hands-on calculation exercises.

Outline

I. **Introduction to bilirubin** **(10 minutes)**
- Define bilirubin and its physiological significance.
- Discuss the sources and metabolism of bilirubin in the body.
- Highlight the clinical importance of monitoring serum bilirubin levels.

II. **Physiology of bilirubin metabolism** **(10 minutes)**
- Describe the formation of bilirubin from heme breakdown.
- Explain the conjugation of bilirubin in the liver and its excretion in bile.
- Discuss the enterohepatic circulation of bilirubin and its implications for bilirubin levels in blood.

III. **Principles of serum bilirubin estimation** **(10 minutes)**
- Discuss laboratory methods for measuring serum bilirubin levels, including direct and indirect bilirubin assays.
- Explain the chemical reactions underlying bilirubin estimation and the principles of Colorimetry or spectrophotometry.
- Describe factors that may affect the accuracy of bilirubin measurements and strategies for quality control.

IV. **Laboratory demonstration of bilirubin estimation** **(15 minutes)**
- Perform a step-by-step demonstration of the laboratory techniques for estimating serum bilirubin levels.
- Explain the procedures for sample preparation, reagent mixing, and absorbance measurement.
- Involve students in the demonstration process by allowing them to observe and ask questions about the techniques used.

V. **Interpretation of results** **(10 minutes)**
- Review sample laboratory reports showing serum bilirubin levels.
- Discuss the clinical significance of total bilirubin, direct bilirubin, and indirect bilirubin measurements.
- Interpret abnormal bilirubin levels in terms of liver function, bile duct obstruction, hemolysis, and other pathological conditions.

VI. **Hands-on activity** **(5 minutes)**
- Provide sample data for serum bilirubin concentrations.
- Guide students through the calculation of total bilirubin, direct bilirubin, and indirect bilirubin levels.
- Encourage students to work in pairs or small groups to analyze and interpret the provided data.

VII. **Clinical applications of bilirubin estimation** **(5 minutes)**
- Describe how serum bilirubin levels are used in clinical practice to diagnose and monitor liver diseases, jaundice, and hemolytic disorders.
- Highlight the importance of serial bilirubin measurements in assessing disease progression and treatment response.

VIII. **Review and summary** **(5 minutes)**
- Summarize the key points covered in the lecture regarding the estimation of serum bilirubin.
- Reinforce the importance of bilirubin monitoring in the evaluation of liver and hematological disorders.
- Provide additional resources for further reading and self-study on bilirubin metabolism and laboratory techniques.

IX. **Conclusion** **(5 minutes)**
- Conclude the lecture by emphasizing the clinical relevance of serum bilirubin estimation in the diagnosis and management of various medical conditions.
- Encourage students to apply the knowledge gained in the lecture to their clinical practice or research endeavors.

Note: Ensure that students have a basic understanding of liver function and bilirubin metabolism before delving into the estimation of serum bilirubin levels. Use real-life examples and case studies to illustrate the clinical relevance of bilirubin monitoring and engage students in active learning throughout the lecture.

DEGRADATION OF HEME AND BILIRUBIN SYNTHESIS

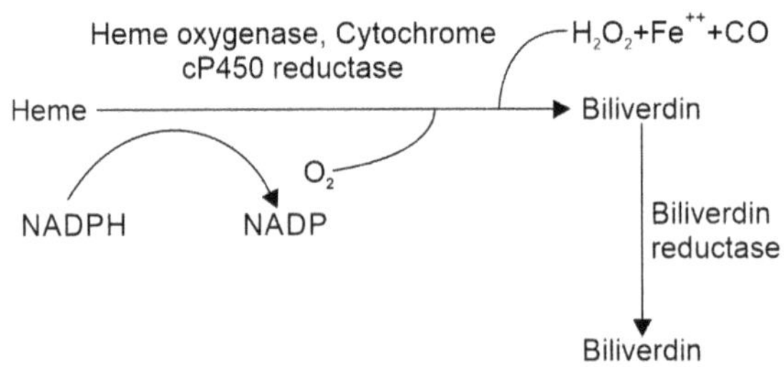

Per day production of bilirubin: 250–300 mg

85% formed from old red blood cells (RBCs)

15% formed from ineffective erythropoiesis in bone marrow

Minute amount of bilirubin formed by breakdown of heme proteins (myoglobin, catalase, peroxidase, cytochromes)

Bilirubin formed from reticuloendothelial cells (liver, spleen) is not conjugated

This fraction is insoluble in plasma

Contd....

Contd....

It needs to bind with albumin for transport

It reaches the liver via a carrier-mediated process, bilirubin is attached to intracellular proteins, such as ligandin and Z protein inside the liver cells, gets conjugated with glucuronic acid by enzyme UDP-glucuronyltransferase

Bilirubin monoglucuronides and bilirubin diglucuronide is formed

This conjugated form of bilirubin is soluble in water and gets secreted in the bile

Bile gets stored in gallbladder and from here it goes to duodenum through cystic and common bile ducts

In the intestine, it gets reduced to urobilinogen by the bacteria, UBG is reabsorbed from large intestine

Most of this is again secreted in the bile by liver via enterohepatic circulation

A small portion is excreted as stercobilinogen in stools and as urobilinogen in urine

Malloy and Evelyn Method

Principle: (van den Bergh)	Plasma/serum bilirubin + diazotized sulfanilic acid → azobilirubin (reddish-purple), color formed is directly proportional to amount of soluble bilirubin, measured colorimetrically at 560 nm
Conjugated/polar/soluble bilirubin: (Direct reaction)	It is measured in the first test before adding methanol
Total bilirubin (conjugated and unconjugated): (Indirect reaction)	It is measured in the second test after the addition of methanol. This is because of conversion of unconjugated bilirubin to soluble/measurable form after adding methanol (accelerator)
Reagents needed	• Diazo reagent made of sulfanilic acid and sodium nitrate in hydrochloric acid • Diazo blank—1.5% HCl • Methanol • Bilirubin standard (280 mg% methyl red is used, which gives OD of 0.32 that is equivalent to 8 mg% of bilirubin concentration)
Precautions	• Bilirubin is photo labile, so artificial standard of methyl red is used • Avoid hemolysis which can give false results

Procedure

Reagents	**T1 (mL) for total bilirubin**	**T2 (mL) for conjugated bilirubin**	**Control (mL)**
Diazo reagent	0.5	0.5	
Diazo blank			0.5
Serum	0.2	0.2	0.2
Methanol	2.5		2.5
DW	1.8	4.3	1.8
Total	5	5	5

Keep in dark for half an hour, OD read at 560 nm

Calculations

- Concentration of total bilirubin in serum = OD of test T1–OD of control/OD of standard × 8
- Concentration of conjugated bilirubin in serum = OD of test T2–OD of control/OD of standard × 8 [OD of standard is 0.32]
- Concentration of unconjugated bilirubin = total bilirubin–conjugated bilirubin

Clinical interpretation

Normal value of total bilirubin: 0.2–1.2 mg%	**Normal value of conjugated bilirubin:** 0.0–0.2 mg%	**Normal value of unconjugated bilirubin:** 0.2–1.0 mg%

Out of total serum bilirubin, 70% is indirect/unconjugated and 30% is direct/conjugated bilirubin

Hyperbilirubinemia	When plasma levels exceed 1 mg/dL
Nonicteric phase/latent jaundice	When the level is between 1 mg/dL to 3 mg/dL
Icteric phase	If the levels exceed 3 mg/dL, then the bilirubin diffuse to the tissues producing yellow discoloration of sclera, conjunctiva, skin and mucous membrane giving rise to jaundice.

Types of Jaundice			
According to cause:	Hemolytic	Hepatic	Obstructive
In newborns	Physiological	Pathological	

Hemolytic jaundice/retention jaundice/acholuric jaundice: Unconjugated hyperbilirubinemia, that is increase in both, total and unconjugated bilirubin

Causes	**Laboratory findings**		
A. Hemolysis of RBC's		**Blood**	
1. In hemolytic anemia, abnormal RBC's are seen which are prone to hemolysis	Conjugated bilirubin	Unconjugated bilirubin	Total bilirubin
2. Abnormal shape of red blood cells	Normal	Very high	Very high
3. Deficient enzymes, such as pyruvate kinase, glucose 6 phosphate dehydrogenase		**Urine**	
B. Mismatched blood transfusion	UBG	Bile salts	Bilirubin
C. Excess bilirubin enters the liver cells, the capacity of liver to conjugate bilirubin is limited, as the hemolysis is in excess, the concentration of unconjugated bilirubin increases in blood, which being water insoluble is not able to get excreted out in urine	High Ehrlich's test +	Nil	Nil
		Stool	
	Excess UBG	Excess stercobilinogen	
D. The concentration of conjugated bilirubin is also more than normal, which forms excess UBG and its excretion in urine and stools, as proportionately more UBG is absorbed in enterohepatic circulation			

Hepatic jaundice: Diminished hepatic functions, common in congenital hepatic jaundice where there is deficiency or complete absence of glucuronosyl transferase enzyme leading to decreased or absent conjugation of bilirubin

	Causes		
1. Acute hepatitis	Hepatitis viruses A, B, C, D and E Swelling of hepatocytes lead to narrow hepatic canaliculi, resulting in intrahepatic obstruction. This may lead to reabsorption of conjugated bilirubin in circulation and excretion in urine as it is water soluble		
2. Alcoholism			
3. Drug induced	Anti TB drugs, chloroform		
4. Congenital abnormalities	Gilbert's syndrome	Crigler–Najjar syndrome	
	Laboratory findings		
Blood	**Conjugated**	**Unconjugated**	**Total**
	Low/normal (due to residual conjugation activity)	High (main metabolic abnormality)	High
Urine	**UBG**	**Bile salts**	**Bilirubin**
	High (there is less hepatic uptake and recirculation of conjugated bilirubin, so relatively more conjugated bilirubin is secreted into the intestines from where it is absorbed and excreted in urine)	Nil	Nil/present

Obstructive jaundice/regurgitation/choluric jaundice: Conjugation in the liver is absolutely normal, main cause being extrahepatic obstruction to the flow of bile, thus conjugated bilirubin is not secreted into the intestines

Causes	**Lab findings—conjugated hyperbilirubinemia with increase in both total and conjugated bilirubin levels**					
1. Common bile duct stones		**Blood**			**Urine**	
2. Bile duct atresia	Conjugated bilirubin	Unconjugated bilirubin	Total bilirubin	UBG	Bile salts	Bilirubin

Contd....

Contd....

3. Carcinoma of the head of pancreas	Very high (conjugated bilirubin does not flow in the bile because of obstruction so it is reabsorbed into the blood and then excreted in urine)	Normal	High	Absent (UBG is not formed in intestines as no conjugated bilirubin is secreted into the intestines, giving pale yellow/ white color to stools)	Present	Present
Stool	No stercobilinogen in stools					

Neonatal jaundice: In newborn infants	
Physiological	**Pathological**
Cause: Immature enzymes of liver	**Cause:** Rh incompatibility between the fetus and the mother during pregnancy
Seen in: Premature babies, almost in 50% newborn babies, child is not born with jaundice, develops within 48–72 hours after birth	Child is born with jaundice, peak comes on seventh or eighth day and hyperbilirubinemia stays longer
Rise is mainly of: Unconjugated bilirubin	**Rise is mainly of:** Unconjugated bilirubin
Rise is moderate up to 15 mg/dL	Rise is critical up to 25 mg/dL
Returns to basal level by maximum 2 weeks	Because of the level of 25 mg/dL, albumin gets saturated, which results in excess free bilirubin, that can cross the blood brain barrier resulting in encephalopathy/kernicterus resulting in damage of brain
Treatment: Phototherapy—UV light changes Z isomers of bilirubin which are insoluble in water to E isomers which are soluble in water Corticosteroids may be given to increase fetal lung maturity and to prevent acute respiratory distress syndrome during pregnancy in cases of preterm labor	1. Needs active monitoring 2. Exchange blood transfusion (blood exchanged with normal blood) 3. Phenobarbital that is inducer of glucuronosyl transferase enzyme thus increasing bilirubin conjugation
Z isomers	**E isomers**
Increase intramolecular bonding, so water fearing property is present making it water insoluble	Do not favor intramolecular bonding, so water loving property is present making it water soluble, thus get excreted out by kidneys
Unconjugated hyperbilirubinemia: *Types:* 1. Physiological jaundice 2. Gilbert's disease 3. Crigler–Najjar syndrome 4. Hemolytic anemia 5. Hepatic jaundice	**Conjugated hyperbilirubinemia:** as conjugated bilirubin is water soluble, it is detectable in urine in such patients *Types:* 1. Dubin–Johnson syndrome 2. Rotor syndrome 3. Obstructive jaundice 4. Hepatic jaundice

Gilbert's disease	
Defect	Inherited defect of bilirubin uptake by hepatocytes

Crigler–Najjar syndrome	
Classification: Two types	
Type I	*Type II*
Congenital nonhemolytic jaundice	Benign condition
Enzyme deficient is UDP glucuronyltransferase	Mild defect in conjugation of bilirubin
Fatal condition, death almost before the age of two years	Mild
Jaundice onset is within one day of birth	–
Finally result in hyperbilirubinemia toxic encephalopathy/ kernicterus	No kernicterus
Unconjugated bilirubin is >20 mg/dL	Bilirubin is >15 mg/dL

	Dubin–Johnson syndrome
Defects	Hepatic secretion of conjugated bilirubin in the bile
Clinical defect	The liver cells of centrilobular area develop an abnormal pigment

OSCE

Case 1: Jaundice in a 48-year-old Man

A 48-year-old man presents with yellow skin/sclerae, serum bilirubin: 5.1 mg/dL (normal range: 0.3–1.2 mg/dL), direct bilirubin: 3.1 mg/dL and indirect bilirubin: 2.1 mg/dL, AST: 68 U/L (normal range: 15–40 U/L), ALT: 65 U/L (normal range: 15–40 U/L), ALP: 255 U/L (normal range: 40–150 U/L).

1. **What is the interpretation of the serum bilirubin?**
   The clinical scenario suggests—Mixed hyperbilirubinemia that is common in hepatocellular damage as indicated by slight raised AST/ALT. The significant rise in direct bilirubin suggests cholestasis, that may be intrahepatic as in liver disease/extrahepatic as in bile duct obstruction. The high ALP further supports the presence of obstructive jaundice. The pattern is consistent with hepatobiliary disease.
2. **What are the causes of the jaundice?**
   Hepatitis, such as viral/alcoholic/drug-induced that can explain the hepatocellular injury due to findings of high AST and high ALT and the mixed hyperbilirubinemia.
   Cholestasis is because of presence of gallstones or biliary strictures/tumors obstructing the bile ducts, resulting in conjugated hyperbilirubinemia as indicated by increased direct bilirubin.
   Cirrhosis or liver failure: Chronic liver diseases can lead to impaired conjugation/excretion of bilirubin, resulting in both direct and indirect bilirubin raise.
   Further investigations, such as ultrasound/hepatitis serology/CT scan.
3. **What additional tests are recommended?**
   Abdominal ultrasound: To check for signs of bile duct obstruction/gallstones.
   Hepatitis panel: To test for hepatitis A/B/C/other viral reasons.
   Imaging studies: CT scan/MRCP for visualization of the biliary tree.
   Liver biopsy: For evaluating degree of liver damage/ruling out cirrhosis and hepatocellular carcinoma.
   Complete blood count: To check for signs of hemolysis when indirect bilirubin is high.
4. **What are the management plans?**
   Management options are to treat underlying cause:
   When the reason is viral hepatitis: Antiviral therapy, such as interferons depends on type of hepatitis virus.
   When there is biliary obstruction: Endoscopic/surgical intervention for relieving obstruction, such as cholecystectomy for gallstones/biliary stent placement.
   Supportive care: Life style changes/medications/liver transplant.

Case 2: Jaundice in a Newborn

A 2-day-old neonate is presenting with jaundice, serum bilirubin: 16 mg/dL (normal range: 0.3–1.2 mg/dL), direct bilirubin: 1.6 mg/dL, indirect bilirubin: 13.9 mg/dL. The baby has no symptoms

1. **What is the interpretation of the bilirubin levels?**
   Unconjugated hyperbilirubinemia that is common in newborns because of immature liver enzymes which are insufficient for conjugating bilirubin during the first few days of life. The jaundice is likely due to physiological jaundice, that is present in 50–60% of full-term neonates and peaks between days 2–3 of life.
   Careful monitoring is required for preventing complications, such as kernicterus.
2. **What are the likely reasons?**
   Physiological jaundice which is characterized by high indirect/unconjugated bilirubin, more common in the first few days of life and generally becomes normal by 1 to 2 weeks.
   Other causes of jaundice in neonates are Hemolytic diseases, such as Rh incompatibility/ABO incompatibility, in which there is high breakdown of erythrocytes, breastfeeding jaundice, because of insufficient milk intake, Gilbert's syndrome (deficiency of the enzyme UDP-glucuronosyltransferase).
3. **What more investigations are recommended?**
   Blood type/Coombs test: To exclude ABO/Rh incompatibility.
   Reticulocyte count: Assess for hemolysis.

G6PD deficiency test: If there is suspected hemolytic anemia.
Liver function tests: If direct bilirubin is elevated.
Complete blood count: To assess anemia/hemolysis.

4. **How would you manage?**
Prevent kernicterus:
Phototherapy: First-line treatment, blue light aids to hydrolyze bilirubin to form water-soluble compounds which are then excreted out in the urine.
Exchange transfusion: When bilirubin >20 mg/dL/if phototherapy does not work.
Supportive care: Focus on adequate hydration/nutrition likely breast milk.

Case 3: Acute Liver Injury with Hyperbilirubinemia

A 51-year-old woman presents with jaundice/abdominal pain, bilirubin: 13 mg/dL (normal range: 0.3–1.2 mg/dL), direct bilirubin: 9.1 mg/dL, indirect bilirubin: 3.1 mg/dL, AST: 157 U/L, ALT: 189 U/L, ALP of 220 U/L.

1. **What is the interpretation of the bilirubin levels?**
Clinical scenario suggests the presence of Cholestatic jaundice, probably because of liver injury. The high AST/ALT suggests hepatocellular injury. The high ALP suggests cholestasis, that may be intrahepatic because of liver disease or extrahepatic because of bile duct obstruction. The clinical picture is indicative of liver-related cause of jaundice.
2. **What are the possible reasons?**
Hepatitis: Viral, such as hepatitis B or C/alcoholic hepatitis can result in hepatocellular injury with cholestasis.
Drug-induced liver injury: Some drugs, such as acetaminophen overdose or antibiotics may lead to hepatocellular injury as well as cholestasis.
Primary biliary cirrhosis/primary sclerosing cholangitis: Chronic liver diseases which might lead to intrahepatic cholestasis.
3. **What further investigations are needed?**
Hepatitis serology: For checking viral hepatitis.
Abdominal ultrasound: For checking signs of bile duct obstruction, such as stones/tumors.
Liver biopsy: When reason of liver injury is not clear after non-invasive investigations.
Serum acetaminophen level: When suspicion is of drug-induced injury is present.
4. **What is the management?**
Supportive care, such as hydration/pain management/monitoring.
Antiviral therapy for viral hepatitis.
Discontinue offending drugs if suspected drug-induced liver damage.
Liver transplantation when significant liver failure/cirrhosis is present.

CLINICAL MCQS

1. **A newborn is presented with jaundice on the second day. The total bilirubin: 15 mg/dL, direct bilirubin: 0.8 mg/dL. What is the most common reason of jaundice?**
   a. Physiological jaundice
   b. Sepsis
   c. Hemolytic disease
   d. Atresia

   Answer: a. Physiological jaundice
2. **A 49-year-old man having jaundice, shows with dark urine, pale stools, total bilirubin: 12 mg/dL direct bilirubin: 8 mg/dL. What is the diagnosis?**
   a. Hepatitis B
   b. Hemolysis
   c. Obstructive jaundice
   d. Neonatal jaundice

   Answer: c. Obstructive jaundice
3. **Which of these following is the key methodology for the estimation of serum bilirubin in the laboratory?**
   a. Colorimetry
   b. Spectrophotometry
   c. Diazo reaction
   d. Jaffe's method

   Answer: c. Diazo reaction

4. **A patient with suspected liver disorder has a total bilirubin: 12 mg/dL direct bilirubin: 7.1 mg/dL. Which enzyme is high?**
   a. ALT
   b. AST
   c. ALP
   d. GGT

   Answer: c. ALP

5. **In the lab, which reagent is commonly used in the diazo method of bilirubin assay?**
   a. Sodium nitrite
   b. Sulfanilic acid
   c. Methanol oxide
   d. Both A and B

   Answer: d. Both A and B

6. **A 63-year-old woman having jaundice reported with lab values: total bilirubin: 15 mg/dL, direct bilirubin: 12 mg/dL, alkaline phosphatase: significantly high. What is the diagnosis?**
   a. Hemolytic anemia
   b. Cholangiocarcinoma
   c. Viral hepatitis
   d. Acute hepatitis

   Answer: b. Cholangiocarcinoma

7. **What is the difference between conjugated, unconjugated bilirubin?**
   a. Conjugated bilirubin is water-soluble.
   b. Conjugated bilirubin is excreted in urine.
   c. Conjugated bilirubin is albumin-bound.
   d. Conjugated bilirubin is formed in the intestines.

   Answer: a. Conjugated bilirubin is water-soluble.

8. **A 3-day-old neonate having jaundice reported, total bilirubin: 19 mg/dL and a direct bilirubin: 0.6 mg/dL. What treatment is suggested?**
   a. Antibiotics treatment
   b. Phototherapy
   c. Transfusion
   d. Phenobarbital medication

   Answer: b. Phototherapy

9. **A patient reported with Gilbert's syndrome has high bilirubin in the fasting state. What type of bilirubin is more and predominantly high?**
   a. Bilirubin
   b. Unconjugated bilirubin
   c. Delta bilirubin
   d. Total bilirubin

   Answer: b. Unconjugated bilirubin

10. **Which of the conditions are linked with high delta bilirubin levels?**
    a. Acute liver failure
    b. Chronic liver disease
    c. Physiological jaundice
    d. Dubin-Johnson syndrome

    Answer: b. Chronic liver disease

VIVA VOCE

Q1. Mention types of bilirubin/how they help differentiate liver disorders?

Bilirubin exists in two forms:

Unconjugated/indirect bilirubin: Bound to albumin/not water-soluble/increased in hemolysis, Gilbert's syndrome, and ineffective erythropoiesis.

Conjugated/direct bilirubin: Water-soluble/processed by the liver/increased in obstructive jaundice, hepatocellular disease/Dubin–Johnson/Rotor syndrome.

Q2. Differentiate between prehepatic, hepatic, and posthepatic jaundice.

Prehepatic jaundice: Raised unconjugated bilirubin, normal liver enzymes, such as hemolysis.

Hepatic jaundice: Mixed elevation of unconjugated/conjugated bilirubin, with high ALT/AST, such as viral hepatitis, cirrhosis.

Posthepatic jaundice: Significantly high conjugated bilirubin, with elevated ALP/GGT, such as biliary obstruction, gallstones, pancreatic cancer.

SPOTTERS

Q1. Show a serum bilirubin report having high indirect bilirubin.

Hemolysis/Gilbert's syndrome.

Additional tests, such as reticulocyte count/haptoglobin/LDH are required to confirm hemolysis.

Q2. Show an MRI/CT scan of obstructive jaundice because of pancreatic head tumor.

Scan may exhibit biliary duct dilation/double duct sign/suggesting extrahepatic cholestasis generally because of pancreatic carcinoma/choledocholithiasis.

REFLECTION

Describe the principle and significance of estimation of serum bilirubin and perform the estimation of serum bilirubin along with clinical interpretation.

CHAPTER 16

Estimation of Calcium

COMPETENCY

BC14.14: Describe estimation of calcium and phosphorus and interpretation of results in clinical scenarios.

LEARNING OBJECTIVES

After reading this chapter, the readers should be able to:
- Describe the significance and principle of estimation of serum calcium estimation.
- Perform the estimation of calcium in blood along with clinical interpretations.

BLUE PRINT

Estimation of Calcium and Phosphorus

Demonstrate estimation of calcium and phosphorous (Chapters 16 and 17).

Objective

By the end of the lecture, students should be able to:
1. Understand the importance of calcium and phosphorus in the body.
2. Describe the principles and laboratory methods for the estimation of calcium and phosphorus.
3. Demonstrate the laboratory techniques for the estimation of serum calcium and phosphorus levels.
4. Interpret laboratory results of serum calcium and phosphorus levels in clinical practice.

Duration: ***75 minutes***

Materials Needed

1. Presentation slides explaining the physiology of calcium and phosphorus metabolism, laboratory techniques, and interpretation of results.
2. Charts or diagrams illustrating the structure and functions of calcium and phosphorus.
3. Examples of laboratory reports showing serum calcium and phosphorus levels.
4. Laboratory equipment and reagents for calcium and phosphorus estimation demonstration.
5. Calculators for students use during hands-on calculation exercises.

Outline

I. **Introduction to calcium and phosphorus** **(10 minutes)**
- Define calcium and phosphorus and their physiological roles in the body.
- Discuss the importance of calcium and phosphorus in bone health, muscle function, and cellular metabolism.
- Highlight the significance of monitoring serum calcium and phosphorus levels in health and disease.

II. **Physiology of calcium and phosphorus metabolism** **(10 minutes)**
- Describe the sources, absorption, distribution, and excretion of calcium and phosphorus in the body.
- Explain the regulatory mechanisms involved in maintaining calcium and phosphorus homeostasis, including hormonal control and bone remodeling.

III. **Principles of serum calcium and phosphorus estimation** **(10 minutes)**
- Discuss laboratory methods for measuring serum calcium and phosphorus levels, including colorimetric assays and complexometric titrations.
- Explain the chemical reactions underlying calcium and phosphorus estimation and the principles of Spectrophotometry.
- Describe factors that may affect the accuracy of calcium and phosphorus measurements and strategies for quality assurance.

IV. **Laboratory demonstration of calcium and phosphorus estimation** **(15 minutes)**
- Perform a step-by-step demonstration of the laboratory techniques for estimating serum calcium and phosphorus levels.
- Explain the procedures for sample preparation, reagent mixing, and absorbance measurement.
- Involve students in the demonstration process by allowing them to observe and ask questions about the techniques used.

V. **Interpretation of results** **(10 minutes)**
- Review sample laboratory reports showing serum calcium and phosphorus levels.
- Discuss the optimal ranges for serum calcium and phosphorus levels in different age groups and clinical conditions.
- Interpret the significance of abnormal calcium and phosphorus levels in terms of bone health, renal function, and metabolic disorders.

VI. **Hands-on activity** **(5 minutes)**
- Provide sample data for serum calcium and phosphorus concentrations.
- Guide students through the calculation of calcium and phosphorus concentrations and the determination of mineral profiles.
- Encourage students to work in pairs or small groups to analyze and interpret the provided data.

VII. **Clinical applications of calcium and phosphorus estimation** **(5 minutes)**
- Describe how serum calcium and phosphorus levels are used in clinical practice to assess bone health, renal function, and metabolic disorders.
- Highlight the role of calcium and phosphorus supplementation in managing hypocalcemia, hypercalcemia, hyperphosphatemia, and hyperphosphatemia.

VIII. **Review and summary** **(5 minutes)**
- Summarize the key points covered in the lecture regarding the estimation of serum calcium and phosphorus.
- Reinforce the importance of calcium and phosphorus monitoring in the diagnosis and management of various medical conditions.
- Provide additional resources for further reading and self-study on calcium and phosphorus metabolism and laboratory techniques.

IX. **Conclusion** **(5 minutes)**
- Conclude the lecture by emphasizing the significance of serum calcium and phosphorus levels in maintaining overall health and wellbeing.
- Encourage students to apply the knowledge gained in the lecture to their clinical practice or research endeavors.

Total body content in a healthy adult	1–1.5 kg
Three forms of plasma calcium	• Free/ionized calcium—active in nature (50% of the total plasma calcium) • Protein bound (albumin/globulin, 40% of the total plasma calcium) • Bound to other anions, such as citrate/bicarbonate/lactate/phosphate/oxalate, 50% of the total plasma calcium)
Effect of pH on the level of calcium: Change in pH also changes the charge on proteins so binding of calcium to the protein is affected	• Ionized calcium is active physiological form • At physiological plasma pH of 7.35–7.45 proteins are negatively charged therefore binds calcium avidly
In alkalosis	Plasma pH is more → proteins get more of positive charge increasing the binding of calcium to them therefore the free or ionized form that is physiologically active form is decreased resulting in hypocalcemia Acidosis–reverse mechanism

Contd....

Contd....

Role of hormones in calcium homeostasis	
Parathyroid hormone (act through vitamin D) and vitamin D	Increase serum calcium by increasing the intestinal and renal absorption of calcium
Calcitonin	Decreases the serum calcium level
Serum phosphate levels vary inversely with serum calcium level	
Effect of concentration of plasma proteins on the level of calcium	In hypoalbuminemia, more calcium is in free/ionized form
Functions	• Muscle contraction • As second messenger • Required for hormones secretion • As a metallic cofactor in enzyme activity • Bones/teeth formation (structural): In bones it combines with phosphorus to form hydroxyapatite crystals • Blood clotting • Membrane integrity • Plasma membrane transport • Excitation of heart • Excitability of nerves • Neuromuscular transmission
Methods of estimation of serum total calcium	• OCPC (o-Cresolphthalein complexone) method/colorimetric method • Calcium–arsenazo III dye method • Titration method of Clark and Collip using $KMnO_4$ • Atomic absorption spectrophotometry sensitive and specific measuring method • Flame photometry—light emission of excited calcium atoms is measured
Methods of estimation of serum ionized calcium	• Ion selective electrode (ISE) • There is a calcium ionizer that uses ion selective calcium electrode • Loss of CO_2 from the samples should be avoided by sealed syringes quickly as, increase in pH results in increased calcium binding by proteins thus decreasing free calcium
Samples	• EDTA and oxalate binds to calcium so not used for estimation • Serum/lithium heparin plasma is preferred

OCPC (o-Cresolphthalein Complexone) Method/Colorimetric Method	
Principle: Calcium + OCPC ⟷ Calcium-cresolphthalein complexone complex of pink color, read at 580 nm	o-Cresolphthalein complexone dye binds the calcium in basis medium to form a pink color complex, intensity of color is measured at 580 nm

Procedure	
Reagents	• Color reagent: pH is basic (11.7) • (o-Cresolphthalein complexone + urea + ethanol + hydroxy quinoline + acetic acid in diethanolamine buffer)
Function of hydroxy quinoline	Improves the efficiency of the reaction by binding with magnesium and preventing the interference
Function of urea	Intensify the color and decreases the turbidity if the serum is lipemic
Function of ethanol	• Reduces blank absorbance • Calcium standard (10 mg/dL)

Reagents	**Blank (mL)**	**Standard (mL)**	**Test (mL)**
Color reagent	5	5	5
Calcium standard (10 mg%)		0.5	
Serum (1: 10 dilution)			0.5
DW	0.5		
Total	5.5	5.5	5.5

Mix well, incubate at room temperature for 5 minutes, read the absorbance at 580 nm

Contd....

Contd....

	Calculation
Serum calcium (mg%)	OD of test/OD of standard × amount of standard (mg)/volume of serum (mL) × 100 To convert mg% to mmol/L, multiply with 0.25
Corrected calcium: Because 40% of total serum calcium is bound to albumin, the variation in the level of albumin affects the total calcium level, the adjusted/corrected calcium level takes into account the serum albumin level	Corrected total calcium is the value where the correction of the protein variation is done
Corrected total calcium (mg%):	Total calcium ←→ serum calcium (mg/dL) + 0.8 (4-serum albumin in g%)

Total and Ionized Calcium in Normal Adults and Children

	Total calcium	Ionized calcium
Adults (mg/dL)	8.6–10	4.6–5.3
Children (mg/dL)	8.8–10.8	4.8–5.5

Hypocalcemia causes	• Deficiency of vitamin D–rickets/osteomalacia • Hypoparathyroidism • Malabsorption—steatorrhea/celiac disease • Chronic renal failure (CRF), nephrosis, nephritis • Nephrotic syndrome • Drugs, such as diuretics, such as furosemide and anti-convulsant drugs • Blood transfusion with citrate • Hypomagnesemia
Hypercalcemia causes	• Hypervitaminosis D • Hyperparathyroidism • Multiple myeloma • Milk alkali syndrome (ingestion of milk in excess and antacids in excess in peptic ulcer) • Secondary metastasis in bones/bone neoplasm • Sarcoidosis • Paget's disease of the bone • Thyrotoxicosis • Polycythemia vera
Symptoms of Hypercalcemia	Anorexia, nausea, constipation, pain abdomen, renal calculi, soft tissue calcium deposits
Tetany: Clinical condition characterized by carpopedal spasm and treated by infusion of calcium gluconate	Decrease in calcium level below 6 mg%
Diet sources of calcium	Milk, and products of milk, beans, leafy vegetables, eggs, sea food

Daily requirement of calcium

Infants	Children	Adult males	Adult females	Pregnant women
400 mg/day	800 mg/day	1000 mg/day	1200 mg/day	1200 mg/day

Titration method of Clark and Collip using $KMnO_4$	• Calcium is precipitated as calcium oxalate by ammonium oxalate • Before doing titration, calcium oxalate is dissolved in 1 N H_2SO_4 to form oxalic acid • Titrated is done with $KMnO_4$ (potassium permanganate) • End point is indicated by pink color, titer value is used to calculate calcium concentration
Precautions of estimation of calcium	• Acid washed glasswares are used • Venous stasis must be avoided during collection of sample • Muscle activity should be avoided during collection of sample • Fasting samples should be taken to avoid diurnal variations and diet induced calcium increase

Age	3-year-old female
Complains	Convulsions (hypocalcemia)
History	Started walking late
On examination	Retarded growth, malnourished, poor muscle tone, protruded abdomen
Diagnosis	Rickets (Less serum calcium, high ALP level, X-ray showed poor calcification of bones)
Mechanism	• Main function of calcium and vitamin D is calcification of bones making them strong • Calcitriol which is the active form of vitamin D is required for calcium absorption from the intestine and stimulate reabsorption of calcium from the kidneys, is deficient due to deficiency of vitamin D in rickets
Renal rickets	Active calcitriol is synthesized in the kidney (25-hydroxy cholecalciferol to 1, 25-dihydroxy cholecalciferol by 1-alpha-hydroxylase enzyme), but in renal failure cases, this is not possible, thus leading to deficient vitamin D and rickets called as renal rickets
Role of UV rays	7-Dehydrocholesterol in the skin is converted to cholecalciferol in presence of sunlight in the skin
Treatment	Calcitriol—50,000 IU/week is given initially for 12 weeks, and then 800 IU/day routinely along with calcium—2 g/day

OSCE

Case 1: Hypercalcemia in a 55-Year-Old Woman

A 50-year-old woman presents with frequent urination, serum calcium: 12.5 mg/dL (normal range: 8.5–10.5 mg/dL), serum albumin: 3.0 g/dL (normal range: 3.5–5.0 g/dL), PTH: 150 pg/mL (normal range: 10–65 pg/mL).

1. **What is the interpretation of the calcium levels?**
   Hypercalcemia
   As the albumin level is decreased the corrected calcium formula:
   Corrected calcium = Total calcium + 0.8 × (4.0 – Serum albumin)
   This formula accounts for the less protein binding of calcium in hypoalbuminemia. However, even without this correction, the calcium is raised indicating primary hyperparathyroidism. The high PTH is in support of this diagnosis, because PTH is responsible to increase calcium levels by stimulating resorption of bone/increasing renal reabsorption of calcium.
2. **What are the possible reasons of hypercalcemia?**
   Primary hyperparathyroidism: Caused by a parathyroid adenoma/hyperplasia.
   Malignancy: Breast cancer/lung cancer, can form parathyroid hormone-related peptide resulting in hypercalcemia of malignancy.
   Vitamin D intoxication: Excess use of vitamin D can result in high calcium absorption in the intestines, though the high PTH makes this probability less likely.
   Sarcoidosis: Granulomatous diseases may increase calcium levels because of production of 1,25-dihydroxyvitamin D by macrophages.
3. **What additional tests would you recommend?**
   24-hour urinary calcium excretion: For evaluating hypercalciuria, that might be present in hyperparathyroidism.
   Neck ultrasound: Parathyroid adenoma/hyperplasia.
   Dual-energy X-ray absorptiometry scan: For osteopenia/osteoporosis because of chronic hyperparathyroidism.
   Serum phosphorus: For checking for decreased phosphorus, that is mainly observed in primary hyperparathyroidism.
   Vitamin D levels: To exclude vitamin D intoxication.
   Serum PTHrP: Suspected malignancy.
4. **What is the management plan?**
   For primary hyperparathyroidism: parathyroidectomy.
   If hypercalcemia is symptomatic, such as fatigue/dehydration then give IV fluids, loop diuretics for promoting calcium excretion, and bisphosphonates for reducing calcium levels.
   Vitamin D/calcium supplementation to avoid unless the patient has secondary hypoparathyroidism.

Case 2: Hypocalcemia in a 67-Year-Old Man

A 67-year-old man with chronic kidney disease presents with tetany/tingling in his fingers, serum calcium: 7.6 mg/dL (normal range: 8.5–10.5 mg/dL), phosphorus: 5.1 mg/dL (normal range: 2.5–4.5 mg/dL), albumin: 3.1 g/dL (normal range: 3.5–5.0 g/dL), PTH: elevated at 128 pg/mL (normal range: 10–65 pg/mL).

1. **What is the interpretation of the calcium levels in this patient?**
   Hypocalcemia, as the elevated phosphorus is present, this pattern is typical in chronic kidney disease in which impaired kidney function results in decreased conversion of vitamin D to calcitriol leading to decreased calcium absorption in the gut. This leads to compensatory high PTH/secondary hyperparathyroidism to increase the calcium levels. The high PTH level confirms this compensatory response towards hypocalcemia.
2. **What are the possible reasons of hypocalcemia?**
   Chronic kidney disease: Impaired kidney function results in less conversion of vitamin D to its active form, leading to less intestinal calcium absorption and secondary hyperparathyroidism.
   Hypoalbuminemia: Although the albumin level is slightly low, it is unlikely to explain the hypocalcemia here because corrected calcium would still be less.
   Vitamin D deficiency: Very common in CKD patients because of decreased renal conversion.
   Magnesium deficiency: Impairs PTH secretion along with PTH action, ultimately contributes to hypocalcemia.
3. **What additional tests are recommended?**
   Serum vitamin D levels: For evaluating vitamin D deficiency.
   Magnesium levels: For ruling out magnesium deficiency, that might exacerbate hypocalcemia.
   24-hour urinary calcium excretion: For checking kidney-related calcium handling.
   Bone mineral density: For To assessing bone loss because of chronic hyperparathyroidism in CKD.
4. **What is the management?**
   Calcium supplementation, Vitamin D supplementation, Phosphate binders: For controlling high phosphate levels, that might further contribute for secondary hyperparathyroidism, Management of CKD, Monitor for hyperparathyroidism.

Case 3: Calcium Imbalance in a Postmenopausal Woman

A 57-year-old postmenopausal woman with no symptom but history of osteopenia was there. Serum calcium: 9.1 mg/dL (normal range: 8.5–10.5 mg/dL), PTH: 26 pg/mL (normal range: 10–65 pg/mL), vitamin D: 14 ng/mL (normal range: 30–100 ng/mL).

1. **What is the interpretation of the calcium levels?**
   The patient has normal serum calcium/normal PTH/low vitamin D levels. The deficiency of vitamin D results in reduced calcium absorption from the gut. This can lead to osteopenia. Vitamin D deficiency can eventually result in secondary hyperparathyroidism also and all the more bone loss.
2. **What are the factors behind her calcium/vitamin D status?**
   Vitamin D deficiency: Improper sun exposure/less dietary intake.
   Postmenopausal changes: Low estrogen results in high bone resorption, that might be exacerbated by vitamin D deficiency.
   Osteopenia: Very common in postmenopausal women because of less bone density.
3. **What additional tests are recommended?**
   Bone mineral density: For assessing degree of osteopenia or osteoporosis.
   Serum phosphorus levels: For checking for associated mineral imbalances.
   Calcium and vitamin D supplementation: For correcting deficiencies and avoid more bone loss.
4. **What is the management?**
   Vitamin D supplementation: Correction of deficiency/increase calcium absorption.
   Calcium supplementation: If dietary intake is not sufficient.
   Weight-bearing exercise: Improve bone density.
   Bone-protective medications: When osteoporosis confirmed.

CLINICAL MCQS

1. **A 38-year-old woman complains of muscle cramps, tingling sensations around mouth. Serum calcium: 6.5 mg/dL. What can be the reason?**
   a. Deficient Vitamin D
   b. Hypoparathyroidism
   c. Acute kidney disease
   d. Hypoparathyroidism
   Answer: d. Hypoparathyroidism
2. **Which of the methods is most common for assay of serum calcium?**
   a. Absorption spectrophotometry
   b. Arsenazo III method

c. Enzymatic colorimetry
d. Ion-selective electrode method

Answer: b. Arsenazo III method

3. **A 68-year-old man having chronic kidney disease presents with total serum calcium: 7.8 mg/dL. His albumin level: 3.0 g/dL (normal: 4.0–5.0 g/dL). What is the corrected calcium level?**
a. 7.6 mg/dL
b. 8.6 mg/dL
c. 8.8 mg/dL
d. 9.8 mg/dL

Answer: c. 8.8 mg/dL
(Corrected calcium = Total calcium + 0.8 × [4 - serum albumin])

4. **A 49-year-old woman having hypercalcemia shows with a serum calcium of 12.5 mg/dL. Which hormone is high?**
a. PTH
b. Calcitriol
c. Calcitonin
d. TSH

Answer: a. PTH

5. **Which is the best indicator of active calcium status?**
a. Unionized calcium
b. Ionized calcium
c. Corrected calcium
d. Urinary calcium

Answer: b. Ionized calcium

6. **A patient comes with symptoms of nephrolithiasis, serum calcium level: 11.5 mg/dL. What other lab test are helpful for confirmation?**
a. Serum calcium
b. Serum PTH
c. Serum Phosphorus
d. Serum ALP

Answer: b. Serum PTH

7. **A 39-year-old man comes with symptoms of fatigue, nausea, confusion. Serum calcium: 14 mg/dL. What is the first step for management?**
a. Bisphosphonates
b. IV fluids
c. Calcitriol
d. Dialysis

Answer: b. IV fluids

8. **A patient having osteoporosis is prescribed with calcium, vitamin D supplements. Which form of calcium is bioavailable for the absorption?**
a. Calcium
b. Calcium citrate
c. Calcium carbonate
d. Gluconate form

Answer: b. Calcium citrate

9. **A 13-year-old boy presents with delayed growth, bow legs. Serum calcium: 7.5 mg/dL, phosphate is very low, alkaline phosphatase is high. What is the diagnosis?**
a. Rickets
b. Osteomalacia
c. Hyperparathyroidism
d. Paget's bone disease

Answer: a. Rickets

10. **Which anticoagulant must be avoided for plasma calcium assay as it can binds calcium?**
a. EDTA
b. Heparin
c. Citrate
d. Both A/C

Answer: d. Both A/C

VIVA VOCE

Q1. Give the normal serum calcium levels/conditions causing hypocalcemia/hypercalcemia.

Normal serum calcium: 8.5–10.5 mg/dL.

Hypocalcemia (<8.5 mg/dL) is observed hypoparathyroidism/vitamin D deficiency/chronic kidney disease/pancreatitis/hypomagnesemia.

Hypercalcemia (>10.5 mg/dL) is observed in primary hyperparathyroidism/malignancy, such as multiple myeloma and bone metastases/vitamin D toxicity/sarcoidosis.

Q2. How albumin levels affect serum calcium/give corrected calcium formula?

Since calcium binds to albumin, total serum calcium should be corrected in cases of hypoalbuminemia.

Formula: Corrected Calcium (mg/dL) = Measured Calcium + 0.8 × (4 - Serum Albumin in g/dL)

This correction helps to avoid misdiagnosing hypocalcemia in low albumin states, such as nephrotic syndrome and liver disease.

SPOTTERS

Q1. Show an ECG of a patient having hypocalcemia.

ECG may show prolonged QT interval, that may result in arrhythmias, such as Torsades de Pointes. Hypocalcemia can cause tetany, muscle spasms, and Chvostek's and Trousseau's signs.

Q2. Show an X-ray of osteolytic lesions in hypercalcemia due to malignancy (e.g., multiple myeloma).

X-ray may show "punched-out" lytic bone lesions, that are characteristic of multiple myeloma. Hypercalcemia in malignancy is because of parathyroid hormone-related protein/bone resorption.

REFLECTION

Describe the significance and principle of estimation of serum Calcium and also perform the estimation and clinically correlate with lab reports and diagnosis.

17

CHAPTER

Estimation of Phosphorus

COMPETENCY

BC14.14: Describe estimation of calcium and phosphorus and interpretation of results in clinical scenarios.

LEARNING OBJECTIVES

After reading this chapter, the readers should be able to:

- Describe the significance and principle of estimation of serum phosphate estimation.
- Perform the estimation of serum phosphorus along with clinical interpretations.

Total body content of phosphorus	500 g
Total content in bones	About 90% of the total content is present in bones
Distribution of blood phosphorus:	
1. Inorganic phosphorus	Phosphates ($H_2PO_4^-$ and HPO_4^{-2}) in combination with cations, such as Na^+, K^+, Ca^{++}, etc.
2. Lipid phosphorus	Phosphorus in combination with lipids, such as phospholipids—lecithin, cephalin, sphingomyelin
3. Organic phosphorus	Phosphorus in combination with organic molecules other than lipids, such as glycerophosphates, nucleoside phosphate
4. Residual phosphorus	Important constituent of proteins, enzymes
Functions	• Bone formation (87% of total body phosphorus is present in bones as a component of bone salt) • Component of phospholipids and nucleic acids • Glycolysis, glycogenolysis • Nucleotide formation, such as ATP, GTP, UTP, CTP • Coenzyme formation, such as TPP, PLP • Acid base balance • Phosphate buffer is the important intracellular buffer • Energy transfer reactions and high energy compounds
	Estimation of serum inorganic phosphorus
Sample	• EDTA, citrate and oxalate binds to phosphorus so not used for estimation • Serum/lithium heparin plasma is preferred • Hemolyzed samples are to be discarded as red blood cells have high amount of phosphorus
	Fisk and Subba Rao method
Reagents	• Acid Molybdate • 10 N H_2SO_4 • 10% (W/V) trichloroacetic acid • Reducing agent (amino-naphthol-sulfonic acid) • Phosphate standard (0.8 mg%)

Contd....

Contd....

Principle	Protein-free filtrate (PFF) is made PFF is reacted with acid Molybdate reagent to form Phosphomolybdic acid Phosphomolybdic acid is reduced to molybdenum blue by 1,2,4 amino-naphtho- sulfonic acid (ANSA) which is of blue color and is measured at 680 nm		
PFF preparation	2 mL serum + 8 mL 10% TCA → centrifuged and supernatant is used for estimation		
Reagents	**Blank (mL)**	**Standard (mL)**	**Test (mL)**
PFF			5
Standard (0.04 mg/5 mL)		5	
Molybdate reagent	1	1	1
DW	5		
Reducing agent	0.4	0.4	0.4
Total	6.4	6.4	6.4
Test tubes are mixed well and incubated at room temperature for 5 minutes, absorbance is read at 680 nm			
Calculation	OD of test/OD of standard × amount of standard (mg)/volume of serum (mL) × 100		
Precautions	• RBC's are rich in phosphate in comparison to plasma, so they should be separated out and also the proteins must be precipitated out • After the performance of the test, quickly take the reading as reoxidation and fading of color may be present • Hemolyzed samples must be avoided as false high levels may be obtained • Tap water has phosphorus so use DW • Use fasting serum • Blank test tube should be colorless		
Estimation of total phosphorus	Estimated in the same way after digesting organic and lipid phosphorus with strong acids		
	Normal range of serum inorganic phosphorus		
Adults	2.5–4.5 mg/dL		
Children	4.0–6.0 mg/dL		
	Clinical interpretation		
Hyperphosphatemia is seen in	• Chronic nephritis • Renal failure • Uremic come (may reach to 20 mg%) • Hypoparathyroidism (moderate decrease with low serum calcium) • Hypervitaminosis D • Chemotherapy • Rhabdomyolysis • Hemolysis • During fracture healing		
Hypophosphatemia is seen in	• Hyperparathyroidism • Fanconi's syndrome (less renal tubular reabsorption) • Vitamin D deficiency causing rickets and osteomalacia • Diabetic coma • Parenteral nutrition • Malabsorption • After taking insulin injection • Antacids, such as aluminum hydroxide		
Regulation of serum phosphate level	• The level of serum phosphate is reciprocally related to the level of serum calcium and is under same hormonal regulation as of calcium • If serum PO_4^{3-} level increases, serum calcium decreases • Produce of serum calcium and phosphorus concentration is equal to 40 [Ca × P = 40]		

Contd....

Contd....

Effect of vitamin D and parathyroid hormone on its level	• Parathyroid hormone decreases tubular reabsorption of PO_4^{3-} in kidneys thus decreasing its level • Vitamin D also decreases the phosphorus level
Effect of calcitonin on its level	It increases the phosphorus level
Pseudohypoparathyroidism	Genetic defect where the target organ receptors for parathyroid hormones are defective and there is end organ resistance, therefore serum phosphate increases even with normal parathyroid hormone level

OSCE

Case 1: Hypophosphatemia in a Diabetic Patient

A 51-year-old male having history of uncontrolled diabetes shows with irritability/confusion, excessive urination, poor appetite:
Serum phosphorus: 1.4 mg/dL (normal range: 2.5–4.5 mg/dL)
Serum calcium: 9.3 mg/dL (normal range: 8.5–10.5 mg/dL)
Blood glucose: 420 mg/dL (normal range: 70–110 mg/dL)
Urine output: high

1. **What is the interpretation of the serum phosphorus level in this patient?**
   The patient has hypophosphatemia: Low phosphorus level is probably associated to insulin therapy in uncontrolled diabetes. In such state the body experiences high excretion of phosphate in urine mainly in hyperglycemia. Insulin therapy, specifically in cases of diabetic ketoacidosis might also cause a shift of phosphate inside cells, exacerbating hypophosphatemia.
2. **What are the main reasons of hypophosphatemia?**
   Diabetic ketoacidosis: Phosphate is shifted into cells when insulin is administered in this condition of ketoacidosis resulting in decreased serum phosphorus.
   Hyperglycemia and osmotic diuresis: Elevated blood glucose levels might lead to osmotic diuresis that excretion of phosphate in urine.
   Refeeding syndrome: If the patient recently initiated eating after a long time that is after starvation, then phosphate will be quickly consumed by cells, resulting in hypophosphatemia.
   Chronic alcohol use: Alcohol impairs phosphate absorption in the gut and leads to high renal excretion.
   Hyperparathyroidism: High PTH can raise renal excretion of phosphate.
3. **What additional tests are recommended?**
   Serum glucose/HbA1c: For evaluating glycemic control.
   Urine phosphate excretion (24-hour urine collection): For evaluating extent of loss of phosphate.
   Serum magnesium levels: Hypomagnesemia is commonly linked with hypophosphatemia.
   Arterial blood gas: For assessing metabolic acidosis as in DKA.
   Vitamin D levels: For excluding possibility of vitamin D that might affect phosphate metabolism.
4. **What is the management plan for this patient?**
   Manage blood glucose levels with insulin for avoiding any more phosphate shifts.
   Phosphate supplementation that can be oral/IV based on severity of hypophosphatemia.
   Monitor electrolytes: Serum phosphate, calcium, and magnesium levels while the patient is on treatment.
   Prevention of refeeding syndrome: Carefully reintroduce nutrition after long starvation period to prevent sudden shift of phosphate inside cells.

Case 2: Hyperphosphatemia in a CKD Patient

A 75-year-old female with end-stage renal disease undergoing hemodialysis shows with pruritus/pain in bone.
Serum phosphorus: 7.7 mg/dL (normal range: 2.5–4.5 mg/dL)
Serum calcium: 8.1 mg/dL (normal range: 8.5–10.5 mg/dL)
Parathyroid hormone: 358 pg/mL (normal range: 10–65 pg/mL)
Creatinine: 5.3 mg/dL (normal range: 0.6–1.2 mg/dL)

1. **What is the interpretation of the serum phosphorus?**
   The patient is suffering from hyperphosphatemia which is common in patients with chronic kidney disease specifically those undergoing hemodialysis. The capacity of kidney for excreting phosphate is compromised in CKD resulting in high phosphate. The impaired kidney functions also reduces conversion of vitamin D to calcitriol resulting in less absorption of calcium and secondary hyperparathyroidism indicated by high PTH. The low calcium levels even more complicate the phosphate management.

2. **What are the main reasons of hyperphosphatemia?**
   Chronic kidney disease: Decreased renal excretion of phosphate because of reduced kidney function.
   Secondary hyperparathyroidism: Because of CKD, less vitamin D activation results in hypocalcemia thus stimulating secretion of PTH and further increasing phosphate release from bones.
   Increased dietary phosphate: It can exacerbate hyperphosphatemia.
   Hemodialysis: Improper phosphate removal during dialysis contribute to high phosphate levels.
3. **What additional tests are recommended?**
   Serum calcium: For assessing hypocalcemia, that can be seen in CKD and contribute to secondary hyperparathyroidism.
   Serum vitamin D: For assessing for deficiency, that is very common in CKD and might worsen phosphate and calcium imbalances.
   Bone mineral density: For checking bone mineralization defects/osteoporosis associated with CKD.
   24-hour urine collection: For assessing phosphate excretion.
4. **What is the management plan?**
   Phosphate binders: Calcium acetate is common for reducing phosphate absorption from the gut.
   Dietary phosphate restriction
   Calcium and vitamin D supplementation: For managing hypocalcemia/secondary hyperparathyroidism.
   Dialysis optimization: For adequate phosphate removal during dialysis.
   Parathyroidectomy: In secondary hyperparathyroidism.

Case 3: Phosphorus Imbalance in a Malnourished Patient

A 39-year-old male with habit of alcohol use presents with muscle weakness/irritability. He has been starving for several days.
Serum phosphorus: 1.7 mg/dL (normal range: 2.5–4.5 mg/dL)
Serum calcium: 8.5 mg/dL (normal range: 8.5–10.5 mg/dL)
Blood glucose: 79 mg/dL (normal range: 70–110 mg/dL)
Serum albumin: 3.0 g/dL (normal range: 3.5–5.0 g/dL)

1. **What is the interpretation of the serum phosphorus level?**
   The patient is suffering from hypophosphatemia due to refeeding syndrome that has resulted in quick shift of phosphorus into cells as compensatory metabolic adaptation, leading to hypophosphatemia. All the more, using alcohol contribute to malnutrition/impaired phosphate metabolism.
2. **What are the main factors of hypophosphatemia?**
   Refeeding syndrome, alcohol can result in reduced dietary intake/impaired phosphate metabolism.
   Hypomagnesemia: This state is commonly linked with malnutrition and may impair phosphate metabolism.
   Chronic malnutrition: results in decreased serum phosphate levels.
3. **What additional tests are recommended?**
   Serum magnesium levels for evaluating hypomagnesemia.
   Serum potassium/calcium levels for assessing other electrolyte imbalances.
   Nutritional assessment for evaluating patient's overall nutritional status.
4. **What is the management plan?**
   Gradual refeeding for preventing any more phosphate shifts.
   Phosphate supplementation for correcting the deficiency.
   Electrolyte monitoring during refeeding.
   Alcohol withdrawal management: Appropriate medications/rehabilitation.

CLINICAL MCQS

1. **A 64-year-old patient with chronic kidney disease presents with bone pain. Serum phosphate: 6.5 mg/dL (normal: 2.5–4.5 mg/dL). What is the reason of hyperphosphatemia?**
   a. Low renal excretion
   b. Impaired phosphate excretion by the kidneys due to decreased GFR
   c. High bone resorption
   d. Hypoparathyroidism
   Answer: b. Impaired phosphate excretion by the kidneys due to decreased GFR
2. **Which of the methods is commonly used for the assay of serum phosphate?**
   a. Molybdate UV method
   b. Jaffe's technique

c. Arsenazo method
d. Biuret technique

Answer: a. Molybdate UV method

3. **A patient presents with: muscle weakness, fatigue. Serum phosphate: 1.5 mg/dL. Which condition is linked with hypophosphatemia?**
   a. Vitamin A toxicity
   b. Hyperparathyroidism
   c. Acute kidney disease
   d. Tumor lysis

   Answer: b. Hyperparathyroidism

4. **What is the main regulator of serum phosphate levels?**
   a. Calcium
   b. Parathyroid hormone
   c. Calcitriol
   d. Insulin

   Answer: b. Parathyroid hormone

5. **A 9-year-old child presents with: delayed growth, bowlegs, low serum phosphate. What is the diagnosis?**
   a. Osteogenesis imperfecta
   b. Rickets
   c. Osteomalacia
   d. Hypophosphatemia

   Answer: b. Rickets

6. **A 59-year-old woman with metastatic cancer has a serum phosphate: 6.0 mg/dL. Which of the following is the most likely mechanism?**
   a. High renal reabsorption of phosphate
   b. High release of phosphate from bone
   c. Low intestinal absorption of phosphate
   d. Low renal excretion of phosphate

   Answer: b. High release of phosphate from bone

7. **In a patient having severe hyperphosphatemia, which clinical finding is present?**
   a. Tetany
   b. Acidosis
   c. Nephrocalcinosis
   d. Liver enlargement

   Answer: c. Nephrocalcinosis

8. **A person presents with hypophosphatemia. What complication is most likely in this condition?**
   a. Respiratory muscle weakness
   b. Gall stones
   c. Hypocalcemia
   d. Osteomalacia

   Answer: a. Respiratory muscle weakness

9. **What is the preferred anticoagulant to collect blood samples for phosphate assay?**
   a. EDTA
   b. Heparin
   c. NaF
   d. Citric acid

   Answer: b. Heparin

10. **A patient presents with hypophosphatemia but normal calcium levels. Which of the following conditions is most likely linked with this presentation?**
    a. Tumor lysis syndrome
    b. Refeeding syndrome
    c. Hypoparathyroidism
    d. Hyperparathyroidism

    Answer: b. Refeeding syndrome

VIVA VOCE

Q1. Give the normal serum phosphorus reference range and discuss the causes of hypophosphatemia/hyperphosphatemia.

Normal serum phosphorus: 2.5–4.5 mg/dL.

Hypophosphatemia (<2.5 mg/dL) causes: Hyperparathyroidism/vitamin D deficiency/refeeding syndrome/chronic alcoholism.

Hyperphosphatemia (>4.5 mg/dL) causes: chronic kidney disease, hypoparathyroidism, tumor lysis syndrome, and excessive phosphate intake.

Q2. What are the clinical manifestations of phosphorus imbalances?

Hypophosphatemia results in muscle weakness/confusion/rhabdomyolysis/hemolysis/osteomalacia because of less ATP production.

Hyperphosphatemia results in calcification of soft tissues/secondary hyperparathyroidism/tetany because of altered calcium-phosphate balance.

SPOTTERS

Q1. Show report having decreased phosphorus levels (<2.5 mg/dL).

The report indicates hypophosphatemia, that may be seen in malnutrition/chronic alcoholism/refeeding syndrome. Further evaluation with parathyroid hormone/vitamin D levels is required

Q2. Show an X-ray/CT scan of metastatic calcification in a patient of CKD.

X-ray may exhibit vascular/soft tissue calcifications, that happen because of hyperphosphatemia in CKD. This is because of secondary hyperparathyroidism/calcium-phosphate imbalance.

REFLECTION

Describe the significance and principle of estimation of serum Phosphorus and also perform the estimation and clinically correlate with lab reports and diagnosis.

18

CHAPTER

Estimation of AST or SGOT and ALT or SGPT

COMPETENCY

BC14.16: Describe the estimation of SGOT or AST and SGPT or ALT and alkaline phosphatase, and interpretation of results in clinical scenarios.

LEARNING OBJECTIVES

After reading this chapter, the readers should be able to:
- Describe the significance and principle of serum SGOT and SGPT estimation.
- Perform the estimation of serum SGOT and SGPT along with the clinical interpretations.

BLUE PRINT

Estimation of SGOT and SGPT

Objective

By the end of the lecture, students should be able to:
1. Understand the concept of serum enzymes and their release into circulation during pathological conditions.
2. Describe the clinical utility of various serum enzymes as diagnostic markers for specific diseases.
3. Discuss the limitations and challenges associated with the use of serum enzymes in clinical practice.

Duration: *90 minutes*

Materials Needed

1. PowerPoint presentation or visual aids
2. Whiteboard and markers
3. Handouts with key points and diagrams
4. Case studies or clinical examples (optional)

Outline

I. **Introduction to serum enzymes as diagnostic markers** **(10 minutes)**
- Brief overview of the lecture's objectives and agenda.
- Explanation of the concept of serum enzymes and their significance in clinical diagnosis.

II. **Mechanisms of serum enzyme release** **(20 minutes)**
- Overview of the mechanisms underlying the release of enzymes into circulation during pathological conditions.
- Discussion on cell damage, membrane permeability changes, and other factors contributing to enzyme leakage.

III. **Common serum enzymes and their clinical utility** **(40 minutes)**
- Description of various serum enzymes commonly used as diagnostic markers, including:
  - Alanine aminotransferase (ALT) and aspartate aminotransferase (AST) for liver damage.
  - Creatine kinase (CK) for muscle injury.
  - Alkaline phosphatase (ALP) for liver and bone disorders.
  - Amylase and lipase for pancreatic diseases.
- Explanation of how changes in enzyme levels correlate with specific pathological conditions.

IV. **Interpretation and clinical application** **(15 minutes)**
- Discussion on the interpretation of serum enzyme levels in clinical practice.
- Explanation of how enzyme assays are used in diagnosis, prognosis, and monitoring of disease progression.
- Illustration of clinical cases or examples to demonstrate the use of serum enzymes in diagnosis.

V. **Limitations and challenges** **(5 minutes)**
- Overview of the limitations and challenges associated with the use of serum enzymes as diagnostic markers.
- Discussion on factors influencing enzyme levels and interpretation of results.

VI. **Conclusion and recap** **(10 minutes)**
- Summary of key points covered in the lecture.
- Emphasis on the clinical relevance of serum enzymes in disease diagnosis and management.
- Encouragement for further exploration of diagnostic techniques and biomarkers.

BLUE PRINT

Demonstration of Estimation of SGOT/SGPT

Objective

By the end of the lecture, students should be able to:
1. Understand the significance of SGOT (serum glutamate-oxaloacetate transaminase) and SGPT (serum glutamate-Pyruvate transaminase) in assessing liver function.
2. Describe the principles and laboratory methods for the estimation of SGOT and SGPT levels.
3. Demonstrate the laboratory techniques for the estimation of SGOT and SGPT.
4. Interpret laboratory results of SGOT and SGPT levels in clinical practice.

Duration: *60 minutes*

Materials Needed

1. Presentation slides explaining the physiology of SGOT and SGPT, laboratory techniques, and interpretation of results.
2. Charts or diagrams illustrating the structure and functions of liver enzymes.
3. Examples of laboratory reports showing SGOT and SGPT levels.
4. Laboratory equipment and reagents for SGOT and SGPT estimation demonstration.
5. Calculators for students use during hands-on calculation exercises.

Outline

I. **Introduction to SGOT and SGPT** **(10 minutes)**
- Define SGOT and SGPT and their roles in liver function assessment.
- Discuss the sources, metabolism, and physiological significance of SGOT and SGPT.
- Explain the clinical relevance of monitoring SGOT and SGPT levels in various liver diseases and conditions.

II. **Physiology of SGOT and SGPT** **(10 minutes)**
- Describe the functions of SGOT and SGPT in cellular metabolism and amino acid metabolism.
- Explain the release of SGOT and SGPT into the bloodstream during liver injury or hepatocellular damage.
- Discuss the diagnostic value of SGOT-to-SGPT ratio (De Ritis ratio) in differentiating liver disorders.

III. **Principles of SGOT and SGPT Estimation** **(10 minutes)**
- Discuss laboratory methods for measuring SGOT and SGPT levels, including enzymatic assays and spectrophotometric techniques.
- Explain the chemical reactions underlying SGOT and SGPT estimation and the principles of enzyme kinetics.
- Describe factors that may influence the accuracy of SGOT and SGPT measurements and strategies for quality control.

IV. **Laboratory demonstration of SGOT and SGPT estimation** **(15 minutes)**
- Perform a step-by-step demonstration of the laboratory techniques for estimating SGOT and SGPT levels.
- Explain the procedures for sample preparation, reagent mixing, enzymatic reaction, and absorbance measurement.
- Involve students in the demonstration process by allowing them to observe and ask questions about the techniques used.

V. **Interpretation of results** **(10 minutes)**
- Review sample laboratory reports showing SGOT and SGPT levels.
- Discuss the optimal ranges for SGOT and SGPT levels in different age groups and clinical conditions.

- Interpret the significance of abnormal SGOT and SGPT levels in terms of liver function, hepatocellular damage, and liver disease severity.

VI. **Hands-on activity** **(5 minutes)**
- Provide sample data for SGOT and SGPT concentrations.
- Guide students through the calculation of enzyme activity and the interpretation of liver function tests.
- Encourage students to work in pairs or small groups to analyze and interpret the provided data.

VII. **Clinical applications of SGOT and SGPT estimation** **(5 minutes)**
- Describe how SGOT and SGPT levels are used in clinical practice to diagnose liver diseases, monitor disease progression, and assess treatment response.
- Highlight the importance of serial monitoring of SGOT and SGPT levels in managing acute and chronic liver conditions.

VIII. **Review and summary** **(5 minutes)**
- Summarize the key points covered in the lecture regarding the estimation of SGOT and SGPT.
- Reinforce the significance of liver enzyme testing in evaluating liver function and diagnosing liver disorders.
- Provide additional resources for further reading and self-study on liver enzymes and their clinical implications.

IX. **Conclusion** **(5 minutes)**
- Conclude the lecture by emphasizing the importance of accurate SGOT and SGPT estimation in clinical decision-making.
- Encourage students to apply the knowledge gained in the lecture to their clinical practice or research endeavors.

BLUE PRINT

Understanding Enzyme Activity in Clinical Diagnosis

Objective

By the end of the lecture, students should be able to:
1. Interpret laboratory results of enzyme activities.
2. Describe the clinical utility of various enzymes as markers of pathological conditions.
3. Understand the significance of enzyme assays in clinical diagnosis and management.

Duration: *90 minutes*

Materials Needed

1. PowerPoint presentation or visual aids
2. Whiteboard and markers
3. Handouts with key points and diagrams
4. Examples of enzyme activity profiles in clinical scenarios (optional)

Outline

I. **Introduction to enzyme activity interpretation** **(10 minutes)**
- Brief overview of the lecture's objectives and agenda.
- Explanation of the importance of enzyme activity interpretation in clinical diagnosis.

II. **Basics of enzyme activity measurement** **(20 minutes)**
- Overview of the methods used to measure enzyme activity in laboratory settings.
- Discussion on the principles of enzyme assays and factors influencing assay results.

III. **Interpretation of laboratory results** **(30 minutes)**
- Explanation of how enzyme activity levels are interpreted in clinical practice.
- Description of reference ranges and cutoff values for normal and abnormal enzyme activity.
- Discussion on the significance of changes in enzyme activity levels in different pathological conditions.

IV. **Clinical utility of various enzymes** **(20 minutes)**
- Description of specific enzymes commonly used as markers of pathological conditions, such as:
  - Creatine kinase (CK) for muscle injury.
  - Alanine aminotransferase (ALT) and aspartate aminotransferase (AST) for liver damage.
  - Amylase and lipase for pancreatic diseases.
- Explanation of how changes in enzyme levels correlate with specific diseases and clinical presentations.

V. **Case studies and examples** **(10 minutes)**
- Presentation of case studies or examples illustrating the interpretation of enzyme activity results in clinical scenarios.
- Discussion on the implications of enzyme activity findings for diagnosis and patient management.

VI. **Conclusion and recap** **(10 minutes)**
- Summary of key points covered in the lecture.
- Emphasis on the clinical relevance of interpreting enzyme activity results.
- Encouragement for further exploration of enzyme assays in clinical practice.

Aminotransferases	Enzymes that catalyze the interconversion of amino acids and alpha keto acids by transfer of amino groups
AST/SGOT	Serum glutamate oxaloacetate transaminase/aspartate transaminase belongs to class II enzymes transferases
Transamination reaction	It's a pyridoxal phosphate (PLP)-dependent reaction: $\text{L-aspartate + Alpha ketoglutarate} \xrightarrow{\text{AST, PLP}} \text{Oxaloacetate + L-glutamate}$

Location of AST [both, cytosolic (present in the plasma in normal conditions) and mitochondrial (present/increased in plasma in cases of cell necrosis):

In high concentration:	Cardiac tissue	Liver	Skeletal muscle
In mild concentration:	Pancreas	Kidney	Red blood cells

Clinical importance: Assess liver and skeletal muscle abnormalities

Pattern in acute myocardial infarction	**Pattern in viral hepatitis**	**Pattern in cirrhosis**
Rises within 6 hours of attack, peak comes at 24 hours and by 5 days it reaches back to normal	May increase up to 100 times of upper limit of normal	May increase up to 4 times of upper limit of normal

Macro SGOT	It is formed from SGOT which is bound to anti-SGOT autoantibody
Clinically	It results in delayed increase of SGOT level even after recovery of patient

Estimation of SGOT level in plasma: (Mohunand Cook,1957)

Principle

$$\text{L-aspartate + Alpha ketoglutarate} \xrightarrow{\text{AST, PLP}} \text{Oxaloacetate + L-glutamate}$$

$$\text{Oxaloacetate + 2, 4, dinitrophenyl hydrazine} \xrightarrow{\text{Alkaline medium}} \text{Hydrazone complex (red-brown) and read at 520 nm}$$

The intensity of the color is directly proportional to oxaloacetate concentration which in turn is directly proportional to the concentration of serum AST

Reagents

Standard: Oxaloacetate solution (2 µmol/L)
- 0.1 M phosphate buffer (pH 7.4)
- 2, 4, dinitrophenyl hydrazine: 1 mM
- 0.4 N sodium hydroxide

Substrate: L-aspartate + alpha keto glutarate in phosphate buffer

Substrate preparation: L-aspartic acid–0.30 g, alpha keto glutarate–50 mg are taken and dissolved in 20 mL phosphate buffer, 10% sodium hydroxide–1.1 mL is mixed for adjusting the pH and finally the volume is made to 100 mL by adding phosphate buffer

Reagents	**Test**	**Standard**	**Control**	**Blank**
Substrate	1 mL	–	1 mL	–
		Incubate at 37° (5 minutes)		
Serum	0.2 mL	–	–	–
		Incubate at 37° (1 hour)		
DNPH	1 mL	1 mL	1 mL	1 mL
Standard	–	0.2 mL	–	–
Serum	–	–	0.2 mL	–

Contd....

Contd....

		Incubate at 37° (20 minutes)		
NaOH	10 mL	10 mL	10 mL	10 mL
		Incubate at RT (10 minutes)		
		Read the OD of all test tubes at 520 nm		
Calculation: Serum AST (IU/L)	• OD test–OD control/OD standard–OD control × Amount of standard (mmol)/volume of serum (mL) × 1000 × 1/incubation time • OD test–OD control/OD standard–OD control × 0.4/0.2 × 1000 × 1/60 • OD test–OD control/OD standard–OD control X 33.3 IU/L			
		Interpretation		
Normal range (serum)	5–30 U/L			
Increased in	• Liver disorder • Liver cirrhosis • Acute myocardial infarction (significantly) • Dystrophy of skeletal muscles • Primary hepatoma • Viral hepatitis (not much rise as ALT, which rises more)			
		De Ritis ration/AST: ALT ratio		
Normal range	1.15			
Ratio of more than 2 (3:1 or 4:1)	Alcoholic liver disease			
Ratio of less than 1	Viral hepatitis	Extrahepatic biliary obstruction		

Spectrophotometric method/UV kinetic method for estimation of AST: They are used in auto analyzers

Principle	L-aspartate + Alpha ketoglutarate $\xrightarrow{\text{AST, PLP}}$ Oxaloacetate + L-glutamate Oxaloacetate + NADH + H^+ forms Malate + NAD^+ (in presence of MDH) • Because the NADH is consumed here, there is decrease in optical density at 340 nm • The change in absorbance per minute is measured (Δ A), and result is given by calculation
Calculation	AST activity (IU/L) = Δ A 340/6.3 × Volume in tube/sample volume × 10^3 (molecular extinction coefficient of NADH is 6.3 × 10^3/mol/cm)

ALT/SGPT	Serum glutamate pyruvate transaminase/alanine transaminase belongs to class II enzymes transferases
Transamination reaction	It's a PLP-dependent reaction: L-alanine + Alpha ketoglutarate $\xrightarrow{\text{ALT, PLP}}$ Pyruvate + L-glutamate
Clinical importance	• It is considered to a more specific enzyme for liver disorders than AST • It is increased more than AST in all inflammatory liver disorders • It remains increased for longer periods than AST

Estimation of SGPT level in plasma: (Mohunand Cook,1957)

Principle	L-alanine + Alpha ketoglutarate $\xrightarrow{\text{ALT, PLP}}$ Pyruvate + L-glutamate Pyruvate + 2, 4, dinitrophenyl hydrazine $\xrightarrow{\text{Alkaline medium}}$ Hydrazone complex (red-brown) and read at 520 nm The intensity of the color is directly proportional to pyruvate concentration which in turn is directly proportional to the concentration of serum ALT
Reagents	**Standard:** Pyruvic acid solution (2 μmol/L) • 0.1 M phosphate buffer (pH 7.4) • 2, 4, dinitrophenyl hydrazine: 1 mM • 0.4 N sodium hydroxide

Contd....

Contd....

Substrate: L-aspartate + alpha ketoglutarate in phosphate buffer

Substrate preparation:	L-alanine–5 gm, alpha ketoglutarate–20 mg are taken and dissolved in 20 mL phosphate buffer, 10% sodium hydroxide–1.1 mL is mixed for adjusting the pH and finally the volume is made to 100 mL by adding phosphate buffer			
Reagents	**Test**	**Standard**	**Control**	**Blank**
Substrate	1 mL	–	1 mL	–
		Incubate at 37° (5 minutes)		
Serum	0.2 mL	–	–	-
		Incubate at 37° (1 hour)		
DNPH	1 mL	1 mL	1 mL	1 mL
Standard	–	0.2 mL	–	–
Serum	–	–	0.2 mL	–
		Incubate at 37° (20 minutes)		
NaOH	10 mL	10 mL	10 mL	10 mL
		Incubate at RT (10 minutes)		
		Read the OD of all test tubes at 520 nm		
Calculation: Serum ALT (IU/L)	• OD test–OD control/OD standard–OD control × Amount of standard (mmol)/Volume of serum (mL) × 1000/30 × 1 • OD test–OD control/OD standard–OD control × 0.4/0.2 × 1000/30 × 1 • OD test–OD control/OD standard–OD control × 66.6 IU/L			
		Interpretation		
Normal range (serum)	5–40 U/L			
Increased in	• Infective liver disorder • Liver cirrhosis			
Very high in	Acute hepatitis (toxic/viral)			
Moderately increased in	Cirrhosis, hepatitis C, nonalcoholic steatohepatitis			
		De Ritis ration/AST: ALT ratio		
Normal range	1.15			
Ratio of more than 2 (3:1 or 4:1)	Alcoholic liver disease			
Ratio of less than 1	Viral hepatitis	Extrahepatic biliary obstruction		

Spectrophotometric method/UV kinetic method for estimation of ALT: They are used in auto analyzers

Principle

$$\text{L-alanine} + \text{Alpha ketoglutarate} \xrightarrow{\text{ALT, PLP}} \text{Pyruvate} + \text{L-glutamate}$$

$$\text{Pyruvate} + \text{NADH} + H^+ \xrightarrow{\text{LDH}} \text{Lactate} + \text{NAD}^+$$

- Because the NADH is consumed here, there is decrease in optical density at 340 nm
- The change in absorbance per minute is measured (Δ A), and result is given by calculation

Calculation: ALT activity (IU/L) = Δ A 340/6.3 × Volume in tube/sample volume × 10^3 (molecular extinction coefficient of NADH is 6.3×10^3/mol/cm)

OSCE

1. **Give normal range of SGOT in serum/what does an increased SGOT suggest?**
Normal range: 8–40 IU/L
Clinical significance of high SGOT:
Liver diseases, such as hepatitis/cirrhosis/fatty liver, myocardial infarction, muscle disorders, such as rhabdomyolysis/muscular dystrophy.
Pancreatitis or other inflammatory conditions
2. **A patient shows with jaundice/high SGOT of 160 IU/L. What is the probable interpretation and what are other investigations?**
Interpretation: The high SGOT is suggestive of liver damage/hepatitis/alcohol-induced liver damage.
Additional tests:
Serum Glutamic-Pyruvic Transaminase
Alkaline phosphatase
Bilirubin both total and direct
Prothrombin time
Imaging, such as ultrasound/CT of liver
3. **In a patient, SGOT is high: 410 IU/L, SGPT is normal. What is the probable cause?**
Likely reason: Muscle involvement along with liver, such as myocardial infarction, muscular dystrophy, rhabdomyolysis.
For confirmation: Creatine kinase/troponin for assessing myocardial damage, and creatine kinase for muscle damage.
4. **A patient with alcoholic hepatitis shows with SGOT: 300 IU/L, SGPT: 100 IU/L. What is the interpretation?**
SGOT/SGPT ratio in alcoholic hepatitis:
A ratio >2 (SGOT > SGPT) is specific of alcoholic liver damage.
This happens because of mitochondrial damage/pyridoxine deficiency in alcoholics that selectively affects formation of SGPT.
5. **What clinical conditions lead to isolated SGOT rise without liver involvement?**
Myocardial infarction, muscle trauma or strenuous exercise, hemolysis, hypothyroidism, certain medications like statins.
Confirmation: CK/CK-MB/troponin/lactate dehydrogenase.
6. **In a patient of viral hepatitis SGOT: 500 IU/L, SGPT: 600 IU/L. What does this pattern indicate?**
Pattern indication: Viral hepatitis presents with elevation of SGOT/SGPT however SGPT is generally more than SGOT.
Implication: Acute hepatocellular injury, such as in viral/toxic hepatitis.
7. **How should we interpret SGOT and SGPT levels in cirrhosis?**
Mild to moderate rise of these 2 enzymes
SGOT generally > SGPT with a ratio >1 (reversal of normal)
This is because of chronic nature of hepatocellular injury/decreased hepatocyte ability to synthesize SGPT.
8. **What is SGOT and what does it indicative of?**
SGOT: Enzyme mainly located in the liver/heart/skeletal muscle/kidneys. It is released into the circulation when tissues get damaged. Elevated SGOT suggest tissue injury and are usually associated with liver disorders/cardiac disorders/muscle injuries.
9. **How do you interpret isolated rise of SGOT in comparison of SGPT in liver disorder?**
SGOT > SGPT: Indicates nonhepatic causes, such as alcoholic liver disease/muscle injury. Alcoholic liver disease generally exhibits AST:ALT ratio > 2:1.
SGPT > SGOT: Suggests primary liver injury such as viral hepatitis/fatty liver.
10. **A 47-year-old patient presents with jaundice and high SGOT: 200 U/L, SGPT: 80 U/L. What is the probable diagnosis?**
The AST:ALT ratio = 200:80 = 2.5, that is >2. This is characteristic of alcoholic liver disease. Alcohol induces damage of mitochondria and raises SGOT
11. **In a suspected myocardial infarction how does SGOT aids in diagnosis?**
High within 6–12 hours of attack
Peaks at 24–48 hours
Returns to normal by 3–5 days
It is used with other markers such as CK-MB/troponins for confirming cardiac damage.
12. **A young male presents with muscle pain after doing exercise. SGOT: 410 U/L, SGPT: 103 U/L. What does this suggest?**
This is exercise-induced muscle injury. SGOT is also present in skeletal muscles therefore its levels can rise after muscle damage, however SGPT remains almost low.
13. **What are the normal ranges for SGOT/what levels are considered significantly high?**
Normal range: 10–40 U/L
Mild rise: 40–100 U/L, such as mild liver injury/muscle strain

Moderate rise: 100–500 U/L, such as hepatitis/myocardial infarction
Severe rise: >500 U/L, such as acute viral hepatitis/rhabdomyolysis

14. **A 61-year-old patient with cirrhosis shows SGOT: 106 U/L, SGPT: 42 U/L. What does this suggest?**
The AST:ALT ratio = 100:40 = 2.5, that is consistent with advanced liver fibrosis/leads to cirrhosis. Chronic liver damage leads to raise SGOT more than SGPT.
15. **How does pyridoxine deficiency affect SGOT levels?**
Vitamin B6: cofactor for SGOT activity. In its deficiency, SGOT activity is decreased significantly resulting in falsely decreased levels even in the presence of liver damage.
16. **What is SGPT, and how is it clinically important?**
SGPT: Enzyme mainly found in the liver. It gets released into the circulation during liver cell injury as it is specific marker for liver functions.
Clinical significance: High levels show liver damage. Monitors hepatotoxicity because of drugs/toxins.
17. **What is the normal range of SGPT, and when is it considered high?**
Normal range: 7–56 U/L.
Mild rise: 56–200 U/L fatty liver/mild hepatitis).
Moderate rise: 200–400 U/L viral hepatitis.
Severe rise: >400 U/L acute viral hepatitis/toxic liver injury.
18. **A 39-year-old patient presents with abdominal discomfort. SGPT: 325 U/L, SGOT: 106 U/L. What does this indicate?**
The SGPT > SGOT ratio indicates acute liver injury, most probably because of viral hepatitis/drug-induced liver damage. SGPT is more specific to the liver in comparison to SGOT.
19. **How is SGPT utilized for differentiating between alcoholic liver disease/nonalcoholic fatty liver disease?**
Alcoholic liver disease: SGOT > SGPT with a ratio >2:1.
NAFLD: SGPT > SGOT/a ratio <1.
20. **A 49-year-old diabetic patient has SGPT: 71 U/L, SGOT: 58 U/L. What is the probable reason?**
Mild rise in SGPT/SGOT in diabetics is usually associated with nonalcoholic fatty liver disease, a common side effect of metabolic syndrome.
21. **In a patient on anti-tuberculosis therapy, SGPT is high (180 U/L). How should this be interpreted?**
High SGPT in a patient on ATT might suggest drug-induced hepatotoxicity usually because of isoniazid/rifampicin.
22. **A 59-year-old male with jaundice shows SGPT: 520 U/L, bilirubin: 8 mg/dL. What is the likely diagnosis?**
Acute viral hepatitis, where hepatocellular damage is the characteristic feature
23. **A patient recovering from viral hepatitis exhibits SGPT levels decreasing from 320 U/L to 54 U/L over two weeks. How should this be interpreted?**
The decreasing SGPT levels suggest liver recovery plus resolution of hepatocellular injury.
24. **A 34-year-old obese female has mild elevation of SGPT: 66 U/L. She says she does not take alcohol. What could be the reason?**
Nonalcoholic steatohepatitis/NAFLD because of high fat deposition in liver.
25. **How does hemolysis affect SGPT?**
Hemolysis can falsely raise SGPT as red blood cells release intracellular enzymes because of destruction. We must focus on accurate sample handling in order to get accurate results.
26. **Why is SGPT more specific to liver damage in comparison to SGOT?**
SGPT is mainly localized in cytosol of liver cells, and SGOT is localized in both, cytosol and mitochondria of liver and also heart and muscle.
Therefore, elevation of SGPT is more liver-specific.

CLINICAL MCQS

1. **A 49-year-old man presents with fatigue, jaundice. AST level: 300 IU/L, ALT: 450 IU/L. What is the diagnosis?**
   a. Nonalcoholic liver disease
   b. Acute viral hepatitis
   c. Fatty liver disease
   d. Hemolysis
   Answer: b. Acute viral hepatitis
2. **Which cofactor is needed for the activity of enzymes AST, ALT?**
   a. Pyridoxal phosphate
   b. Coenzyme A

c. B12
d. FAD

Answer: a. Pyridoxal phosphate

3. **A 63-year-old alcoholic individual presents with high liver enzymes: AST: 250 IU/L, ALT: 120 IU/L. How do you explain for the AST:ALT ratio > 2?**
a. Viral hepatitis
b. Alcoholic liver disease
c. Hypothyroidism
d. Hepatitis

Answer: b. Alcoholic liver disease

4. **A 39-year-old pregnant woman has high ALT/AST levels with symptoms of vomiting along with abdominal pain. What is the most likely diagnosis?**
a. HELLP syndrome
b. Acute fatty liver of pregnancy
c. Toxic hepatitis
d. Preeclampsia

Answer: b. Acute fatty liver of pregnancy

5. **A patient complains of right upper quadrant pain, high AST, ALT levels. Alkaline phosphatase is high. What additional test can help differentiate liver disorder from bile duct obstruction?**
a. Gamma-glutamyl transferase
b. ALP
c. LDH
d. PT

Answer: a. Gamma-glutamyl transferase

6. **Which of the conditions show a disproportionate elevation of AST in comparison to ALT?**
a. Acute myocardial infarction
b. Viral hepatitis
c. NAFLD
d. Acute hepatitis B

Answer: a. Acute myocardial infarction

7. **A 67-year-old diabetic patient has moderately high ALT levels. What is the cause?**
a. Hepatitis C attack
b. Nonalcoholic fatty liver disease
c. Hypercalcemia
d. Alcoholic fatty liver

Answer: b. Nonalcoholic fatty liver disease

8. **Which tissue, in addition to liver, is a key source of AST?**
a. Heart
b. Skin
c. Pituitary glands
d. Pancreas

Answer: a. Heart

9. **A 39-year-old man comes with history of muscle injury, has high AST and normal ALT. What is the source of the high AST?**
a. Pancreas
b. Skeletal muscle
c. Kidney
d. Heart

Answer: b. Skeletal muscle

10. **What is the key principle that is made use of for the assay of AST and ALT levels?**
a. Colorimetric method by oxaloacetate
b. Kinetic method using NADH and its conversion to NAD^+
c. ELISA method: enzyme quantification
d. Immunoassay: enzyme detection

Answer: b. Kinetic method using NADH and its conversion to NAD^+

VIVA VOCE

Q1. What is the clinical significance of ALT/AST in LFT?

ALT/AST are liver enzymes for assessing liver function. ALT is more specific to liver injury, and AST is found in the liver, heart, muscle, and kidneys. High ALT indicates liver-specific damage, and high AST/ALT ratio (>2:1) is generally observed in alcoholic liver disease.

Q2. Differentiate between hepatocellular/cholestatic liver injury on basis of liver enzyme patterns?

Hepatocellular injury, such as in hepatitis, liver cirrhosis exhibits significant elevation in ALT and AST, whereas cholestatic injury, such as in biliary obstruction, primary biliary cholangitis exhibits predominant rise in ALP and GGT with only mild rise in ALT/AST.

SPOTTERS

Q1. Show a liver function test report having high ALT and AST.

Liver damage is suggested. If ALT is disproportionately high it suggests viral hepatitis/fatty liver. If AST is significantly increased than ALT (AST/ALT ratio >2), this indicates alcoholic liver disease.

Q2. Show liver biopsy image of viral hepatitis showing enzyme elevation.

Biopsy shows hepatocyte necrosis, inflammation, and ballooning degeneration. ALT and AST levels would be significantly high in acute viral hepatitis, with ALT > AST.

REFLECTION

Describe the significance and principle of estimation of SGOT and SGPT also perform and write about the clinical interpretation of estimation of both.

19

CHAPTER

Estimation of Alkaline Phosphatase (ALP)

COMPETENCY

BC14.16: Describe the estimation of SGOT or AST and SGPT or ALT and alkaline phosphatase and interpretation of results in clinical scenarios.

LEARNING OBJECTIVES

After reading this chapter, the readers should be able to:
- Describe the significance and principle of serum ALP estimation.
- Perform the estimation of serum ALP along with the clinical interpretations.

BLUE PRINT

Demonstration of the Estimation of Alkaline Phosphatase

Objective

By the end of the lecture, students should be able to:
1. Understand the significance of alkaline phosphatase (ALP) in clinical diagnosis.
2. Describe the principles and laboratory methods for the estimation of ALP levels.
3. Demonstrate the laboratory techniques for the estimation of ALP.
4. Interpret laboratory results of ALP levels in clinical practice.

Duration: *75 minutes*

Materials Needed

1. Presentation slides explaining the physiology of ALP, laboratory methods, and interpretation of results.
2. Charts or diagrams illustrating the structure and functions of ALP.
3. Examples of laboratory reports showing ALP levels.
4. Laboratory equipment and reagents for ALP estimation demonstration.
5. Calculators for students use during hands-on calculation exercises.

Outline

I. **Introduction to alkaline phosphatase (ALP)** **(10 minutes)**
- Define ALP and its physiological functions in the body.
- Discuss the sources and distribution of ALP in tissues and organs.
- Explain the clinical significance of ALP in diagnosing liver and bone disorders.

II. **Physiology of alkaline phosphatase** **(10 minutes)**
- Describe the enzymatic activity of ALP and its role in catalyzing phosphate hydrolysis.
- Explain the mechanisms of ALP regulation and its involvement in bone mineralization and liver function.
- Discuss the variations in ALP levels across different age groups and physiological conditions.

III. **Principles of ALP estimation** **(10 minutes)**
- Discuss laboratory methods for measuring ALP levels, including colorimetric and enzymatic assays.
- Explain the chemical reactions underlying ALP estimation and the principles of spectrophotometry.
- Describe factors affecting ALP measurement accuracy and strategies for quality assurance.

IV. **Laboratory demonstration of ALP estimation** **(15 minutes)**
- Perform a step-by-step demonstration of the laboratory techniques for estimating ALP levels.
- Explain the procedures for sample preparation, reagent mixing, enzymatic reaction, and absorbance measurement.
- Involve students in the demonstration process by allowing them to observe and ask questions about the techniques used.

V. **Interpretation of results** **(10 minutes)**
- Review sample laboratory reports showing ALP levels.
- Discuss the optimal ranges for ALP levels in different age groups and clinical conditions.
- Interpret the significance of abnormal ALP levels in terms of liver function, bone metabolism, and disease states.

VI. **Hands-on activity** **(5 minutes)**
- Provide sample data for ALP concentrations.
- Guide students through the calculation of enzyme activity and the interpretation of ALP test results.
- Encourage students to work in pairs or small groups to analyze and interpret the provided data.

VII. **Clinical applications of ALP estimation** **(5 minutes)**
- Describe how ALP levels are used in clinical practice to diagnose liver diseases, bone disorders, and other medical conditions.
- Highlight the importance of serial monitoring of ALP levels in managing hepatic and skeletal diseases.

VIII. **Review and summary** **(5 minutes)**
- Summarize the key points covered in the lecture regarding the estimation of ALP.
- Reinforce the significance of ALP testing in diagnosing and monitoring liver and bone disorders.
- Provide additional resources for further reading and self-study on ALP and its clinical implications.

IX. **Conclusion** **(5 minutes)**
- Conclude the lecture by emphasizing the importance of accurate ALP estimation in clinical decision-making.
- Encourage students to apply the knowledge gained in the lecture to their clinical practice or research endeavors.

Phosphatases	Enzymes catalyzing hydrolytic removal of phosphoric acid from phosphoric esters, for example, glycerophosphates and phenyl phosphates				
Types	Acid phosphatase (for assessing prostate disorders)		Alkaline phosphatase		
	Act in acid pH of 5 to 6		Act in alkaline pH of 10		
Alkaline phosphatase	This enzyme hydrolyzes phosphate monoesters at optimum pH of 10				
Location	Found at the surface of the cells of tissues like: Liver, bones, placenta, intestine, kidney, spleen				
Clinical importance	Increased in hepatobiliary diseases, such as hepatic and obstructive conditions and osteoblasts related bone diseases				
	Four times increased activity of ALP is seen in gallstones, carcinoma of the head of pancreas and atresia of common bile duct, rickets, osteomalacia, Paget's disease, metastasis of cancers in bones, liver cirrhosis, healing fractures, hyperparathyroidism, tumors of uterus and intestinal tract disorders				
Decreased level of ALP	Achondroplasia, cretinism, scurvy, anemia, kwashiorkor and hypophosphatasia (inherited autosomal disorder)				
Isoenzymes	Liver/alpha 2 ALP	Bone/pre beta ALP	Intestine/gamma ALP	Placenta/alpha 2 ALP	Biliary/alpha 1 ALP
Characteristics of isoenzymes	Move fastest in electrophoresis	Most heat labile isoenzyme	Move slowest in electrophoresis	Most stable in heat, can resist heat of 65° for half hour	Source is biliary canaliculi
% of total isoenzymes in serum	25% of total is present in serum	50% of total is present in serum	10% of total is present in serum	1% of total is present in serum	10% of total is present in serum
Importance of isoenzymes	–	Increase	Increase in ulcerative colitis	Increase in pregnancy	Increase in obstructive liver disorder
Regan isoenzyme/ carcinoplacental ALP	Found in cancer patients, used for assessing the response towards therapy				
Normal blood level	40–125 IU/L or 3–13 KA units/Dl				
Physiological causes of increased ALP in serum	In growing children because of increasing osteoblastic activity		Second and third trimester of pregnancy because of increased isoenzyme of placenta		

Assessment of ALP	
Procedures	• King and Armstrong • Bowers and McComb
King and Armstrong	
Principle	Disodium phenyl phosphate $\xrightarrow{\text{ALP}}$ Phenol + Sodium phosphate Phenol + 4-aminoantipyrine $\xrightarrow{\text{Potassium Ferricyanide}}$ Purple color complex read at 525 nm
Reagents	• *4-aminoantipyrine*: 0.5% • *Potassium Ferricyanide*: 2.4% • *Substrate*: Disodium phenyl phosphate: 0.01 M • *Sodium carbonate/bicarbonate buffer*: 0.1 M and pH 10 • *NaOH*: 0.5 N • *$NaHCO_3$*: 0.5 M • *Phenol standard*: 1 mg/dL
Estimation of ALP	
Test (T)	• Bicarbonate buffer: 1.0 mL + Substrate: 1.0 mL • Incubate for 5 minutes at 37°C • Add 0.1 mL serum, mix, incubate for 15 minutes at 37°C • Stop the reaction by adding 0.8 mL of 0.5 N NaOH
Control (C)	• Bicarbonate buffer: 1.0 mL + Substrate: 1.0 mL + 0.8 mL of 0.5 N NaOH (for stopping the reaction) + 0.1 mL serum • Incubate for 15 minutes at 37°C
Blank (B)	• Buffer: 1.1 mL + DW: 1.0 mL + NaOH: 0.8 mL • Incubate for 15 minutes at 37°C
Standard	Buffer: 1.1 mL + phenol standard: 1.0 mL + NaOH: 0.8 mL
For color development	
Add 0.5 N sodium bicarbonate: 1.2 mL and amino-antipyrine reagent: 1 mL and potassium ferricyanide: 1 mL to all the test tubes, mix and take OD at 525 nm	
Calculation	1 King Armstrong unit is that activity of 100 mL enzyme that liberates 1 mg of phenol in 15 minutes
Concentration of ALP in serum (KA/dL)	• OD test–OD control/OD standard–OD blank × amount of standard/volume of serum × 100 • OD test–OD control/OD standard–OD blank × .01/0.1 × 100 • OD test–OD control/OD standard–OD blank × 10
Serum ALP in IU/L	• OD test–OD control/OD standard–OD blank × 10 × 7.1 [(since 1 KA unit/dL = 7.1 µmol/minute/L) = 7.1 IU/L)] • 1 International unit is the amount of enzyme activity present in 1 L that liberates 1 micromole of phenol per minute
Explanation	1 KA unit/dL = 1 mg of phenol/15 min/dL = 100 µg of phenol/15 min/dL = 1000/15 µg of phenol/min/dL = 1000/15 × 94 µg of phenol/min/dL (MW of phenol is 94) = 1000/15 × 94 = 0.71 µg of phenol/min/L

OSCE

Q1. What is ALP, and what does its elevation indicate?

Ans: ALP: enzyme mainly located in the liver/bone/kidneys/bile ducts. High ALP level is suggestive of:

Hepatobiliary diseases: Obstruction of bile flow, such as in cholestasis/biliary obstruction.

Bone disorders: States of increased bone turnover, such as in Paget's disease/osteomalacia/rickets.

Pregnancy: Placental ALP might result in physiological rise during third trimester.

Hyperparathyroidism/bone metastases/fractures.

Q2. A patient shows with jaundice a/high ALP. What is the most probable likely reason?

Ans: High ALP in a jaundice case is suggestive of posthepatic/obstructive reason like Biliary obstruction for example gallstones/bile duct stricture/tumors, such as cholangiocarcinoma, primary biliary cirrhosis/primary sclerosing cholangitis.

Additional diagnostic steps:

Gamma-Glutamyl Transferase: High GGT plus ALP supports diagnosis is of hepatobiliary origin.

Imaging studies: Ultrasound/CT scan for confirmation of biliary obstruction.

Q3. A child shows with bowlegs/high ALP. What is your interpretation?

Ans: The scenario of the case is suggestive of rickets, which is state that is characterized by defective mineralization of bones in children, usually because of vitamin D deficiency.

ALP is high because of excess osteoblastic activity.

Serum calcium/phosphorus concentration is commonly decreased however parathyroid hormone level gets high.

Q4. An elderly patient suffering from bone pain/high ALP but normal GGT. What is the diagnosis?

Ans: This scenario indicates Paget's disease of bone that is characterized by high bone remodeling.

Normal GGT was present so it excludes hepatobiliary reasons.

ALP elevation reflects increased bone turnover.

Confirmatory test: Bone scan

Q5. A pregnant woman in third trimester presents with high ALP. Is this normal?

Ans: Yes, physiological rise of ALP is usual during pregnancy, specifically in third trimester, because of placental ALP isoenzyme.

Focus on: Liver function tests, such as bilirubin/ALT.

Q6. A patient having chronic liver disease shows persistently rise in ALP. What additional investigations would be suggested?

Ans: Persistently raised ALP in chronic liver disease can suggest:

Biliary obstruction/primary biliary cirrhosis.

Investigations: Autoantibodies: anti-mitochondrial antibodies for primary biliary cirrhosis.

Imaging: MRCP/ERCP for biliary tract evaluation.

Q7. How can ALP isoenzyme studies aid in differential diagnosis?

Ans: ALP isoenzyme assay aids to localize the source of raise or elevation:

Bone origin: Raised in bone disorders, such as Paget's/rickets, associated by high serum calcium plus phosphate abnormalities.

Liver origin: Raised in hepatobiliary diseases, correlates with high GGT, bilirubin.

Q8. What is the function of ALP for diagnosing metabolic bone disorders?

Ans: ALP is a marker for bone formation, its rise in conditions with high bone turnover like:

Osteomalacia or Rickets: Vitamin D deficiency.

Paget's disease: Localized disease of bone remodeling.

CLINICAL MCQS

1. **A 49-year-old woman presents with joint pain/bone tenderness, high alkaline phosphatase: 300 U/L (normal range: 44–147 U/L, AST, ALT, bilirubin are normal, diagnosis will be?**
   a. Osteoarthritis
   b. Hepatitis B
   c. Hypoparathyroidism
   d. Paget's disease of bone

   Answer: d. Paget's disease of bone

2. **A 75-year-old male is suffering from bone pain/palpable mass over his low spine, ALP: 450 U/L, calcium, phosphate levels are normal. Which of the following is next step?**
   a. Biopsy
   b. Serum calcium assay
   c. Isotope bone scan
   d. Kidney ultrasound

   Answer: c. Isotope bone scan

3. **A 49-year-old woman comes with history of chronic alcohol consumption and presents with jaundice, ALP: 500 U/L, AST = 250 U/L, ALT = 350 U/L. What is the cause of the high ALP?**
   a. Cholestasis due to alcohol-induced liver disease
   b. Secondary biliary cirrhosis

c. Metastatic bone disorder
d. Hypoparathyroidism

Answer: a. Cholestasis due to alcohol-induced liver disease

4. **A 36-year-old woman presents with a history of bone fractures high ALP: 451 U/L, serum calcium and phosphate levels: normal. X-rays: bow long bones/decreased bone density. What is the diagnosis?**
a. Osteomalacia
b. Hypoparathyroidism
c. Arthritis
d. Rickets

Answer: a. Osteomalacia

5. **A 51-year-old male with a history of chronic kidney disease presents with bone pain, ALP: 452 U/L, low serum calcium and phosphate levels. What is the most likely explanation/cause for the elevated ALP?**
a. Secondary hyperparathyroidism due to chronic kidney disease
b. Primary cirrhosis
c. Osteomalacia
d. Rickets

Answer: a. Secondary hyperparathyroidism due to chronic kidney disease

6. **A 68-year-old woman presents with unexplained weight loss/bone pain, ALP: 610 U/L, calcium: 11.7 mg/dL/low phosphate. What is the diagnosis?**
a. Hyperparathyroidism
b. Osteoarthritis
c. Paget's disease
d. Myeloma

Answer: a. Hyperparathyroidism

7. **A 28-year-old woman comes with history of anorexia nervosa/fractures. ALP level: 500 U/L, low calcium, low phosphate. What is the reason for the high ALP?**
a. Osteomalacia due to malnutrition
b. Hypoparathyroidism
c. Liver disorder
d. Metastases of bone

Answer: a. Osteomalacia due to malnutrition

8. **A 63-year-old male with a history of chronic alcohol consumption/jaundice/right upper quadrant abdominal pain, High AST high ALT levels, ALP: 400 U/L. What is the reason of the elevated ALP?**
a. Alcoholic liver disease with cholestasis
b. Secondary biliary cirrhosis
c. Hepatitis C
d. Gallstones

Answer: a. Alcoholic liver disease with cholestasis

9. **A 34-year-old man presents with weight loss, back pain, ALP level: 810 U/L, normal calcium and normal phosphate, lytic lesion in the vertebral body. What is the reason of the high ALP?**
a. Biliary cirrhosis
b. Metastatic cancer to bone
c. Osteoarthritis
d. Paget's disease

Answer: b. Metastatic cancer to bone

10. **A 58-year-old male presents with abdominal pain/yellow skin. Normal AST, ALT, ALP is 356 U/L. Ultrasound: gallstones/no liver metastasis. What is the reason of the high ALP?**
a. Cholelithiasis with cholestasis
b. Hepatitis A
c. Cirrhosis
d. Secondary sclerosing cholangitis

Answer: a. Cholelithiasis with cholestasis

VIVA VOCE

Q1. What is alkaline phosphatase/what is the location?

ALP is an enzyme found in liver, bones, kidneys, and bile ducts. It breaks down proteins. High levels of ALP might suggest liver disease/bone disorders/bile duct obstruction.

Q2. What are the causes of high ALP level/differentiate between liver and bone causes?

High ALP levels may be caused by liver diseases, bone diseases, and other conditions like pregnancy.

To differentiate, advise for ALT, AST and assess hepatic involvement. Bone-related ALP elevation generally occurs without significant changes in liver enzymes, but a liver cause often correlates with abnormal liver function tests.

SPOTTERS

Q1. Show sample of blood with high ALP levels/mention possible causes.

High ALP levels may be suggestive of liver pathology like biliary obstruction/cirrhosis or bone pathology like Paget's disease/bone metastasis.

Assays of gamma-glutamyl transferase or bone-specific ALP will aid in differential diagnosis.

Q2. Show an X-ray of a patient with Paget's disease

In Paget's disease, the X-ray exhibits characteristic bone changes, such as thickening/deformities/"cotton wool" appearance of the skull. The ALP level in these cases is elevated because of high bone turnover.

REFLECTION

Describe the significance and principle of estimation of serum ALP and also perform the estimation and correlate with lab reports and diagnosis.

CHAPTER 20

Cerebrospinal Fluid Analysis

COMPETENCY

BC14.17: Describe briefly various body fluids and discuss the composition of CSF.

LEARNING OBJECTIVES

After reading this chapter, the readers should be able to:

- Describe the CSF composition along with clinical significance of constituents, such as sugar, proteins and chlorides in CSF.

BLUE PRINT

Composition of Cerebrospinal Fluid (CSF)

Describe and discuss the composition of CSF.

Objective

By the end of the lecture, students should be able to:

1. Understand the physiological importance of cerebrospinal fluid (CSF).
2. Describe the composition of CSF, including its physical properties and chemical constituents.
3. Discuss the formation, circulation, and functions of CSF in the central nervous system.
4. Explain the clinical significance of CSF analysis in diagnosing neurological disorders.

Duration: *80 minutes*

Materials Needed

1. Presentation slides outlining the structure, formation, and composition of CSF.
2. Diagrams or illustrations depicting the circulation of CSF within the central nervous system.
3. Examples of CSF analysis reports showing normal and abnormal findings.
4. Models or visual aids representing the ventricular system and subarachnoid space.
5. Whiteboard or flipchart for interactive discussions and brainstorming.

Outline

I. **Introduction to cerebrospinal fluid (CSF)** **(10 minutes)**
   - Define CSF and its anatomical location within the central nervous system.
   - Discuss the physiological functions of CSF in protecting and nourishing the brain and spinal cord.
   - Introduce the importance of CSF analysis in diagnosing neurological disorders.

II. **Formation and circulation of CSF** **(15 minutes)**
   - Describe the process of CSF formation in the choroid plexus of the brain's ventricles.
   - Explain the pathways of CSF circulation through the ventricular system and into the subarachnoid space.
   - Discuss the role of arachnoid villi and granulations in CSF absorption into the venous system.

III. **Physical properties of CSF** **(10 minutes)**
   - Explain the volume and pressure regulation of CSF within the intracranial space.
   - Discuss the clear and colorless appearance of normal CSF and the significance of turbidity or discoloration.
   - Describe the specific gravity, viscosity, and osmolality of CSF and their clinical relevance.

IV. **Composition of CSF** **(15 minutes)**
- Outline the chemical constituents of CSF, including electrolytes, proteins, glucose, and cellular elements.
- Discuss the normal ranges and variations in CSF composition based on age, gender, and physiological state.
- Highlight the blood-brain barrier's role in regulating the transfer of substances between blood and CSF.

V. **Clinical significance of CSF analysis** **(10 minutes)**
- Explain the diagnostic value of CSF analysis in evaluating neurological disorders such as meningitis, encephalitis, and hydrocephalus.
- Review common CSF abnormalities observed in various pathological conditions.
- Discuss the techniques and indications for performing lumbar puncture and CSF sampling in clinical practice.

VI. **Interactive discussion and case studies** **(10 minutes)**
- Engage students in a discussion about real-life cases involving CSF analysis and interpretation.
- Present case scenarios or clinical vignettes for students to analyze and discuss potential CSF findings.
- Encourage critical thinking and problem-solving skills in correlating CSF results with clinical presentations.

VII. **Review and summary** **(5 minutes)**
- Summarize the key points covered in the lecture regarding the composition and clinical significance of CSF.
- Reinforce the importance of CSF analysis as a diagnostic tool in neurology and neurosurgery.
- Provide additional resources for further reading and self-study on CSF physiology and pathology.

VIII. **Conclusion** **(5 minutes)**
- Conclude the lecture by emphasizing the essential role of CSF in maintaining central nervous system homeostasis.
- Encourage students to apply the knowledge gained in the lecture to their future clinical practice or research endeavors.

Cerebrospinal fluid (CSF)	• Fluid is produced from the choroid plexus cells in the brain ventricles • It is ultra filtrate of plasma surrounding the brain and spinal cord
Location	Present in the cavity (subarachnoid space) surrounding the brain and spinal cord between the pia and arachnoid matters in the brain
Total volume of CSF	130 mL (25 mL is present in ventricles)
Per day secretion	750 mL due to selective ultra filtration of plasma and also an active secretion by epithelial membrane
Clinical significance	Important for diseases in brain, spinal cord and meninges
Indications	• Infection of CNS (acute/sub-acute/chronic/bacterial/viral/fungal leading to meningitis, encephalitis and myelitis) • Demyelination disorders (sub-acute sclerosing panencephalitis called SSPE and multiple sclerosis) • Central nervous system (CNS) hemorrhage (vascular diseases, thrombosis) • Cancer/tumors (meningiomas/gliomas/tuberculoma/secondary metastatic deposits) • Inflammatory states where meninges are irritated by tumors/trauma/disc prolapse) • Post infective polyneuritis • Trauma (head injuries with subdural hematoma, intervertebral disc prolapse)
	Functions of CSF
1. Physical support/ protection	Acts like a cushion around the brain and spinal cord preventing any thrust/shock
2. Gives a controlled chemical environment	The tissues are supplied with nutrients and wastes are removed by CSF
3. Intracerebral/ extracerebral transport	Distribution of hypophyseal hormones within the brain and clearing of hormone from the brain and then sent to cell is done by CSF
Collection of sample	• It is collected by lumbar punctures, normally between L3 and L4 vertebrae under all aseptic conditions, analyzed for biochemical, bacteriological examination, serological and hematology (20 mL is enough for analysis) • Bacteriological examination for cell count and microbes identification by culture studies
Precautions	• Blood sample must be taken 4 hours before collection of CSF for perfect interpretations • Physical characteristics must be studied in CSF before centrifugation • Consumption of glucose by bacteria can give false results in vitro so immediate estimation of glucose must be done after collection of sample

	Biochemical analysis
Physical examination:	
1. Pressure	100–200 mm H_2O
Variation in pressure	Increased flow indicates increased pressure because of obstruction by tumors
2. Appearance	• Clear • Colorless • No sediments • No turbidity • No coagulum
Variations:	
Bacterial/viral/fungal CNS infections	Cloudy appearance
Traumatic puncture/subarachnoid hemorrhage	Red/yellow/brown due to presence of blood, bilirubin
3. pH	7.4–7.6
4. Specific gravity	1.006–1.007
Chemical composition:	
Protein: Generally albumin	15–45 mg/dL (much <serum)
Glucose	45–100 mg/dL (almost similar to blood levels)
Chlorides	120–130 mEq/L (>blood levels)
Calcium	5.5–6.0 mg/dL
Inorganic phosphate	1.0–2.4 mg/dL
Urea	20–40 mg/dL
Immunoglobulins	IgG: 30 mg/L
	IgA: 4 mg/L
Cells:	Mainly lymphocytes: 0–4 cells/mm^3
Variation:	Increased cells result in turbidity
	Protein Estimation in CSF
Method:	Turbidimetric by use of sulfosalicylic acid
Principle:	There is appearance of turbidity due to precipitation and denaturation of proteins by sulfosalicylic acid
	The turbidity leads to incident light scattering
	The intensity of the emergent light decreases in proportion to the content of protein, which is measured in photo metrically at 660 nm
	Test for Globulin in CSF
Method: Pandy's test	Pandy's reagent (10 g phenol in 150 mL H_2O) + 2 drops CSF
	Note the degree of turbidity
Increased turbidity is seen due to increased globulins in	Multiple sclerosis Neurosyphilis
Sugar estimation in CSF	Estimated by glucose oxidase method
Chloride estimation in CSF	Done by electronic chloridometer
Principle	The instrument has ion selective chloride electrode that gives direct result
CSF chloride decreases in	Meningitis (102–120 mEq/L)

Serological parameters in CSF analysis	
Glucose	• Specific carriers take glucose to CSF fluid • CSF glucose level is normally two-third of plasma glucose • It ranges between 45–100 mg/dL based on plasma glucose • For a good clinical diagnosis, we need to do blood glucose estimation also
Increased glucose in CSF	Denotes hyperglycemia but still lower than blood levels
Decreased glucose in CSF	Hypoglycorrhachia
Causes of Hypoglycorrhachia	• Active glucose metabolism • Bacterial (septic)/fungal/amebic microorganisms may lead to active metabolism of glucose • Diseases of carrier-mediated transport, such as tuberculosis, sarcoidosis • Carcinomatous infiltration of brain and spinal cord • Consumption of CSF by CNS because of excess metabolism as in case of tumors of brain, diffuse meningeal malignancies
Glucose in bacterial meningitis	40 mg/dL
Glucose in viral meningitis	Normal
Glucose in TB meningitis	<50 mg/dL
Lactate:	Glucose consumption by cells/microorganisms may lead to increased levels of lactate
Bacterial meningitis	Increased level of lactate and decreased level of glucose indicates bacterial meningitis
Proteins	• CSF total protein is 0.5% of that of plasma (15–45 mg/dL) • Out of these total proteins, 80% of proteins come from ultrafiltrate of plasma and 20% comes from intrathecal synthesis • The proteins pass from brain to CSF by active process
Increased proteins in CSF seen in	• The active process increases in inflammation conditions and CSF flow obstruction, blood brain barrier breaks leading to excess proteins in CSF • Bacterial meningitis (>100 mg/dL) • Viral meningitis (20–80 mg/dL) • Spinal tumor causing mechanical obstruction (>100–2000 mg/dL) • Tuberculous (TB) meningitis • Hemorrhage • Multiple sclerosis
Decreased proteins in CSF seen in	• Tearing of duramater may result in leakage of CSF • Decreased dialysis from plasma • Removal of excess CSF
Glutamine in CSF	The levels of plasma ammonia and CSF glutamine are the indicators of hepatic encephalopathy (both are increased), where excess formation of glutamine takes place in brain

CSF in different types of meningitis

WBC (per micro L):	Normal CSF	Bacterial meningitis	Viral meningitis	TB meningitis
	<5	>1,000	25–500	25–500

Opening pressure	Normal	Bacterial	Viral	Fungal	Tubercular
	80–200 mm H_2O	Increased	Normal	Varies	Varies

Appearance	Normal	Bacterial	Viral	Fungal	Tubercular
	Clear	Cloudy	Clear	Varies	Coagulated

WBC	Normal	Bacterial	Viral	Fungal	Tubercular
	<5 cells/µL	>1,000 per µL	<100 per µL	Varies	Varies

Contd...

Contd...

Cell differential	Normal	Bacterial	Viral	Fungal	Tubercular
	No red cells, no neutrophils	High neutrophils	Many 100/μL, mainly mononuclear cells, high lymphocytes	Occasional mild high mononuclear cells, high lymphocytes	Mixed, mainly mononuclear high lymphocytes
Protein (g/dL)	Normal	Bacterial	Viral	Fungal	Tubercular
	0.15–0.1	Mild to marked increase	Normal to high	High	Mild to marked increase
Glucose	Normal	Bacterial	Viral	Fungal	Tubercular
	50–70% serum	Highly low	Normal mainly	Low	Low
Lactate (mmol/L) and other test	Normal	Bacterial	Viral	Fungal	Tubercular
	Lactate <2.1	Lactate >3.5 Gram positive stain	Lactate <2.1	–	Lactate >3.5 Ziehl–Neelson stain acid fast bacilli

OSCE

Q1. Discuss about the normal biochemical parameters of CSF?

Ans: *Appearance*: Clear/colorless
Protein: 15–45 mg/dL
Glucose: 50–80 mg/dL
Lactate: <2.0 mmol/L
Cells: 0–5 lymphocytes/μL
Chloride: 116–130 mmol/L

Q2. A patient has cloudy CSF with raised protein decreased glucose/neutrophilic pleocytosis. What is the probable diagnosis?

Ans: Acute bacterial meningitis.
Important findings:
High protein (>100 mg/dL).
Decreased glucose (<40 mg/dL or CSF: serum glucose ratio <0.4).
Neutrophilic pleocytosis (>1000 cells/μL).
Next step: Gram stain and culture for bacterial identification.

Q3. A patient presents with fever/CSF findings of lymphocytic pleocytosis/normal protein/normal glucose. What is the likely diagnosis?

Ans: Viral meningitis.
Important findings:
Lymphocytic pleocytosis (10–500 cells/μL).
Normal/slightly high protein (<100 mg/dL).
Normal glucose.
Next step: PCR for common viruses (e.g., enteroviruses, HSV).

Q4. A patient has xanthochromic CSF with raised protein (>150 mg/dL)/normal glucose. What could this suggest?

Ans: Possible causes:
Subarachnoid hemorrhage (SAH): Xanthochromia due to RBC lysis.
Guillain-Barré Syndrome (GBS): Elevated protein with normal glucose (albuminocytologic dissociation).
Next step:
For SAH: CT scan or CSF spectrophotometry.
For GBS: Electrophysiological studies.

Q5. How does tuberculous meningitis present in CSF analysis?

Ans: *Appearance*: Clear/mild turbid.
Protein: High (100–500 mg/dL).
Glucose: decreased (<45 mg/dL or CSF: serum glucose ratio <0.4).
Cells: Lymphocytic pleocytosis (50–300 cells/μL).
Chloride: low.
Next step: CSF AFB staining/GeneXpert/culture for Mycobacterium tuberculosis.

Q6. What does raise CSF lactate indicate?

Ans: *High lactate (>3.5 mmol/L) indicates*:
Bacterial meningitis because of anaerobic metabolism.
Hypoxic brain injury.
Mitochondrial disorders.
Rare malignancy in CSF.
Normal lactate in viral meningitis helps differentiate it from bacterial meningitis.

Q7. A patient with suspected fungal meningitis shows what CSF findings?

Ans: *Appearance*: Clear/mild cloudy.
Protein: High (>50 mg/dL).
Glucose: Decreased (<40 mg/dL).
Cells: Lymphocytic pleocytosis.
Specific test: CSF India ink/cryptococcal antigen test for Cryptococcus.

Q8. What is albuminocytologic dissociation, and where is it seen?

Ans: *Definition*: Elevated CSF protein (>45 mg/dL) with normal or low cell count (<10 cells/μL).
Observed in: Guillain-Barré syndrome/chronic inflammatory demyelinating polyneuropathy (CIDP).

Q9. What is the importance of oligoclonal bands in CSF?

Ans: Presence of oligoclonal bands is indicative of intrathecal IgG synthesis
Observed in: Multiple sclerosis/Neuroinfections, such as neurosyphilis/HIV encephalopathy/Autoimmune diseases, such as lupus cerebritis.
Test: Electrophoresis/isoelectric focusing.

Q10. How can traumatic tap be differentiated from subarachnoid hemorrhage?

Ans: *Traumatic tap*: RBC count decreased in sequentially collected tubes.
Supernatant is clear.
SAH: RBC count is constant.
Xanthochromia present/not clear.

CLINICAL MCQS

1. **A 37-year-old man presents with symptoms of headache/neck stiffness. CSF analysis: high protein/low glucose/elevated neutrophil count. What is the diagnosis?**
   a. Bacterial meningitis
   b. Meningitis
   c. Viral meningitis
   d. Tubercular meningitis

   Answer: a. Bacterial meningitis
2. **Which of the methods is usually used for estimating glucose levels in CSF?**
   a. Glucose oxidase-peroxidase method
   b. Jaffe's method
   c. Arsenazo method
   d. Glucokinase method

   Answer: a. Glucose oxidase-peroxidase method
3. **CSF sample: high opening pressure, elevated lymphocyte count, high protein, and very low glucose levels. Which is the condition?**
   a. Viral meningitis
   b. Tubercular meningitis

c. Meningitis
d. Guillain-Barré syndrome

Answer: b. Tubercular meningitis

4. **What is the normal reference range of glucose concentration in CSF in comparison to blood glucose levels?**
   a. 50–60% of blood glucose
   b. 75–80% of blood glucose
   c. Equal to blood glucose
   d. 25–30% of blood glucose

   Answer: a. 50–60% of blood glucose

5. **A 56-year-old man presents with headache/altered consciousness. CSF analysis: xanthochromia. What is the diagnosis?**
   a. Subarachnoid hemorrhage
   b. Fungal meningitis
   c. Viral meningitis
   d. Multiple sclerosis

   Answer: a. Subarachnoid hemorrhage

6. **A patient of multiple sclerosis goes for CSF analysis. Which of the following findings is suspected?**
   a. Oligoclonal bands
   b. Raised neutrophil count
   c. Low protein concentration
   d. High glucose levels

   Answer: a. Oligoclonal bands

7. **A 46-year-old patient comes with symmetric ascending paralysis. CSF analysis: high protein, normal glucose, normal cell count. What is the diagnosis?**
   a. Guillain-Barré syndrome
   b. Fungal meningitis
   c. Bacterial meningitis
   d. Viral meningitis

   Answer: a. Guillain-Barré syndrome

8. **Which of the enzymes is elevated in CSF of patients having bacterial meningitis?**
   a. Lactate dehydrogenase
   b. ACP
   c. Lipase
   d. GGT

   Answer: a. Lactate dehydrogenase

9. **A neonate presents with: fever, irritability. CSF analysis: glucose: 20 mg/dL (normal: 40–70 mg/dL), protein: 150 mg/dL (normal: 15–45 mg/dL), neutrophilic pleocytosis. What is the causative organism?**
   a. Escherichia coli
   b. Mycobacterium tuberculosis
   c. Herpes simplex
   d. Cryptococcus

   Answer: a. Escherichia coli

10. **A 65-year-old patient having fever, confusion goes for CSF analysis. CSF lactate: elevated. What is the clinical significance?**
    a. Suggests bacterial or fungal meningitis
    b. Indicates toxic etiology
    c. Confirms Guillain-Barré syndrome
    d. Suggests normal physiology

    Answer: a. Suggests bacterial or fungal meningitis

VIVA VOCE

Q1. What is the composition of CSF and how it is different from plasma?

CSF is a clear, colorless fluid which surrounds the brain/spinal cord.
It has water, electrolytes, such as sodium/chloride/potassium, glucose, protein, and a very low concentration of cells mainly lymphocytes.
It has low protein concentration, low glucose levels, and few/no cells compared to plasma.
The low protein content/absence of red blood cells in normal CSF differentiates it from plasma.

Q2. What does high white blood cell count in CSF suggest?

High white blood cell count/pleocytosis in the CSF typically suggests inflammation/infection of the CNS because of meningitis/encephalitis/multiple sclerosis. The differential count/percentage of different white blood cells may aid in differentiating between bacterial/viral/infections.
Neutrophils indicates bacterial infections.
Lymphocytes suggest viral/fungal infections.

Q3. What is the importance of low glucose level in CSF?

Bacterial meningitis where pathogens consume glucose decreasing its concentration. Normal CSF glucose levels are typically 60–70% of the plasma glucose concentration. Decreased glucose can also be seen for tuberculous meningitis/fungal infections/cancer affecting CNS.

Q4. Differentiate between viral/bacterial meningitis based on CSF analysis?

White blood cell count:
In bacterial meningitis, there is a raised neutrophil count commonly >1000 cells/μL.
In viral meningitis, the WBC is typically lower like 10–500 cells/μL with lymphocytes predominating.
Glucose levels:
In bacterial meningitis, glucose is reduced may be <40 mg/dL.
In viral meningitis, glucose levels are commonly normal (40–70 mg/dL).
Protein levels:
In bacterial meningitis, protein levels are generally high may be >100 mg/dL.
In viral meningitis, protein levels may be slightly high/normal.

Q5. What is the importance of CSF analysis in diagnoses of multiple sclerosis?

Oligoclonal bands: These bands can be detected by electrophoresis and are a hallmark of MS and suggest intrathecal antibody formation in the CNS.
Mildly high protein levels: Protein can be slightly high in some cases of MS.
Normal glucose/cell count: Glucose/cell count are normal in MS, aiding to differentiate it from infectious causes of CNS inflammation.

SPOTTERS

Q1. Show an image of clear, colorless CSF sample in a tube. What are the characteristics of a normal CSF sample?

Clear/colorless.
Low protein content/20-45 mg/dL, normal glucose levels/60-70% of plasma glucose/very few or no cells/usually <5 white blood cells/μL. The absence of red blood cells is normal, suggesting no recent hemorrhage.

Q2. Show an image of cloudy CSF sample in a test tube. What cloudy CSF indicate?

Infection/inflammation. The turbidity is because of white blood cells/pleocytosis/protein. It may indicate bacterial meningitis/tuberculous meningitis/fungal infections.

Q3. Show image of CSF sample with reddish color. Possible cause?

Xanthochromic CSF sample indicates presence of hemorrhage/subarachnoid/intraventricular. This color is because of hemoglobin/bilirubin in the fluid. The presence of blood may be due to trauma during lumbar puncture/from conditions, such as subarachnoid hemorrhage/intracranial hemorrhage.

Q4. Show an image of CSF electrophoresis with oligoclonal bands. Significance of presence of oligoclonal bands in CSF?

Multiple sclerosis where the bands suggest intrathecal antibody formation/are considered a diagnostic hallmark for MS.

Q5. Show a scenario of CSF with markedly increased white blood cell count/predominantly neutrophils/low glucose. Interpret this CSF profile?

Bacterial meningitis may be suggested which lead to significant inflammation in the CSF, resulting in increased white blood cell count, low glucose due to consumption by bacteria, and high protein levels.

REFLECTION

Describe the clinical significance of sugar, chlorides and proteins in CSF.

21 CHAPTER

Electrophoresis of Serum Proteins

COMPETENCY

BC14.18: Observe use of commonly used equipments/techniques in biochemistry laboratory including: Protein electrophoresis, TLC, PAGE.

LEARNING OBJECTIVES

After reading this chapter, the readers should be able to:
- Describe the principle and applications of electrophoresis.
- Describe the separation of serum proteins by Agarose gel electrophoresis along with its applications.

BLUE PRINT

Observe use of Commonly used Equipments/Techniques in Biochemistry Laboratory including: Protein Electrophoresis, TLC, PAGE

Objective

By the end of the lecture, students should be able to:
1. Understand the principles and applications of various commonly used equipments and techniques in biochemistry laboratory.
2. Familiarize themselves with the operation and maintenance of laboratory instruments.
3. Gain practical knowledge of performing biochemical assays and analyses.
4. Learn about quality control measures to ensure accurate and reliable laboratory results.

Duration: ***90 minutes***

Materials Needed

1. Presentation slides illustrating each equipment and technique.
2. Demonstration models or actual laboratory instruments for hands-on learning.
3. Samples or reagents required for practical demonstrations.
4. Whiteboard or flipchart for interactive discussions and note-taking.

Outline

I. **Introduction to biochemistry laboratory techniques** **(10 minutes)**
- Overview of the role of biochemistry laboratory in biomedical research and clinical diagnostics.
- Importance of accurate and reliable laboratory techniques in biochemical analysis.

II. **Protein electrophoresis** **(50 minutes)**
- Overview of protein electrophoresis principles and gel electrophoresis techniques.
- Demonstration of protein separation by SDS-PAGE or agarose gel electrophoresis.

III. **Thin layer chromatography (TLC) and polyacrylamide gel electrophoresis (PAGE)** **(30 minutes)**
- Introduction to TLC and PAGE techniques for analyzing biomolecules.
- Practical demonstration of sample application, development, and visualization.

Objective	Separation of serum proteins by agarose gel electrophoresis			
Definition of electrophoresis	• Migration of charged particles in an electric field • Negative ions migrate toward anode and vice versa • Proteins become negatively charged in basic solution so will move towards the anode • In case the connections become wrong, they can move in the opposite direction and the length of the gel will not be enough for full and proper separation			
Factors on which the migration in electric field depends	Ion charge (high ion strength decreases the migration)	Size of the charged particle (large size decreases the migration)	pH of the medium	Electric field strength

Normally bands observed starting farthest from the origin

Bands	Their fractions	Their normal%
Albumin	3.5–5.5 g/dL	55–70% of the total
Alpha-1 globulin	0.1–0.4 g/dL	1.5–5.5% of the total
Alpha-2 globulin	0.4–0.8 g/dL	6–10% of the total
Beta globulin	0.5–1.2 g/dL	8–15% of the total
Gamma globulin	0.7–1.5 g/dL	2–20% of the total
When we use plasma and not serum, we get an extra band	Added band in beta globulin—fibrinogen	
Other uses of electrophoresis	• Separation of isoenzymes—PAGE is done where isoenzymes are separated by vertical disc gel and horizontal slide gel • Separation of lipoproteins	
Examples of various globulins	Alpha-1 globulin	Alpha-1 antitrypsin
	Alpha-2 globulin	Ceruloplasmin
	Beta globulin	Transferrin, fibrinogen
	Gamma globulin	Immunoglobulins

Types of electrophoresis

1. Horizontal	
2. Vertical	
3. Agarose gel (with different molecular sizes)	• Separation is faster and good • Agarose is made of agarobiose which is made of D galactose and 3,6-Anhydro-L-galactose
4. Polyacrylamide gel (act as molecular sieves decreasing the movement of large particles)	• The support media is polyacrylamide which is made of acrylamide and methylene bis acrylamide as the cross-linking support • Different pore sizes are available based on different concentrations of acrylamide and BIS
5. Capillary	Made of fused silica
6. SDS-PAGE (sodium dodecyl sulfate—PAGE)	
7. Two dimensional	

LOG ACTIVITY

Separation of serum proteins by agarose gel

Reagents needed	• 1% agarose gel • Barbitone sodium acetate buffer pH 8.6 • Amino black 10B stain • Acetone to fix the solution • 2% glacial acetic acid to destain

Contd....

Contd....

Method	
1. Slide preparation	• Prepare a homogenous mixture of 200 mg pure agarose in 20 mL buffer by boiling in water bath • Keep 5 slides on a glass plate • Now pour 2.5 mL of gel on each slide and spread uniformly with the help of a warmed delivery pipette • The gel gets set, then store in a moist Petri dish covered with a filter paper
2. Sample loading	• Take 2 slides and make a well of 5 mm at one end of both the slides 1 cm away from the margin • Wipe the excess fluid with a filter paper from the wells • Put 5 μL serum samples in the well of both the slides by a micropipette
3. Electrophoresis run	• Fill the buffer in 2 compartments of the electrophoresis chamber • Place the bridge in the electrophoresis chamber and cover with the layer of filter paper soaked in buffer • Now keep the slides inverted on the bridge and cover the chamber by the lid • Connect the electrode on the side of the slide having the sample well to the cathode and other electrode to the anode of the power supply • Current setting is 7 ampere/slide for 45 minutes, after which remove the slides
Slide staining	• Put the slides in fixing solution for 15 minutes • Now put the slides in staining solution for 2 minutes, after which some bands are seen • Wash the extra stain by destaining solution for few minutes • Dry the slides at room temperature for 12 hours and scan the slides with a densitometer and quantitate the various bands
Principle	• In alkaline pH of 8.6 the proteins will migrate towards the anode when arranged an electric field • Because of different mobility based on charge to size ratio, the various proteins are separated during the migration
Clinical interpretation	
Multiple myeloma	• Use the serum and urine of the patient • There are malignant changes in a single plasma cell which forms a clone of identical cells • These cell form monoclonal antibodies that forms a sharp and intense band known as M band in the region of gamma globulin • This M band protein is generally IgG in 60% cases and also IgA • There is excess formation of light chains of immunoglobulins by the malignant plasma cells which start get excreting out in urine as Bence-Jones proteins • Same band is seen for urine sample also • They get precipitated when we heat the urine to 50–60°C, get dissolved on boiling the urine, and reappear back on cooling • Multiple myeloma is type of monoclonal gammopathy where a sharp, intense and good defined M band is formed
Total protein in multiple myeloma	10–12 g/dL (increased)
Globulin in multiple myeloma	4–10 g/dL (increased)
Albumin in multiple myeloma	Low – 2 g/dL
Polyclonal gammopathy	Generalized increase in IgG of different types formed by various clones of plasma cells, forming a diffused band in the gamma globulin region
Alpha-1 antitrypsin deficiency: (antiprotease that can hydrolyze elastin)	Observed in emphysema Here alpha 1 band is decreased/absent
Cirrhosis	Less albumin formation so its peak is low along with low alpha and beta bands also
Acute inflammation	Here there is formation of acute phase proteins, such as CRP, haptoglobin, ceruloplasmin, they belong to alpha 1 and alpha 2 bands so these bands get increased
Congenital hypogammaglobulinemia	Here there is decreased level of globulins that are observed as gamma band so they can be seen as less dense band with small peak
Chronic inflammation	Because of increased globulin formation, there is a band which looks like polyclonal gammopathy

OSPE

1. **Explain the principle of serum protein electrophoresis?**
   Serum proteins are separated on the basis of their charge/size in an electric field.
   Proteins are distributed in five regions:
   1. *Albumin*: Largest peak/migrates fastest.
   2. *α1-globulin*: α1-antitrypsin.
   3. *α2-globulin*: Haptoglobin/ceruloplasmin.
   4. *β-globulin*: Transferrin/C3 complement.
   5. *γ-globulin*: Immunoglobulins that is IgG/IgA/IgM.
2. **A patient's SPEP exhibits monoclonal spike in the γ-globulin region. What is the probable diagnosis?**
   Multiple myeloma.
   Important findings:
   Monoclonal protein M spike in γ-globulin region.
   Might have raised total protein with less albumin/reversed A:G ratio.
   Confirmation: Serum immunofixation electrophoresis for identifying specific immunoglobulin/Free light chain assay.
3. **How does SPEP looks like in nephrotic syndrome?**
   Important findings:
   Markedly low albumin peak.
   Elevated α2-globulin because of haptoglobin/macroglobulin.
   Normal/decreased γ-globulin levels.
   Explanation: Loss of albumin along with immunoglobulins via urine and there is a compensatory formation of α2-macroglobulin.
4. **What changes can be observed in SPEP in chronic inflammation?**
   Important findings:
   Low albumin because of negative acute-phase reaction.
   Elevated α1-globulin like α1-antitrypsin.
   Elevated α2-globulin like haptoglobin or ceruloplasmin.
   Polyclonal rise in the γ-globulin region because of chronic immune activation.
5. **A patient has a broad-based rise in the γ-globulin region. What does this interpret?**
   Polyclonal gammopathy.
   Observed for: Chronic infections like tuberculosis/HIV.
   Autoimmune diseases, such as rheumatoid arthritis or systemic lupus erythematosus
   Chronic liver diseases, such as cirrhosis.
   Differentiation: Unlike monoclonal gammopathy, polyclonal gammopathy exhibits broad-based elevation and not a sharp spike.
6. **What are the characteristic SPEP findings in liver cirrhosis?**
   Important findings:
   Low albumin.
   Polyclonal rise in γ-globulin that is β-γ bridging because of IgA raise.
   Low α1-globulin/α2-globulin.
7. **How does SPEP help in diagnosing α1-antitrypsin deficiency?**
   Important findings:
   Low/absent α1-globulin band.
   Confirmatory test: Serum α1-antitrypsin concentration/genetic testing for SERPINA1 mutations.
8. **In what conditions is an increased β-globulin region seen on SPEP?**
   Important causes:
   Hyperlipidemia: High β-lipoproteins (LDL).
   Iron deficiency anemia: High transferrin.
   Multiple myeloma: β-globulin spike may be seen with monoclonal proteins.
9. **A patient's SPEP shows hypogammaglobulinemia. What conditions can this indicate?**
   Primary immunodeficiency disorders: Common variable immunodeficiency/X-linked agammaglobulinemia.
   Secondary causes: Immunosuppressive therapy.
   Nephrotic syndrome that is loss of immunoglobulins in urine.
   Protein-losing enteropathy.
10. **What are the findings on SPEP in Waldenström's macroglobulinemia?**
    Important findings:
    Monoclonal spike in the γ-globulin region generally IgM.

High serum viscosity
Differentiation from multiple myeloma: IgM monoclonal protein along with no lytic bone lesions.

11. **How is SPEP useful in amyloidosis?**
Important findings:
Monoclonal protein that is light chains that can be κ or λ.
Might exhibit low albumin.
Further assay: Serum free light chain test/tissue biopsy along with Congo red stain for amyloid deposition.

12. **How is SPEP interpreted in acute phase response?**
Important findings:
Low albumin/negative acute-phase reactant.
Elevated α1-globulin/α1-antitrypsin.
Elevated α2-globulin/haptoglobin/ceruloplasmin.
Normal/slightly low γ-globulin.

CLINICAL MCQS

1. **A 67-year-old man comes with complains of bone pain/frequent infections, serum protein electrophoresis: sharp M spike in gamma region. What is the likely diagnosis?**
   a. Multiple myeloma
   b. Macroglobulinemia
   c. Lymphocytic leukemia
   d. Amyloidosis

   Answer: a. Multiple myeloma

2. **Which of these is the key principle of serum protein electrophoresis?**
   a. Separation of proteins on basis of molecular weight
   b. Separation of proteins on basis of charge and size
   c. Detection of complexes
   d. Quantification of total protein

   Answer: b. Separation of proteins on basis of charge and size

3. **Which protein fraction migrates closest to the anode in serum protein electrophoresis?**
   a. Albumin
   b. Alpha globulins
   c. Beta globulins
   d. Gamma globulins

   Answer: a. Albumin

4. **A 56-year-old woman presents with nephrotic syndrome and takes up serum protein electrophoresis. Which of the following findings is suspected?**
   a. Low albumin/increased alpha-2 globulin
   b. Low gamma globulin/high albumin
   c. High beta globulin/normal albumin
   d. Low alpha-1 globulin/high gamma globulin

   Answer: a. Low albumin/increased alpha-2 globulin

5. **A patient having liver cirrhosis exhibits beta-gamma bridging pattern. What is the likely underlying reason?**
   a. Polyclonal gammopathy
   b. Gammopathy
   c. Hypoalbuminemia
   d. Nephrotic syndrome

   Answer: a. Polyclonal gammopathy

6. **Which condition is linked with a decreased alpha-1 globulin fraction?**
   a. Alpha-1 antitrypsin deficiency
   b. Multiple myeloma
   c. Acute inflammation
   d. Acute liver disorder

   Answer: a. Alpha-1 antitrypsin deficiency

7. **A 78-year-old man presents with chronic inflammation/high alpha-2 globulins. What is the most suspected protein that is responsible for the rise?**
   a. Haptoglobin
   b. Globulin
   c. IgM
   d. CRP

   Answer: a. Haptoglobin

8. **A monoclonal gammopathy is characterized by?**
   a. Broad-based rise in the gamma region
   b. Sharp and narrow band in gamma region
   c. Low albumin with high alpha-2 globulins
   d. Normal electrophoretic pattern

   Answer: b. Sharp and narrow band in gamma region

9. **A 62-year-old patient presents with multiple myeloma, and a sharp monoclonal spike in the gamma region. Which technique confirms the identity of the monoclonal protein?**
   a. Immunofixation electrophoresis
   b. Colorimetry
   c. Southern blot
   d. Western blot

   Answer: a. Immunofixation electrophoresis

10. **A 66-year-old patient with CKD takes up serum protein electrophoresis. Which of the following findings is most likely?**
    a. Decreased albumin and increased beta globulin
    b. Elevated alpha-1 and alpha-2 globulins
    c. Low gamma globulin and increased albumin
    d. Abnormal electrophoretic pattern

    Answer: a. Decreased albumin and increased beta globulin

VIVA VOCE

Q1. What is the principle of electrophoresis, and how is it used to separate serum proteins?

Q2. Explain the significance of the different bands observed in serum protein electrophoresis.

Q3. What is the significance of the albumin to globulin ratio (A/G ratio) in serum protein electrophoresis?

Q4. What could cause an abnormal increase in gamma globulins in serum protein electrophoresis?

Q5. Why is it important to interpret serum protein electrophoresis in conjunction with the patient's clinical history and other laboratory tests?

SPOTTERS

Q1. Image: A serum protein electrophoresis gel with distinct bands for albumin, alpha-1 globulins, alpha-2 globulins, beta globulins, and gamma globulins. What does these bands represent?

They show separation of serum proteins based on their charge and size:
Albumin: The largest/most negatively charged, migrating the furthest towards the positive electrode.
Alpha-1 globulins: A group of proteins which migrate just behind albumin.
Alpha-2 globulins: Further down, before the beta globulins.
Beta globulins: Including proteins such as transferrin.
Gamma globulins: The slowest-migrating proteins, having immunoglobulins/antibodies.

Q2. Scenario: A serum sample with increased band intensity in gamma region. Give the potential cause of an increased gamma globulin band?

Increased band in the gamma region indicates high concentration of immunoglobulins which can be because of chronic inflammation/autoimmune diseases/monoclonal gammopathies like multiple myeloma/Waldenström's macroglobulinemia.

Q3. Image: A serum protein electrophoresis pattern with reduced albumin band and increased alpha-2 globulin band. Cause of such pattern?

Decreased albumin band while increased alpha-2 globulin band indicates nephrotic syndrome/liver disease. Decreased albumin suggests loss of proteins and increase in alpha-2 globulins may suggest acute phase response like during inflammation/infection.

Q4. Scenario: Monoclonal band in the gamma region. Significance of a monoclonal band?

M spike in the gamma region indicates monoclonal gammopathy, mainly observed for multiple myeloma/Waldenström's macroglobulinemia. This suggests the over formation of a single type of immunoglobulin/M protein by the plasma cells.

Q5. Image: Abnormal pattern with a broad gamma region. Cause of broadening of the gamma region?

Broadening of the gamma region may be suggestive of polyclonal gammopathy, that is seen in chronic infection/autoimmune diseases/liver disease. It reflects the over formation of multiple different immunoglobulins, in contrast to sharp monoclonal band observed for monoclonal gammopathy.

REFLECTION

Observations, results and comments.

22

CHAPTER

Estimation of Serum Electrolytes by Ion Selective Electrodes

COMPETENCY

BC14.18: Observe use of commonly used equipments/techniques in biochemistry laboratory including: Electrolyte analysis by ISE.

LEARNING OBJECTIVES

After reading this chapter, the readers should be able to:

- Describe the basis of ISE in measurement of electrolytes and their clinical significance.
- Describe the use of serum electrolyte measurement by this process.

BLUE PRINT

Estimation of Serum Electrolytes by Ion Selective Electrodes

Objective

By the end of the lecture, students should be able to:

1. Understand the principles and applications of various commonly used equipments and techniques in biochemistry laboratory.
2. Familiarize themselves with the operation and maintenance of laboratory instruments.
3. Gain practical knowledge of performing biochemical assays and analyses.
4. Learn about quality control measures to ensure accurate and reliable laboratory results.

Duration: ***60 minutes***

Materials Needed

1. Presentation slides illustrating each equipment and technique.
2. Demonstration models or actual laboratory instruments for hands-on learning.
3. Samples or reagents required for practical demonstrations.
4. Whiteboard or flipchart for interactive discussions and note-taking.

Outline

I. **Introduction to biochemistry laboratory techniques** **(10 minutes)**
- Overview of the role of biochemistry laboratory in biomedical research and clinical diagnostics.
- Importance of accurate and reliable laboratory techniques in biochemical analysis.

II. **Electrolyte analysis by ion-selective electrode (ISE)** **(50 minutes)**
- Explanation of ISE principles and applications in electrolyte analysis.
- Demonstration of electrolyte measurement using ISE instrument.

Objective	Demonstrate the measurement of serum electrolytes by ion selective electrode analyzer
Serum electrolytes	Na^+, K^+, Cl^-, Ca^{++}, Mg^{++}, HCO_3, lactate in the blood
Their estimation is important for assessing functions, such as:	• Acid base balance • Maintaining volume of fluid in various compartments • Maintenance of osmolality • Nerve impulse transmission • Muscle contraction
Ion selective electrodes	These electrodes consist of a glass membrane having a particular/specific permeability to one ion, rather than the other ion
Composition of glass membrane	Main component is silicon dioxide (SiO_2) Other components are calcium oxide (CaO), sodium oxide (Na_2O), aluminum trioxide (Al_2O_3)
How ion selectivity is created:	By varying the above stated composition, like by increasing the ion selectivity to sodium or by increasing the Al_2O_3 with respect to Na_2O and if we want to increase ion selectivity to K^+, we can increase $Na_2O > Al_2O_3$
Types of ion selective electrode	**Membrane** **Liquid** **Solid**
Principle: (same as that of H^+ specific electrode)	• The movement of only one specific ion is allowed by ion selective electrodes • Solid state electrodes are very common, made from materials, such as carboxylated polyvinyl chloride or indium tin oxide • There is a particular ionophore on the membrane for making it ion sensitive, such as sodium ionophore is put on the membrane for making it sodium specific • This system is then attached to an internal potential measuring electrode • The above system is then connected to a reference electrode • When a sample of different sodium concentration comes in contact with the electrode, the movement of specific ion takes place across the membrane which has ionophore and the sample • Because of the activity the specific ion there is development of an equilibrium potential at the membrane • This potential is finally measured by internal electrode
Potential (E)	$= EO \times 0.0591 \times \log Ax$ Here EO = constant for electrode Ax = ion activity 59.1 Mv
Method	• They are fully automated and should be calibrated daily • The sample is fed into the instrument • A timed inlet capillary takes in the needed sample • Processing takes place and printer gives the final result • Internal standards are present and are readymade, normally 2 standards (one high and one low) are used for fixed concentration of analyte for calibration

Standard	**A**	**B**
Sodium	150 mmol/L	100 mmol/L
Potassium	5 mmol/L	1.8 mmol/L
Chloride	115 mmol/L	72 mmol/L

Precautions	• Clear sample is used, it should not be hemolyzed • No suspended particle should be present in the sample • For collection, red vial with no anticoagulant is used • If plasma is taken, then instead of oxalate, heparin should be used • Instrument should be properly maintained with appropriate instructions

Clinical interpretation

Normal ranges:

Na^+	135–145 mEq/L
K^+	3.6–5.4 mEq/L
Cl^-	96–106 mEq/L

Contd....

Contd....

Hyponatremia	**Causes** • Heat exhaustion • Burns • Diarrhea • Vomiting • Repeated gastric aspiration • Addison's disease
Hypernatremia	**Causes** • Repeated corticosteroid therapy • Diabetic ketoacidosis • Cushing's syndrome • Conn's syndrome/primary aldosteronism due to excess aldosterone because of adrenal hyperplasia, carcinoma or Cushing's syndrome
Hypokalemia	**Causes** • Diarrhea • Cushing's syndrome • Primary aldosteronism
Hyperkalemia	**Causes** • Renal failure • Diabetic coma • Addison's disease • Dehydration
Serious effects of hyperkalemia	**Arrhythmia** • Tachycardia • Ventricular fibrillation • Diastolic cardiac arrest

OSCE

1. **Scenario: Hyponatremia**
   Case: A patient shows with seizures. Serum sodium: 125 mEq/L.
   Causes: SIADH, fluid overload like CHF/cirrhosis/renal failure/thiazide diuretics.
   Interpretation: Hyponatremia is linked with water retention/focus on hypovolemic/euvolemic/hypervolemic to confirm.
2. **Scenario: Hypernatremia**
   Case: A 71-year-old with altered mental status presents with serum sodium of 157 mEq/L.
   Significance: Hypernatremia indicative of water deficit.
   Causes: Improper intake of water/diabetes insipidus/osmotic diuresis.
   Management: Hypotonic fluids for preventing cerebral edema.
3. **Scenario: Hypokalemia**
   Case: A patient presents with muscular weakness/ECG shows U waves and serum potassium: 2.9 mEq/L.
   Causes: Vomiting/diarrhea/diuretics/hyperaldosteronism.
   Treatment: Oral/IV potassium replacement.
4. **Scenario: Hyperkalemia**
   Case: A patient on ACE inhibitors shows with fatigue/ECG shows peaked T wave and serum potassium: 6.2 mEq/L.
   Interpretation: Decreased renal excretion/cell lysis like hemolysis or rhabdomyolysis.
   Management: Calcium gluconate that is cardioprotective/insulin with glucose/dialysis
5. **Scenario: Hypocalcemia**
   Case: A postthyroidectomy patient shows with tetany/positive Chvostek sign and serum calcium: 6 mg/dL.
   Causes: Hypoparathyroidism/vitamin D deficiency/chronic renal disease.
   Interpretation: Hypocalcemia results in neuromuscular irritability.
   Management: Correction of calcium/focus parathyroid hormone.
6. **Scenario: Hypercalcemia**
   Case: A 56-year-old with bone pain/serum calcium: 12.9 mg/dL.
   Causes: Primary hyperparathyroidism/malignancy like multiple myeloma/vitamin D toxication.
   Next steps: PTH assay/25(OH)D assay rule out malignancy.

7. **Scenario: Metabolic acidosis with anion gap**
Case: A diabetic patient with Kussmaul respiration: Na^+ 140, Cl^- 104, HCO_3^- 12.
Calculation: Anion gap = $Na^+ - (Cl^- + HCO_3^-) = 140 - (104 + 12) = 24$.
Interpretation: High anion gap suggestive of lactic acidosis/renal failure.

8. **Scenario: Hypomagnesemia**
Case: A chronic alcoholic presents with seizures and serum magnesium: 1.0 mg/dL.
Causes: Poor diet/GI loss/diuretics.
Management: IV magnesium replacement/focus coexisting hypocalcemia/hypokalemia.

CLINICAL MCQS

1. **A 71-year-old man presents with confusion/serum sodium: 120 mmol/L (normal: 135–145 mmol/L). Which condition is present?**
a. Hypoaldosteronism
b. Syndrome of inappropriate antidiuretic hormone (SIADH)
c. Diabetes mellitus
d. Hypocalcemia
Answer: b. Syndrome of inappropriate antidiuretic hormone (SIADH)

2. **Which method is commonly used for the assay of serum electrolytes?**
a. Colorimetry
b. Flame photometry
c. Ion-selective electrode method
d. Spectrophotometry
Answer: c. Ion-selective electrode method

3. **A patient with CKD has serum potassium: 6.5 mmol/L (normal: 3.5–5.0 mmol/L). Which ECG finding is linked with hyperkalaemia?**
a. U waves
b. Tall peaked T waves
c. Prolonged PR interval
d. ST-segment depression
Answer: b. Tall peaked T waves

4. **A 57-year-old woman complains of carpopedal spasms and serum calcium: 7.0 mg/dL (normal: 8.5–10.5 mg/dL). What is the reason?**
a. Hyperkalaemia
b. Hypoparathyroidism
c. Hypocalcaemia
d. Hypomagnesemia
Answer: c. Hypocalcaemia

5. **A 75-year-old diabetic patient complains of metabolic acidosis/serum anion gap: 21 mEq/L (normal: 8–12 mEq/L). Which condition can be suspected?**
a. Diabetic ketoacidosis
b. Diarrhea
c. Renal tubular acidosis
d. Hyperalbuminemia
Answer: a. Diabetic ketoacidosis

6. **A 31-year-old man presents with paralysis and serum potassium: 2.0 mmol/L. Which condition is the most likely cause?**
a. Hypocalcemia
b. Loop diuretic use
c. Malignancy
d. Tumor lysis syndrome
Answer: b. Loop diuretic use

7. **A patient complains of seizures and serum sodium: 156 mmol/L. What is the underlying condition?**
a. SIADH
b. Dehydration

c. Adrenal overactivity
d. Overhydration

Answer: b. Dehydration

8. **Which of these is a common reason behind hypermagnesemia?**
   a. Chronic kidney disease
   b. Vomiting
   c. Hyperparathyroidism
   d. Diuretics

   Answer: a. Chronic kidney disease

9. **A patient presents with severe diarrhea low serum bicarbonate, potassium. What is the acid-base disturbance?**
   a. Alkalosis
   b. Renal acidosis
   c. Metabolic acidosis
   d. Mixed acidosis

   Answer: c. Metabolic acidosis

10. **A 59-year-old woman with a history of chronic alcoholism complains of changed mental status. Serum magnesium: 0.8 mg/dL (normal: 1.7–2.2 mg/dL). What complication can be linked with this situation of electrolyte disorder?**
    a. Hyperparathyroidism
    b. Cardiac arrhythmias
    c. Osteomalacia
    d. Renal stones

    Answer: b. Cardiac arrhythmias

VIVA VOCE

Q1. What is the principle of ion-selective electrodes?
Selective ion interaction, where electrode is designed to be sensitive to a specific ion like sodium/potassium/chloride. When a sample is introduced, the electrode measures voltage between the ISE and a reference electrode which is directly proportional to the concentration of the specific ion in the sample, allowing for its quantification.

Q2. Mention advantages of ion-selective electrodes for electrolyte estimation?
ISEs are selective for specific ions and give accurate/direct measurements without interference from other ions.
Minimum sample volume
Quick results
Continuous monitoring

Q3. How a potassium ISE measure the concentration of potassium in serum?
Potassium ISE is made with a membrane that is selective for potassium ions. When serum is kept in contact with the electrode, potassium ions interact with the membrane, and generate potential difference which is measured by electrode and, by using a calibration curve we can get concentration of potassium ions in the sample. It is based on the Nernst equation, that relates ion concentration to the measured potential.

Q4. What are the components of an ion-selective electrode system?
Ion-selective membrane: This interacts with the target ion.
Internal reference solution: Has stable reference ion concentration for maintaining a constant potential.
Reference electrode: Stable electrode which measures potential difference between the ISE/sample.
Signal amplifier/readout system: Converts potential difference into voltage, displays the corresponding ion concentration.

Q5. What factors affect the accuracy of electrolyte estimation?
Interference from other ions, temperature variations, calibration errors, contamination, electrode condition

SPOTTERS

Q1. Show an image: A sodium ion-selective electrode connected to a serum sample. Give the principle of operation of this sodium ISE?

It is a sodium ion-selective electrode which measures the concentration of sodium ions in the serum sample. The electrode has a membrane that is selectively permeable to sodium ions/it generates a potential difference in response to the concentration of sodium ions in the sample. The voltage is finally measured and linked and correlated to the sodium concentration.

Q2. Show a scenario: A lab technician is doing potassium measurement using an ISE, and the electrode has been calibrated with standard potassium solutions. What is the need to calibrate?

Calibration ensures that the ion-selective electrode responds accurately to the target ion here potassium within the range of expected concentrations. It creates relationship between the measured potential and the actual ion concentration, thus improving accuracy and precision.

Q3. Show an image of graph exhibiting relationship between the voltage measured by an ion-selective electrode and the concentration of specific ion in serum. What does the graph show?

It represents calibration curve of the ion-selective electrode. It reflects linear relationship between the measured voltage and the ion concentration. By measuring the potential from a serum sample, we can use the calibration curve to interpolate/calculate the ion concentration.

Q4. Show a scenario: During the analysis, a serum sample exhibits high chloride concentration. Explain potential reasons of high chloride levels in the serum?

Elevated chloride levels are observed in hyperchloremia, that may be due to dehydration/kidney dysfunction/more consumption of saline solutions. High chloride may affect acid-base balance/metabolic acidosis.

Q5. Show scenario: After measuring sodium and potassium by ion-selective electrodes, the technician sees that there is abnormally low potassium level in the serum sample. What factors can lead to inaccurate measurement?

Electrode contamination, improper calibration, sample interference, temperature fluctuations.

REFLECTION

Describe the basis of ISE in measurement of electrolytes and their clinical significance. Describe the use of serum electrolyte measurement by this process.

23

CHAPTER

Enzyme-linked Immunosorbent Assay (ELISA)

COMPETENCY

BC14.18: Observe use of commonly used equipments/techniques in biochemistry laboratory including: ELISA.

LEARNING OBJECTIVES

After reading this chapter, the readers should be able to:
- Describe the principle, types and applications of ELISA.
- Describe the estimation of serum hCG level by sandwich ELISA along with the interpretation of the results.

BLUE PRINT

Observe use of commonly used equipments/techniques in biochemistry laboratory including: ELISA

Commonly Used Equipments/Techniques in Biochemistry Laboratory

Objective

By the end of the lecture, students should be able to:

1. Understand the principles and applications of various commonly used equipments and techniques in biochemistry laboratory.
2. Familiarize themselves with the operation and maintenance of laboratory instruments.
3. Gain practical knowledge of performing biochemical assays and analyses.
4. Learn about quality control measures to ensure accurate and reliable laboratory results.

Duration: *60 minutes*

Materials Needed

1. Presentation slides illustrating each equipment and technique.
2. Demonstration models or actual laboratory instruments for hands-on learning.
3. Samples or reagents required for practical demonstrations.
4. Whiteboard or flipchart for interactive discussions and note-taking.

Outline

I. **Introduction to biochemistry laboratory techniques** **(10 minutes)**
   - Overview of the role of biochemistry laboratory in biomedical research and clinical diagnostics.
   - Importance of accurate and reliable laboratory techniques in biochemical analysis.

II. **Enzyme-linked immunosorbent assay (ELISA)** **(50 minutes)**
   - Introduction to ELISA technique for quantifying antigens or antibodies.
   - Demonstration of ELISA procedure including plate coating, incubation, and detection.

BLUE PRINT

BI2.6: Use of enzymes in laboratory investigations (enzyme-based assays).

Exploring Enzyme-based Assays in Laboratory Investigations

Objective

By the end of the lecture, students should be able to:

1. Understand the principles of enzyme-based assays.
2. Describe common enzyme-based assays used in laboratory investigations.
3. Explain the applications and limitations of enzyme-based assays in various fields.

Duration: *90 minutes*

Materials Needed

1. PowerPoint presentation or visual aids
2. Whiteboard and markers
3. Handouts with key points and diagrams
4. Examples of enzyme-based assay protocols (optional)

Outline

I. **Introduction to enzyme-based assays** **(10 minutes)**
- Brief overview of the lecture's objectives and agenda.
- Explanation of the principles underlying enzyme-based assays.

II. **Principles of enzyme-based assays** **(20 minutes)**
- Overview of the basic principles of enzyme-substrate interactions.
- Discussion on how enzyme activity can be measured quantitatively in laboratory settings.
- Explanation of the factors influencing enzyme assays, including temperature, pH, and substrate concentration.

III. **Common enzyme-based assays** **(40 minutes)**
- Description of common enzyme-based assays used in laboratory investigations, including:
  - Enzyme-linked Immunosorbent assay (ELISA) for detecting antigens or antibodies.
  - Enzyme activity assays for quantifying specific enzyme activity levels.
  - Enzyme immunoassays (EIA) for detecting and quantifying molecules in biological samples.
- Explanation of the procedures involved in each assay and their applications in research and diagnostics.

IV. **Applications and limitations** **(15 minutes)**
- Discussion on the applications of enzyme-based assays in various fields, including clinical diagnostics, drug discovery, and environmental monitoring.
- Explanation of the limitations and challenges associated with enzyme-based assays, such as assay sensitivity, specificity, and interference.

V. **Case studies and examples** **(5 minutes)**
- Presentation of case studies or examples illustrating the use of enzyme-based assays in real-world scenarios.
- Discussion on the interpretation of assay results and their implications in research or clinical practice.

VI. **Conclusion and recap** **(10 minutes)**
- Summary of key points covered in the lecture.
- Emphasis on the importance of enzyme-based assays in laboratory investigations.
- Encouragement for further exploration of enzyme assay techniques and applications.

Objective	Estimation of serum human chorionic gonadotrophin hormone level by ELISA
Human chorionic gonadotropin (hCG)	Glycoprotein of weight 40 kD secreted by placenta required for maintaining normal pregnancy, made of 2 subunits called alpha and beta
Significance	• After fertilization it starts rising after 10 days • It reaches maximum by the end of 12 weeks of pregnancy (50,000–1,50,000 mIU/L) • Then it starts decreasing to around 20,000 mIU/L and remains at this level throughout the pregnancy
Clinical variation	Abnormally excess levels are found in chorionic tumors

Contd....

Contd....

Principle of ELISA	• Based on the principle of antigen-antibody interaction • Required for qualitative and quantitative estimations • Sensitive and comfortable operation • A solid plastic plate has micro well on it • Either antigen or antibody gets bound to these micro wells • If the antibodies get bound to the plate then start the antigen antibody reaction by adding antigen • If the antigen get bound to the plate then start the antigen antibody reaction by adding antibodies
To detect the antigen-antibody reaction	Couple this reaction by a colored reaction
Colored reaction	• A substrate and enzyme are mixed to form a color, the intensity of which is proportional to the antigen antibody reaction • The color in all the wells is read out by ELISA reader
Result	Plot a standard curve for the parameter to be detected and then result of unknown sample is calculated from the curve
Types of ELISA	Two types, Indirect and sandwich
1. Indirect	• Antigen is bound to the plate • This antigen reacts with antibody A1
Color reaction	• The A1 binding is indirectly detected by another antibody A2 • A2 binds to A1 • It is tagged with enzyme peroxidase • A2 is detected after adding substrate of the enzyme peroxidase • The color formed is measured
2. Sandwich ELISA	• Antigen gets sandwiched between 2 antibodies, A1 and A2 • A1 and A2 binds with same antigen but at different sites • Color forms after binding of A2 and is measured for final result

LOG ACTIVITY

Estimation of hCG by ELISA	• hCG (antigen) is sandwiched by two monoclonal antibodies A1 and A2 • A1 is bound to one binding site of hCG antigen and A2 binds with another binding site on hCG antigen • The second antibody A2 is tagged with peroxidase enzyme–horseradish peroxidase (HRP) • The wells of ELISA plate are coated with antibody A1 • After adding serum, antigen hCG present in serum binds to the antibody A1 • Then antibody A2 tagged with HRP is added along with substrate of HRP • Excess of/unbound hCG/A1/A2, is wiped off • The color is formed when the enzyme acts on the substrate • The intensity of the color is proportional to the concentration of antibody A2 which in turn is proportional to hCG concentration • For the final result of hCG the color is measured
Reagents	• Micro well strips coated with hCG and antibody A1 • Standards of hCG of concentrations 0, 5, 25, 50, 100 and 200 milli units/mL • Anti-hCG enzyme conjugate (antibody A2 bound to HRP) • Substrate—tetramethylbenzidine • Stop solution—1.8 N H_2SO_4 • Wash buffer—phosphate buffered saline

Method

- Pipette 50 µL of hCG standards, controls, samples
- Add 100 µL of enzyme conjugate to all the wells
- Cover the plate
- Incubate for 1 hour at room temperature
- Remove the liquid from the wells
- Put wash buffer in the wells and wash thrice
- Blot on absorbent paper towels
- Add 100 µL of tetramethylbenzidine substrate in all wells

Contd....

Contd....

- Incubate for 10 minutes at room temperature (RT)
- Add 50 µL of stop solution to each well
- Mix by shaking the well plate slowly
- Read the absorbance at 450 nm by ELISA reader by 20 minutes after addition of stop solution
- Make a standard curve by plotting the absorbance of hCG standards on Y axis and their concentrations at X axis
- Read the absorbance of the controls and all unknown samples from the curve
- Precautions:
  - Samples, controls and standards should not be frozen many times
  - Lipemic samples must not be used
  - High value samples must be diluted
  - Mixing and washing must be well done
  - Preservative—sodium azide interferes/inhibits the enzyme hence should be avoided
  - Run the serum samples in duplicate

Clinical interpretation	
Normal range of hCG	<5 mIU/L
In malignancy/chorionic tumors	Increased level is seen
Used as tumor marker	For those malignancies that produce ectopic hCG (testicular, pancreatic, bronchogenic pulmonary malignancies)

OSCE

1. **Scenario: HIV diagnosis**
   Case: A 29-year-old patient with a history of unprotected sexual contact undergoes an HIV ELISA test and result comes positive.
   Interpretation: A positive ELISA indicative of **possible** HIV infection.
   Next step: Confirm by Western blot/nucleic acid test.
2. **Scenario: Hepatitis B diagnosis**
   Case: A patient presents with jaundice. Hepatitis B surface antigen (HBsAg) ELISA comes positive.
   Interpretation: Positive HBsAg indicative of active hepatitis B infection that can be acute/chronic .
   Next step: Anti-HBc IgM/anti-HB/HBV DNA for differentiating acute/chronic infection.
3. **Scenario: Autoimmune disease (anti-dsDNA antibodies)**
   Case: A 39-year-old female with joint pain undergoes ELISA testing for anti-dsDNA antibodies and result comes positive.
   Interpretation: Positive result of anti-dsDNA antibodies suggestive of systemic lupus erythematosus.
   Next step: Correlate clinically and with other lab findings (e.g., ANA, complement levels).
4. **Scenario: Food allergy testing**
   Case: A child with recurrent urticaria undergoes ELISA testing for specific IgE antibodies against peanuts and test comes positive.
   Interpretation: Positive specific IgE antibodies suggestive of peanut allergy.
   Next step: Skin prick test/oral food challenge/dietary counseling.
5. **Scenario: Dengue diagnosis**
   Case: A patient with rash/myalgia undergoes ELISA for dengue NS1 antigen that comes positive.
   Interpretation: Positive dengue NS1 antigen indicative of acute dengue infection.
   Next step: Monitoring of platelet count/hematocrit for severity monitoring.
6. **Scenario: COVID-19 serology**
   Case: A patient shows positive ELISA test for IgG antibodies against SARS-CoV-2.
   Interpretation: IgG positivity suggestive of past exposure/vaccination against SARS-CoV-2.
   Next step: No action is required unless has symptoms of active infection.
7. **Scenario: Celiac disease**
   Case: A patient with GIT infection/weight loss undergoes ELISA for anti-tissue transglutaminase IgA, that comes positive.
   Interpretation: Positive anti-tTG IgA suggestive of celiac disease.
   Management: Duodenal biopsy/No gluten diet.
8. **Scenario: H. Pylori infection**
   Case: A 65-year-old with dyspepsia takes up ELISA test for anti-H. pylori IgG antibodies. Result: positive.
   Interpretation: Positive IgG suggestive of past/current H. pylori infection.
   Next step: Urea breath test/stool antigen test.

9. **Scenario: Leptospirosis**
   Case: A patient with myalgia is investigated for anti-Leptospira IgM by ELISA. Result: positive.
   Interpretation: Positive IgM indicative of recent leptospirosis infection.
   Next step: Antibiotic therapy.

10. **Scenario: Rubella immunity in pregnancy**
    Case: A pregnant woman undergoes an ELISA test for rubella IgG antibodies that is positive.
    Interpretation: Positive IgG indicative of immunity to rubella may be from past infection/vaccination.
    Clinical relevance: No risk to fetus by rubella.

CLINICAL MCQS

1. **A 37-year-old man complains of fever, weight loss. An ELISA test for HIV-1 and HIV-2 antibodies is positive. How to confirm the diagnosis?**
   a. Western blot
   b. Polymerase chain reaction
   c. Flow cytometry
   d. Repeat with control

   Answer: a. Western blot

2. **What is the principle of ELISA technique?**
   a. Antigen-antibody binding detected with enzyme-mediated color change
   b. Separating proteins based on charges
   c. DNA amplification
   d. Radioisotope labelling

   Answer: a. Antigen-antibody binding detected with enzyme-mediated color change

3. **Which is a clinical application of ELISA?**
   a. Detection of hepatitis B surface antigen
   b. Measuring blood glucose
   c. Quantifying serum electrolytes
   d. Identifying bacterial growth

   Answer: a. Detection of hepatitis B surface antigen

4. **A patient suspects of having dengue fever takes up ELISA test. Which type of ELISA is most commonly used for detecting dengue IgM antibodies?**
   a. Indirect
   b. Competitive
   c. Sandwich
   d. Direct

   Answer: a. Indirect

5. **What enzyme is used in ELISA to catalyze the colorimetric reaction?**
   a. Horseradish peroxidase
   b. PDH
   c. PK
   d. GOD-POD

   Answer: a. Horseradish peroxidase

6. **A technician does sandwich ELISA for detecting a particular antigen. What is the function of capture antibody?**
   a. To bind the antigen and immobilize it on the plate
   b. For detecting enzyme action
   c. For amplifying signal
   d. For blocking binding sites

   Answer: a. To bind the antigen and immobilize it on the plate

7. **A patient with autoimmune disorder undergoes an ELISA test for antinuclear antibodies. Which ELISA is the most appropriate for detection of antibodies?**
   a. Indirect
   b. Direct
   c. Competitive
   d. Sandwich

   Answer: a. Indirect

8. **In competitive ELISA, what happens to the signal when concentration of target antigen in the sample is elevated?**
   a. Signal intensity decreases
   b. Signal intensity high
   c. Signal remains remain constant
   d. Signal is not detectable

   Answer: a. Signal intensity decreases
9. **Which is a limitation of ELISA?**
   a. Highly sensitive
   b. Low specificity
   c. Needs specialized equipment
   d. Can detect only antigens

   Answer: c. Needs specialized equipment
10. **A 7-year-old child shows with recurrent infections. ELISA test was done to quantify serum immunoglobulin levels. Which type of ELISA is suitable?**
    a. Sandwich
    b. Competitive
    c. Direct
    d. Indirect

    Answer: a. Sandwich

VIVA VOCE

Q1. Discuss principle behind ELISA?

ELISA is based on the principle of antigen-antibody interaction. It uses an enzyme-labeled antibody/antigen to bind to the target molecule, and after substrate addition, the enzyme catalyzes a reaction which forms detectable signal that is like color change. This signal is proportional to the amount of antigen or antibody present in the given sample, allowing for quantitative or qualitative analysis.

Q2. Discuss types of ELISA methods.

Direct ELISA: Antigen is immobilized on a solid surface/enzyme-labeled antibody is made use of to detect it.

Indirect ELISA: The antigen is immobilized, and the primary antibody binds to it. Then enzyme-labeled secondary antibody (directed against the primary antibody) is utilized to amplify the signal.

Sandwich ELISA: Antigen is "sandwiched" between two antibodies—one that is immobilized on the surface and one that is enzyme-labeled. It commonly detects large antigens such as cytokines.

Competitive ELISA: Antigen in the sample competes with a labeled antigen for binding sites on the antibody. The amount of bound labeled antigen inversely correlates with amount of antigen in the sample.

Q3. What is the importance of substrate in ELISA assay?

Substrate is important to detect enzyme activity in the final step of ELISA. When substrate reacts with the enzyme, such as horseradish peroxidase/alkaline phosphatase then color changes, fluorescence, or chemiluminescence happens. The intensity of the signal is proportional to the concentration of the target antigen/antibody in the sample. The selection of substrate depends on the enzyme used.

Q4. Interpret the results of ELISA?

Results are interpreted by measuring the optical density at a specific wavelength by using a spectrophotometer. A higher OD suggests higher concentration of the antigen/antibody in the sample. The results are compared to standard curve created from known concentrations of the analyte to quantify the concentration of the target in the sample.

Positive result: A significant color change suggests presence of the target.

Negative result: No color change suggests absence/very low concentration of the target.

Q5. Mention clinical significance of ELISA?

Detecting infectious diseases, such as HIV/Hepatitis B/C/COVID-19 antibodies
Measuring hormones, such as insulin/thyroid hormones
Quantifying cytokines/biomarkers in inflammation/autoimmune diseases
Detecting allergens in food/environmental samples
Pregnancy tests, such as detection of human chorionic gonadotropin

SPOTTERS

Q1. Show an image: A sandwich ELISA with antigen immobilized on a microplate/labeled antibody added. Which ELISA is depicted and mention its working?

Sandwich ELISA, where the antigen is "sandwiched" between two antibodies—one immobilized on the plate and the other labeled with an enzyme. The enzyme reacts with substrate to form detectable signal, that is proportional to the concentration of antigen in the sample.

Q2. Show a scenario: In an indirect ELISA, the OD of a sample is measured at 450 nm, result is compared to a standard curve. Give significance of the OD value?

OD value at 450 nm is directly related to the concentration of antibody in the sample. A high OD shows high concentration of the antibody, and the sample's concentration may be determined by comparing it to the standard curve.

Q3. Show a scenario: A laboratory technician performs a direct ELISA for detecting an antigen in a sample. It gives clear color change after substrate addition. Give the role of the substrate in this ELISA?

Substrate reacts with the enzyme conjugated to the antibody, leading to color change. Intensity of color is proportional to amount of antigen in sample, allowing for qualitative or quantitative analysis.

Q4. Show an image: A graph exhibiting standard curve for an ELISA test, with OD values plotted against known antigen concentrations. How is this standard curve used in an ELISA?

Standard curve allows for the quantification of antigen in an unknown sample. By measuring the optical density of the sample, its concentration can be interpolated from the standard curve.

Q5. Show a scenario: A competitive ELISA test done for detecting a specific antigen. Result shows a weak signal after the addition of the substrate. What does weak signal in a competitive ELISA indicate?

Weak signal in a competitive ELISA indicates that there is a high concentration of the target antigen in the sample. The antigen competes with the labeled antigen for binding sites on the antibody, therefore more antigen in the sample results in less labeled antigen binding, resulting in a weak signal.

REFLECTION

Describe the principle, types and applications of ELISA. Describe the estimation of serum hCG level by sandwich ELISA along with the interpretation of the results.

24

CHAPTER

Immunodiffusion

COMPETENCY

BC14.18: Observe use of commonly used equipments/techniques in biochemistry laboratory including: Immunodiffusion.

LEARNING OBJECTIVES

After reading this chapter, the readers should be able to:
- Describe the principle, types and uses of immunodiffusion.
- Describe the procedure of immunodiffusion on slide using agarose gel.

BLUE PRINT

Commonly Used Equipments/Techniques in Biochemistry Laboratory

Objective

By the end of the lecture, students should be able to:
1. Understand the principles and applications of various commonly used equipments and techniques in biochemistry laboratory.
2. Familiarize themselves with the operation and maintenance of laboratory instruments.
3. Gain practical knowledge of performing biochemical assays and analyses.
4. Learn about quality control measures to ensure accurate and reliable laboratory results.

Duration: ***60 minutes***

Materials Needed

1. Presentation slides illustrating each equipment and technique.
2. Demonstration models or actual laboratory instruments for hands-on learning.
3. Samples or reagents required for practical demonstrations.
4. Whiteboard or flipchart for interactive discussions and note-taking.

Outline

I. **Introduction to biochemistry laboratory techniques** **(10 minutes)**
- Overview of the role of biochemistry laboratory in biomedical research and clinical diagnostics.
- Importance of accurate and reliable laboratory techniques in biochemical analysis.

II. **Immunodiffusion** **(50 minutes)**
- Overview of Immunodiffusion techniques such as radial Immunodiffusion and Ouchterlony method.
- Practical demonstration of antigen-antibody interaction and precipitation reactions.

Immunodiffusion	Process of diffusion of an antigen or an antibody or both in medium
Immunodiffusion technique	• Qualitative and quantitative techniques based on the principle of antigen-antibody reaction in vitro, after their diffusion are known as immunodiffusion techniques • There is formation of a antigen-antibody complex that is then used to quantitate or detect the antigen or the antibody
Two types of reactions	Precipitation and agglutination reactions are present based on the nature of antigen an size of antigen-antibody complex
Precipitation reaction	• We need a soluble antigen • The antigen must have at least two or more antibody binding sites • It reacts with a corresponding antibody (called as precipitins) and result in producing a large antigen-antibody complex that is easily seen by naked eye as a precipitate • The precipitate appears as a line or ring or zone at the place of antigen antibody reaction • If we want a large complex formation, there has to be a optimum amount of antigen and antibody, less or more amounts will not make a proper antigen antibody complex • Zone of optimal ratio of antigen and antibodies is known as equivalence zone
Agglutination reaction (like regular blood group testing)	A particulate natured antigen reacts with the antibodies resulting in visible clumping
Types of immunodiffusion techniques	Two types: 1. Single/Mancini technique 2. Double/Ouchterlony technique
1. Single/Mancini technique	There is formation of a precipitate of disc shape at the zone of equivalence due to radial diffusion of antigen into the antibody containing gel
	1. There is a microscopic slide coated with gel
	2. The antigen is kept in a well
	3. The antigen shows radial diffusion into the gel-containing antibody resulting in formation of a circular spot at the radial precipitation zone
	Ring diameter square is directly proportional to the concentration of the antigen
	A standard curve is plotted for quantitative estimation of antigens and antibodies, by taking a known antigen concentration and measuring the diameter of the ring
Clinical interpretation	• Technique measures the IgG in agammaglobulinemia • Technique measures the IgM in multiple myeloma • It estimates the concentration of transferrin and alpha fetoproteins
2. Double/Ouchterlony technique:	• Here the antigen as well as antibody are allowed to diffuse in the gel • There is formation of a thin sharp line at the zone of diffusion • There are different wells cut in the gel where antigen and antibodies are placed • They diffuse towards each other to form the precipitation line • The pattern of sharp lines depend on nature and number of Ag/Ab • The slow diffusing substance is generally antibody • The shape of the lines is generally hyperbolic with concavity towards the slow diffusing substance (Ab)
Clinical significance	• The technique is used for identifying antigens and antibodies, to decide the optimum concentration of antigens and antibodies for testing, characterization of antigens and antibodies • Technique can differentiate between homologous and heterologous antigen antibody reactions • When two antigens diffuse and react with the antiserum-containing antibodies, they can be qualitatively identified
When the two antigens are identical	• They react with the antibodies in the antiserum with same epitopes • A smooth, merged line of confluence is produced
When the two antigens are not identical	• They do not share common epitopes, and the antiserum has antibodies for both • Two independent sharp lines crossing over each other are seen
When the two antigens are partially identical	There may be some shared epitopes between two antigens, but the antibody to it has to be present in the serum
	It is observed as 'Spur' due to the presence of some unique epitope present in one of the antigen

Contd....

Contd....

Method	• Make 1% agarose gel in phosphate buffer saline (pH 7.4) • Using a glass pipette, put molten agarose on a clean glass slide • Allow the agarose to get hard, then keep a template of position of holes under the slide, punching three sets of wells with the gel punch, place the slide in a moist chamber • We have total three sets, in each set, antiserum is added in single wells and antigens are added in double wells • In the first set of wells, add 20 µL of antiserum I and 20 µL of antigen A and 20 µL of antigen B • In the second set of wells, add 20 µL of antiserum II and 20 µL of antigen C and 20 µL of antigen D • In the third set of wells, add 20 µL of antiserum III and 20 µL of antigen × and 20 µL of antigen Y • All are kept in a moist chamber for 1 night at 37°C • After incubation period of 16 hours, see the pattern of precipitation lines
Precautions	• Flat leveled surface is used for keeping glass slide • Do not over fill the wells • Take care while handling hot molten agarose • The agarose should not be dry • The pipette should be properly washed for pipetting agarose onto the slide

OSCE

1. **Scenario: Detection of fungal infection (aspergillosis)**
   Case: A patient presents with symptoms of weight loss/hemoptysis. Immunodiffusion for *Aspergillus* precipitins exhibits two distinct bands.
   Interpretation: Presence of two distinct bands suggests specific antibodies against *Aspergillus*, indicating chronic pulmonary aspergillosis.
   Next steps: Clinical correlation/confirm with imaging/galactomannan assay
2. **Scenario: Diagnosis of coccidioidomycosis**
   Case: A patient with fever/respiratory symptoms tests positive on immunodiffusion for IgM and IgG antibodies against *Coccidioides spp.*
   Interpretation:
   IgM positivity: Recent/acute infection
   IgG positivity: Established/disseminated infection
   Next steps: Confirmation to be done by culture/molecular testing/to start antifungal therapy
3. **Scenario: Identification of hypogammaglobulinemia**
   Case: A child with recurrent infections undergoes immunodiffusion testing for immunoglobulin levels. There is development of very faint/no precipitation bands for IgG, IgA, and IgM.
   Interpretation: Hypogammaglobulinemia/agammaglobulinemia/indicating a primary immunodeficiency disorder such as Bruton's agammaglobulinemia
   Next steps: Quantitative immunoglobulin assay/genetic testing
4. **Scenario: Autoimmune disease (rheumatoid arthritis)**
   Case: A patient with joint pain/stiffness undergoes immunodiffusion for rheumatoid factor that exhibits strong precipitation band.
   Interpretation: Positive RF is suggestive of rheumatoid arthritis
   Next steps: Correlate with clinical findings/additional tests like anti-CCP antibodies/CRP.
5. **Scenario: Diagnosis of paraproteinemia (multiple myeloma)**
   Case: Immunodiffusion done for serum proteins exhibits a sharp monoclonal band for IgG kappa.
   Interpretation: A monoclonal IgG kappa band suggestive of paraprotein, consistent with multiple myeloma/monoclonal gammopathy of undetermined significance.
   Next steps: Serum protein electrophoresis/immunofixation/bone marrow biopsy
6. **Scenario: Diagnosis of alpha-1 antitrypsin deficiency**
   Case: A patient with early-onset emphysema undergoes immunodiffusion for alpha-1 antitrypsin that exhibits reduced precipitation bands.
   Interpretation: Absent bands suggestive of alpha-1 antitrypsin deficiency that is a genetic disease.
   Next steps: Serum alpha-1 antitrypsin levels assay/genotyping

7. **Scenario: Detection of specific antigens in infections (histoplasmosis)**
   Case: A patient with hepatosplenomegaly and fever undergoes immunodiffusion for *Histoplasma* antigen exhibiting precipitin bands.
   Interpretation: Positive precipitation bands indicative of active/past *Histoplasma* infection.
   Next steps: Antigen detection tests in serum/urine
8. **Scenario: Diagnosis of pernicious anemia**
   Case: A patient with anemia and neurological signs undergoes immunodiffusion assay for antibodies against intrinsic factor that is positive.
   Interpretation: Positive antibodies are confirmatory for pernicious anemia because of deficient vitamin B12 might be a result of deficient intrinsic factor.
   Next steps: Vitamin B12 replacement therapy
9. **Scenario: Detection of antibodies in systemic lupus erythematosus (SLE)**
   Case: Immunodiffusion done for anti-Sm/anti-RNP antibodies exhibiting distinct precipitation lines for both.
   Interpretation:
   Anti-Sm: Specific for SLE.
   Anti-RNP: Seen in SLE/mixed connective tissue disease
   Next steps: Other investigations like ANA.
10. **Scenario: Diagnosis of allergic bronchopulmonary aspergillosis (ABPA)**
    Case: A patient with asthma/lung infiltrates undergoes immunodiffusion for *Aspergillus* IgE, that exhibits strong bands.
    Interpretation: Positive IgE antibodies against *Aspergillus* suggestive of ABPA.
    Next steps: Do total IgE level assay/imaging studies.

CLINICAL MCQS

1. **A patient having autoimmune disease goes for Ouchterlony double immunodiffusion assay. What result exhibits presence of multiple antigen-antibody reactions?**
   a. Precipitation line
   b. Crossing lines
   c. Single—merged lines
   d. Spurred lines
   Answer: b. Crossing lines
2. **Which of this exhibit principle of double immunodiffusion?**
   a. Both antigen/antibodies diffuse toward each other in a gel and form a visible precipitate at equivalence.
   b. Only antigen diffuses
   c. Antigen-antibody complexes are separated by size
   d. Antigen is immobilized
   Answer: a. Both antigen/antibodies diffuse toward each other in a gel and form a visible precipitate at equivalence.
3. **What is clinical use of single radial immunodiffusion?**
   a. Quantification of immunoglobulin levels
   b. Assay of autoimmune antibodies
   c. Diagnosis of fungal disorders
   d. Assay of monoclonal proteins
   Answer: a. Quantification of immunoglobulin levels
4. **A patient had fungal infection. Double immunodiffusion is used to detect which fungal antigens?**
   a. *Aspergillus*
   b. *Histoplasma capsulatum*
   c. *Candida albicans*
   d. *Cryptococcus*
   Answer: b. *Histoplasma capsulatum*
5. **In Ouchterlony immunodiffusion, what does a line of identity between two wells suggestive of?**
   a. The antigens are identical or share common epitopes.
   b. The antigens are not related.
   c. The antigens are little bit related.
   d. Excess antibody is present.
   Answer: a. The antigens are identical or share common epitopes.

6. **A 55-year-old man having frequent infections goes for radial immunodiffusion. Which principle explains best the diameter of the precipitation ring?**
   a. It is proportional to the antigen concentration.
   b. It is proportional to antibody level.
   c. It is inversely proportional to antigen-antibody complex.
   d. It depends on the molecular weight.

   Answer: a. It is proportional to the antigen concentration.

7. **Which component is needed in the gel for double immunodiffusion?**
   a. Agar or agarose
   b. Polyacrylamide
   c. Nitrocellulose
   d. Chromatography sheet

   Answer: a. Agar or agarose

8. **A spurred precipitation line in double immunodiffusion is indicative of:**
   a. Partial antigenic identity
   b. Incomplete antigenic identity
   c. Antigen-antibody complex
   d. No relationship

   Answer: a. Partial antigenic identity

9. **What is the limitation of immunodiffusion techniques?**
   a. Needs large sample volumes
   b. Time-consuming and less sensitive
   c. Inability to detect multiple antigens
   d. High cost

   Answer: b. Time-consuming and less sensitive

10. **A patient complains of symptoms of systemic lupus erythematosus. Immunodiffusion test is done for detecting specific antibodies. Which antibody is mainly tested in SLE?**
    a. Anti-dsDNA
    b. Anti-Sm
    c. Anti-CCP
    d. Anti-Ro/SSA

    Answer: b. Anti-Sm

VIVA VOCE

Q1. What is immunodiffusion?

A laboratory technique that is used for detecting and quantifying specific antigens/antibodies in a sample. There is diffusion of antigens and antibodies in an agar gel, where they make visible precipitates when they react.

Significance: used for diagnosing infections like fungal/bacteria), identifying antibodies like in autoimmune diseases, and determining serological profiles.

Q2. Give principle behind the radial immunodiffusion method.

Antigen is diffused radially through an agar gel which has the antibody. The antigen-antibody reaction makes precipitin ring around the well/diameter of the ring is proportional to the concentration of the antigen in the sample.

Use: For quantifying antigen levels, like in serum proteins for example IgG.

Q3. Differentiate between immunoelectrophoresis/double immunodiffusion.

Immunoelectrophoresis combines electrophoresis and immunodiffusion. First antigen mixture is separated by electrophoresis based on charge, secondly antibodies are applied to the gel, allowing antigen-antibody precipitates to be formed.

It is utilized for analyzing complex mixtures of proteins.

Double immunodiffusion (Ouchterlony method) involves two sets of wells: one for antigen and the other for antibody. Both antigens and antibodies diffuse radially, and precipitin lines are produced where they meet.

It is utilized to identify/compare analysis of antigens.

Q4. Limitations of the immunodiffusion technique.

Diffusion is a slow process, so immunodiffusion techniques take hours to days to give results.

Immunodiffusion is less sensitive in comparison to ELISA/Western blot.

Interpretation of results is challenging when complex antigens are present, because false positives/weak precipitin lines might occur.

This method is typically used for soluble antigens and is not suited for detection of cell-bound antigens.

Q5. How is the Ouchterlony double immunodiffusion method interpreted?

Identity (same antigen): If antigen and antibody form a single precipitin line, it indicates that they are identical.

Nonidentity (different antigens): When two precipitin lines form and do not merge, this suggests that the antigens are different.

Partial identity (related antigens): When one precipitin line merges with another but forms a spur, this indicates that the antigens are partially similar or cross-reacting.

SPOTTERS

Q1. Immunodiffusion test

A lab test where antigens and antibodies are allowed to diffuse through agar gel, producing precipitin lines which suggest presence of specific antibodies or antigens.

Q2. Single radial immunodiffusion

Technique where antibodies are placed in an agar gel/antigen diffusion creates a precipitation ring. Size of the ring correlates with the concentration of antigen.

Q3. Double immunodiffusion/Ouchterlony test

Test involving two wells in an agar plate: one for antigen and another for antibody. The production of a precipitin line between them suggests antigen-antibody reaction.

Q4. Hepatitis B surface antigen immunodiffusion

Used for diagnosing hepatitis B infections by detecting HBsAg in the serum of the patient, where a precipitin line is made between the antigen and antibody in an agar gel.

Q5. Ring test/immunodiffusion

Technique where a well is made in an agar plate and an antigen is placed in the center. The antibody is applied around the well/ visible ring of precipitation forms when antigen-antibody interaction happens.

REFLECTION

Explain the principle, types and uses of immunodiffusion and also explain this procedure on slide using agarose gel.

25

CHAPTER

DNA Isolation and Quantification

COMPETENCY

BC14.18: Observe use of commonly used equipments/techniques in biochemistry laboratory including: DNA isolation and quantification.

LEARNING OBJECTIVES

After reading this chapter, the readers should be able to:

- Describe the principle and significance of isolation and quantification of DNA.
- Describe the procedure of the isolation and quantification of DNA.

BLUE PRINT

Commonly Used Equipments/Techniques in Biochemistry Laboratory

Objective

By the end of the lecture, students should be able to:

1. Understand the principles and applications of various commonly used equipments and techniques in biochemistry laboratory.
2. Familiarize themselves with the operation and maintenance of laboratory instruments.
3. Gain practical knowledge of performing biochemical assays and analyses.
4. Learn about quality control measures to ensure accurate and reliable laboratory results.

Duration: ***90 minutes***

Materials Needed

1. Presentation slides illustrating each equipment and technique.
2. Demonstration models or actual laboratory instruments for hands-on learning.
3. Samples or reagents required for practical demonstrations.
4. Whiteboard or flipchart for interactive discussions and note-taking.

Outline

I. **Introduction to biochemistry laboratory techniques** **(10 minutes)**
- Overview of the role of biochemistry laboratory in biomedical research and clinical diagnostics.
- Importance of accurate and reliable laboratory techniques in biochemical analysis.

II. **DNA isolation from blood/tissue** **(50 minutes)**
- Overview of DNA isolation techniques such as phenol-chloroform extraction and column- based purification.

III. **Practical demonstration of DNA extraction from blood or tissue samples** **(30 minutes)**

Objective	Isolation of DNA from blood and quantitate it by Spectrophotometric measurement
Importance of molecular medicine	• For diagnosis of some diseases like molecular level diagnosis of leukemias, and some congenital disorders prior to implantation or in antenatal duration • To come to any conclusion for such diagnosis, we need to isolate pure DNA from blood/cells
Procedures	Steps of DNA extraction: 1. Lysis of the cell/disruption of the cell membrane 2. Cellular proteins are removed 3. DNA precipitation by ethanol 4. Quantification and measurement of purity
Sample	Whole blood in EDTA (freshly taken)
Short-term storage temperature	2–8°C
Long-term storage temperature	–20°C

Chloroform-phenol extraction procedure

Principle	Liquid phase based method where DNA is separated in one phase and proteins or lipids are separated in a different phase

Method

Step 1	Lysis of cells is done by detergents and proteinase K in aqueous solution
Step 2	Make a biphasic mixture by adding saturated chloroform-phenol mixture
Step 3	Proteins are present in the organic phase
	The DNA is present in the aqueous phase
Step 4	Precipitation of DNA present in the upper supernatant is done by ethanol/isopropanol
Step 5	Let it dry
Step 6	The DNA sample is reconstituted in tris EDTA buffer
Step 7	Quantification and purity assessment is done
Advantages	Can be wide range done on wide range of samples and can extract large amounts of DNA
Disadvantage	Tedious method which uses toxic chemicals like chloroform and phenol

DNA extraction in nonorganic phase with salting out

Principle	Lysis of cells is done, protein denaturation is done with detergents like SDS/triton X, RNAase removes the RNA, salts precipitate the proteins and extraction of DNA is done by alcohol

Reagents required

1. RBC lysis solution	Ammonium chloride: 8.29 g
	Potassium bicarbonate: 1 g
	Na_2EDTA: 0.034 g
	All are added to DW
	pH: 7.4
2. Cell lysis buffer	Sodium dodecyl sulfate in tris EDTA buffer (tris—10 mm and EDTA—1 mM, pH—8.0)
3. Ethanol	70%
4. Isopropanol	–
5. Ammonium acetate	3 M

Method

- Take 1.5 mL micro centrifuge tube
- Take 450 μL of red blood cell (RBC) lysis buffer
- Add 150 μL of fresh whole blood in ethylenediaminetetraacetic acid (EDTA)
- The blood should be at room temperature (RT)
- The blood is used after half an hour of collection
- Invert at least 10 times for proper mixing
- Incubate at RT for 5 minutes
- Centrifuge for 3 minutes
- Discard the supernatant leaving white blood cell (WBC) pellet with 10 μL of liquid
- Add 150 μL of cell lysis buffer and vortex for 10 seconds
- Add 50 μL of ammonium acetate for protein precipitation and vortex for 20 seconds at good speed
- Centrifuge for 2 minutes to make protein pellet
- Add supernatant to another tube having 300 μL of Isopropanol
- Invert at least 50 times for proper mixing till you see a thread/clump of DNA
- Centrifuge and drain the supernatant on an absorbent paper
- Pellet should remain in the tube
- Wash the DNA pellet by 300 μL of 70% ethanol (mixing and inverting)
- Centrifuge and drain the supernatant leaving the DNA pellet in the tube
- For few seconds air dry the pellet
- Add 50 μL of tris E buffer and vortex for 5 seconds at medium speed
- To dissolve the DNA, incubate at 65°C for 15 minutes
- Incubate at RT for full night by gentle shaking

Extraction of DNA using solid phase silica spin column for determining the purity and concentration

Principle

- Nucleic acid undergoes reversible binding with silica (solid phase) under optimum conditions
- Ultimately the DNA can be eluted from silica (reversible binding), uses chaotropic agent–geranium hydrochloride which aids in binding of DNA to silica membrane

Method

Step 1: Cell lysis
Step 2: Extraction of DNA by binding to silica from lysate
Step 3: Wash the nucleic acid bound to silica
Step 4: Elution of nucleic acid

- DNA from blood can be separated in 2 hours by this method
- Use proper solution for cell lysis
- The binding lysate is made by adding ethanol for DNA precipitation
- To remove the RNA from the DNA containing lysate we can use RNAase initially
- The binding solution is transferred to a column which is centrifuged
- This forces the binding solution through the silica gel membrane that is in the spin column
- In optimum pH and salt concentration, the DNA binds to the membrane
- The bound DNA is washed and eluted by use of buffers and solutions
- The DNA is collected from the bottom of the column

Advantage

Fast, simple technique, nontoxic chemicals are used and extraction is high quality

Quantification of DNA

- Dilute the DNA in DW and mix well
- The reference cell of spectrophotometer is filled with DW and TE buffer
- Fill the sample cell with diluted DNA
- Adjust the spectrophotometer to measure optical density at 260 nm and 280 nm

Precautions

- DNA should not be allowed to get sheared so do not vigorously mix/pipette
- Autoclave all glasswares before use
- Corrosive phenol should be carefully handled

LOG ACTIVITY

Calculations

OD at 260 nm	....
OD at 280 nm	....
Quantification: DNA concentration in the sample is calculated by taking the OD of DNA sample and dilution factor in consideration	Done by taking the OD equal to 1.0 of a DNA sample of concentration–50 µg/mL at 260 nm, path length of 1 cm
Unit:	µg or ng/mL of sample
Purity: A ratio of absorbance at 260 nm to absorbance at 280 nm shows the purity of the DNA sample	Absorbance at 280 nm is because of proteins and at 260 nm, absorbance is due to DNA
Ratio of a pure DNA sample	1.8

OSCE

1. **Scenario: Diagnosis of genetic disorder (Thalassemia)**
   Case: A child having anemia undergoes DNA isolation from peripheral blood. Quantification exhibits sufficient DNA concentration/PCR identifies a mutation in the HBB gene.
   Interpretation: Mutation in HBB gene is conclusive of beta-thalassemia.
   Next steps: Genetic counseling/supportive treatment/transfusion therapy.
2. **Scenario: Prenatal diagnosis of down syndrome**
   Case: DNA is isolated from amniotic fluid. Quantitative PCR exhibits trisomy 21.
   Interpretation: Trisomy 21 is suggestive of Down syndrome in fetus.
   Next steps: Counselling to family members for diagnosis and prognosis.
3. **Scenario: Quantification for PCR optimization**
   Case: DNA isolated from a blood sample shows concentration of 5 ng/µL and A260/A280 ratio of 1.8.
   Interpretation: The DNA concentration and purity (A260/A280 ratio) both are acceptable for PCR.
   Next steps: Adjust DNA concentration as needed for PCR that is use 10–100 ng per reaction.
4. **Scenario: Molecular diagnosis of cystic fibrosis**
   Case: A patient with recurrent respiratory infections has DNA isolated and quantified. Mutation analysis identifies a delta-F508 mutation in the CFTR gene.
   Interpretation: The delta-F508 mutation is conclusive of cystic fibrosis.
   Next steps: Nutritional management/genetic counseling.
5. **Scenario: Detection of BRCA mutations in breast cancer**
   Case: A woman having family history of breast cancer has DNA isolated from blood, and sequencing identifies a BRCA1 mutation.
   Interpretation: The BRCA1 mutation is suggestive of higher risk for breast/ovarian cancers.
   Next steps: Focus on preventive measures like surveillance/prophylactic surgery.
6. **Scenario: DNA yield and purity check**
   Case: DNA is isolated from a tissue biopsy, and spectrophotometric analysis provides A260/A280 ratio of 1.2.
   Interpretation: A ratio of 1.2 is indicative of protein contamination. The sample is not appropriate for applications such as PCR/sequencing.
   Next steps: Re-purify DNA by making use of phenol-chloroform extraction/column-based purification.
7. **Scenario: Forensic identification**
   Case: DNA isolated from a hair follicle is quantified at 2 ng/µL. STR analysis matches the DNA to a suspect.
   Interpretation: STR analysis confirms identity of the individual.
   Next steps: Use evidence in the legal investigation.
8. **Scenario: Diagnosis of viral infection (HPV)**
   Case: DNA is isolated from a cervical swab and quantified. PCR detects high-risk HPV DNA.
   Interpretation: High-risk HPV DNA is suggestive of potential risk for cervical dysplasia or cancer.
   Next steps: Pap smear/colposcopy for further assessment.
9. **Scenario: Contamination during DNA isolation**
   Case: DNA isolated from blood exhibits a low A260/A230 ratio (<1.5).
   Interpretation: A decreased A260/A230 ratio suggests contamination with salts or organic solvents.
   Next steps: Re-purify the DNA to remove contaminants before use in downstream applications.

10. **Scenario: Gene expression studies (qPCR)**
Case: DNA isolated from tissue has a concentration of 50 ng/μL. RNA contamination is suspected.
Interpretation: RNA contamination might interfere with DNA quantification and downstream applications.
Next steps: Treat sample with RNase before proceeding with qPCR.

CLINICAL MCQS

1. **A patient comes with suspected genetic disease. DNA isolation was done from peripheral blood. Which method is generally utilized to isolate genomic DNA from the blood**
   a. Phenol extraction
   b. Silica gel-based column extraction
   c. Ethanol precipitation
   d. Cesium chloride centrifugation

   Answer: b. Silica gel-based column extraction
2. **In DNA quantification, which method uses absorbance at 260 nm for measuring DNA concentration?**
   a. Fluorometric methodology
   b. Agarose gel electrophoresis
   c. Spectrophotometry method
   d. Southern blotting technique

   Answer: c. Spectrophotometry method
3. **Which reagent is used for lyses of cells/releasing DNA for/during the DNA extraction technique?**
   a. Ethanol
   b. Sodium dodecyl sulfate
   c. Propanol
   d. Formaldehyde

   Answer: b. Sodium dodecyl sulfate
4. **A 39-year-old woman having family history of Huntington's disease takes up DNA extraction in order to do genetic testing. What is the main challenge in the isolation of high-quality DNA from the blood samples?**
   a. Contamination with RNA
   b. DNA degradation due to proteases
   c. Low yield of DNA from blood
   d. Presence of inhibitors such as hemoglobin

   Answer: b. DNA degradation due to proteases
5. **A technician measures the concentration of DNA in a sample. A260/A280 ratio of sample is 1.8. What does this suggest?**
   a. The sample is contaminated
   b. The DNA sample is of high purity
   c. The sample has RNA contamination
   d. The sample is very diluted

   Answer: b. The DNA sample is of high purity
6. **A clinical laboratory performs DNA extraction by patient's biopsy sample. Which is the key factor for ensuring high-quality DNA isolation?**
   a. Minimizing exposure to sunlight
   b. Using fresh reagents
   c. Proper sample storage and handling
   d. Using peripheral blood samples

   Answer: c. Proper sample storage and handling
7. **In DNA quantification by fluorometric methods, what dye is utilized to stain DNA?**
   a. Ethidium bromide dye
   b. SYBR Green
   c. Methylene blue dye
   d. Crystal violet dye

   Answer: b. SYBR Green

8. **What is the application of using spectrophotometer over gel electrophoresis for the technique of DNA quantification?**
   a. Spectrophotometry provides more accurate sizing of DNA fragments.
   b. Spectrophotometry is more sensitive and quicker for quantification.
   c. Gel electrophoresis is better for quantifying small DNA amounts.
   d. Spectrophotometry does not require DNA staining agents.

   Answer: b. Spectrophotometry is more sensitive and quicker for quantification.

9. **Which is the key step in DNA extraction for ensuring that DNA remains intact and free from the degradation?**
   a. Incubation
   b. Use of a protease inhibitor
   c. Addition of a buffer
   d. Centrifugation at slow speed

   Answer: b. Use of a protease inhibitor

10. **A sample DNA was quantified by using the absorbance at 260 nm. Reading of 1.0 corresponds to 50 μg/mL of DNA. If the sample has an absorbance of 0.8, what is the concentration of DNA?**
    a. 40 μg/mL
    b. 55 μg/mL
    c. 85 μg/mL
    d. 60 μg/mL

    Answer: a. 40 μg/mL

VIVA VOCE

Q1. Mention main steps of DNA isolation from a biological sample?

1. Cell lysis for breaking open the cell membrane and releasing DNA by the use of detergents/enzymes.
2. Remove proteins by the use of proteases/organic solvents.
3. DNA precipitation using alcohol (ethanol or isopropanol) to isolate DNA.
4. Wash for removing contaminants.
5. Resuspension in a suitable buffer like TE buffer for further use.

Q2. How to quantify DNA after isolation?

UV spectrophotometry at 260 nm (A260)—Absorbance is proportional to the concentration of DNA.

Fluorometric methods using intercalating dyes like PicoGreen which binds specifically to DNA and fluoresce when exposed to UV light.

Agarose gel electrophoresis by comparing the sample with a DNA ladder for estimating concentration visually.

Q3. Give principle of UV spectrophotometry for DNA quantification?

DNA absorbs UV light maximally at wavelength of 260 nm. The absorbance (A260) is proportional to the concentration of nucleic acids in the given sample. The DNA concentration is calculated.

Q4. How to assess purity of isolated DNA?

Purity can be assessed by measuring the A260/A280 ratio by use of UV spectrophotometry.

A ratio of 1.8–2.0 suggests pure DNA.

A lower ratio indicates protein contamination and higher ratio is suggestive of RNA contamination.

The A260/A230 ratio can also be checked, with a value close to 2.0 suggesting minimal contamination by organic solvents/salts.

Q5. Discuss common methods for DNA extraction from plant tissues?

Plant DNA extraction needs more stringent protocols because of presence of cell walls.

Cetyltrimethylammonium bromide method, that aids break down plant cell walls/remove polysaccharides.

DNeasy kits which use silica-based columns for DNA purification.

Use of liquid nitrogen for grinding tissues to aid break down tough cell walls.

SPOTTERS

Q1. Show image: Agarose gel electrophoresis exhibiting DNA sample with a faint band at the 1 kb marker/no visible contamination. What can you confirm about the quality and quantity of the DNA sample?

The faint band indicates low DNA concentration, but the absence of smearing suggests that the DNA is of high quality without any degradation.

Q2. Show a scenario: A DNA sample is quantified by fluorometric method with PicoGreen dye. Reading: concentration of 200 ng/µL. What are the advantages of fluorometric method over UV spectrophotometry for DNA quantification?

Fluorometric method is more sensitive/specific for DNA, as the dye selectively binds to DNA and fluoresces. It is less prone to interference from contaminants such as RNA and proteins, that might affect UV readings.

Q3. Show a scenario: A technician isolates DNA from plant tissue by CTAB method. After extraction, sample is seen to be viscous/turbid. What does turbidity show/cause?

Turbidity shows presence of polysaccharides/plant debris, that might co-precipitate with DNA. The CTAB method aids in removing the impurities, but more purification might be required like phenol-chloroform extraction.

Q4. Show a scenario: DNA isolation from a bacterial culture was done, then the technician measures the A260/A280 ratio and observes to be 1.6. What does this suggest regarding purity of the DNA/how to correct?

An A260/A280 ratio of 1.6 indicates protein contamination. The sample must be more purified by proteinase K treatment/phenol-chloroform extraction for removing proteins.

REFLECTION

26

CHAPTER

Autoanalyzers

COMPETENCY

BC14.18: Observe use of commonly used equipments/techniques in biochemistry laboratory including: Autoanalyzer.

LEARNING OBJECTIVES

After reading this chapter, the readers should be able to:

- Describe the concepts, principle, and significance of automatic analyzers.
- Describe the operation of autoanalyzers along with the advantages.

BLUE PRINT

Observe use of Commonly used Equipments/Techniques in Biochemistry Laboratory including: Autoanalyzer

Objective

By the end of the lecture, students should be able to:

1. Understand the principles and applications of various commonly used equipments and techniques in biochemistry laboratory.
2. Familiarize themselves with the operation and maintenance of laboratory instruments.
3. Gain practical knowledge of performing biochemical assays and analyses.
4. Learn about quality control measures to ensure accurate and reliable laboratory results.

Duration: ***60 minutes***

Materials Needed

1. Presentation slides illustrating each equipment and technique.
2. Demonstration models or actual laboratory instruments for hands-on learning.
3. Samples or reagents required for practical demonstrations.
4. Whiteboard or flipchart for interactive discussions and note-taking.

Outline

I. **Introduction to biochemistry laboratory techniques** **(10 minutes)**
- Overview of the role of biochemistry laboratory in biomedical research and clinical diagnostics.
- Importance of accurate and reliable laboratory techniques in biochemical analysis.

II. **Automated analyzer (autoanalyzer)** **(50 minutes)**
- Explanation of automated analyzers for high-throughput biochemical analysis.
- Demonstration of sample loading, analysis, and result interpretation using an autoanalyzer.

Autoanalyzers	Automatic machines used in clinical laboratory for analysis of various test parameters in various samples
Advantages	• Workload is less • Saves time/analysis • Increase the total number of tests in decreased time • Improvement of accuracy is there as human error chances are not there • Improvement of reproducibility • Minimum amount of sample and reagent requirement is there • Quality is improved
Disadvantages	Trained technicians are needed to perform Cost of maintenance is high (system upgrading/servicing/trained engineers)

Six types:
1. Open system
2. Closed system
3. Modular system
4. Integrated system
5. Random access analyzer
6. Centrifugal analyzer

Open system	Proper reagents from any manufacturer can be used, so save a lot of money and the cost of test is also low
Closed system (high degree of automation but costly)	Mandatory to use the reagents provided in unique containers/formats of a specific company recommended by the manufacturer of the instrument
Modular system	Advantage is that if one part of the instrument goes out of order, it can be replaced without affecting the whole instrument because, the whole system in these are divided into multiple modules, assembling together in one instrument
Integrated system (provides good communication and good data exchange between various softwares and the machines)	One integrated unit is made by merging functionally different parts and softwares
Disadvantage	Service and maintenance is costly, depend on company engineers for minute servicing
Random access analyzer	A list of tests is available in the machine, and the instrument can select the required tests randomly
Advantages	• Simple steps are there like loading the sample, and give proper commands • Versatile—one sample can be tested for multiple tests, multiple samples can be tested for one test • One sample requires renal profile, another sample needs lipid, and calcium estimation, third sample requires only glucose estimation, then we can load all three samples and by giving proper commands, we get the results
Centrifugal (part of space program as can be performed in a zero gravity environment)	• There are various chambers on a rotor • Samples and reagents are pipette into different chambers • For mixing of samples and reagents, centrifugal force is used • The final product is moved from the rotor to an optical system for final results
Advantage	Saves time as all the cuvettes are read at one time, but only suitable for batch analysis of a specific parameter like lipid profile
Disadvantage	One test can be performed at one time—suitable for batch analysis of a specific parameter like lipid profile
	Six parts of autoanalyzer
Sampler	• There is a circular tray on which there are separate cups to hold the batch of samples • The tray rotates at intervals • There is a probe connected by plastic tube to proportionating pump to enter each sample serially • Volume of the aspirated sample depends on the pumping rats and adjustable dwell time of the probe in the sample
Proportionating pump	• Does the functions of different sized pipettes in manual methods • It determines the relative flow rates of samples and all reagents

Contd....

Contd....

Dialyzer	To separate small and large molecules by allowing the smaller molecules to pass through the semipermeable membrane from the sample to the stream of reagents
Constant temperature module	Maintains the reaction mixture at a constant temperature for a specific time period resulting in the required chemical changes under optimum temperature Generally the incubator baths are set at 37°C/95°C/120°C
Flow through colorimeter	There is selected wavelength in the colorimeter that can measure the color intensity in the reaction and gives us a graph which shows color change with time
Potentiometer recorder	For recording the responses to the intensity of light reaching the detectors
	Identification of specimen
Step 1	Unique identity is generated for the patient
Step 2	A bar code for the laboratory sample is generated
Step 3	The details are pasted on the vacutainers containing the sample
Delivery of the sample	Delivered to the laboratory via pneumatic tube system/messenger
Preparation of the sample	After received in laboratory, they are centrifuged for either serum or plasma on which processing has to be done
Loading of sample on machine:	Manual/automated track/conveyer belt system
Processing of the sample: Done by either of the two ways:	
1. Continuous flow processing	• The sample is injected into a flowing carrier solution • The sample gets mixed well with diluents and reagents and it is sent through the small tubes and mixing coils • There is a continuous flow of the flowing solution in the small tubes • Carry over effect between different samples is prevented by injecting air bubbles
2. Discrete processing	• Every sample is given a discrete space • Specific amount of sample and reagent is aspirated and mixed
Advantages	• There is no loss of excess reagents • No carry over effect is seen as every sample is processed in a different cup and read in different cuvette • Reagent cost is saved • 60–300 samples per hour can be processed
Operation of the autoanalyzers	Requires daily preparation, maintenance and calibration
1. Maintenance check	• Clean the probes • Check the fluid levels of the calibrating fluids • Check the optical reading for assessing the suitability of the cuvettes • Temperature check • Humidity check • After refilling the chemicals or reagents, inventory check of all the chemicals is also required
2. Loading of the reagents	Refrigerated reagent trays are present
3. Calibration (for quality assurance)	Done daily
4. Quality check	Running of quality control samples for checking the system/corrective measures are taken if needed
5. Sample processing	Load the samples
Proportionating pumps	• They will aspirate the samples through sample probe and also dilute the samples • Dilutes samples are led through dialyzer unit • The proportionating pump will introduce the proper reagents through the reagent probe to other side of dialyzer • The flow of the stream is directed by plastic tubing from one module to another • The samples are loaded in the cup of sampler, and the proportionating pump aspirates and dilute them also • In this way, diluted serum samples are led through one of the dialyzer unit and the pump introduces suitable reagents through the other side of the dialyzer • The two streams run side by side, being separated by dialyzing membrane • A part of dialyzable constituents of serum pass across the membrane to the reagent stream • Constant temperature bath provides incubation • Color intensity formed is measured by colorimeter and recorded in recorder • Treat the standards in the same way

OSCE

1. **Scenario: Hyperglycemia diagnosis**
   Case: A patient presents with symptoms of polyuria/polydipsia. Blood glucose: (fasting glucose) 140 mg/dL.
   Interpretation: Fasting glucose ≥126 mg/dL confirms diabetes mellitus.
   Next steps: Confirm with HbA1c test (≥6.5% for diabetes diagnosis).
2. **Scenario: Hyperlipidemia**
   Case: Lipid profile analyzed by autoanalyzer shows the following results:
   Total cholesterol: 258 mg/dL
   LDL cholesterol: 189 mg/dL
   HDL cholesterol: 34 mg/dL
   Triglycerides: 205 mg/dL
   Interpretation: Hyperlipidemia with high total as well as LDL cholesterol/less HDL cholesterol/high triglycerides leading to high cardiovascular risk.
   Next steps: Lifestyle changes/statin therapy
3. **Scenario: Acute kidney injury (AKI)**
   Case: Serum creatinine measured by autoanalyzer is 2.6 mg/dL (normal: 0.7–1.3 mg/dL), blood urea nitrogen: 45 mg/dL (normal: 7–20 mg/dL).
   Interpretation: High creatinine/BUN indicative of AKI.
   Next steps: Focus on BUN/creatinine ratio go for urinalysis/imaging for determining reason, such as prerenal/intrinsic/postrenal AKI.
4. **Scenario: Liver function test (LFT) abnormality**
   Case: LFT results by autoanalyzer show:
   ALT: 152 U/L (normal: <40 U/L)
   AST: 141 U/L (normal: <40 U/L)
   ALP: 121 U/L (normal: 40–130 U/L)
   Total bilirubin: 2.6 mg/dL (normal: <1.2 mg/dL)
   Interpretation: High ALT/AST and high bilirubin indicates hepatocellular injury most likely hepatitis
   Next steps: Assess viral hepatitis/alcohol consumption as other reasons of liver injury.
5. **Scenario: Electrolyte imbalance**
   Case: Serum electrolytes analyzed using an autoanalyzer show:
   Sodium: 138 mmol/L (normal: 135–145 mmol/L)
   Potassium: 5.6 mmol/L (normal: 3.5–5.0 mmol/L)
   Interpretation: Hyponatremia/hyperkalemia indicates potential adrenal insufficiency/renal dysfunction.
   Next steps: Assess aldosterone along with cortisol/renal function tests
6. **Scenario: Thyroid function test (TFT)**
   Case: TFT results by autoanalyzer show:
   TSH: 10 μIU/mL (normal: 0.5–5 μIU/mL)
   Free T4: 0.5 ng/dL (normal: 0.8–2.0 ng/dL)
   Interpretation: High TSH/low free T4 suggests primary hypothyroidism.
   Next steps: Initiate thyroid hormone replacement therapy/monitoring of TSH levels
7. **Scenario: Cardiac enzyme analysis**
   Case: A patient with chest pain has cardiac biomarkers measured by autoanalyzer:
   Troponin I: 2.1 ng/mL (normal: <0.04 ng/mL)
   Interpretation: Raised troponin shows myocardial injury indicating acute myocardial infarction.
   Next steps: Cardiac care/treat for acute coronary syndrome.
8. **Scenario: Anemia evaluation**
   Case: A complete blood count using autoanalyzer reveals:
   Hemoglobin: 7 g/dL (normal: 13–17 g/dL for males)
   MCV: 71 fL (normal: 80–100 fL)
   Ferritin: 11 ng/mL (normal: 30–300 ng/mL)
   Interpretation: Microcytic anemia along with decreased ferritin indicating iron-deficiency anemia.
   Next steps: Assess the cause which can be dietary deficiency/blood loss/iron supplementation
9. **Scenario: Pancreatitis diagnosis**
   Case: Serum amylase and lipase levels measured by autoanalyzer are high
   Amylase: 310 U/L (normal: 30–110 U/L)
   Lipase: 520 U/L (normal: 10–140 U/L)

Interpretation: High amylase plus lipase indicating acute pancreatitis.
Next steps: CT abdomen along with focus on underlying causes that can be gallstones/alcohol.

10. **Scenario: Monitoring diabetes control**
Case: HbA1c measured by autoanalyzer is 9.1% (normal: <5.7%, diabetic control target: <7%).
Interpretation: Poor glycemic control in a diagnosed diabetic patient.
Next steps: Manage diabetes/lifestyle changes/adjust medications.

11. **Scenario: Monitoring renal function in chronic kidney disease (CKD)**
Case: A patient diagnosed with CKD has following lab results using autoanalyzer:
Serum creatinine: 4.1 mg/dL (normal: 0.7–1.3 mg/dL)
Blood urea nitrogen: 71 mg/dL (normal: 7–20 mg/dL)
eGFR: 21 mL/min/1.74 m^2 (normal: >60 mL/min/1.73 m^2)
Interpretation: eGFR suggests Stage 4 CKD that is severely impaired kidney functions
Next steps: Manage complications that can be anemia/electrolyte imbalance/potential renal replacement therapy.

12. **Scenario: Electrolyte monitoring in dehydration**
Case: Serum electrolyte levels measured in a case with diarrhea/omitting:
Sodium: 149 mmol/L (normal: 135–145 mmol/L)
Potassium: 3.1 mmol/L (normal: 3.5–5.0 mmol/L)
Interpretation: Hypernatremia/hypokalemia indicates dehydration/potassium loss because of fluid loss.
Next steps: Start oral/intravenous rehydration and potassium supplementation.

13. **Scenario: Evaluation of hyperbilirubinemia in a neonate**
Case: Total and direct bilirubin levels analyzed:
Total bilirubin: 19 mg/dL (normal: <5 mg/dL in neonates)
Direct bilirubin: 1.5 mg/dL (normal: <1 mg/dL)
Interpretation: Unconjugated hyperbilirubinemia probably because of physiological jaundice/hemolysis.
Next steps: Monitoring of bilirubin level/phototherapy/exchange transfusion.

14. **Scenario: Acid-base imbalance**
Case: Arterial blood gas analysis by autoanalyzer shows:
pH: 7.15 (normal: 7.35–7.45)
pCO_2: 52 mmHg (normal: 35–45 mmHg)
HCO_3^-: 23 mEq/L (normal: 22–26 mEq/L)
Interpretation: Respiratory acidosis because of high pCO_2.
Next steps: Investigate main causes that can be COPD/ventilatory support if required.

15. **Scenario: Diagnosis of gout**
Case: Serum uric acid measured by autoanalyzer is 8.6 mg/dL (normal: 3.4–7.0 mg/dL).
Interpretation: Hyperuricemia indicating gout/high risk of gout flares.
Next steps: Dietary modification/NSAIDs for acute flare/urate-lowering therapy

16. **Scenario: Diagnosis of myopathy**
Case: Serum creatine kinase levels analyzed are 1,210 U/L (normal: 30–200 U/L).
Interpretation: High CK indicates muscle damage, likely because of myopathy/rhabdomyolysis/muscular dystrophy.
Next steps: Identify the cause and manage electrolyte imbalances and renal complications.

17. **Scenario: Hypercalcemia workup**
Case: Serum calcium and parathyroid hormone:
Calcium: 13 mg/dL (normal: 8.5–10.5 mg/dL)
PTH: 88 pg/mL (normal: 10–65 pg/mL)
Interpretation: Hypercalcemia and high PTH is suggestive of primary hyperparathyroidism.
Next steps: Imaging of the parathyroid glands/surgical intervention

18. **Scenario: Hypoglycemia in a diabetic patient**
Case: Random blood glucose measured by autoanalyzer is 51 mg/dL (normal: >70 mg/dL).
Interpretation: Hypoglycemia in a diabetic patient might be because of excess insulin/excess oral hypoglycemic drugs.
Next steps: Administration of glucose urgently/adjust antidiabetic therapy.

19. **Scenario: Proteinuria in kidney disease**
Case: Urine protein/creatinine ratio analyzed by autoanalyzer is 5.1 (normal: <0.2).
Interpretation: Marked proteinuria indicating nephrotic syndrome/glomerular disease.
Next steps: Kidney biopsy/focus on main cause.

20. **Scenario: Hypoalbuminemia in liver cirrhosis**
Case: Serum albumin measured by autoanalyzer is 2.1 g/dL (normal: 3.5–5.0 g/dL).
Interpretation: Hypoalbuminemia indicating liver dysfunction, such as in cirrhosis/protein loss because of nephrotic syndrome/malnutrition.
Next steps: Manage the main cause/albumin infusion if clinically required

CLINICAL MCQS

1. **A 47-year-old patient is taking up routine lab investigations by using an autoanalyzer. What is the main function of an autoanalyzer?**
   a. To automate pipetting
   b. To do enzyme-linked immunosorbent assays
   c. To automate the analysis of substances in blood or urine samples
   d. To perform cell count

   Answer: c. To automate the analysis of substances in blood or urine samples
2. **Which is a significant application of using an autoanalyzer in clinical biochemistry labs?**
   a. Reduced testing time and high throughput
   b. Requires less sample handling than manual methods
   c. Involves complex reagents
   d. Limited to quantitative testing

   Answer: a. Reduced testing time and high throughput
3. **In an autoanalyzer, which is actually required to measure light absorbance of any sample?**
   a. Photodiode
   b. Centrifuge machine
   c. Sample injector
   d. Sample dispenser

   Answer: a. Photodiode
4. **What is commonly measured by autoanalyzer in clinical chemistry?**
   a. ABG
   b. Serum glucose and cholesterol levels
   c. Hemoglobin electrophoresis
   d. Urinary flow rate

   Answer: b. Serum glucose and cholesterol levels
5. **A clinical laboratory person calibrates autoanalyzer to measure a serum sodium level. What step is required for calibration process?**
   a. Running a blank sample
   b. Using a standard solution with a known concentration of sodium
   c. Adjusting the pH
   d. Adjusting the sample volume

   Answer: b. Using a standard solution with a known concentration of sodium
6. **During an autoanalyzer test for creatinine level assay one sample is incorrectly done and processed because of malfunction. What can be the complication?**
   a. Pseudo negative result for creatinine
   b. Inaccurate measurement of the serum creatinine concentration
   c. High reagent consumption
   d. Increase in the volume of the sample

   Answer: b. Inaccurate measurement of the serum creatinine concentration
7. **Which assay is used in autoanalyzer for measuring glucose level in blood samples?**
   a. Enzymatic assay
   b. Nephelometry
   c. Absorption mass spectrometry
   d. Immunoassay

   Answer: a. Enzymatic assay

8. **Which could result in erroneous results in an autoanalyzer's biochemical assay?**
   a. Proper sample handling
   b. Contamination of reagents
   c. Use of standardized buffers
   d. Routine maintenance

   Answer: b. Contamination of reagents

9. **A patient's lipid profile was done. Which component is required to measure total cholesterol, triglycerides in the sample?**
   a. Reagents that convert cholesterol into a colored complex
   b. Ion-selective electrode
   c. Measurement of light scattering
   d. HPLC

   Answer: a. Reagents that convert cholesterol into a colored complex

10. **What is function of sample injector in an autoanalyzer?**
   a. For mixing sample with reagents
   b. To accurately transfer a precise volume of sample into the analyzer
   c. Measurement of light absorbance
   d. To separate serum and plasma

   Answer: b. To accurately transfer a precise volume of sample into the analyzer

VIVA VOCE

Q1. What is an autoanalyzer?

Autoanalyzer: Automated instrument utilized in clinical biochemistry for performing multiple tests on biological samples quickly/efficiently. It improves accuracy/precision/reproducibility/throughput/reducing manual errors along with workload.

Q2. What are the types of autoanalyzers?

Discrete analyzers: They perform individual tests in separate reaction chambers like Cobas, Architect.
Continuous flow analyzers: They use a continuous stream of liquid for analyzing multiple samples like Technicon autoanalyzer.
Dry chemistry analyzers: They use dry reagent slides/strips like Vitros analyzers.

Q3. What are the components of an autoanalyzer?

Sample handling system that is pipettor, probe, sample trays.
Reagent dispensing unit that is mixing and reaction chambers.
Incubation system that is temperature control for reactions.
Detection system that is photometers/fluorometers/ion-selective electrodes.
Data processing unit that is software for result calculation and reporting.

Q4. What are the advantages/limitations of autoanalyzers?

Advantages:
High throughput, decreased turnaround time.
Improved precision along with accuracy.
Less reagent wastage/human errors.
Limitations:
High cost initially.
Needs regular calibration/maintenance.
May not be suitable for low-volume/specialized tests.

Q5. How is quality control maintained in autoanalyzers?

Running internal QC samples/daily/shift-wise.
Calibrate analyzer regularly using standard solutions.
Using Levey-Jennings charts/Westgard rules for monitoring precision/accuracy.
Performing preventive maintenance/reagent lot verification.

SPOTTERS

Q1. Show an image: A diagram of a discrete autoanalyzer with labeled components like sample tray/reagent dispenser/mixing chamber/detection unit. Identify which type of autoanalyzer is this.

Discrete autoanalyzer to perform individual tests separately and commonly used in modern labs.

Q2. Show a scenario: A lab technician reports that an autoanalyzer is consistently giving low glucose readings despite normal patient values. What can be the reason?

Calibration error/reagent deterioration and requires recalibration plus reagent check.

Q3. Show an image: A Levey-Jennings chart with a trend where control values gradually shift downward over several days. Interpret.

Systematic error/trend error—might be because of instrument drift/reagent aging/calibration issues.

Q4. Show a scenario: A lab receives an external QC sample for sodium estimation. The autoanalyzer reports 170 mmol/L, but the expected value was 140 mmol/L. What error does this suggest?

Instrument calibration/ion-selective electrode malfunction—needs recalibration/electrode check.

Q5. Show an image: A continuous flow autoanalyzer with multiple samples moving through the tubing. What is the type of analyzer and its disadvantage?

Continuous flow autoanalyzer—risk of sample carryover plus reagent wastage.

REFLECTION

Visit to the hospital laboratory, observe the operation and principle of working of the auto analyzer and write the reflection.

27

CHAPTER

Quality Control in Laboratory

COMPETENCIES

BC14.20: Describe and identify preanalytical (especially order of draw and tourniquet technique), analytical and postanalytical errors.
BC14.21: Describe quality control and identify basic LJ charts in clinical Biochemistry lab.

LEARNING OBJECTIVES

After reading this chapter, the readers should be able to:
- Describe the basis and concepts of quality control in biochemistry laboratory.
- Describe the main approach required to ensure quality of tests performed in biochemistry laboratory.
- Understand the principles and applications of various commonly used equipments and techniques in biochemistry laboratory.
- Familiarize themselves with the operation and maintenance of laboratory instruments.
- Gain practical knowledge of performing biochemical assays and analyses.
- Learn about quality control measures to ensure accurate and reliable laboratory results.

BLUE PRINT

BC14.21: Describe quality control and identify basic LJ charts in clinical Biochemistry lab.

Objective

By the end of the lecture, students should be able to:
1. Understand the principles and applications of various commonly used equipments and techniques in biochemistry laboratory.
2. Familiarize themselves with the operation and maintenance of laboratory instruments.
3. Gain practical knowledge of performing biochemical assays and analyses.
4. Learn about quality control measures to ensure accurate and reliable laboratory results.

Duration: ***60 minutes***

Materials Needed

1. Presentation slides illustrating each equipment and technique.
2. Demonstration models or actual laboratory instruments for hands-on learning.
3. Samples or reagents required for practical demonstrations.
4. Whiteboard or flipchart for interactive discussions and note-taking.

Outline

I. **Introduction to biochemistry laboratory techniques** **(10 minutes)**
   - Overview of the role of biochemistry laboratory in biomedical research and clinical diagnostics.
   - Importance of accurate and reliable laboratory techniques in biochemical analysis.

II. Quality control in biochemistry laboratory (50 minutes)

- Importance of quality control measures in ensuring accurate and reliable laboratory results.
- Discussion of internal quality control (QC) and external proficiency testing.

Quality control system	It is the process which ensures that the results reported to the patients under all conditions are correct, that is the quality and reliability of the results is mainly due to a quality control system
Parameters of basic quality	Accuracy Precision Specificity Sensitivity When the test is specific, precise, accurate, and sensitive that means the results are within the reliable quality
Accuracy	• When the estimated value of an analyte is close to/near to its actual value in a sample, the report is said to be accurate • Accuracy depends on the method adopted in the laboratory
Example of accuracy	• True fasting glucose concentration of a sample comes to be 110 mg% • The estimated value of the same in the laboratory comes to be 108 mg% by a good method, which is closer to the actual value of 110 mg% (true value) • The estimated value of the same in the laboratory by another method comes to be 85 mg% • The value of 85 mg% is not closer to the actual value (110 mg%), so it is not accurate
Precision	• Repeated estimated values of the same parameter and on the same sample decides the precision • A test is precise if there is no wide variation in the repeated estimations of the same parameter in the same sample
Example of precision	• True fasting glucose concentration of a sample comes to be 110 mg% • Thus, the repeated values of 103, 105, 108 are relatively close values to each other as well as to the actual true value of 110 mg%, so the repeatability of the test is precise • But the repeated values of 96, 98, 100 are relatively not close to the actual true value of 110 mg%, so the repeatability of the test is not precise by this test
Accurate and precise results	When a specific test gives accurate and precise results, this signifies that the result is near the actual value and repeated estimations does not affect it significantly
Specificity	Ability of a particular test by which it can distinguish between same substances that it can measure
Example of specificity	• Glucose estimation can be done by two methods: (1) enzymatic, and (2) reduction • Enzymatic method uses glucose oxidase enzyme which is very specific and acts on glucose and not on other hexoses • Reduction methods are based on reducing property of all sugars, so these are nonspecific, and give false positive tests for all substances in the sample that show reducing nature
Sensitivity	Ability of a test to estimate very minute concentration of the required parameter present in the sample
Work flow/path	All the activities taking place in the laboratory during testing
Preanalytical phase: Operating procedure stages before the analysis of the sample	Begins from collection of sample —Transport→ to sample put to analysis There may be a time lag between the collection of sample and analysis of the sample
Stages of sample collection	• Perfect antiseptic care • Perfect container • Preservation in perfect conditions • Perfect labeling • Perfect details put on the label • Perfect time and date of collection on the label
Transport	Reaching to the laboratory
Analysis	Done by appropriate methods and standardized instruments

Preanalytical errors	**Errors occurring during preanalytical phase**
Example of preanalytical errors:	Requisition of a test: • Patient selection may be wrong • Patient details may be wrong • Poor/erroneous writing • The patient is wrongly prepared (not adequately fasting/taken milk or tea) In sample collection: • Improper container of the sample • Insufficient collection • Hemolyzed sample • Wrong time of collection
Analytical phase: All the stages in analytical phase must be duly verified and validated to give accurate and precise results	• Sample preparation (centrifuging to separate serum/plasma, avoiding hemolysis, noting hemolysis if present, especially in electrolyte estimation, otherwise high value can be obtained for K^+ in a hemolyzed sample) • Analysis requires methods which use good quality reagents, perfectly calibrated instruments, and by well trained technicians
Analytical errors	• Errors during analytical stages • Sample mixing • Improper calibration • Improper quality of reagents • Improper washing results in analysis of interfering substances • Improper preparation of reagents • No trained technicians • Autoanalyzers should be properly calibrated and regularly monitored otherwise they can give errors too
Postanalytical errors	• Errors after analytical phase • Errors in transcription of reports (report of patient A goes to patient B by mistake) • Mixing of results • Delayed reporting (critically ill patients may suffer)
Types of errors	Systemic errors; Random errors
Systemic errors	There is a shift in the mean value of a test monitored on a daily basis
Cause	Calibration problems
Rectified	Check the test reagents, instruments and follow proper protocols
Random errors	Inefficient methodology resulting in large standard deviation values without much change in the mean value, indicating a reproducibility problem
Causes	• Poor precision • Pipetting errors • Timing variations • Temperature variations
Quality assurance	Some regimens are there to be followed for perfect quality results
1. Use standards and quality control serum samples	They indicate the accuracy of a result We should use standards and QC samples of normal and abnormal results (higher and lower values)
Standards	• While performing a test, we have to first standardize the test by using standard protocol of using standards • The running of standards on daily basis ensure that same absorbance values are obtained under similar conditions by the test samples
Quality control samples	They are also used in the same manner for monitoring the test performance
2. Monitoring of precision	• We can monitor standards and QC samples over a period of time • We can also divide the sample into several separate samples and mixed into other sample lots without telling the laboratory staff, but with proper labels • If the tests are done properly, not much variations are seen
3. Checking on wide fluctuations	If the fluctuations in results persists on a longer basis, they need to be checked by examining the range of results over a period of time on a day-to-day basis, so that we can compare and rectify

Contd....

Contd....

Statistical methods	Monitoring the results on a daily basis
Plot Levey–Jennings chart	• Calculate the mean and standard deviation of all the results of a particular test in a day (100 blood urea estimations) for 20 days • Then take daily mean and SD values and see if they are within mean + –3SD values or not • If they fall in this range, the test is in control • Daily man values must lie around the mean level or within mean + –2SD or mean + –3SD • Also, they must be uniformly distributed on both the sides of the mean value and not much drifted in any one particular way
Internal quality assurance service (IQAS)	Internal quality control samples are run for identifying errors and monitoring accuracy and precision
Quality control serum: They are available for normal, high and low ranges	• It is a sample that has known amount of substance to be tested • It is tested along with the patients samples so that we can assess the analysis performance • They should be within range, mean values must not change on a daily basis and should conform to Levey–Jennings chart • In case of any abnormal result, corrective measures should be immediately taken
External quality assurance service (EQAS)	• There is an external agency which gives quality samples • The agency designs a format of documented results • We run the control samples in our laboratory, following the desired procedure given by the agency along with patients samples and the results are documented as per the agency format • Then we send our results to the agency, which are then compiled and analyzed by the external agency, which then finally apprises the laboratory about the quality and level of performance

OSCE

1. **Scenario: High CV (coefficient of variation) in glucose analysis**
   Case: During internal QC for blood glucose assay the CV is 10% (acceptable CV for glucose: <5%).
   Question: What does this result suggest?
   Interpretation: A elevated CV is indicative of imprecision in the glucose assay, leading to unreliable results.
   Possible causes: Malfunctioning of instrument/degradation of reagent/error by operator.
   Next steps:
   1. Recalibrate analyzer
   2. Verify reagents/replace if needed
   3. Train staff for corrections

2. **Scenario: Levey-Jennings chart outlier**
   Case: A Levey-Jennings chart for a lipid profile exhibits one data point outside the ±2 SD range for cholesterol.
   Question: What does this result indicate/what action must be taken?
   Interpretation: A single outlier might indicate a random error, that might be because of pipetting error/reagent inconsistency.
   Next steps:
   1. Repeat test for control sample.
   2. If the repeat value is within range, no more action is needed.
   3. If value goes out of range, investigate source of error a/resolve it.

3. **Scenario: Westgard rules violation**
   Case: During enzyme investigation QC data violates the 4-1s rule that is four consecutive values comes within ±1 SD on the same side of the mean.
   Question: What does violation suggest/how can it be addressed?
   Interpretation: A systematic error is there likely because of deterioration of reagent/calibration drift/instrument bias.
   Next steps:
   1. Check calibration of the analyzer.
   2. Review the storage states of the reagent/replace if required.
   3. Perform preventive maintenance on instrument.

4. **Scenario: Shift in QC data**
   Case: Over 7 days the QC values for serum creatinine assay are consistently more than mean but within ±2 SD.
   Question: What is the interpretation?

Interpretation: This shift suggests potential systematic error. However, results are but acceptable but error might deteriorate.
Next steps:
1. Find out potential causes, like reagent lot changes/calibration errors.
2. Recalibration/monitor further quality control results.

5. **Scenario: Trends in QC data**
Case: A Levey-Jennings chart for albumin exhibits gradual upward trend over 10 consecutive times.
Question: What does this trend suggest?
Interpretation: A gradual trend indicates systematic drift, likely because of instrument wear/reagent degradation with time.
Next steps:
1. Focus on instrument maintenance/recalibrate
2. Verify integrity of all reagents.
3. Run additional QC samples for confirming the stability.

6. **Scenario: Failure of external quality assurance (EQA)**
Case: An EQA program for LFT's reports that the lab's ALT values are consistently elevated than the peer group mean.
Question: What may be the cause/what actions to be taken?
Interpretation: Consistently elevated ALT values suggest a bias in the lab's results, likely because of calibration error/reagent issues/analytical interference.
Next steps:
1. Review calibration/reagent preparation.
2. Analyze method's performance against a reference standard.
3. Participate in more proficiency testing of parameter for validating corrective actions.

7. **Scenario: Random error in QC**
Case: QC data for urea exhibits sporadic points outside ±2 SD without a consistent pattern.
Question: What does this suggest?
Interpretation: Random errors, such as inaccurate pipetting/formation of air bubbles/sample handling problems
Next steps:
1. Check all pipettes in context of accuracy/precision.
2. Make sure proper mixing of reagents/samples.
3. Train all staff for following standardized operating methodologies.

8. **Scenario: Bias in QC results**
Case: A new reagent lot for calcium assay consistently provides QC results 5% lower than the previous lot.
Question: What does this interpret?
Interpretation: The new reagent lot introduces a systematic bias in this parameter measurements.
Next steps:
1. Verify performance of new reagent lot by making use of patient sample comparisons.
2. Adjust calibration curve
3. Notify reagent supplier.

9. **Scenario: Delta check alert**
Case: A patient's current potassium report is 2.0 mmol/L, but the previous result was 4.5 mmol/L. A delta check triggers alert for this significant change.
Question: How can this be interpreted?
Interpretation: The result might indicate a true critical change, such as hypokalemia/preanalytical error, such as hemolysis/improper sample handling.
Next steps:
1. Repeat test for confirmation of result.
2. Verify sample integrity/collection procedure.
3. Focus on clinical reason behind hypokalemia

10. **Scenario: Use of two levels of QC**
Case: A lab runs two levels of QC that is both low and high for glucose analysis every day. The low QC level consistently meets acceptable criteria however high QC level fails repeatedly.
Question: What does this suggest?
Interpretation: The failure at the high QC level indicates problem with assay linearity/calibration at higher concentrations.
Next steps:
1. Verify linearity of the glucose measurements.
2. Recalibrate analyzer across the entire reportable range.
3. Check for reagent/instrument problems if any affecting high concentrations.

OSPE

1. **Scenario: Analytical quality control**
   Case: A biochemistry laboratory is noticing inconsistent results for serum glucose assays. The technician runs the same sample multiple times, and the readings vary significantly each time. The laboratory participates in an external quality assessment program, and its results have been in the acceptable range.
   Laboratory results:
   Sample A, glucose (test 1): 98 mg/dL
   Sample A, glucose (test 2): 110 mg/dL
   Sample A, glucose (test 3): 105 mg/dL
   Question: What does the variation in glucose test results suggest, and what steps should be taken now?
   Interpretation: The significant variation in test results for the same sample indicates a precision issue in the glucose assay procedure. This suggests a possible instrument malfunction, reagent instability, or operator error.
   Diagnosis: The laboratory is facing issues with within-run precision.
   Next steps:
   Check calibration of the instrument and reagents.
   Perform maintenance on the analyzer, ensuring all equipment is functioning properly.
   Review sample handling procedures to ensure consistency.
   Conduct regular internal quality control tests and participate in the external quality assessment program to monitor performance.
2. **Scenario: External quality control participation**
   Case: A laboratory receives its external quality control results for liver function tests. The laboratory's results for serum alanine aminotransferase (ALT) are significantly different from the EQA reference values.
   EQA Results:
   Serum ALT (reference value): 35 U/L
   Laboratory ALT result: 65 U/L (out of acceptable range)
   Question: What does the discrepancy between the laboratory result and the EQA reference value suggest, and what steps should the laboratory take?
   Interpretation: The laboratory's serum ALT result is outside the acceptable range for the EQA results, indicating a potential systematic error in the ALT assay.
   Diagnosis: This suggests a possible calibration or method error with the ALT testing system.
   Next steps:
   Recalibrate the equipment used for ALT testing.
   Review the assay procedure to identify potential sources of error (e.g., reagent expiration, incorrect procedure).
   Run internal quality control (QC) tests on known samples to check for consistency.
   Compare methods with other laboratories or external sources if the issue persists.
3. **Scenario: Control charts and acceptable range**
   Case: A laboratory technician notices that the results for serum cholesterol levels appear to be stable, but a review of the control chart shows that the results have begun to drift slightly upward over the past week.
   Control chart data:
   Day 1: 185 mg/dL
   Day 2: 186 mg/dL
   Day 3: 188 mg/dL
   Day 4: 191 mg/dL
   Day 5: 195 mg/dL
   Question: What does the upward trend in control chart results suggest, and how should the laboratory address this?
   Interpretation: The upward drift in the control chart data suggests a potential calibration or reagent issue, where the analytical system is becoming less accurate over time.
   Diagnosis: The results are exhibiting a bias or systematic error.
   Next steps:
   Recheck calibration and perform calibration adjustment if necessary.
   Check reagent quality for degradation or expiration.
   Review procedural consistency, ensuring that the method and handling of samples are correct.
   Investigate external environmental factors, such as changes in temperature or humidity, that may affect instrument performance.
4. **Scenario: Acceptable error limits in QC**
   Case: A biochemistry laboratory technician is reviewing the results of an internal quality control (QC) for serum creatinine. The QC samples have fallen outside the acceptable error limits defined by the laboratory.
   Internal QC results:
   QC sample (expected value): 1.2 mg/dL

QC sample (test result): 1.4 mg/dL (outside acceptable range)
Error limit: ±10%
Question: What does the result outside the error limit indicate, and what steps should be taken?
Interpretation: The QC result for serum creatinine is outside the acceptable range (within ±10%), indicating a potential systematic error. This could be due to issues like reagent instability, calibration drift, or operator error.
Diagnosis: Quality control failure for serum creatinine testing.
Next steps:
Troubleshoot the equipment by performing calibration checks and running a maintenance cycle on the analyzer.
Test the reagent to ensure it is not expired or compromised.
Review the protocol for the test to confirm that all steps were followed properly.
Repeat QC tests and reassess performance before testing patient samples.

5. **Scenario: Interference in laboratory testing**
Case: A laboratory technician notices that the serum bilirubin test results for a particular patient are unusually high. The patient is being treated with a medication known to interfere with bilirubin assays.
Laboratory results:
Serum total bilirubin: 10 mg/dL (elevated, normal: 0.2–1.2 mg/dL)
Direct bilirubin: 8.5 mg/dL (elevated)
Question: How should the laboratory address this potential interference?
Interpretation: The elevated bilirubin levels could be due to medication interference with the bilirubin assay. Some substances (e.g., certain drugs, lipemia, hemolysis) can interfere with the accuracy of bilirubin measurements.
Diagnosis: Assay interference due to medication or sample contamination.
Next steps:
Verify with the clinical team whether the patient is on any medication known to interfere with the bilirubin assay.
Repeat the test with a modified method or use an alternate method that is not affected by the interference (e.g., a different reagent or technique).
Document the potential interference and alert the clinical team about it.

6. **Scenario: Proficiency testing**
Case: A laboratory has completed an annual proficiency testing program for serum protein electrophoresis. The laboratory's results are consistent with the external reference laboratory's results for most cases, except for a few with marginal differences in the interpretation of band patterns.
Proficiency testing results:
Laboratory result: Correct for 18 out of 20 samples
External reference: Correct for 20 out of 20 samples
Question: What should the laboratory do after receiving these proficiency testing results?
Interpretation: The laboratory's results are generally accurate, but the marginal differences in interpretation for a few samples suggest areas for improvement in test accuracy or interpretation.
Diagnosis: Minor discrepancy in interpretation of results.
Next steps:
Review the test procedures and band interpretation criteria for serum protein electrophoresis.
Provide additional training for laboratory personnel on the proper interpretation of electrophoresis patterns.
Repeat proficiency testing to assess the accuracy and consistency of results and track improvement over time.

CLINICAL MCQS

1. **Which is the key reason of quality control in clinical biochemistry laboratories?**
   a. For ensuring accurate/reproducible results
   b. For minimizing number of tests done
   c. To decrease workload of lab personnel
   d. For improving patient comfort at the time of blood collection

   Answer: a. For ensuring accurate/reproducible results

2. **Which control material is used for quality control in order to monitor laboratory performance over time?**
   a. Calibration standards
   b. Samples from patients
   c. External quality assessment samples
   d. Blank

   Answer: c. External quality assessment samples

3. **What is the main reason of using internal quality control in a clinical laboratory?**
   a. For verifying the laboratory is complying with proper standards
   b. For monitoring precision/accuracy of results on a day-to-day basis
   c. For confirming identity of the patient samples
   d. For evaluating sensitivity of equipments

   Answer: b. For monitoring precision/accuracy of results on a day-to-day basis

4. **A technician of lab observes a control sample is consistently falling out of the acceptable range. What step should be taken?**
   a. Ignore the result
   b. Investigate potential sources of error and re-run the control sample
   c. Repeat the patient tests
   d. Adjust instrument calibration

   Answer: b. Investigate potential sources of error and re-run the control sample

5. **In quality control charts, what do we mean by "Westgard rule"?**
   a. Need for calibrating equipment
   b. Random errors and systematic errors in test results
   c. The quality of reagent
   d. The amount of blood samples collected

   Answer: b. Random errors and systematic errors in test results

6. **What is the reason to perform calibration checks on analytical instruments?**
   a. For monitoring temperature
   b. For making sure the accuracy and precision of analytical results
   c. For maintaining cleanliness
   d. For evaluating shelf life

   Answer: b. For making sure the accuracy and precision of analytical results

7. **Which is method to assess the precision of laboratory tests?**
   a. Running control samples with known concentrations at proper intervals
   b. Performing only one test
   c. Using one reagent batch
   d. Testing negative patient samples

   Answer: a. Running control samples with known concentrations at proper intervals

8. **What type of external quality control program includes comparison of lab results with the results of other labs?**
   a. Internal quality control
   b. Proficiency testing
   c. Calibration
   d. Lab accreditation

   Answer: b. Proficiency testing

9. **Which is example of a systematic error in laboratory assay?**
   a. Random fluctuation
   b. A constant error due to incorrect calibration of equipment
   c. Varied patient sample collection procedures
   d. Contamination

   Answer: b. A constant error due to incorrect calibration of equipment

10. **What is the reason to use "Levey-Jenning's chart" in quality control?**
    a. For tracking test results over time
    b. To graphically display the precision and accuracy of laboratory test results
    c. To calibrate equipments
    d. For assessing performance of external quality control programs

    Answer: b. To graphically display the precision and accuracy of laboratory test results

11. **Which is the purpose of quality control?**
    a. To reduce the workload of technicians
    b. To ensure accurate and reliable test results
    c. To comply with legal requirements
    d. To identify new testing methods

    Answer: b. To ensure accurate and reliable test results

12. **What is the main reason of the Westgard rules?**
   a. To identify systematic and random errors
   b. To calculate the mean and standard deviation of test results
   c. To determine the turnaround time for tests
   d. To compare results with external laboratories

   Answer: a. To identify systematic and random errors

13. **Which defines precision?**
   a. The ability to obtain similar results on repeated testing
   b. The closeness of the result to the true value
   c. The comparison of test results to a reference standard
   d. The time taken to perform the test

   Answer: a. The ability to obtain similar results on repeated testing

14. **What does a Levey-Jennings chart monitor?**
   a. The linearity of an assay
   b. The stability and variability of control results over time
   c. The reagent inventory levels
   d. The calibration of laboratory equipment

   Answer: b. The stability and variability of control results over time

15. **A laboratory control sample consistently gives results which are very low than expected. Which type of error is present?**
   a. Random error
   b. Systematic error
   c. Analytical error
   d. Preanalytical error

   Answer: b. Systematic error

16. **The control values for a assay are within acceptable limits but shows high variability over time. What should be done now?**
   a. Ignore the trend since values are acceptable
   b. Recalibrate the instrument and review reagent stability
   c. Increase the number of control runs
   d. Repeat the control using the same reagents

   Answer: b. Recalibrate the instrument and review reagent stability

17. **What is an example of an internal quality control?**
   a. Sending the samples for external proficiency investigations
   b. Regularly analyzing the control materials alongside patient samples
   c. Participating in an inter-laboratory comparison events
   d. Monitoring the performance of the staff

   Answer: b. Regularly analyzing the control materials alongside patient samples

18. **What is the primary goal of the program of EQA?**
   a. To assess the lab test accuracy in comparison to other laboratories
   b. To monitor cost-effectiveness of lab investigations
   c. To ensure patient samples are processed well on time
   d. To train lab faculty and staff

   Answer: a. To assess the lab test accuracy in comparison to other laboratories

19. **What is the acceptable range for a control result when mean: 100, standard deviation: 5?**
   a. 90 to 111
   b. 95 to 106
   c. 85 to 115
   d. 80 to 121

   Answer: c. 85 to 115

20. **Which error is associated with improper sample collection/handling?**
   a. Preanalytical error
   b. Analytical error
   c. Postanalytical error
   d. Random error

   Answer: a. Preanalytical error

VIVA VOCE

Q1. Discuss QC in a laboratory.

Quality control in a laboratory ensures accuracy/precision/reliability of test results by the use of control materials/monitoring performance/identifying errors.

Types: Internal QC/daily checks, external QC/proficiency testing by external agencies.

Q2. Differentiate between accuracy and precision in laboratory testing.

Accuracy: How close a test result is to the true/accepted value.

Precision: How consistently a test gives the same results when repeated again under the same conditions.

Q3. Discuss Levey–Jennings charts, and their importance.

Levey-Jennings charts: Graphical representations of QC data over time, they plot test values against control limits for detecting errors. Result beyond ±2 SD indicates warning, and ±3 SD suggests a significant error needing corrective action.

Q4. What are Westgard rules?

Westgard rules are statistical criteria done for detecting errors in laboratory QC.

1-2s rule: Warning when one value exceeds ±2 SD.

1-3s rule: Reject when one value exceeds ±3 SD/random error.

2-2s rule: Reject when two consecutive values exceed ±2 SD on the same side/systematic error.

R-4s rule: Reject when there is a 4 SD difference between two controls/random error.

Q5. How can preanalytical errors affect laboratory QC?

Preanalytical errors occur prior testing, can affect QC such as:

- Improper sample collection such as hemolysis/wrong anticoagulant.
- Delayed sample transport/storage such as glucose degradation.
- Incorrect patient identification resulting in misinterpretation of results.

Q6. Differentiate between internal/external quality control in laboratory.

Next question/Follow-up: Why internal QC is performed daily, and external QC is periodic?

Q7. Discuss Levey–Jennings charts, and their utility in quality control.

Next question/Follow-up: What do 2SD and 3SD rule violations suggest?

Q8. Discuss Westgard rules, and how do they aid in laboratory quality control?

Next question/Follow-up: Give example of a critical violation utilizing Westgard rules?

Q9. What is the effect of preanalytical, analytical, and postanalytical errors on laboratory quality?

Next question/Follow-up: Which of these errors is in a clinical lab?

Q10. What is proficiency testing, why is it used for laboratory accreditation?

Next question/Follow-up: Name some international organizations which regulate laboratory quality standards.

SPOTTERS

Q1. Show image of Levey–Jennings chart with data point beyond +3 SD. What does this suggest?

A significant error (1-3s rule violation) needing investigation plus corrective action.

Q2. Show scenario: Technician does glucose test on the same sample twice. Results are: 150 mg/dL and 180 mg/dL. What does this suggest?

Poor precision because there is a large variation in repeated measurements. Possible reasons may be instrument malfunction/reagent issue/pipetting errors.

Q3. Show a scenario: A lab receives external QC samples from an accredited agency. The reported values consistently deviate from the expected range. What does this suggest?

Systematic error/that could be because of calibration errors/reagent deterioration/instrument malfunction.

Q4. Show a scenario: A technician notices a trend in the QC results, with values gradually increasing over time. What type of error this is?

Systematic error/trend error generally because of reagent aging/instrument wear/environmental changes.

Q5. Show an image: A Westgard rules table with a marked violation of the 2-2s rule. What does this show?

Systematic error that means two consecutive QC values exceeded ±2 SD on the same side, needs investigation.

Q6. Show an image of a Levey–Jennings chart with a shift/trend.

Identify this chart and describe the abnormality shown.

Q7. Show picture of different types of QC samples, such as normal/high/low controls in test tubes.

What are these, and why are they used in laboratory quality control?

Q8. Westgard rules chart with an example of a violation like 2-2s/R-4s rule.

Identify quality control rule being violated and also discuss its importance.

Q9. Show a graph with preanalytical/analytical/postanalytical errors in lab testing

Give the classification of errors shown with example of each.

Q10. Show certificate of accreditation by NABL/CAP/ISO 15189.

What do you understand by certificate, and what is its significance in a clinical laboratory?

REFLECTION

Visit the hospital laboratory, observe the quality control techniques and write reflections.

28

CHAPTER

Biochemical Tests in Diabetes Mellitus

COMPETENCY

BC14.19: Explain the basis and rationale of tests done in Diabetes mellitus

LEARNING OBJECTIVES

After reading this chapter, the readers should be able to:

- Describe the etiopathogenesis of diabetes mellitus and its biochemical basis.
- Describe the biochemical tests performed in diabetes mellitus.
- Describe the diagnostic basis of diabetes mellitus.
- Describe the principles of glycemic control and complications of diabetes mellitus.
- Understand the biochemical basis and rationale behind diagnostic tests used in various medical conditions.
- Explain how specific laboratory parameters are utilized in the diagnosis, monitoring, and management of different diseases.
- Interpret the results of biochemical tests in the context of specific clinical scenarios.
- Appreciate the role of biochemical investigations in understanding the pathophysiology of different medical conditions.

BLUE PRINT

Explanation of Biochemical Tests in Various Medical Conditions

Objective

By the end of the lecture, students should be able to:

1. Understand the biochemical basis and rationale behind diagnostic tests used in various medical conditions.
2. Explain how specific laboratory parameters are utilized in the diagnosis, monitoring, and management of different diseases.
3. Interpret the results of biochemical tests in the context of specific clinical scenarios.
4. Appreciate the role of biochemical investigations in understanding the pathophysiology of different medical conditions.

Duration: ***70 minutes***

Materials Needed

1. Presentation slides illustrating the biochemical tests and their interpretation in different medical conditions.
2. Case studies or clinical vignettes representing each medical condition for interactive discussion.
3. Whiteboard or flipchart for drawing biochemical pathways and explaining concepts.
4. Handouts summarizing the biochemical tests and their significance in each medical condition.

Outline

I. **Introduction to biochemical testing in medicine** **(10 minutes)**
   - Overview of the role of biochemical tests in the diagnosis and management of medical conditions.
   - Importance of understanding the underlying biochemical mechanisms for interpretation of test results.

II. **Diabetes mellitus** **(50 minutes)**
- Explanation of biochemical tests such as fasting blood glucose, oral glucose tolerance test (OGTT), glycated hemoglobin (HbA1c), and serum insulin.
- Interpretation of test results in diagnosing diabetes, assessing glycemic control, and monitoring treatment efficacy.

III. **Conclusion and recap** **(5 minutes)**
- Summarize key points covered in the lecture regarding the biochemical tests used in various medical conditions.
- Emphasize the importance of interdisciplinary collaboration between clinicians and laboratory professionals in interpreting test results.

IV. **Question and answer session** **(5 minutes)**
- Encourage students to ask questions and seek clarification on any aspects of the lecture.
- Foster discussion on practical applications of biochemical tests in clinical practice.

BLUE PRINT

Interpretation of Laboratory Results in Carbohydrate Metabolism

Understanding Laboratory Results in Carbohydrate Metabolism

Objective

By the end of the lecture, students should be able to:
1. Understand the significance of laboratory tests related to carbohydrate metabolism.
2. Interpret common analytes associated with carbohydrate metabolism.
3. Discuss the clinical implications of abnormal laboratory results in carbohydrate metabolism.

Duration: ***90 minutes***

Materials Needed

1. PowerPoint presentation or visual aids
2. Whiteboard and markers
3. Handouts with key points and diagrams
4. Examples of laboratory reports illustrating analytes associated with carbohydrate metabolism (optional)

Outline

I. **Introduction to laboratory tests in carbohydrate metabolism** **(10 minutes)**
- Overview of the lecture's objectives and agenda.
- Introduction to the importance of laboratory tests in assessing carbohydrate metabolism.

II. **Overview of analytes** **(20 minutes)**
- Description of common analytes associated with carbohydrate metabolism (e.g., glucose, insulin, HbA1c, lactate).
- Explanation of the physiological significance of each analyte.

III. **Interpretation of laboratory results** **(30 minutes)**
- Discussion on normal ranges and interpretation of laboratory results for each analyte.
- Explanation of how abnormal results may indicate underlying metabolic disorders.

IV. **Clinical case studies** **(20 minutes)**
- Presentation of clinical case studies or examples of laboratory reports related to carbohydrate metabolism.
- Group discussion on interpreting laboratory results and determining possible diagnoses.

V. **Management and follow-up** **(5 minutes)**
- Brief overview of management strategies for abnormalities detected in carbohydrate metabolism laboratory tests.
- Discussion on the importance of follow-up monitoring.

VI. **Conclusion and recap** **(5 minutes)**
- Summary of key points covered in the lecture.
- Emphasis on the importance of understanding laboratory results in carbohydrate metabolism.
- Encouragement for further exploration of clinical aspects of carbohydrate metabolism.

BLUE PRINT

Mechanism and Significance of Blood Glucose Regulation

Understanding Blood Glucose Regulation

Objective

By the end of the lecture, students should be able to:

1. Explain the mechanisms involved in blood glucose regulation.
2. Discuss the significance of maintaining blood glucose homeostasis in health and disease.
3. Understand the pathophysiology of common disorders related to blood glucose regulation.

Duration: *90 minutes*

Materials Needed

1. PowerPoint presentation or visual aids
2. Whiteboard and markers
3. Handouts with key points and diagrams
4. Examples of blood glucose regulation mechanisms in health and disease (optional)

Outline

I. **Introduction to blood glucose regulation** **(10 minutes)**
   - Overview of the lecture's objectives and agenda.
   - Introduction to the importance of blood glucose homeostasis.

II. **Mechanisms of blood glucose regulation** **(30 minutes)**
   - Discussion on the role of hormones (insulin, glucagon, cortisol, epinephrine) in blood glucose regulation.
   - Explanation of the mechanisms of glucose uptake, storage, and release by liver, muscle, and adipose tissue.
   - Overview of the counter regulatory response to hypoglycemia.

III. **Significance of blood glucose regulation** **(30 minutes)**
   - Discussion on the importance of maintaining blood glucose levels within a narrow range.
   - Explanation of the physiological effects of hyperglycemia and hypoglycemia.
   - Description of the impact of dysregulated blood glucose on various organ systems.

IV. **Disorders of blood glucose regulation** **(15 minutes)**
   - Overview of common disorders related to blood glucose regulation (e.g., diabetes mellitus, hypoglycemia).
   - Discussion on the pathophysiology and clinical manifestations of these disorders.

V. **Clinical case studies** **(5 minutes)**
   - Presentation of clinical case studies illustrating blood glucose regulation mechanisms in health and disease.
   - Group discussion on interpreting case studies and determining appropriate management strategies.

VI. **Conclusion and recap** **(10 minutes)**
   - Summary of key points covered in the lecture.
   - Emphasis on the significance of blood glucose regulation for overall health.
   - Encouragement for further exploration of blood glucose regulation mechanisms in clinical practice.

BLUE PRINT

Interpretation of Blood Glucose Levels and Carbohydrate Metabolism Disorders

Understanding Blood Glucose Levels and Carbohydrate Metabolism Disorders

Objective

By the end of the lecture, students should be able to:

1. Interpret the results of blood glucose levels and other laboratory investigations related to disorders of carbohydrate metabolism.
2. Explain the pathophysiology of common carbohydrate metabolism disorders.
3. Understand the clinical implications and management strategies for these disorders.

Duration: ***90 minutes***

Materials Needed

1. PowerPoint presentation or visual aids
2. Whiteboard and markers
3. Handouts with key points and diagrams
4. Clinical cases or scenarios related to carbohydrate metabolism disorders

Outline

I. **Introduction to carbohydrate metabolism** **(10 minutes)**
   - Overview of the lecture's objectives and agenda.
   - Explanation of the importance of carbohydrate metabolism in energy production and maintenance of blood glucose levels.

II. **Blood glucose regulation** **(20 minutes)**
   - Description of the normal regulation of blood glucose levels, including:
     - Role of insulin, glucagon, and other hormones
     - Mechanisms of glucose uptake and storage
     - Factors affecting blood glucose homeostasis
   - Discussion on the significance of maintaining blood glucose within normal range.

III. **Laboratory investigations for carbohydrate metabolism disorders** **(30 minutes)**
   - Explanation of common laboratory tests for assessing carbohydrate metabolism disorders, including:
     - Fasting blood glucose (FBG) levels
     - Oral glucose tolerance test (OGTT)
     - Glycated hemoglobin (HbA1c)
     - Serum insulin levels
   - Interpretation of test results and clinical significance.

IV. **Disorders of carbohydrate metabolism** **(20 minutes)**
   - Description of common disorders, including:
     - Diabetes mellitus (type 1 and type 2)
     - Hypoglycemia
     - Metabolic syndrome
   - Discussion on the pathophysiology, clinical manifestations, and management of these disorders.

V. **Case studies and application** **(10 minutes)**
   - Present case studies or clinical scenarios related to carbohydrate metabolism disorders.
   - Facilitate a discussion on the interpretation of laboratory results and treatment options for each case.

VI. **Conclusion and recap** **(10 minutes)**
   - Summary of key points covered in the lecture.
   - Emphasis on the importance of laboratory investigations in diagnosing and managing carbohydrate metabolism disorders.
   - Encouragement for further study and research in the field of metabolic diseases.

Diabetes mellitus (DM)	Group of metabolic disorders comprising of hyperglycemia due to insulin deficiency or decreased utilization of glucose and increased production of glucose, leading to secondary pathophysiological alterations in multiple organ systems causing increased morbidity and mortality
Type I A DM/brittle diabetes	• Commonly found in people aged below 30 years • There is pancreatic beta cell destruction causing insulin deficiency • The patients are genetically susceptible and prone to develop ketosis • Patients are insulin dependent
Type I B DM/idiopathic disorder	Immunological markers are not seen
Type II DM characterized by	• Variable degree of insulin resistance, impaired secretion of insulin and increased glucose production • Mainly develops in increased age but can also be seen in obese children

Contd....

Contd....

This condition of type II DM is preceded by a period of abnormal glucose homeostasis which is mainly of two types	1. Impaired fasting glycemia (IFG) 2. Impaired glucose tolerance (IGT)
Impaired fasting glycemia (IFG)	Fasting plasma sugar is above normal (normal range: 110–126 mg%), but 2 hour post glucose value is within normal range (<140 mg%)
Impaired glucose tolerance (IGT)	• Blood sugar values are >normal, but below diabetic levels • *FPG*:110–126 mg% • *2 hour PP*: 140–200 mg% • IGT can progress to frank diabetes or rarely revert to normal • Dietary control and physical exercise is recommended
Gestational diabetes/frank diabetes	• Mainly due to insulin resistance in late pregnancy resulting in impaired glucose tolerance, and may revert to normal glucose tolerance after delivery but at more risk of developing DM in future • *FPG*: >126 mg% • Increased risk of neonatal mortality, fetus secretes more insulin, excess fetal growth is seen along with excess birth weight

Clinical manifestations due to hyperglycemia	
Polyuria	Frequent and increased output of urine at short intervals
Cause of polyuria	• Blood glucose levels cross the renal threshold level of glucose which is 180 mg% thus excreting glucose in urine • The urine output is large and frequent because the excretion of glucose requires water that it draws from the vascular compartment because of osmotic effect
Polydipsia	Excess thirst and frequent water intake
Cause of polydipsia	Dehydration due to polyuria
Polyphagia	Frequent intake of food
Cause of polyphagia	Deficiency of insulin leads to decreased entry of glucose in the cell called cellular hypoglycemia which is manifesting as hunger

Diagnosis of DM	**ADA guidelines for diagnosing DM**
Fasting blood glucose	>126 mg%
2 hours PP blood glucose	>200 mg%
Random blood glucose	>200 mg% with symptoms of DM
HbA1c	>6.5%
Normal blood glucose	
FBG	<100 mg%
PPBG	After 75 g glucose load, 140 mg/dL
Normal HbA1c	6%
Impaired glucose tolerance	
FBG	101–126 mg%
2 hours PPBG	After 75 g oral glucose load 140–200 mg%

Treatment approach	
Type I DM	Patient needs insulin from the beginning
Type II DM	After diagnosis, diet regulation and weight management, followed by antidiabetic drugs and ultimately insulin
Glycemic control	1. Once the hyperglycemia is under control, the patient is advised to monitor this control 2. If proper regulation of blood glucose is maintained, the complications of DM are delayed and severity is not resent 3. Proper and regular assessment of blood glucose and detection of any complication are parts of long-term management of DM

Insulin resistance syndrome/metabolic syndrome/syndrome X	**Prediabetic state**
Characteristics	• Excess blood glucose in spite of increased insulin called insulin resistance • High blood pressure • Less HDL and more TG called dyslipidemia • Central obesity • Cardiovascular disease (CVD)
Cause of insulin resistance	Post receptor signaling defect in target tissues like skeletal muscles

Complications of DM	Poor glycemic control because of improper treatment or compliance
Acute complications	Diabetic ketoacidosis
Chronic complications	
Fine vessels complications/micro vascular complications	• Retinopathy/macular edema causing blindness • Sensory/autonomic/motor neuropathy • Renal disease/nephropathy
Major vessels complications/Macro vascular complications	• Coronary artery disease • Myocardial infarction • Cerebrovascular disorder like stroke • Peripheral vascular disorder
Miscellaneous	• Cataract/glaucoma • Foot ulcer/osteomyelitis • Candida/fungal infections

Diabetic ketoacidosis	Acute medical emergency condition with severe acute complications of uncontrolled DM
Characteristics	Severe hyperglycemia, dehydration, hyponatremia, hyperkalemia, acidosis, decreased bicarbonate of <15 mEq/L, increased anion gap
Clinical symptoms	Nausea, vomiting, abdomen pain, tachycardia, lethargy, depression, hyperventilation, fruity breath of acetone, urine test positive for ketone body
Treatment	Intravenous/intramuscular injections, fluids, electrolytes are given for correcting dehydration and electrolyte imbalance.

Biochemical basis of diabetic complications

Complication	**Mechanism**
1. Atherosclerosis	Underlying cause is excess glycosylation of intracellular proteins, such as Hb, collagen, albumin and cell matrix proteins, etc.
2. Endothelial dysfunctions	
3. Alteration of matrix protein structure and functions	
4. Increased cell osmolality	Aldose reductase pathway Excess glucose → Sorbitol → Alteration of redox potential → Reactive oxygen species production
5. Alteration of gene expression of collagen, contractile proteins and extracellular matrix proteins	Hyperglycemia → excess formation of diacylglycerol → stimulation of protein kinase C → abnormal cell functions
6. Transformation of growth factor beta (TGF beta)	Alteration of endothelial nitric oxide synthetase
7. Transformation of vascular endothelial growth factors	

Biochemical basis of tests done for DM

Blood glucose estimation	Glycated Hb estimation	Glucose tolerance test	Tests for various complications

Blood glucose

It is the important investigation?	Deficiency of insulin/insulin resistance → Hyperglycemia (increased blood glucose level)
Clinical importance	• Diagnosis of DM • Monitor glycemic control

Contd....

Contd....

Method	• Venous fasting blood sample is taken in a vial having NaF and potassium oxalate • Specific enzymatic methods are done • Repeated samples are then taken at normal carbohydrate diet
	Glycated Hb
What is glycated Hb/GHb?	Amino groups of the beta globin chain of Hb + Sugar residues $\xrightarrow{\text{Non enzymatically}}$ GHb
Types of adult Hb:	HbA1 (97%) HbA2 (2.5%) HbF (0.5%) HbA1a HbA1b HbA1c
Glucose gets attached to HbA1c nonenzymatically to form glycated Hb	
Clinical importance of glycated Hb	• Formation of GHb is irreversible • Its concentration depends on life of red blood cells and blood glucose level to which it is directly proportional • HbA1c level in the blood gives an estimate of blood glucose level over the preceding 2 to 3 months
	Estimation of HbA1c
Separation	Electrophoresis/ion exchange chromatography/high performance liquid chromatography (HPLC)
Principle of separation	• Cation exchange resin is present to separate HbA1c which is positively charged • Sample is hemolyzed, aliquot is applied to column packed with resin • HbA1c is less positively charged than HbA so it binds weakly to the column as compared to HbA • Elution is done with a buffer, absorbance read at 415 nm • Total HbA is determined from the hemolysate directly • HbA1c is expressed as a percentage of total Hb
Normal HbA1c	6%
Diagnosis of DM	>6.5%
Desirable in DM	7%
Poor glycemic control	7.5%

Glucose tolerance test (GTT): Body's ability to absorb and metabolize glucose by secreting enough inulin

Importance	• To assess the tolerance degree toward a glucose load under standard conditions • A normal person shows a characteristic time related blood glucose response after taking a known amount of glucose load
Indications	• Diagnosis of DM and IGT in doubtful cases • Assessment of nondiabetic glycosuria • Confirm gestational diabetes
Preparation	• Patient is asked to take a normal unrestricted diet having minimum 150 grams carbohydrate for 3 days, no smoking before the test • Test is done in the morning after an overnight fast on empty stomach • Patient should be relaxed, seated and not involved in physical activity • Insulin, antidiabetic drugs, steroids, thyroxine, thiazide, diuretics, salicylates, oral contraceptives should be stopped
Procedure	Oral GTT Intravenous GTT

Oral GTT

1. After overnight fasting, a fasting blood and urine sample is taken
2. A glucose load of 75 g is given in adults dissolved in 300 mL of water to be taken in 5 minutes
3. The load for children is 1.75 g/kg body weight, up to a maximum of 75 g
4. For pregnant women the glucose load is 100 g
5. Blood and urine samples are collected after every half hour interval from the time of taking glucose load, for two and a half hours
6. Quantitative estimation is done in blood samples and urine is qualitatively tested for glucose presence by Benedict's test
7. Plot a curve between the blood glucose level and time of sampling

Glucose levels in GTT curves: + – shows the presence or absence of sugar in the respective sample

GTT	Blood glucose at different times (hour)					
Response	0	½	1	1 .5	2	2.5
Normal	90	135	145	100	70	90
	–	–	–	–	–	–
Diabetic curve	170	210	270	240	220	190
	+ -	+	++	++	++	+
Lag curve	70	220	190	115	80	70
	–	++	+	–	–	–
Renal glycosuria	85	130	140	105	95	85
	–	+	+	–	–	–
Flat curve	75	90	115	95	85	80
	–	–	–	–	–	–

Normal curve

- Fasting level is within the normal limit (<100 mg%)
- Peak is reached at 1 hour and is below the renal threshold of 180 mg% (usually below 150 mg%)
- It returns to the fasting levels by 2 hours
- Dip is when there is a greater decrease at 2 hours even <the original fasting level
- It returns to normal fasting level by 2.5 hours
- All urine samples test negative for the presence of glucose

Impaired glucose tolerance curve (IGT)

- Fasting level is between 100–126 mg%
- Peak is >renal threshold of 180 mg%
- 2 hour values are between 140–200 mg%
- There are traces of glycosuria at the peak and 2 hour samples

Diabetes mellitus curve (DM)

- Maximum intolerance is exhibited in this curve
- The fasting levels are >126 mg%
- The level steadily increases to significant more values than the RT level
- The value reaches a peak at 1 hour
- The value gradually decreases, but the 2 hour level is always >200 mg%
- Glycosuria is present for most of the urine samples

Lag curve/alimentary glycosuria (lag/delay in secretion of insulin)

- The GTT curve is almost normal, except that there is an abnormal more level at the peak along with transient glycosuria during that time
- The fasting level is within the normal limit
- The 2 hour glucose level is within normal limit
- Abnormally high peak is present
- The return of the peak is almost normal
- The condition is benign

Renal Glycosuria curve

Lowered renal threshold	Raised renal threshold
Peak is reached a little lower than normal curve	Glycosuria is not seen even at very high levels than the normal RT of 160–180 mg% (sometimes blood glucose of 200 mg% is seen without glycosuria)
At this lowered peak also, there is transient glycosuria due to reabsorption defect in the renal tubules, which is the renal threshold level for such kind of people	Mechanism is because of decreased glomerular filtration rate, which can be due to glomerular arteriosclerosis, at decreased GFR, an increased glucose concentration may be reached before the saturation of tubular re absorptive capacity of glucose
Harmless, mostly seen in late pregnancy	Mostly observed in elders and diabetics

Flat curve/increased glucose tolerance

Fasting values are normal

Peak values are relatively low

Glycosuria is not seen in any of the sample

Mechanism is due to endocrinal glands hypo activity, such as hypothyroidism, hypoadrenalism (Addison's disease), hypopituitarism (Simmond's disease) and malabsorption like steatorrhea

GTT in GDM (Gestational DM)

Requirement of GTT	• In pregnancy of women >25 years of age • Family history of DM • History of DM in previous pregnancy • Advanced age of pregnant women
Method 1	Fasting sample is taken, 75 g glucose is given and 3 samples are taken hourly
Normal range	• Fasting—90 mg% • 1 hour—180 mg% • 2 hours—155 mg% • 3 hours—145 mg%

Minimum 2 values must exceed the above mentioned values

Method 2	75 g oral GTT and 2 hour blood glucose level of >140 mg% is taken to be diagnostic for gestational DM

Intravenous GTT

Required in	• Patients who are unable to take oral glucose • Malabsorption syndrome of the intestine • Partial gastrectomy (inadequate absorption of glucose)
Method	• Glucose load of 0.5 g/kg body weight is given as a 25 g% solution IV • Blood samples are taken at 30, 60, 90 and 120 minutes after injection
Normal range	• At 30 minutes–peak levels are got • In 60 minutes, value returns to basal level
In diabetic patients	The basal level comes after 2 hours or even beyond

Extended GTT

Required in	• In patients with a transient postprandial hypoglycemia due to rapid emptying of stomach and excess secretion of insulin which is corrected by taking glucose • In patients of partial gastrectomy • In patients with beta cell islet tumor like Insulinoma
Method	The test is done for 5 hours instead of 2.5 hours

Aims/goals of assessment of glycemic control

To maintain:
1. FPG: 90–130 mg% (frequent measurements are recommended)
2. Two hours PP glucose levels: <180 mg%
3. HbA1c: <7% of total Hb (at least twice a year is recommended)

Assessments of DM complications

Acute complications	• Hypoglycemia • Ketoacidosis
Hypoglycemia	Blood glucose level below 60 mg%
Cause	• Self-intervention in ongoing treatment • Irregular medicines, excess of medicines, missing meals, more time interval between the meals

Contd....

Contd....

Warning signs	• Excess sweating • Weakness • Giddiness
Immediate attention	Take sugar/sweet beverages/chocolates
In hospital	Patient is given IV glucose immediately
If untreated	Fatal
	Ketoacidosis
Clinical manifestations:	• Metabolic acidosis (due to beta hydroxybutyrate and acetoacetate) • Hyperglycemia • Ketonemia • Ketonuria • Hyperkalemia
Investigations required	• Blood glucose (for hyperglycemia) • Urinary ketone bodies (for ketonuria) • Serum electrolytes (for hyperkalemia) • Arterial blood gas (ABG) analysis (for acidosis)
Hospitalization required	Yes
	Chronic complications
Renal complications	Decreased glomerular filtration rate (GFR) and kidney failure
Atherosclerosis	Causing myocardial infarction and cerebral stroke
Blindness	Loss of vision
Investigations required	*RFT*: Blood urea, creatinine, creatinine clearance for GFR, urinary and serum proteins for proteinuria, electrolytes *Atherosclerosis*: Lipid profile including serum total cholesterol, LDL-cholesterol, HDL- cholesterol and triglycerides

OSCE

1. **Scenario: Diagnosis of diabetes mellitus**
   Case: A 46-year-old male shows with fatigue/increased thirst.
   Fasting plasma glucose: 144 mg/dL (normal: <100 mg/dL)
   HbA1c: 7.3% (normal: <5.7%)
   Interpretation: FPG ≥126 mg/dL/HbA1c ≥6.5% confirms diabetes mellitus.
   Next steps: Start lifestyle modifications/pharmacological therapy/monitor glycemic control by assay of HbA1c.
2. **Scenario: Acute complications—diabetic ketoacidosis (DKA)**
   Case: A 29-year-old type 1 diabetic presents with abdominal pain/rapid breathing.
   Blood glucose: 358 mg/dL (normal: 70–110 mg/dL)
   Arterial blood gas: pH 7.16 (normal: 7.35–7.45)
   Serum bicarbonate: 12 mEq/L (normal: 22–26 mEq/L)
   Serum ketones: Positive
   Interpretation: The patient is having DKA that is involving hyperglycemia along with metabolic acidosis/ketonemia.
   Next steps: Urgent treatment with IV fluids/insulin therapy/correction of electrolyte imbalances, such as potassium.
3. **Scenario: Monitoring long-term glycemic control**
   Case: A diabetic patient presents with
   HbA1c: 9.1% (goal for diabetics: <7.0%)
   Fasting glucose: 186 mg/dL
   Interpretation: Poor glycemic control
   Next steps: Adjust treatment regimen again focus on dietary management/increase walking and physical activity/Reassess HbA1c every 3 months.

4. **Scenario: Hypoglycemia**
   Case: A diabetic patient on insulin therapy presents with sweating and confusion.
   Blood glucose: 51 mg/dL (normal: >70 mg/dL)
   Interpretation: Hypoglycemia because of excessive insulin/fasting
   Next steps: Give oral glucose/IV dextrose/review insulin dose counsel him on prevention of hypoglycemia.
5. **Scenario: Gestational diabetes mellitus (GDM)**
   Case: A pregnant woman undergoes an oral glucose tolerance test (OGTT):
   Fasting glucose: 96 mg/dL (normal: <92 mg/dL)
   1-hour glucose: 191 mg/dL (normal: <180 mg/dL)
   2-hour glucose: 161 mg/dL (normal: <153 mg/dL)
   Interpretation: Two abnormal values in OGTT confirms GDM.
   Next steps: Start dietary modifications/monitor glucose levels/consider insulin if condition worsens.
6. **Scenario: Nonketotic hyperosmolar hyperglycemia (HHS)**
   Case: A 71-year-old type 2 diabetic presents with dehydration and mental confusion.
   Blood glucose: 705 mg/dL
   Serum osmolality: 331 mOsm/kg (normal: 275–295 mOsm/kg)
   Serum ketones: Negative
   Interpretation: HHS is characterized by severe hyperglycemia/hyperosmolality/absence of significant ketonemia.
   Next steps: Administration of IV fluids for correction of dehydration/start insulin therapy/monitor electrolytes.
7. **Scenario: Lipid profile in diabetes**
   Case: A type 2 diabetic has the following lipid profile:
   Total cholesterol: 258 mg/dL (normal: <200 mg/dL)
   LDL cholesterol: 164 mg/dL (normal: <100 mg/dL)
   HDL cholesterol: 34 mg/dL (normal: >40 mg/dL)
   Triglycerides: 222mg/dL (normal: <150 mg/dL)
   Interpretation: Dyslipidemia very commonly linked with diabetes, enhancing cardiovascular risk.
   Next steps: Advise lifestyle changes/statins/set lipid targets.
8. **Scenario: Microalbuminuria in diabetic nephropathy**
   Case: A diabetic patient undergoes urine tests:
   Urine albumin: 46 mg/day (normal: <30 mg/day)
   Interpretation: Microalbuminuria suggestive of early diabetic nephropathy.
   Next steps: Optimize glycemic plus blood pressure control/monitor regular renal functions
9. **Scenario: C-peptide test for diabetes classification**
   Case: A patient with hyperglycemia undergoes a C-peptide test:
   C-peptide: 0.1 ng/mL (normal: 0.8–3.1 ng/mL)
   Interpretation: Less C-peptide is indicative of insulin deficiency/consistent with type 1 diabetes.
   Next steps: Start insulin therapy/glucose monitoring.
10. **Scenario: Fructosamine for short-term glycemic control**
    Case: A diabetic patient with anemia has an HbA1c of 6.8%, but fructosamine is on higher side at 350 μmol/L (normal: 200–285 μmol/L).
    Interpretation: Fructosamine reflects short-term glycemic control (2–3 weeks). High fructosamine is suggestive of poor glycemic control.
    Next steps: Adjust ongoing treatment/monitor fructosamine levels regularly.

CLINICAL MCQS

1. **Which test is commonly used for diagnosing diabetes mellitus?**
   a. Serum creatinine
   b. Fasting blood glucose
   c. Serum urea
   d. AST

   Answer: b. Fasting blood glucose
2. **A 54-year-old patient complains of elevated blood glucose levels. Which is the best method for assessing long-term glucose control?**
   a. Fasting blood glucose
   b. Hemoglobin A1c

c. Urine ketones
d. Post prandial blood glucose

Answer: b. Hemoglobin A1c

3. **A 33-year-old patient with type 2 diabetes and takes an oral glucose tolerance test. What is the diagnostic criterion for diabetes that is based on the 2-hour plasma glucose value?**
   a. 141 mg/dL
   b. 161 mg/dL
   c. 200 mg/dL
   d. 224 mg/dL

   Answer: c. 200 mg/dL

4. **In patients having uncontrolled diabetes, which biochemical marker is high because of diabetic nephropathy?**
   a. Serum urea
   b. Urinary albumin
   c. Serum calcium
   d. Serum sodium

   Answer: b. Urinary albumin

5. **What is the importance of measuring C-peptide concentration in a diabetic patient?**
   a. It indicates the insulin resistance
   b. It helps assess beta-cell function and insulin secretion
   c. It determines the renal disorder
   d. It monitors kidney function

   Answer: b. It helps assess beta-cell function and insulin secretion

6. **Which investigation is used for detecting ketone bodies in urine in patients suffering from DKA?**
   a. Dipstick for glucose
   b. Urinary albumen
   c. Urinary ketone bodies
   d. Urinary globulin

   Answer: c. Urinary ketone bodies

7. **In patients having type 1 diabetes, the presence of which antibodies might suggest autoimmune destruction of pancreatic beta cells?**
   a. Anti-glutamic acid decarboxylase antibody
   b. Anti-insulin receptor antibody
   c. Anti-thyroid peroxidase antibody
   d. Anti-cyclic citrullinated peptide antibody

   Answer: a. Anti-glutamic acid decarboxylase antibody

8. **Which biochemical abnormality is very commonly observed in a diabetic patient who has poorly control of blood glucose level?**
   a. Hyperkalemia
   b. Hypernatremia
   c. Hypophosphatemia
   d. Hyperlipidemia

   Answer: d. Hyperlipidemia

9. **A patient having diabetes mellitus presents with HbA1c level: 8.5%. What does this suggest?**
   a. Good long-term glucose control
   b. Poorly long-term glucose control
   c. Type 1 diabetes
   d. Immediate requirement for insulin therapy

   Answer: b. Poorly long-term glucose control

10. **A diabetic patient complains of excessive thirst/frequent urination. Which test aids to assess for diabetic ketoacidosis?**
    a. Blood glucose and pH
    b. Serum creatinine and urea
    c. Serum potassium and bicarbonate
    d. HbA1c and C-peptide

    Answer: a. Blood glucose and pH

VIVA VOCE

Q1. Discuss biochemical tests performed for diagnosing diabetes mellitus.

Fasting plasma glucose (FPG) ≥126 mg/dL (≥7.0 mmol/L)
Random blood glucose (RBG) ≥200 mg/dL (≥11.1 mmol/L) with symptoms
Oral glucose tolerance test (OGTT, 2-hour plasma glucose) ≥200 mg/dL
HbA1c ≥6.5%

Q2. Why is HbA1c preferred for long-term control of diabetes mellitus?

This parameter reflects average blood glucose levels over 2–3 months because it measures glycation of hemoglobin and is not affected by short-term fluctuations plus does not require fasting.

Q3. Give significance of the C-peptide test in diabetes mellitus.

C-peptide aids differentiate type 1 from type 2 diabetes:
Low C-peptide: Indicates type 1 diabetes because of β-cell destruction.
Normal/high C-peptide: Indicates type 2 diabetes/insulin resistance.

Q4. How does the OGTT aids in diagnoses of diabetes?

In an oral glucose tolerance test: Patient takes 75g of glucose/1.75 g/kg in children, blood glucose is measured at 0 hours/fasting and 2 hours.
Diabetes: When 2-hour plasma glucose is ≥200 mg/dL.
Impaired glucose tolerance: When 140–199 mg/dL.

Q5. What is the importance of urinary ketone assay in diabetes mellitus?

Urinary ketone test detects ketonuria, that is significant in:
Diabetic ketoacidosis in type 1 DM.
Starvation ketosis in prolonged fasting.
It aids in early detection of metabolic decompensation in diabetes.

SPOTTERS

Q1. Show a lab report:
FPG: 134 mg/dL
HbA1c: 7.1%
What is diagnosis?

Diabetes mellitus (FPG ≥126 mg/dL and HbA1c ≥6.5%).

Q2. Show a scenario: A patient having recurrent hypoglycemia:
Blood glucose: 41 mg/dL
Insulin: 31 µU/mL
C-peptide: 0.1 ng/mL
What is the condition?

Factitious hypoglycemia/exogenous insulin use, because C-peptide is low and insulin is elevated.

Q3. Show a lab report:
RBG: 292 mg/dL
Urine Ketones: Positive (+++)
pH: 7.1
HCO_3^-: 11 mEq/L
What is the diagnosis?

Diabetic ketoacidosis that is because there is elevated glucose ketonuria and metabolic acidosis.

Q4. Show a lab report:
2-hour OGTT: 166 mg/dL
FBG: 96 mg/dL
HbA1c: 5.9%
Interpretation?

Impaired glucose tolerance (OGTT: 140–199 mg/dL, HbA1c: 5.7–6.4%).

Q5. Show a clinical scenario: A diabetic patient taking metformin medication comes with fatigue/breathlessness.
Serum lactate: 6.8 mmol/L
Blood pH: 7.2
Condition?

Metformin-induced lactic acidosis.

REFLECTION

Describe the etiopathogenesis of diabetes mellitus and its biochemical basis; describe the biochemical tests performed in diabetes mellitus. Describe the diagnostic basis of diabetes mellitus; describe the principles of glycemic control and complications of diabetes mellitus.

29

CHAPTER

Interpretation of Laboratory Result: Carbohydrate Metabolism

COMPETENCY

BC14.19: Explain the basis and rationale of biochemical tests done in diabetes mellitus.

LEARNING OBJECTIVES

After reading this chapter, the readers should be able to:
- Describe the clinical interpretation related to tests done in carbohydrate metabolism.

BLUE PRINT

Lesson Plan: Interpretation of Lab Results in Carbohydrate Metabolism

Objective

By the end of this lesson, the student shall be able to:
1. Understand important lab tests linked with carbohydrate metabolism.
2. Interpret abnormal values/clinical significance.
3. Correlate lab findings with clinical conditions, such as diabetes, hypoglycemia, and metabolic disorders.

Outline

I. **Introduction** **(5 minutes)**
   - Brief introduction of carbohydrate metabolism.
   - Significance of lab tests in diagnoses of metabolic disorders.

II. **Key laboratory tests** **(15 minutes)**
   A. *Blood glucose tests*:
      1. *Fasting blood glucose*:
         Normal: 70–100 mg/dL
         Prediabetes: 100–125 mg/dL
         Diabetes: ≥126 mg/dL
      2. *Random blood glucose*:
         Normal: <140 mg/dL
         Diabetes: ≥200 mg/dL with symptoms
      3. *Postprandial Blood Glucose*:
         Normal: <140 mg/dL
         Diabetes: >200 mg/dL
      4. *Oral glucose tolerance test—2 hours after 75 g glucose)*:
         Normal: <140 mg/dL
         Impaired glucose tolerance (IGT): 140–199 mg/dL
         Diabetes: ≥200 mg/dL
   B. *HbA1c (glycated hemoglobin)—for long-term control of blood glucose*:
      Normal: <5.7%
      Prediabetes: 5.7–6.4%
      Diabetes: ≥6.5%

C. *Insulin/C-peptide levels*:
Raised insulin + raised C-peptide → insulinoma/sulfonylurea use
Raised insulin + reduced C-peptide → exogenous insulin use
Reduced insulin + reduced C-peptide → type 1 DM
D. Ketone bodies (serum/urine ketones)
Positive in diabetic ketoacidosis
Negative in hyperosmolar hyperglycemic state
E. Lactate levels (lactic acidosis)
Increased in metformin toxicity/shock/sepsis/hypoxia

III. **Interpretation of abnormal results** **(15 minutes)**

IV. **Case-based discussions** **(15 minutes)**
Case 1: A patient presents with polyuria/polydipsia/weight loss, FBG: 142 mg/dL, HbA1c is 7.3%.
Diagnosis: Diabetes mellitus
Next step: Initiate lifestyle modification/medications.
Case 2: A patient with a history of diabetes is found unconscious and sweating, RBG: 41 mg/dL.
Diagnosis: Hypoglycemia (possible insulin overdose)
Next step: Give IV dextrose.

V. **Summary and quick recap** **(5 minutes)**
Glucose tests: diagnosis and monitoring.
HbA1c: long-term glucose control.
Ketones for identifying DKA.
Insulin and C-peptide: distinguishing endogenous vs. exogenous insulin.

SPOTS/CLINICAL CASES

CASE 1: McARDLE'S DISEASE

Age, gender	10 years, male
Complains	Lethargy, exercise intolerance, muscle cramps
Blood report	
Blood glucose	100 mg%
Blood lactate	0.3 mmol/L (0.5-1 mmol/L)
Muscle biopsy	>4% glycogen
What is the diagnosis?	McArdle's Disease
Reasons	• Excess glycogen in muscles (normal glycogen: <1%) • Decreased level of lactate in blood
Mechanism	There is deficiency of enzyme muscle glycogen phosphorylase, therefore, muscle glycogen will not be able to give the needed glucose-6-phosphate required for glycolysis thus causing exercise intolerance
Why blood lactate is low after exercise?	Due to the reason that there is lack of glucose-6-phosphate enzyme in muscle so no glycolysis is taking place in the muscle
Characteristic features of McArdle's patients	
Second wind phenomenon	Patient has a better tolerance for walking and cycling after 10 minutes of continuous exercise
Mechanism	Increased blood flow during those 10 minutes leading to good fuel energy by glucose and fatty acids for sustaining the muscular exercise

CASE 2: VON GIERKE'S DISEASE

Age, gender	8 years, male
Complains	Lethargy, weakness, tremors, sweating, delayed developing milestones
On examination	Enlarged liver
	Blood report
Fasting blood glucose	50 mg% (hypoglycemia)
Blood lactate	4.9 mmol/L (0.5–1 mmol/L) ↑
Ketone bodies in urine	++
pH	7.30
Uric acid	9.5 mg% ↑
What is the diagnosis?	Von Gierke's disease
Reasons	• It is a glycogen storage disease type Ia • Here there is deficiency of enzyme glucose-6-phosphatase which is a very important enzyme for liver glycogenolysis as well as gluconeogenesis, indicated by severe hypoglycemia in the child
Why ketone bodies are present in urine?	Hypoglycemia results in free fatty acid mobilization from adipose tissue TAG because of the activity of hormone sensitive lipase enzyme, so excess oxidation of fatty acids in liver result in formation of ketone bodies in excess
Crabtree effect	• Due to accumulated glucose-6-phosphate in liver, this excess glucose-6-phosphate goes to glycolysis and results in anaerobic increase of glycolysis, resulting in lactic acidosis • Overproduction and under excretion of uric acid results in high serum levels

CASE 3: CORI DISEASE (LIMIT DEXTRINOSIS)

Age, gender	5 years, male
Complains	Early morning hypoglycemia
On examination	Enlarged liver
	Blood report
Blood glucose	58 mg% (hypoglycemia)
Renal function tests	Normal
Liver function tests	Normal
Muscle biopsy	Limit dextrin (glycogen with less branches)
What is the diagnosis?	Cori disease
Reasons	• It is a glycogen storage disease–limit dextrinosis • Here there is deficiency of debranching enzyme in liver as well as in muscles (IIIA) or in liver alone (IIIB) • The disease has a feature of delayed hypoglycemia and exercise intolerance in case of involvement of muscles

CASE 4: CLASSICAL GALACTOSEMIA

Age, gender	5 months, male child
Complains	Improper feeding, vomiting, hypoglycemia, low body weight
On examination	Enlarged liver, bilateral cataract
	Blood report
Random blood glucose	65 mg% (hypoglycemia)
Serum uric acid	8 mg%

Contd....

Contd....

Lactic acid	Higher side
What is the diagnosis?	Classical galactosemia
Reasons	• Baby has classical galactosemia symptoms • There is deficiency of galactose-1-phosphate uridyltransferase, a very important enzyme of galactose metabolism • Hepatomegaly occurs due to accumulation of galactose 1 phosphate in liver cells • Also, galactose-1-phosphate inhibits the enzyme glycogen phosphorylase required for glycogen breakdown, resulting in hypoglycemia • Hyperuricemia is due to sequestration of ATP for converting galactose to galactose-1-phosphate leading to excess purine nucleotide biosynthesis, so excess breakdown of purine nucleotides results in high level of uric acid (ATP inhibits biosynthesis of purine nucleotides)

CASE 5: DIABETES MELLITUS

Age, gender	55 years, female
Complains	Increased thirst, excess appetite, increased urine frequency for the last 3 months (polydipsia, polyphagia, polyuria)
	Blood report
Fasting blood glucose	150 mg%
Postprandial blood sugar	212 mg%
HbA1c	7%
Dipstick test (urine)	Positive
What is the diagnosis?	Diabetes mellitus
Reasons	Fasting blood glucose of >126 mg% and HbA1c value of >6.5% is suggestive of diabetes mellitus
Diagnostic criterion of diagnosis of diabetes (ADA members, European association for the study of diabetes and IDF)	HbA1c >6.5% FPG >126 mg% 2 hour postprandial blood glucose >200 mg% after oral glucose tolerance test that is 75 g glucose dissolved in water Random blood glucose >200 mg% plus symptoms of diabetes mellitus
Other recommended investigations:	• Urine must be tested for microalbuminuria for possibility of diabetic neuropathy • Dyslipidemia should be ruled out by lipid profile • Advised oral hypoglycemic treatment, dietary changes and physical exercise

CASE 6: DIABETIC KETOACIDOSIS

Age, gender	16 years, male
On admission	In state of coma, fruity odor from breath
Past history	Diabetic for last 7 years, on insulin treatment but not regularly taking insulin
	Blood report
Random blood glucose	450 mg%
Pulse	115/min
Blood pressure	90/60 mm Hg
pH	7.05
	Urine report
Proteins	–
Ketone bodies	++++

Contd....

Contd....

Sugar	++++
What is the diagnosis?	Diabetes ketoacidosis
Reasons	• A characteristic feature of diabetic ketoacidosis is presence of ketone bodies in the body fluid (urine) and also in breath as evident by acetone like fruity smell • Ketoacidosis is aggravated by lack of insulin leading to excess mobilization of fatty acid from adipose tissue

CASE 7: DEFICIENCY OF GLUCOSE-6-PHOSPHATE DEHYDROGENASE

Age, gender	26 years, male
Complains	History of fever, chills, rigors, was taking antimalarial drug primaquine before, presented with mild yellow discoloration of conjunctiva, breathlessness
On examination	Pale skin, pale mucous membrane
	Blood report
Hb	6 g%
Total bilirubin	5 mg%
Direct bilirubin	1 mg%
Indirect bilirubin	4 mg%
Fouchet's test	–
Liver enzymes	Normal
What is the diagnosis?	Glucose-6-phosphate dehydrogenase (G6PD) deficiency
Reasons	• Deficiency of G6PD, a very important enzyme of hexose monophosphate (HMP) shunt, leads to decreased generation of nicotinamide adenine dinucleotide phosphate (NADPH), leading to oxidative stress of all cells and red blood cells (RBCs), causing hemolysis • Primaquine drug treatment increases the oxidative stress in the cells leading to excess hemolysis • Patient is presenting with jaundice that can be due to hemolysis (hemolytic jaundice)

CASE 8: LACTOSE INTOLERANCE

Age, gender	3 months old baby
Complains	Pain in abdomen after feed, tolerates fruit juices well
On examination	Swelling in abdomen
What is the diagnosis?	Lactose intolerance
Reasons	• Lactose does not get digested to glucose and galactose due to deficiency of enzyme lactase in the intestinal mucosa • Intestinal bacteria changes this undigested and unabsorbed lactose to harmful gases like CO_2 and methane, causing distension and flatulence
Advised mother	Lactose and galactose free diet must be given to the baby

OSCE

1. **Scenario: Diagnosis of lactose intolerance**
   Case: A 26-year-old boy complains of bloating/diarrhea after consuming dairy products. Lab assay of hydrogen breath test was done.
   Baseline hydrogen: 11 ppm
   Post-lactose hydrogen (at 2 hours): 51 ppm

Question: What do this interpret?
Interpretation: The marked elevation in hydrogen levels is suggestive of lactose intolerance because of malabsorption of lactose.
Next steps: Advised lactose-free diet/lactase enzyme supplements.

2. **Scenario: Glycogen storage disease (GSD)**
   Case: A 7-month-old baby shows with hepatomegaly along with hypoglycemia.
   Blood glucose (fasting): 44 mg/dL (normal: 70–110 mg/dL)
   Serum lactate: High
   Ketones: Less
   Question: What does this interpret?
   Interpretation: Lab findings are suggestive of glycogen storage disorder most likely Von Gierke's disease.
   Next steps: Confirmation to be done by enzyme assay of glucose-6-phosphatase activity/genetic testing/start frequent feeding by cornstarch therapy.

3. **Scenario: Galactosemia**
   Case: A 3-week-old infant has jaundice/hepatomegaly.
   Reducing substances in urine: Positive
   Galactose-1-phosphate uridyltransferase activity: Absent
   Question: What is the interpretation?
   Interpretation: Classic galactosemia due to absence of GALT activity.
   Next steps: Stop lactose and galactose/go for soy-based formula

4. **Scenario: Hyperglycemia in stress**
   Case: A 51-year-old nondiabetic patient undergoing surgery with following results:
   Fasting glucose: 121 mg/dL
   Random glucose: 210 mg/dL
   HbA1c: 5.5%
   Question: Interpret the results
   Interpretation: High glucose concentration is mostly because of stress-induced hyperglycemia, as HbA1c is suggesting normal long-term glycemic control.
   Next steps: Monitor blood glucose regularly/insulin therapy if hyperglycemia persists even after the surgery

5. **Scenario: Fructose intolerance**
   Case: A child presents with hypoglycemia/vomiting after drinking fruit juice.
   Blood glucose: 51 mg/dL
   Serum fructose: High
   Question: What is the interpretation?
   Interpretation: High serum fructose is suggestive of hereditary fructose intolerance because of deficiency of enzyme—aldolase B.
   Next steps: Remove fructose/sucrose/sorbitol from the diet.

6. **Scenario: Insulinoma**
   Case: A 41-year-old woman presents with sweating/confusion/hunger.
   Blood glucose: 41 mg/dL
   Serum insulin: 21 µIU/mL (normal: <6 µIU/mL during hypoglycemia)
   C-peptide: High
   Question: What is the interpretation?
   Interpretation: High insulin/C-peptide during hypoglycemia has confirmed insulinoma.
   Next steps: Localize tumor by CT/MRI/consider surgical excision.

7. **Scenario: Pyruvate kinase deficiency**
   Case: A child with chronic hemolytic anemia has testing:
   Blood glucose: Normal
   Pyruvate kinase activity: Less
   Question: What does this interpret?
   Interpretation: Pyruvate kinase deficiency, that is a glycolytic enzyme defect leading to hemolysis/anemia.
   Next steps: Folic acid supplementation.

8. **Scenario: Diabetes and ketosis**
   Case: A Type 1 diabetic presents with abdominal pain.
   Blood glucose: 309 mg/dL
   Serum bicarbonate: 17 mEq/L (normal: 22–26 mEq/L)
   Serum ketones: Positive
   Question: What does this interpret?
   Interpretation: The patient has diabetic ketoacidosis.
   Next steps: Urgent IV fluid replacement/insulin therapy/correction of electrolyte imbalance.

9. **Scenario: Hypoglycemia in alcoholism**
   Case: A chronic alcoholic presents with sweating.
   Blood glucose: 51 mg/dL
   Serum lactate: High
   Question: What is the interpretation?
   Interpretation: Hypoglycemia is because of impaired gluconeogenesis due to alcohol-induced decreased level of NAD+.
   Next steps: Administration of IV glucose/thiamine for avoiding Wernicke's encephalopathy.

10. **Scenario: Postprandial hypoglycemia**
    Case: A 31-year-old man shows with dizziness/sweating 2 hours after taking meals.
    Blood glucose: 51 mg/dL
    Serum insulin: High
    C-peptide: High
    Question: What is the interpretation?
    Interpretation: Postprandial hypoglycemia, likely because of reactive hypoglycemia/early diabetes.
    Next steps: Go for OGTT/advise small and frequent diet having low glycemic index.

11. **Scenario: Lactic acidosis in glycolytic disorders**
    Case: A patient faces muscle cramps during exercise:
    Serum lactate: High
    Blood glucose: Normal
    Muscle biopsy: Decreased phosphofructokinase activity
    Question: What is the interpretation?
    Interpretation: Decreased PFK activity is indicating Tarui disease/GSD type VII/disorder of glycolysis
    Next steps: Prevention from strenuous exercise/adopt a high-protein diet for minimizing symptoms.

CLINICAL MCQS

1. **A 53-year-old patient complains of excessive thirst/frequent urination. Blood fasting glucose: 199 mg/dl. Which interpretations is most likely?**
   a. Hypoglycemia
   b. Abnormal glucose
   c. Impaired fasting glucose
   d. Diabetes mellitus

   Answer: d. Diabetes mellitus

2. **A patient takes up oral glucose tolerance test. The 2-hour plasma glucose level: 181 mg/dL. What is the interpretation?**
   a. Normal
   b. Impaired glucose tolerance
   c. Diabetes mellitus type 1
   d. Hyperglycemia

   Answer: b. Impaired glucose tolerance

3. **A 31-year-old patient complains of hypoglycemia after fasting. The serum insulin: high/C-peptide levels: low. What is reason of hypoglycemia?**
   a. Insulinoma
   b. Hypopituitarism
   c. Type 1 diabetes mellitus
   d. Hyperpituitarism

   Answer: a. Insulinoma

4. **A patient with uncontrolled diabetes admitted with symptoms of diabetic ketoacidosis and show high blood glucose/low bicarbonate/high anion gap. What is the key reason of the metabolic acidosis?**
   a. Lactose intolerance
   b. Diabetic ketoacidosis
   c. Renal damage
   d. Respiratory alkalosis

   Answer: b. Diabetic ketoacidosis

5. **A 46-year-old male with uncontrolled diabetes presents with random blood glucose: 354 mg/dL. What is the next key lab investigation for assessing his long-term glucose control?**
   a. Fasting glucose
   b. Hemoglobin A1c (HbA1c)
   c. Urinary ketone bodies
   d. Serum ketones

   Answer: b. Hemoglobin A1c (HbA1c)

6. **In a patient with hypoglycemia, which lab findings are consistent with insulin overdose and not insulinoma?**
   a. High serum insulin and low C-peptide levels
   b. Low serum insulin and high C-peptide levels
   c. Low blood glucose levels
   d. Low serum cortisol levels

   Answer: a. High serum insulin and low C-peptide levels

7. **A 64-year-old diabetic patient complains of blurred vision/excessive thirst. HbA1c: 9%. What does this value indicates?**
   a. Excellent control
   b. Poor control
   c. Normal glucose level
   d. Prediabetic

   Answer: b. Poor control

8. **A patient presents with fasting blood glucose: 111 mg/dL, 2-hour postprandial glucose: 141 mg/dL on a GTT. What is the diagnosis?**
   a. Normal sugar tolerance
   b. Type 1 diabetes
   c. Impaired glucose tolerance
   d. Type 2 diabetes

   Answer: c. Impaired glucose tolerance

9. **A 56-year-old male suffering from type 2 diabetes has a blood glucose level of 420 mg/dL and high serum ketones. What does presence of ketones suggest?**
   a. Diabetic ketoacidosis
   b. Hyperosmolar hyperglycemia
   c. Hypoglycemic
   d. Abnormal response to stress

   Answer: a. Diabetic ketoacidosis

10. **A patient has a high fasting blood glucose: 165 mg/dL, HbA1c: 5.8%. What is the inference?**
    a. Diabetes mellitus
    b. Impaired fasting glucose
    c. Normal glucose concentration
    d. Impaired glucose tolerance

    Answer: b. Impaired fasting glucose

VIVA VOCE

Q1. A patient shows with FBG: 132 mg/dL, HbA1c: 7.3%. Interpret these findings.
The fasting blood glucose is more the normal range (70–99 mg/dL), HbA1c is high (normal <5.7%). This indicates diabetes mellitus, probably Type 2 when there are no other indications of type 1/secondary diabetes.

Q2. A 24-year-old patient presents with FBG: 81 mg/dL, postprandial glucose level: 222 mg/dL. Explain underlying cause.
This clinical scenario is suggestive of IGT/early diabetes. A glucose tolerance test is required to confirm. It will suggest reduced first-phase insulin secretion.

Q3. A patient's serum fructosamine: 2801µmol/L, HbA1c: normal. What does this suggest?
Fructosamine shows/reflects short-term glucose control (2-3 weeks), and HbA1c reflects long-term control (2-3 months). Elevated fructosamine with normal HbA1c may indicate recent hyperglycemia/quick changes in glycemic control/condition that might affect HbA1c measurement like hemolytic anemia.

Q4. What is the importance of high lactate level in a diabetic patient taking metformin?
High lactate (>4 mmol/L) in a diabetic patient taking this medication indicates lactic acidosis, that is rare but serious complication of metformin use, mainly in renal failure/hypoxic conditions.

Q5. A patient with recurrent hypoglycemia shows insulin level: 26 µU/mL/C-peptide of 0.1 ng/m. Interpret the results.
High insulin and low C-peptide indicates exogenous insulin administration that is factitious hypoglycemia because endogenous insulin production releases equimolar C-peptide.

SPOTTERS

Q1. Show a lab report:
Fasting blood glucose: 111 mg/dL
Postprandial blood glucose: 161 mg/dL
HbA1c: 6.1%
What is diagnosis?

→ Prediabetes (impaired fasting glucose and impaired glucose tolerance).

Q2. Show a lab report:
Glucose: 44 mg/dL
Insulin: 31 µU/mL
C-Peptide: 3.5 ng/mL
What is the probable cause?

→ Insulinoma that is endogenous hyperinsulinemic hypoglycemia.

Q3. Show a lab report:
Serum lactate: 6.6 mmol/L
Blood pH: 7.2
History: Patient taking metformin and has renal impairment.
What is the probable condition?

→ Metformin-induced lactic acidosis.

Q4. Show a lab report:
RBG: 328 mg/dL
Serum ketones: Positive
pH: 7.1
HCO_3^-: 13 mEq/L
What is the probable diagnosis?

→ Diabetic ketoacidosis.

Q5. Show a lab report:
FBG: 10 mg/dL
Fructosamine: 281 µmol/L
HbA1c: 4.4%
Interpret?

→ Recent hyperglycemia/fructosamine reflects 2–3 weeks of glycemic control/HbA1c reflects 2–3 months.

REFLECTION

Discuss and interpret laboratory results of analytes associated with metabolism of carbohydrates.
Interpret the results of blood glucose levels and other laboratory investigations related to disorders of carbohydrate metabolism.

30

CHAPTER

Interpretation of Laboratory Result: Oral Glucose Tolerance Test

COMPETENCY

BC14.22: Describe performance of OGTT glucose challenge test and HbA1c and interpretation of results with clinical scenarios.

LEARNING OBJECTIVES

After reading this chapter, the readers should be able to:
- Describe the clinical interpretation related to oral glucose tolerance tests.

BLUE PRINT

Lesson: Oral Glucose Tolerance Test

Objectives

By the end of this session, students should be able to:
1. Understand principle of OGTT.
2. Explain indications/contraindications of OGTT.
3. Describe procedure of OGTT.
4. Interpret OGTT results on basis of diagnostic criteria.
5. Discuss factors that affect OGTT.

Duration: *45–60 minutes*

Outline

I. **Introduction** **(10 minutes)**
   - Definition
   - History/importance in diabetes diagnosis
   - Significance in screening gestational diabetes mellitus

II. **Principle of OGTT** **(5 minutes)**
   - Concept behind glucose metabolism/insulin response
   - Basis of diagnosing DM/IGT

III. **Indications and contraindications** **(5 minutes)**
   - *Indications*: Diagnosis of diabetes mellitus, screening for gestational diabetes mellitus, assessment of impaired glucose tolerance, contraindications, such as critically sick patients, known diabetes mellitus, patients on interfering medications

IV. **OGTT procedure** **(10 minutes)**
   1. *Preparation*:
      - Patient to be on fasting (8–12 hours).
      - Avoid heavy exercise/stress
   2. *Procedure*:
      - Measure fasting plasma glucose.
      - Administer 75 g oral glucose dissolved in 300 mL water, intake in 5 minutes.
      - Measure blood glucose at 0, 1, and 2 hours as WHO criteria.
   3. *Modifications in pregnancy*: DIPSI method—single-step 75g OGTT at 2 hours.

V. **Interpretation of OGTT results** **(10 minutes)**
Gestational diabetes mellitus criteria: 2-hour plasma glucose ≥140 mg/dL.

VI. **Factors affecting OGTT** **(5 minutes)**
- *Physiological*: Stress, pregnancy, exercise
- *Pathological*: Malabsorption, gastric bypass surgery
- *Medications*: Steroids, beta-blockers, diuretics

VII. **Clinical applications and case scenarios** **(10 minutes)**
- Case-based discussion on interpreting OGTT results
- Importance of OGTT in diagnosing GDM/prediabetes

Assessment and Conclusion (5 minutes)

Quiz/Viva:
1. Give standard glucose load for OGTT?
2. Discuss diagnostic cutoff for diabetes on OGTT?
3. Why is OGTT preferred in pregnant women?
4. What factors can result in false positive/negative OGTT?
5. How is OGTT different in DIPSI?

Summary of key points

Oral glucose tolerance tests (OGTT)	• Evaluation of a person's ability to metabolize the load of glucose under specific standard conditions • There is serial measurement of blood glucose along with examination of urine for glucose
Indications	• For diagnosis of gestational diabetes mellitus (DM) • Postpartum screening of females for type II DM who earlier had gestational diabetes mellitus (GDM) • For diagnosing impaired glucose tolerance • For patients with unexplained neuropathy, nephropathy and retinopathy with abnormal blood glucose values • For epidemiological study
Optimum conditions for the test	• 3 days before the test, the patient should take minimum 150 g carbohydrates in one day • Ideal timing of the test is between 7 AM to 9 AM • Overnight fast of 12 hours is mandatory • The patient must be ambulatory • No smoking during last 3 days and on the day of test
Method	• Collect fasting sample of blood and urine • Then ask the patient to drink 75 g of anhydrous glucose in 300 mL water over a period of 5 minutes • After this, blood as well as urine samples are collected every 1/2 hour till 2 hours (total 4 samples after giving glucose—half hour, 1 hour, 1.5 hours, 2 hours) • Plasma glucose in all 6 samples is done, and urine is checked for positive or negative test for glucose by dipstick • Graph is plotted using plasma glucose values

Diagnostic criterion for diabetes according to WHO

Characteristic	**Fasting glucose (mg%)**	**2 hour glucose (mg%)**	**HbA1c**	
			Mmol/mol	Diabetes control and complications trial (DCCT)%
Normal	<110	<140	<42	<6
Impaired fasting glycemia	>110 and <126	<140	42–46	6–6.4
Impaired glucose tolerance	<126	>140	42–46	6–6.4
Diabetes mellitus	>126	>200	>48	>6.5

CASE 1

OGTT values of a 50-year-old female: What is your clinical interpretation?

Time (minutes)	Plasma glucose (mg%)	Benedict's test for urinary sugar
F	80	–
30	120	–
60	136	–
90	125	–
120	94	–

- Plot a graph taking time (min) on x-axis and plasma glucose values (mg%) on y-axis
- It is a normal curve
- Fasting plasma glucose (FPG) is <110 mg%, peak is <160 mg%, return to basal fasting level by 2 hours is <140 mg%

CASE 2

OGTT values of a 60-year-old female: What is your clinical interpretation?

Time (minutes)	Plasma glucose (mg%)	Benedict's test for urinary sugar
F	152	–
30	178	–
60	266	++
90	250	++
120	217	+

- Plot a graph taking time (min) on x-axis and plasma glucose values (mg%) on y-axis
- It is a diabetic curve
- Fasting plasma glucose (FPG) is >126 mg%, and 2 hour postprandial value of plasma glucose is >200 mg%

CASE 3

OGTT values of a 67-year-old female: What is your clinical interpretation?

Time (minutes)	Plasma glucose (mg%)	Benedict's test for urinary sugar
F	119	–
30	127	–
60	124	–
90	137	–
120	140	–

- Plot a graph taking time (min) on x-axis and plasma glucose values (mg%) on y-axis
- It is a impaired fasting glycemia curve
- Fasting plasma glucose (FPG) is between 110 mg% and 125 mg%

CASE 4

OGTT values of a 57-year-old female: What is your clinical interpretation?

Time (minutes)	Plasma glucose (mg%)	Benedict's test for urinary sugar
F	90	–
30	115	–
60	133	–
90	145	–
120	190	+

- Plot a graph taking time (min) on x-axis and plasma glucose values (mg%) on y-axis
- It is a impaired glucose tolerance curve
- Two hour postprandial plasma glucose value is 190 (>140–<200 mg%)

CASE 5

OGTT values of a 69-year-old female: What is your clinical interpretation?

Time (minutes)	Plasma glucose (mg%)	Benedict's test for urinary sugar
F	95	–
30	122	++
60	130	++
90	102	–
120	98	–

- Plot a graph taking time (min) on x-axis and plasma glucose values (mg%) on y-axis
- It is a renal glycosuria curve
- Normal renal threshold for glucose–180 mg% (urine will be positive for glucose only when the plasma glucose rises above 180 mg%)
- In renal glycosuria, even at low plasma glucose levels, glucose comes out in the urine
- Generally observed in 3 trimester of pregnancy, reabsorption defect in tubules of kidney

CASE 6

OGTT values of a 50-year-old female: What is your clinical interpretation?

Time (minutes)	Plasma glucose (mg%)	Benedict's test for urinary sugar
F	82	–
30	115	–
60	199	+
90	125	–
120	65	–

- Plot a graph taking time (min) on x-axis and plasma glucose values (mg%) on y-axis
- It is alimentary glycosuria or lag curve (there is lag in secretion of insulin leading to high glucose level at 1 hour time)
- There is abnormally high response to glucose loading, so the 1 hour sample shows high value, even exceeding the threshold value and urine is positive for glucose also (glycosuria)
- Thereafter fast metabolism of glucose results in a normal level/sometimes below-normal also by the end of 2 hours
- This type of graph is generally observed for hyperthyroid patients and partial gastrectomy patients

CASE 7

OGTT values of a 40-year-old female: What is your clinical interpretation?

Time (minutes)	Plasma glucose (mg%)	Benedict's test for urinary sugar
F	80	–
30	82	–
60	84	–
90	81	–
120	79	–

- Plot a graph taking time (min) on x-axis and plasma glucose values (mg%) on y-axis
- It is a increased glucose tolerance curve (flat curve)
- In patients with malabsorption syndrome, hypothyroidism, hypopituitarism, hypoadrenalism, there is very minimum or zero effect of glucose loading on blood glucose, so even at 1 hour, the level of plasma glucose are at fasting values in normal limits

CASE 8

OGTT in pregnant woman to rule out GDM: These are taken as upper normal limits

100 g of anhydrous glucose is given in such cases

Time (hour)	Plasma glucose (mg%)
F	105
1	190
2	165
3	145

- Clinical significance is that it is done in high risk pregnant woman having a family history of diabetes mellitus/had diabetes mellitus in one pregnancy/more maternal age
- If any of the two values are greater than the values mentioned here, then this is indicative of GDM

LOG ACTIVITY

Make graphs:

1. Normal OGTT
2. OGTT in diabetes mellitus
3. OGTT in impaired fasting glycemia
4. OGTT in impaired glucose tolerance
5. OGTT in renal glycosuria
6. OGTT in alimentary glycosuria (lag curve)
7. Flat curve of increased glucose tolerance

OSCE

1. **Scenario: Diagnosis of diabetes mellitus**
   Case: A 48-year-old woman undergoes a 75 g oral glucose tolerance test (OGTT). Results:
   Fasting glucose: 135 mg/dL (normal: <100 mg/dL)
   2-hour glucose: 255 mg/dL (normal: <140 mg/dL)
   Question: What is the interpretation?
   Interpretation: The fasting glucose level ≥126 mg/dL/2-hour glucose ≥200 mg/dL that confirms diabetes mellitus.
   Next steps: Diabetes management by lifestyle changes/pharmacological treatment
2. **Scenario: Impaired glucose tolerance (IGT)**
   Case: A 45-year-old man undergoes a 75 g OGTT. Results:
   Fasting glucose: 106 mg/dL (normal: <100 mg/dL)
   2-hour glucose: 169 mg/dL (normal: <140 mg/dL)
   Question: How should these results be interpreted?
   Interpretation: The fasting glucose is suggestive of impaired fasting glucose (100–125 mg/dL), and the 2-hour glucose level (140–199 mg/dL) confirms impaired glucose tolerance (IGT).
   Next steps: Patient advised to lose weight/dietary changes/increase exercises or physical activity and decrease further risk of progression to diabetes.
3. **Scenario: Gestational diabetes mellitus (GDM)**
   Case: A 29-year-old pregnant woman at 24 weeks gestation undergoes a 75 g OGTT. Results:
   Fasting glucose: 97 mg/dL (normal: <92 mg/dL)
   1-hour glucose: 189 mg/dL (normal: <180 mg/dL)
   2-hour glucose: 159 mg/dL (normal: <153 mg/dL)
   Question: Does the patient have GDM?
   Interpretation: Two abnormal values in the OGTT confirm gestational diabetes mellitus
   Next steps: Manage the disorder of GDM with diet modifications/regular glucose monitoring/insulin therapy if needed.
4. **Scenario: Reactive hypoglycemia**
   Case: A 31-year-old man undergoes a GTT for evaluation of postprandial symptoms. Results:
   Fasting glucose: 86 mg/dL
   1-hour glucose: 163 mg/dL

2-hour glucose: 92 mg/dL
3-hour glucose: 54 mg/dL
Question: What does this indicate?
Interpretation: The drop in glucose at 3 hours is suggestive of reactive hypoglycemia, probably because of exaggerated insulin secretion after the meals.
Next steps: Advise small, frequent meals with low-glycemic index foods for stabilizing blood glucose concentration.

5. **Scenario: Early diabetes detection**
Case: A patient with a family history of diabetes undergoes a 75 g OGTT. Results:
Fasting glucose: 117 mg/dL (normal: <100 mg/dL)
1-hour glucose: 187 mg/dL (normal: <180 mg/dL)
2-hour glucose: 198 mg/dL (normal: <140 mg/dL)
Question: What do these results suggest?
Interpretation: The fasting glucose is suggestive of impaired fasting glucose/the 2-hour glucose value (140–199 mg/dL) confirms impaired glucose tolerance keeping patient at a higher risk for diabetes.
Next steps: Advise lifestyle changes to avoid progression to diabetes.

6. **Scenario: Glucose malabsorption**
Case: A patient undergoing a GTT for evaluation of unexplained lethargy and fatigue:
Fasting glucose: 901mg/dL
1-hour glucose: 61 mg/dL
2-hour glucose: 52 mg/dL
Question: What do these results indicate?
Interpretation: A drop in glucose levels after ingestion is suggestive of malabsorption/exaggerated insulin response.
Next steps: Evaluate for gastrointestinal disorders/insulinoma plus consider a mixed-meal tolerance test

7. **Scenario: GTT in polycystic ovary syndrome (PCOS)**
Case: A 31-year-old woman with irregular periods undergoes a 2-hour OGTT. Results:
Fasting glucose: 111 mg/dL
2-hour glucose: 151 mg/dL
Question: How should these results be interpreted in relation to PCOS?
Interpretation: The patient has impaired glucose tolerance (2-hour glucose 140–199 mg/dL), that is usual feature in PCOS and increases the risk of diabetes.
Next steps: Advise weight loss, lifestyle changes/consider metformin therapy in order to improve insulin sensitivity.

8. **Scenario: Normal GTT**
Case: A healthy individual undergoes a 75 g OGTT for screening. Results:
Fasting glucose: 84 mg/dL
1-hour glucose: 141 mg/dL
2-hour glucose: 111 mg/dL
Question: How should these results be interpreted?
Interpretation: All values are within the normal range, indicating normal glucose tolerance.
Next steps: No further intervention is advised

9. **Scenario: Pediatric GTT for type 2 diabetes**
Case: A 11-year-old obese child undergoes a 2-hour OGTT. Results:
Fasting glucose: 101 mg/dL
2-hour glucose: 146 mg/dL
Question: What do these results suggest?
Interpretation: Impaired fasting glucose (100–125 mg/dL)/impaired glucose tolerance (140–199 mg/dL) is suggestive of prediabetes.
Next steps: Advised weight/dietary changes/physical activity to prevent progression to Type 2 diabetes.

10. **Scenario: GTT in suspected secondary diabetes**
Case: A 51-year-old with acromegaly undergoes a GTT. Results:
Fasting glucose: 117 mg/dL
2-hour glucose: 161 mg/dL
Question: What does this indicate?
Interpretation: Impaired glucose tolerance because of insulin resistance due to high growth hormone levels.
Next steps: Treat the main cause like surgery for pituitary adenoma/monitor glucose levels frequently

CLINICAL MCQS

1. **A 48-year-old patient goes for OGTT. Fasting blood glucose: 97 mg/dL, 2-hour post-glucose level: 179 mg/dL. What can be the diagnosis?**
   a. Normal glucose tolerance
   b. Diabetes insipidus
   c. Impaired glucose tolerance
   d. Diabetes mellitus type 1

   Answer: c. Impaired glucose tolerance

2. **During an OGTT, a patient's 2-hour post-glucose level is: 222 mg/dL. What does this suggest?**
   a. Normal fructose tolerance
   b. IGT
   c. Diabetes mellitus
   d. Hypoglycemia

   Answer: c. Diabetes mellitus

3. **A 37-year-old pregnant woman undergoes a 75 g OGTT. Fasting glucose: 95 mg/dL, 1-hour post-glucose level: 200 mg/dL. What does this result indicate?**
   a. Normal glucose tolerance
   b. GDM
   c. Type 1 diabetes
   d. Type 2 diabetes

   Answer: b. GDM

4. **A 45-year-old male having family history of diabetes got her OGTT done. Fasting blood glucose: 107 mg/dL, 2-hour post-glucose: 154 mg/dL. What is the interpretation?**
   a. Normal glucose tolerance
   b. IFG
   c. Impaired glucose tolerance
   d. Diabetes mellitus type 1

   Answer: c. Impaired glucose tolerance

5. **A patient shows OGTT results as: Fasting glucose: 96 mg/dL, 1-hour glucose: 186 mg/dL, 2-hour glucose: 121 mg/dL. Which is accurate conclusion?**
   a. Normal glucose tolerance
   b. Impaired glucose tolerance
   c. Hyperglycemia
   d. Impaired fasting glucose

   Answer: a. Normal glucose tolerance

6. **A 27-year-old woman goes for OGTT. Her fasting blood glucose: 91 mg/dL, 2-hour post-glucose: 149 mg/dL. How would you interpret?**
   a. Normal glucose tolerance
   b. Impaired glucose tolerance
   c. Gestational diabetes
   d. Diabetes mellitus

   Answer: b. Impaired glucose tolerance

7. **In a patient with a fasting blood glucose: 110 mg/dL 2-hour post-glucose: 190 mg/dL on OGTT, what is the diagnosis?**
   a. Normal glucose tolerance
   b. Diabetes mellitus
   c. Impaired fasting glucose
   d. Impaired glucose tolerance

   Answer: b. Diabetes mellitus

8. **A 65-year-old male shows OGTT results: fasting glucose: 131 mg/dL, 1-hour glucose: 211 mg/dL, 2-hour glucose: 176 mg/dL. What do these results indicate?**
   a. Type 2 diabetes
   b. Type 1 diabetes
   c. Normal glucose tolerance
   d. Abnormal glucose tolerance

   Answer: a. Type 2 diabetes

9. A 49-year-old patient shows obesity got OGTT done. Fasting glucose: 99 mg/dL, 1-hour glucose: 211 mg/dL, 2-hour glucose: 149 mg/dL. What is interpretation?
   a. Normal glucose tolerance
   b. Diabetes mellitus
   c. Hyperglycemia
   d. Impaired glucose tolerance

   Answer: d. Impaired glucose tolerance

10. A patient has following OGTT results: fasting glucose: 101 mg/dL, 1-hour glucose: 191 mg/dL, 2-hour glucose: 141 mg/dL. What is management?
   a. No treatment required, just routine care
   b. Insulin therapy
   c. Lifestyle modifications for impaired glucose tolerance
   d. Urgent referral for diabetes management

   Answer: c. Lifestyle modifications for impaired glucose tolerance

VIVA VOCE

Q1. Discuss the principle of OGTT.

Q2. Explain the indications for performing this assay.

Q3. How is an OGTT performed/what are the standard glucose load and time intervals?

Q4. Discuss about the diagnostic criteria for gestational diabetes mellitus/diabetes mellitus using OGTT.

Q5. What factors affect results of OGTT?

SPOTTERS

Q1. 75 g glucose powder sachet: Identify/explain its application in OGT.

Q2. OGTT graph exhibiting normal/impaired/diabetic curves: Identify/interpret the importance of different curves.

Q3. Fasting blood sugar/2-hour post-glucose blood sugar report: Identify the diagnostic cutoffs for diabetes/impaired glucose tolerance.

Q4. Glycosuria on urine dipstick test post-OGTT: Explain mechanism of glycosuria/significance.

Q5. Pregnant woman undergoing OGTT (with glucose drink/serial blood samples drawn): Identify the procedure/explain its significance in pregnancy.

REFLECTION

31

CHAPTER

Biochemical Tests in Gout, Thyroid Disorders, Pancreatitis, Acid Base Disorders and Edema

COMPETENCY

BC14.19: Explain the basis and rationale of biochemical tests done in the following conditions: Gout, edema, pancreatitis, disorders of acid base balance, thyroid disorders.

LEARNING OBJECTIVES

After reading this chapter, the readers should be able to:

- Describe the pathogenesis and clinical features of gout, thyroid disorders, pancreatitis, acid base disorders and edema.
- Describe the biochemical basis of the tests performed in these conditions.
- Explain how specific laboratory parameters are utilized in the diagnosis, monitoring, and management of different diseases.
- Interpret the results of biochemical tests in the context of specific clinical scenarios.
- Appreciate the role of biochemical investigations in understanding the pathophysiology of different medical conditions.

BLUE PRINT

Explanation of Biochemical Tests in Various Medical Conditions

Objective

By the end of the lecture, students should be able to:

1. Understand the biochemical basis and rationale behind diagnostic tests used in various medical conditions.
2. Explain how specific laboratory parameters are utilized in the diagnosis, monitoring, and management of different diseases.
3. Interpret the results of biochemical tests in the context of specific clinical scenarios.
4. Appreciate the role of biochemical investigations in understanding the pathophysiology of different medical conditions.

Duration: ***55 minutes***

Materials Needed

1. Presentation slides illustrating the biochemical tests and their interpretation in different medical conditions.
2. Case studies or clinical vignettes representing each medical condition for interactive discussion.
3. Whiteboard or flipchart for drawing biochemical pathways and explaining concepts.
4. Handouts summarizing the biochemical tests and their significance in each medical condition.

Outline

I. **Introduction to biochemical testing in medicine** **(10 minutes)**
   - Overview of the role of biochemical tests in the diagnosis and management of medical conditions.
   - Importance of understanding the underlying biochemical mechanisms for interpretation of test results.

II. **Renal failure and gout** **(10 minutes)**
   - Explanation of renal function tests including serum creatinine, blood urea nitrogen (BUN), and uric acid.
   - Relationship between renal function tests and the development of gout in renal failure.

III. **Edema** **(5 minutes)**
- Brief explanation of electrolyte tests such as serum sodium, potassium, and chloride.
- Understanding the role of electrolyte imbalances in the pathophysiology of edema.

IV. **Pancreatitis** **(5 minutes)**
- Discussion of pancreatic enzymes such as serum amylase and lipase.
- Utility of pancreatic enzyme tests in diagnosing acute pancreatitis.

V. **Disorders of acid-base balance** **(5 minutes)**
- Overview of arterial blood gas (ABG) analysis and serum bicarbonate measurement.
- Interpretation of ABG parameters in assessing acid-base status and identifying metabolic acidosis or alkalosis.

VI. **Thyroid disorders** **(10 minutes)**
- Explanation of thyroid function tests including TSH, free T4, and total or free T3.
- Use of thyroid function tests in diagnosing thyroid dysfunction and monitoring thyroid hormone replacement therapy.

VII. **Conclusion and recap** **(5 minutes)**
- Summarize key points covered in the lecture regarding the biochemical tests used in various medical conditions.
- Emphasize the importance of interdisciplinary collaboration between clinicians and laboratory professionals in interpreting test results.

VIII. **Question and answer session** **(5 minutes)**
- Encourage students to ask questions and seek clarification on any aspects of the lecture.
- Foster discussion on practical applications of biochemical tests in clinical practice.

BLUE PRINT

Test to Diagnose Gout and Lesch-Nyhan Syndrome

Objective

By the end of the lecture, students should be able to:
1. Understand the laboratory tests used in the diagnosis of gout and Lesch-Nyhan syndrome.
2. Interpret the results of these tests in the context of the biochemical abnormalities associated with each condition.
3. Discuss the clinical implications of abnormal laboratory findings in patients with gout and Lesch-Nyhan syndrome.

Duration: *60 minutes*

Materials Needed

1. Presentation slides outlining laboratory tests and results for gout and Lesch-Nyhan syndrome.
2. Handouts summarizing key points and case studies.
3. Whiteboard and markers.

Outline

I. **Introduction to gout and Lesch-Nyhan syndrome** **(5 minutes)**
- Introduction to the biochemical basis and clinical manifestations of gout and Lesch-Nyhan syndrome.
- Overview of the objectives and structure of the lecture.

II. **Laboratory tests for gout** **(20 minutes)**
- Description of laboratory tests used in the diagnosis of gout, including serum uric acid levels, synovial fluid analysis, and imaging studies.
- Interpretation of abnormal laboratory findings and their significance in the diagnosis and management of gout.
- Discussion of differential diagnoses and potential confounding factors.

III. **Laboratory tests for Lesch-Nyhan syndrome** **(20 minutes)**
- Overview of laboratory tests used in the diagnosis of Lesch-Nyhan syndrome, including urine uric acid levels, hypoxanthine-guanine phosphoribosyltransferase (HGPRT) enzyme activity assay, and genetic testing.
- Interpretation of abnormal laboratory results and their implications for the diagnosis and management of Lesch-Nyhan syndrome.
- Discussion of genetic counseling and family screening considerations.

IV. **Case studies and examples** **(10 minutes)**
- Presentation of case studies or examples illustrating laboratory findings in patients with gout and Lesch-Nyhan syndrome.
- Facilitation of discussion on the interpretation of laboratory results and their clinical significance.

V. **Clinical management and follow-up** **(5 minutes)**
- Overview of treatment options and management strategies for patients with gout and Lesch- Nyhan syndrome.
- Discussion of the role of laboratory monitoring in disease management and follow-up care.

VI. **Recap and application** **(5 minutes)**
- Summary of key points covered in the lecture.
- Application of knowledge through case-based questions or scenarios.

VII. **Conclusion** **(5 minutes)**
- Concluding remarks on the importance of laboratory testing in the diagnosis and management of gout and Lesch-Nyhan syndrome.
- Encouragement for further study and research in the field of metabolic disorders.

Gout	Clinical condition due to chronic hyperuricemia beyond the saturation limit of monosodium urate, characterized by deposition of urate crystals in joints, inflammation and deformity followed by destruction of joints
Hyperuricemia (excess catabolism of purines leads to hyperuricemia)	• Major abnormality causing gout • Increased blood uric acid levels >2–7 mg%
Uric acid	End product of the purine that is adenine and guanine bases, the bases are present in nucleic acids in various nucleotides, such as ATP, GTP, cyclic AMP, cGMP, hypoxanthine, xanthines found in tea/coffee, etc.
Two types of gout:	Primary and secondary
1. Primary gout	Defective purine metabolism
a. Lesch–Nyhan syndrome due to deficient enzyme HGPRTase (hypoxanthine-guanine phosphoribosyl transferase)	This leads to increased accumulation of hypoxanthine and guanine and then their catabolism
b. Over activity of enzyme PRPP synthetase	Increased concentration of AMP and GMP are formed
c. Deficiency of enzyme adenosine deaminase	Excess catabolism and excess uric acid formation
2. Secondary gout	• Due to causes other than those related to metabolism of uric acid directly, so excess uric acid is formed but as a result of other diseases where there is excess breakdown of tissues, including nucleic acids leading to gout-like: • Psoriasis • Leukemia • Von-Gierke's disease

Excretion of uric acid

Uric acid as a dibasic acid	• Uric acid has 2 pK values of 9.8 and 5.5 • The pH of blood is 7.4 • At pK of 5.75, uric acid exist in undissociated form as uric acid only • At blood pH of 7.4 uric acid exists in partially dissociated form as monosodium urate
Characteristic of monosodium urate	It is 10 times more soluble than uric acid and is present in synovial fluid and glomerular filtrate
Monosodium urate in synovial fluid (plasma filtrate)	When monosodium urate is present in excess in synovial fluid, it gets precipitated here and accumulates in joint spaces as crystals resulting in inflammatory arthritis
Uric acid form in kidney tubules	In the tubules, acid pH (5.75) leads to conversion of monosodium urate to uric acid form which is less soluble, so easily precipitated and form stones
Effect of alcohol	It increase the tendency of gout because alcohol consumption increases $NADH^+$ H^+ due to metabolism of alcohol to acetaldehyde and acetyl CoA, which decreases the pH and excess formation of uric acid is there which is less soluble in comparison to monosodium urate
Acidic urine (normally)	Leads to excretion of uric acid
If the urine is alkaline	Excretion of uric acid in form of monosodium urate is enhanced

Contd....

Contd....

Causes of gout	• Obesity (excess visceral fat causes inflammatory milleu) • Dyslipidemia • Hypertension (decreases glomerular filtration of uric acid) • Red meat and shellfish in diet which are excellent sources of purines • Excess alcohol • Diuretics (increases output of urine causing dehydration, which can result in increases concentration of uric acid in blood
Symptoms	• Joint pain (knee, wrist, elbow) • Excess pain in metatarsophalangeal joints • Deformation and destruction of big toe • Renal colicky pain because of renal stones
Biochemical basis of investigations	
Blood uric acid level	Levels >7 mg% is hyperuricemia The monosodium urate of plasma exceeds its solubility limit
Urine analysis	For detection of acidic pH and uric acid crystals
Aspiration and analysis of synovial fluid	Analyzed for tophi as negative birefringent needle shaped crystals in wet smear of synovial fluid
Serum urea, creatinine, GFR, proteinuria, electrolytes	Evaluation of renal functions
X-rays	Evaluation of joint destruction
Ultrasound	Renal stones detection
Treatment approach	
Increase excretion of uric acid	Make urine alkaline by considering alkalinizing agents Increased consumption of water/fluids
Decrease the intake of food rich in purines	Decrease use of Nonvegetarian food
Drugs	Allopurinol that inhibits xanthine oxidase enzyme thus decreasing purine catabolism and uric acid
Analgesics	Prevent acute attacks
Avoidance of alcohol	
Weight control	
Thyroid gland	It secretes thyroid hormone (for metabolism and neurological development) and calcitonin (for calcium metabolism)
Thyroid hormones	Triiodothyronine (T3) and tetraiodothyronine (T4)
Thyroglobulin	Glycoprotein containing 2769 amino acids and MW of 660 KDa in the thyroid follicle rich in tyrosine, major binding protein for thyroid hormones also (responsible for 80% of thyroid hormone binding)
Synthesis of thyroid hormones	• Synthesized in the thyroglobulin protein (TG) by iodination of tyrosine residues of TG • Monoiodotyrosine (MIT) and diiodotyrosine (DIT) are formed which are coupled in presence of enzyme thyroperoxidase to form T3 and T4
Amount of bound and free thyroid hormones	• T4 (99.9%) and T3 (99.7%) are bound to proteins in the plasma (not metabolically active) • T4 (0.02–0.03%) and T3 (0.2–0.3%) are free
Thyroid hormone binding proteins	• Thyroxine-binding globulin (TBG) • Thyroxine- binding Prealbumin (TBPA) • Albumin
Free T3 and free T4 (FT3, FT4):	Metabolically active
T3 is more active than T4	T3 has less affinity for binding to proteins and more affinity to nuclear receptor binding

Contd....

Contd....

Regulation of thyroid hormones secretion	Pituitary and hypothalamus
Function of enzyme deiodinase	Conversion of T4 to T3
Functions of thyroid hormones	• Increases basal metabolic rate leading to increased cell metabolism • Increased oxidation of carbohydrates • Increased gluconeogenesis • Increased oxidation of fatty acids • Increased oxidation of cholesterol • Protein catabolism is increased at high concentrations • Protein synthesis is increased at low concentrations • Produces heat by uncoupling oxidative phosphorylation generating thermogenic effect • Cell growth and development
Thyroid diseases	
Hypothyroidism: More common in females and increases with age	Thyroid gland disease, where there is less production of T3 and T4
Hypothyroidism in children	Cretinism
Hypothyroidism in adults	Myxedema
Causes of hypothyroidism	• Hashimoto's disease • Iodine deficiency goiter • Graves' disease
Symptoms of hypothyroidism	• Weight gain • Intolerance to cold • Constipation • Bradycardia • Face puffiness and nonpitting edema on legs and around the ankle • Dry skin • Menorrhagia • Diastolic hypertension • Periorbital edema • Delayed deep tendon reflex
Biochemical parameters	• Low FT3 and FT4 • High/normal TSH • High anti-TPO antibodies
Treatment of hypothyroidism	**Synthetic T4 replacement therapy**
Types of hypothyroidism	
Primary hypothyroidism	Thyroid gland is damaged leading to less production of thyroid hormones and hypothyroidism
Causes of primary hypothyroidism	• Iodine deficiency • Chronic autoimmune thyroiditis (atrophic along with goitrous form) • Total/subtotal thyroidectomy • Infiltrative disorders, such as sarcoidosis, amyloidosis, lymphoma • Thyroid dysgenesis • Lithium • Congenital defect in thyroid hormone synthesis
Investigations	Low FT3, FT4 with compensatory increase in TSH
Secondary hypothyroidism	• Thyroid gland is otherwise normal but cannot produce enough T3, T4 due to insufficient stimulation by TSH due to defect in pituitary gland, when TSH is not secreted adequately • TSH, T3 and T4 are low
Tertiary hypothyroidism	Defect in hypothalamus leading to inadequate production of thyrotropin release hormone (TRH), which is then reflected as low TSH and low FT3, FT4
TRH evaluation	Differentiates between secondary and tertiary hypothyroidism

Contd....

	Normal range
TSH	0.35–5.0 mIU/mL
FT3	1.8–4.20 pg/mL
FT4	0.50–1.40 ng/dL
Overt hypothyroidism	Subclinical hypothyroidism
Low serum FT4 and high serum TSH	Normal serum FT4 and high serum TSH (even >10 mIU/mL)
Treatment of hypothyroidism	Treat the underlying cause and supplementing levothyroxine sodium
Hyperthyroidism/thyrotoxicosis/ hyper- metabolic state	Sustained excess levels of T3 and T4 and low/normal TSH
Graves' disease	Long-acting thyroid stimulator (LATS)/production of thyroid stimulator antibody (TSH R stimulating antibody) leads to hyperthyroidism
Symptoms of hyperthyroidism	• Weight loss • Increased heart rate • Dyspnea (breathless condition) • Hands tremors • Diarrhea • Anxiety/emotional disturbances/irritation • Increased sensitivity towards heat • Ophthalmopathy
Causes of hyperthyroidism	• Graves' disease • Toxic goiter • Hypothyroid patient may take increased thyroxin • TSH secreting tumor • Toxic adenoma
Biochemical parameters	Low TSH and high FT3 and FT4
Treatment of hyperthyroidism	Anti-thyroid drugs (methimazole)
	Surgical partial removal of thyroid gland
Euthyroid goiter	Hyperplasia of thyroid gland
Cause of Euthyroid goiter	• Iodine deficiency • Patient is clinically normal except for goiter because there is a compensatory increase in TSH to maintain almost normal T3 and T4
Thyroid carcinoma	Malignancy of thyroid
Treatment of thyroid carcinoma	Surgical removal of tumor

Thyroid function tests

A. **Assay of T3, T4 (Total and free):** 1. Only free T3 and free T4 are active 2. Diagnosis which is made on the basis of total T3 and T4 can be false because in situations, such as pregnancy or using of OCP, there may be increased concentration of Thyroglobulin increases which results in increased concentration of bound T3 and T4, although, free T3 and free T4 remains normal	Radioimmunoassay ELISA Chemiluminescence immuno-assay (CLIA): Very sensitive method (detection limit is 0.01 mIU/L)
B. **Assay of TSH:** By CLIA 1. The thyroid profile is actually combination of TSH, FT3 FT4 2. TSH is produced by pituitary land 3. TSH is responsible for the feedback regulation of FT3, FT4 4. FT3/FT4 suppression of TSH 5. Decreased FT3/FT4 leads to stimulation of TSH	
C. **T3 resin uptake**	
D. **Thyroid antibodies:** 1. *Anti-TPO*: Antibodies to thyroperoxidase are found in Hashimoto's disease which is a autoimmune disease and a very major cause of hypothyroidism 2. *Long-acting thyroid stimulators (LATS)*: They are thyroid stimulating antibodies to TSH receptors and are found in graves' disease	

Contd....

Contd....

E. **TRH response test:** For assessing the hypothalamus-pituitary axis
   1. TRH act as stimulator of pituitary to make more TSH, and this leads to increased T3 and T4
   2. Thus, when the hypothalamus-pituitary axis is normal, TRH leads to increased TSH and increased T3 and T4
   3. *In hyperthyroidism*: It will not exhibit major changes as T3 and T4 are already more and TSH is already stimulated
   4. *In primary hypothyroidism*: Exaggerated response is observed T3 and T4 are low but TSH will be high
   5. *In Hypopituitarism*: Increased TRH will not result in increased TSH, so T3 and T4 also remain low

Pancreas	Consists of exocrine acinar cells and endocrine islets of Langerhans
Function of acinar cells	Produce digestive enzymes, and to prevent autolysis of tissue of origin, the proteolytic enzymes are secreted in an inactive form and are activated after the release
Function of endocrine tissue	Produce hormones, such as inulin, glucagon, Insulin, such as growth factors I and II, somatostatin, etc.
Alpha amylase	• MW–60 kDa • Produced by pancreas and salivary glands • Calcium requiring metalloenzyme
Function	Acts on alpha 1, 4 glucosidic bonds of starch and glycogen and form simpler glucose, maltose and isomaltose
Acute pancreatitis	Inflammatory mild, self-limiting disease because of mild swelling of the pancreas
Symptoms	Abdominal pain
Nature of abdominal pain	• Dull, mild pain or severe pain in the epigastrium which may radiate to back, low part of chest and flanks • Nausea • Vomiting • Distension of abdomen • Fever • Jaundice due to swelling of the head of pancreas may compress bile duct
Causes	• Biliary tract diseases • Gallstones • Alcoholism increases hypertriglyceridemia • Hypertriglyceridemia • Drugs, such as sulfonamides, estrogens, azathioprine, 6-mercaptopurine • Abdominal injury leading to pancreatic damage
Pathogenesis	Autodigestion of pancreatic tissue
	Ideally the activation of enzymes should be in the intestinal lumen after secretion, but here, they get activated in pancreas itself due to viral infections, ischemia, anoxia, endogenous and exogenous toxins
Mechanism	• Enzymes, such as trypsin, chymotrypsinogen, proelastase, phospholipase A, get activated and cause autodigestion • This results in injury of acinar cells of the pancreas • There is inflammation with accumulated neutrophils and inflammatory cells which release mediators causing damage to various organs, clotting disorders, respiratory distress, shock, etc. • Decreased insulin secretion causes hyperglycemia • There is increased secretion of glucocorticoids, epinephrine, etc.
Diagnosis	• Serum amylase (50–150 IU/L) • Serum lipase (0–50 IU/L) • There is increase in both >three times • Amylase level comes back to normal by 3 days
Treatment principles	Treat the pain and associated abnormalities Oral intake should be avoided IV fluids, Nasogastric suction
Biochemical investigations:	Normal serum contains 60% pancreatic amylase and 40% from salivary glands
Serum amylase	Increased due to autodigestion of the pancreas

Contd....

Contd....

Diseases of salivary gland are ruled out	Mumps
Urinary excretion of amylase	3000–3500 IU/L
Macroamylasemia	Amylase binds to a circulating protein forming a macromolecule which is not filtered by the kidneys so accumulates in the plasma, less excretion of amylase in urine supports it, as in actual rise of serum amylase, both, serum amylase and urinary amylase excretion increases
Test for blood glucose, TG and bilirubin	To assess hyperglycemia, hypertriglyceridemia and hyperbilirubinemia
Other tests	For associated disorders

pH of blood	7.4 ± 0.04
pH of gastric juice	1 to 3
pH of saliva	6.8–8.6
pH of urine	4.8–8.0
pH of bile	7.7

pH regulation

pH Regulation by buffers	• Bicarbonate buffer • Phosphate buffer • Hb buffer • Protein buffer
pH regulation by renal mechanism	The regulation of acid base balance by the kidneys is by: • Reabsorption of HCO_3^- ions from filtrate by renal tubules • New bicarbonate synthesis • Secretion of H^+ ions in metabolic acidosis
pH regulation by respiratory mechanism	• Rate of ventilation regulates blood pCO_2 level • pCO_2 level regulates the concentration of HCO_3^- which regulates the pH
In acidosis	Increased ventilation decreases pCO_2 and H_2CO_3 so pH is increased
In alkalosis	Decreased ventilation retains more CO_2 thus increasing pCO_2 and H_2CO_3 and H^+

Disorders of acid base balance	Normal pH of blood ranges between 7.35–7.45
Acidosis	Clinical state where blood pH is <7.35
Alkalosis	Clinical state where blood pH is >7.35
Two types of acidosis and alkalosis	Metabolic acidosis and alkalosis Respiratory acidosis and alkalosis

Metabolic acidosis and alkalosis	***Respiratory acidosis and alkalosis***
Normal HCO_3^- level in blood is 22 to 26 mEq/L	Normal pCO_2 level in blood is 35 to 45 mm Hg
Acidosis or alkalosis because of changes in (HCO_3^-)	Acidosis or alkalosis because of changes in pCO_2
In metabolic acidosis (HCO_3^-) is low	In respiratory acidosis pCO_2 is high
In metabolic alkalosis (HCO_3^-) is high	In respiratory alkalosis pCO_2 is low

Metabolic acidosis	Low plasma (HCO_3^-)	Low pH	Normal/low pCO_2 Low $PaCO_2$ due to compensatory hyperventilation (increased tidal volume: Kussmaul respiration)

Causes	1. Excess endogenous acid production
Mechanism	In some clinical states, nonvolatile acids are formed because of metabolic reactions which decrease the bicarbonates because the bicarbonates get used up to neutralize the protons liberated from acids
Examples	• DM with ketoacidosis (beta hydroxybutyrate causes acidosis) • Lactic acidosis in ischemia (shock, cardiac arrest) • Poisoning (ethanol, methanol, paracetamol, salicylates) 2. Excess loss of HCO_3^-
Mechanism	Some clinical disorders cause increased loss of HCO_3^- ions (diarrhea)

Contd....

Contd....

Examples	• Renal tubular acidosis where HCO_3^- reclamation and new HCO_3^- generation is defective/renal defect in Na^- H^+ antiport system • Intestinal fistula due to intestinal surgery/trauma can result in loss of alkaline duodenal secretions • with high HCO_3^- amount • Low excretion of acid by the kidney as in CRD
Anion gap	Difference between the major cations and anions in the blood, it can change in acidosis, hyperkalemia, medications with lithium, bromide, hypoalbuminemia
Major cations of blood	Na^+ and K^+
Major anions of blood	Cl^- and HCO_3^-
AG	$= (Na^+ + K^+) - (Cl^- + HCO_3^-)$ $= (140 + 4 - (100 + 25)$ $=144–125$ $=19$ mmoles/L
Normal range	15–20 mEq/L
Importance of anion gap	In acidosis, anion gap can Increase or can be normal
Thus, the 2 types of metabolic acidosis is	1. High anion gap acidosis 2. Normal anion gap acidosis
	High anion gap acidosis
Anion gap is increased in	• Diabetic ketoacidosis • Lactic acidosis
Mechanism of increased anion gap in acidosis	HCO_3^- is used up to neutralize the acids
	Causes
Lactic acidosis	In anemia or asphyxia, there is low O_2 given to muscles, conditions which decrease the muscle perfusion, cardiac failure or shock can lead to lactic acidosis
Renal disorders (acute/chronic)	• Glomerular dysfunction resulting in no filtered Na^+, which is not available for exchange with H^+, which is formed during the new HCO_3^- generation. Thus it decreases HCO_3^- generation • Tubular defects resulting in defective H^+ secretion, which results in decreased HCO_3^- generation forming high anion gap
Excess unmeasured anions	There is no filtration of phosphates, sulfates, etc., which on retaining in the body can lead to high anion gap
Ketoacidosis	In diabetes, starvation and alcohol use
Toxins	Ethylene glycol, salicylate, propylene glycol
	Normal anion gap acidosis and hyperchloremic acidosis
Hyperchloremic acidosis	Low (HCO_3^-) and high (Cl^-) concentration
Mechanism	There is increased HCO_3^- loss, and to maintain the electrical neutrality and anion gap there is increased chloride retention
	Causes
1. Bladder carcinoma	Implanting ureter into ileum in patients of bladder carcinoma results in increased retention of chloride from urine by the ileum
2. Duodenal fistula	There is increased HCO_3^- loss
3. Renal tubular acidosis type 1 and type 2	There is less HCO_3^- formation and H^+ secretion by renal tubules
4. Acetazolamide (used as a treatment in glaucoma to decrease the intraocular pressure)	It decreases the aqueous humor formation and inhibits renal tubular carbonic anhydrase thus decreasing formation of HCO_3^- and H^+ ion secretion
5. Diarrhea, magnesium sulfate therapy	Loss of HCO_3^- by intestine
6. Drug induced	NSAIDs, potassium sparing diuretics, trimethoprim

	Metabolic acidosis compensation
1. Respiratory compensation: $H^+ + HCO_3^- \rightarrow H_2CO_3 \rightarrow CO_2 + H_2O$	• There is stimulation of the respiratory center by the high H^+ ions concentration in acidosis resulting in hyperventilation • This removes the carbon dioxide and decreases the PCO_2 and H_2CO_3 concentration to take back the ratio of $HCO_3^- : H_2CO_3$ back to normal • There may be added response by the kidneys to increase the (HCO_3^-) ion concentration
2. Renal compensation	• (HCO_3^-) reclamation as well as new HCO_3^- formation are increased, as less (HCO_3^-) stimulates the renal tubular carbonic anhydrase which restores the (HCO_3^-) back to normal • The anion of the acids, such as lactate or sulfates are either metabolized or excreted • Kidneys also excrete H^+ ions buffered by phosphates and NH_3^+
Metabolic acidosis: Arterial blood findings	• Low pH • Low HCO_3^- concentration with high/normal anion gap • Low PCO_2 because of compensation • Normal/high Cl^- ions
	Respiratory acidosis
Causes 1. Emphysema 2. Bronchial asthma 3. Chronic obstructive pulmonary disease	• Hypoventilation caused by lung disorders • PCO_2 rises giving rise to low ratio of $HCO_3^- : H_2CO_3$
Renal compensation	• Increased HCO_3^- reclamation and H^+ ion excretion • Urine becomes acidic because of H^+ ion excretion
Blood findings in respiratory acidosis	• Low pH • High PCO_2 • Normal/slightly increased HCO_3^- because of compensation
Metabolic alkalosis	High pH High HCO_3^- High $PaCO_2$ due to compensatory alveolar hypoventilation Accompanied by hypokalemia and hypochloremia
Causes:	1. Addition of alkali in the body 2. Loss of nonvolatile acid (vomiting/pyloric stenosis/Nasogastric suction), results in alkaline tide, the loss of HCl is exchanged by HCO_3^- retention which causes alkaline tide In normal conditions, it is compensated by increased HCO_3^- excretion but because of renal disorders, it can sometimes lead to uremic alkalosis 3. Loop diuretics, such as furosemide can inhibit absorption of Na^+ from the ascending loop of Henle, excess Na^+ is then absorbed from distal tubules in exchange for K^+ and H^+ resulting in hypokalemia Increased H^+ excretion is accompanied by increased HCO_3^- generation which is absorbed resulting in alkalosis
	Compensation
Respiratory compensation	• Maximum PCO_2 can be augmented up to 50 mm Hg • There is a respiratory adjustment where ventilation is depressed by high pH leading to accumulation of CO_2 and increase of PCO_2, ultimately forming more H_2CO_3 which decreases the ratio of $HCO_3^- : H_2CO_3$
Renal compensation	• Occurs by retention of H^+ ions and excretion of HCO_3^- • Main condition required here is correction of hypokalemia • Availability of K^+, stops the loss of H^+ in exchange for Na^+ reabsorption • Retention of H^+ ions also decreases the HCO_3^- generation
Respiratory alkalosis	Decrease in PCO_2 and increase in pH
Causes	• Hyperventilation which removes excess CO_2 decreasing PCO_2 resulting in alkalosis • Hyperventilation can be due to anemia, decreased availability of oxygen at high altitudes, sepsis, shock or tissue hypoxia

Contd....

Contd....

Compensation	• Renal correction is by kidneys which decrease HCO_3^- generation so that the ratio of (HCO_3^-) : (H_2CO_3) returns to normal • Decrease in (HCO_3^-) occurs because of decrease activity of carbonic anhydrase cause by low PCO_2
Plasma findings	• Low PCO_2 • High pH • Slight low HCO_3^-
Final correction needs correction of the cause	
Acid base disturbances	Blood changes
Metabolic acidosis	• Decreased pH • Decreased HCO_3^-
Common cause of metabolic acidosis	Diabetic ketoacidosis because of excess formation of beta-hydroxybutyrate
Compensation of metabolic acidosis	• Respiratory by hyperventilation to remove H^+ ions • Renal reclamation and new HCO_3^- synthesis
Metabolic alkalosis	• Increased pH • Increased HCO_3^-
Common causes of metabolic alkalosis	• Prolonged vomiting • Nasogastric suction as in pyloric stenosis
Compensation of metabolic alkalosis	• Respiratory by hypoventilation to retain H^+ ions and CO_2 • Renal compensation by increased (HCO_3^-) excretion
Respiratory acidosis	• Decreased pH • Increased PCO_2 due to severe respiratory disorder, muscle fatigue • High plasma bicarbonate as a compensatory mechanism
Common causes of respiratory acidosis	• Emphysema • Bronchial asthma resulting in retention of CO_2 • Sedatives • Head injury • Intracranial tumors • Airway obstruction • Polio • Myasthenia • Obesity hypoventilation syndrome • Hypoventilation
Compensation of respiratory acidosis	Renal by increased reclamation of HCO_3^-
Respiratory alkalosis	• Increased pH • Decreased PCO_2 • Low plasma bicarbonate (HCO_3^-)
Common causes of respiratory alkalosis	• Shock/trauma • Ischemia resulting in hyperventilation • Anxiety • Pain • Fever • Tumor • High altitude • Pulmonary embolism • Septicemia
Compensation of respiratory alkalosis	Renal compensation by decreasing HCO_3^- reclamation and regeneration

Contd....

Contd....

Blood gas analysis: Automated blood gas analyzer, using particular ion selective electrodes for measuring various parameters

Sample	Arterial blood sample
Anticoagulant used	Heparin
Precautions in collection and storage	• Stored at 0–4°C and tested by 1 hour • Tourniquet is not used • As the needle enters the artery, the arterial blood pressure should be allowed to push the plunger of the syringe and fill it which is required to prevent the blood to mix with air
pH	To check for acidosis/alkalosis
Normal pH	7.36–7.44
PO_2	To check for ischemia/blood oxygen saturation
Normal saturation	95–98%
Normal PO_2	83–108 mm Hg
PCO_2	To check the retention of CO_2
Normal PCO_2	• 35–48 mm Hg • Variations occur in respiratory disorders
HCO_3^-	22–28 mM/L
Electrolytes	Na^+, K^+, Ca^{++}, Cl^- ions are estimated to assess the anion gap which gets altered in acid base disturbances
Normal Na^+	135–145 mEq/L
Normal K^+	3.5–5.5 mEq/L
Normal Ca^{++}	96–105 mEq/L
Normal Cl^-	9–11 mg%

Edema	Visible swelling because of increased interstitial fluid volume
Types	• Generalized (all over the body) • Localized (some parts of the body, such as face, Periorbital that is around the eyes, feet, legs, around the ankles)
Anasarca	Generalized edema
Pitting edema	Indentation of the skin persists for a few minutes after applying pressure due to accumulation of fluid, commonly around ankles and legs
	Pathophysiology
What leads to edema?	Migration of fluid from plasma to interstitial compartment
What is the key of control?	Edema is controlled by: 1. Hydrostatic pressure due to fluid volume 2. Oncotic pressure due to plasma proteins
Regulation of fluid balance at the capillary network	• There is net outward fluid movement when: The hydrostatic pressure is higher than the oncotic pressure at the arterial end of the capillary network • There is net inward fluid movement when: The hydrostatic pressure is $<$ the oncotic pressure at the venous end of the capillary network
At what state edema is not seen?	When there is balance between the outward fluid movement at the arterial end and the inward fluid movement at the venous end
At what state edema is seen?	When there is decrease in plasma oncotic pressure because of hypoproteinemia or increase in hydrostatic pressure
Causes of edema	• CHD • Nephrotic syndrome • Liver cirrhosis • Obstruction to the venous drainage of a limb • Drugs

Contd....

Contd....

Lab reports–ABG (arterial blood gas)

Case 1: Diabetic female, 75 years, hospitalized with state of Kussmaul type breathing

Blood glucose	400 mg%
Urinary ketone bodies	+
ABG	
pH (Normal: 7.35–7.45)	Low
Plasma bicarbonates (Normal: 22–26 mmol/L)	Low
$PaCO_2$ (partial pressure of CO_2) (Normal: 35–45 mm Hg)	Low because of compensatory hyperventilation (increased tidal volume: Kussmaul respiration)
H_2CO_3 (Normal: 1.2 mEq/L)	Normal
PaO_2 (partial pressure of oxygen) (Normal: 85–105 mm Hg)	Normal
O_2 saturation (Normal: 95–100%)	Normal
Na^+ (Normal: 135–145 mEq/L)	Normal
K^+ (Normal: 3.5–4.5 mEq/L)	Normal
Cl^- (Normal: 95–105 mEq/L)	Normal
Interpret the ABG report	The patient is in a state of uncompensated metabolic acidosis due to diabetic ketoacidosis (above stated ABG report)
Anion gap $[Na^+ + K^+]^- [Cl^- + HCO_3^-]$: (Normal: 10–12 mmol/L)	27 (high) so it is a case of high anion gap acidosis

Case 2: Patient of duodenal ulcer hospitalized for altered sensorium

ABG	
pH (Normal: 7.35–7.45)	High
Plasma bicarbonates (Normal: 22–26 mmol/L)	High
$PaCO_2$ (Partial pressure of CO_2) (Normal: 35–45 mm Hg)	High (because of compensatory alveolar hypoventilation)
H_2CO_3 (Normal: 1.2 mEq/L)	Normal
PaO_2 (Partial pressure of oxygen) (Normal: 85–105 mm Hg)	Normal
O_2 saturation (Normal: 95–100%)	Normal
Interpret the ABG report	The patient is in a state of uncompensated metabolic alkalosis (above stated ABG report)

Case 3: Road accident patient in a coma state

ABG	
pH (Normal: 7.35–7.45)	Low
Plasma bicarbonates (Normal: 22–26 mmol/L)	High (due to compensatory mechanism)
$PaCO_2$ (Partial pressure of CO_2) (Normal: 35–45 mm Hg)	High
H_2CO_3 (Normal: 1.2 mEq/L)	High
PaO_2 (Partial pressure of oxygen) (Normal: 85–105 mm Hg)	Normal
O_2 saturation (Normal: 95–100%)	Normal
Interpret the ABG report	Uncompensated respiratory acidosis

Case 4: Casualty admission of a female 15-year-old patient with hyperventilation, carpopedal spasm in fingers

ABG	
pH (Normal: 7.35–7.45)	High
Plasma bicarbonates (Normal: 22–26 mmol/L)	Low
$PaCO_2$ (Partial pressure of CO_2) (Normal: 35–45 mm Hg)	Low
H_2CO_3 (Normal: 1.2 mEq/L)	Low

Contd....

Contd....

PaO_2 (Partial pressure of oxygen) (Normal: 85–105 mm Hg)	Normal
O_2 saturation (Normal: 95–100%)	Normal
Interpret the ABG report	Uncompensated respiratory alkalosis because of hyperventilation and CO_2 wash off
Reason behind carpopedal spasm	Increased pH leads to more binding of calcium ions to albumin so ionized calcium level becomes low

	Congestive heart failure
Causes	• Chronic obstructive pulmonary disease • Chronic bronchitis • Bronchial asthma • Smoking
Symptoms	• Breathlessness • Edema is more on legs and feet • Edema is more in the evening due to gravity
Mechanism	Poor contractility of ventricular muscles → right ventricular failure → impaired pumping of blood into the aorta → blood accumulates in the venous circulation → increased hydrostatic pressure → movement of fluid from the plasma into the interstitial spaces (edema)
	Nephrotic syndrome
Causes	• Glomerulonephritis • Diabetic nephropathy • Hypertensive nephropathy
Characteristic feature	Proteinuria (>3 g per day)
Symptoms	Edema is seen around the eyes, more in the morning
Mechanism	Proteinuria → hypoproteinemia → decreased plasma oncotic pressure → prevention of inward movement of fluid into the venous network → edema
Liver cirrhosis	Hepatic injury resulting in replacement of hepatic cells with fibrous tissue
Causes	• Alcohol intake • Fatty infiltration of liver • Chronic hepatitis
Symptoms	Edema in abdominal cavity (ascites)
Mechanism	Cirrhosis → liver cannot synthesize albumin → hypoalbuminemia → decreased plasma oncotic pressure → edema
	Venous obstruction in the limb
Cause	Filariasis caused by worm called *Wuchereria bancrofti* infecting the lymphatic system and spreading through mosquito bite
Symptom	Localized edema
Mechanism	Hydrostatic pressure in the venous bed upstream to obstruction increases → abnormal fluid is transferred to interstitial compartment from the plasma
	Drugs
1. Nonsteroidal anti-inflammatory drugs, such as aspirin, brufen causing renal vasoconstriction resulting in edema	They inhibit cyclooxygenase enzyme thus decreasing the synthesis of prostaglandins which normally cause renal arteriolar vasodilation
2. Steroids	Increase edema by causing sodium and water reabsorption

Biochemical investigations for edema diagnosis	
1. Evaluation of hypoalbuminemia	Decreased total proteins and albumin
2. Evaluation of proteinuria	Urinary protein and albumin is done in a 24 hour urine sample
Normal excretion	
Total proteins	<150 mg/day
Albumin	<30 mg/day
Microalbuminuria	• Albumin excretion of up to 300 mg/day • Early sign of diabetic and hypertensive nephropathy
Evaluation of hepatic functions	Cirrhosis (associated with ascites) is majorly responsible for decreased synthesis of proteins, the tests are done to evaluate the liver functions: • Serum bilirubin total and direct • Serum ALT and AST • Serum ALP • Serum cholesterol • Serum proteins and A:G ratio • Urine bile pigments • Test for the cause of cirrhosis
Evaluation of renal functions	The kidneys cause hypoalbuminemia because of glomerular as well as tubular damage, thus we do some tests, such as: • Blood urea • Serum creatinine and glomerular filtration rate • Serum electrolytes • Urinary proteins excretion • Tests for the cause of renal disease
Evaluation of heart	CHF presents with symptoms, such as: • Breathlessness • Tachycardia • Increased jugular venous pressure • Crepitations in bases of lungs • Pedal edema
Biochemical marker indicating heart failure	Pro-BNP level (brain natriuretic peptide) of >125 pg/mL

Age	48 years female
Complains	Pain and swelled right big toe
History	HIV positive taking therapy, had earlier given allopurinol but not diagnosed properly mostly was acute gout
On examination	Swelling in 1st metatarsophalangeal joint
X-ray	No anomalies
Blood report	Uric acid—9 mg%
Diagnosis	Secondary gout
Mechanism	Due to antiretroviral therapy there was increased cell turnover
	Excess cell turnover causes excess catabolism of nucleic acids resulting in hyperuricemia and gout
Effect of alcohol	• Metabolism of alcohol varies the NADH/NAD ratio resulting in excess formation of lactate • The transporter for lactate and uric acid is same for excretion in the renal tubules • Monosodium urate is more soluble and excretable form of uric acid, but the level of uric acid synthesis is more in comparison to monosodium urate
Effect of allopurinol	Suicide inhibition of the enzyme xanthine oxidase required for forming uric acid
Reason behind joint pain	Uric acid crystal deposits in big toe due to gravity effect and less temperature at the extremities

Age	60 years female
Complains	Constipation, lethargy, weakness, weight gain, pain in joints movements
History	Brother had some thyroid disorder
On examination	Dull, obese, faces showed puffiness, thyroid palpable but not enlarged, reflexes were slow
What investigations to suggest?	Hb, FBS, T, FT4, TSH, Anti-TPO, TLC, DLC, PS, X-ray chest, ECG
Hb	Normal
TLC	6400/cc
DLC	P72 L40 M1 E1
PS	Normochromic, normocytic red blood cells
TSH (N: 0.34–4.37 mIU/L)	25 mIU/L
FT4 (10.3–21.9 p mol/L)	3 pmol/L
Anti-TPO	++++ (N: traces)
X-ray chest	Normal
ECG	Bradycardia
Diagnosis	Primary hypothyroidism (less FT4, high TSH and symptoms)
Reason behind obesity	There is excess of stored carbohydrates and fats due to their impaired oxidations
Reason behind reduced tolerance to cold and lethargy	A very important function of thyroid hormones is to increase the BMR and formation of heat that is calorigenic action, so when there is deficiency of thyroid hormones, there will be reduced metabolism of oxidation and fats resulting in low energy and less heat formation
Reason behind anemia	Excess menstrual bleeding can lead to iron deficiency anemia, hypocellularity of bone marrow and reduced erythropoietin results in normocytic and normochromic anemia, hypochlorhydria can lead to pernicious anemia
T3 activity is >T4	1. Free thyroid hormones are more metabolically active The binding affinity of T3 to the carrier proteins is ten times < that of T4 Thus more of T3 is freely present in plasma than T4 2. Secondly the binding affinity to nuclear receptors is 10 times more of T3 than T4
Synthesis of thyroid hormones	• Synthesis of T3 and T4 takes place in Thyroglobulin protein (dimeric protein having 2768 amino acids, most important being tyrosine) • Tyrosine reacts with iodine to form monoiodotyrosine (MIT) and diiodotyrosine (DIT) • There is coupling reaction between MIT and DIT to form T3 and T4 in presence of enzyme thyroperoxidase • Deiodinase enzyme can also remove iodine from T4 to form T3
FT4 and FT3 are good markers for evaluation of thyroid	• In normal people, 80% of T4 and T3 is bond to Thyroglobulin • 20% of T4 and T3 is bound to thyroxine binding globulin and transthyretin • Concentration of free T3 is around 0.2–0.3% • Concentration of free T4 is around 0.02–0.03% • Concentration of total T4 is inclusive of bound T4 plus free T4 • Concentration of total T3 is inclusive of bound T3 plus free T3 • If there is a change in the concentration of Thyroglobulin due to any reason, then there will be a definite change in the concentration of total T4 and total T3 • If there is a change in the concentration of Thyroglobulin due to any reason, then there will be no change in the concentration of FT4 and FT3 • For example, due to the effect of estrogen, Thyroglobulin increases during pregnancy and in women who take OCP's; in these cases, total T4 and total T3 will also increase, but FT3 and FT4 will not increase • Other factors, such as genetic disorders, acute infections, corticosteroids, androgens, [nephrotic syndrome (by decreasing Thyroglobulin in plasma)] can alter the total T3 and T4 levels
Causes of hypothyroidism	• Deficient iodine in the diet • Autoimmune disorder called Hashimoto's disease where thyroid gland destruction occurs because of cytotoxic T lymphocytic infiltration • Graves' disorder where there is surgical removal of thyroid gland takes place in severe hyperthyroidism • Antithyroid drugs, such as thiourea, etc.

Contd....

Contd....

Euthyroid goiter	Due to deficient iodine in diet, hypothyroidism may occur where there is enlarged thyroid gland but the thyroid functions remain normal	
Differences between primary and secondary hypothyroidism	Primary hypothyroidism	Secondary hypothyroidism
	Deficiency of thyroid gland hormones	Defect of pituitary gland
	Increased TSH, decreased FT3 and FT4	Decreased TSH, decreased FT3 and FT4
Management	Replacement therapy with synthetic levothyroxine	
Goitrogens	Thiocyanates present in cabbage and cauliflower, interfere in the uptake of iodine by the thyroid gland, thus formation of thyroid hormones is deranged	
Cretinism	Congenital hypothyroidism presenting with neurological abnormalities, such as mental retardation	

Age	40 years female
Complains	Breathless, palpitation
History	Weight loss, intolerance for heat
On examination	High blood pressure—150/100, RR–24/min, pulse—120/min, sweating, diffuse goiter and a positive bruit
	Investigations
TSH (N: 0.45–4.5 mIU/L)	<0.02 mIU/L
FT3 (N: 2.6–5.7 p mol/L)	>50 p mol/L
FT4 (N: 9–20 p mol/L)	60 p mol/L
Antithyroid peroxidase (TPO) (N: <35 IU/L)	1005 IU/L
Thyroglobulin antibody (N: 0–40 IU/L)	602 IU/L
Thyroid receptor antibody (N: 0–10 IU/L)	42 IU/L
ESR, CRP, leukocytes	Normal
Diagnosis	Graves' disease (symptoms are typical if Graves' disease, such as breathlessness, weight loss, low tolerance for heat exophthalmoses, tremors, and thyroid profile clearly indicates it, such as low TSH, high FT3 and FT4, presence of antithyroid receptor antibody likely proves the diagnosis)
Reason behind low heat tolerance, sweating, breathlessness	There is excess basal metabolic rate due to high level of thyroid hormones
	Due to increased BMR, there is excess formation of heat
	Due to increased BMR, there is excess need for O_2
Reason behind swelling around eyes (proptosis)	The muscles of the eye are attacked by the immune system
Increased antibody profile	It is an autoimmune disease, and autoantibodies are formed against the receptor of TSH, resulting in an active TSH receptor and ultimately hyperthyroidism, all the more, when the thyroid gland shows hypertrophy because of continuous stimulation of the receptor, ends up in goiter
Treatment	Antithyroid drugs, and partial thyroidectomy

Age	42 years male, alcoholic
Complains	Nausea, vomiting, upper abdomen pain radiates at the back
On examination	High pulse, moderate jaundice, tenderness in epigastrium and hypochondrium
	Investigations
Serum amylase	Raised
Serum lipase	Raised
Diagnosis	Acute pancreatitis (symptoms and investigations)
Cause of acute pancreatitis	Alcohol consumption (inflammation caused by the end products of alcohol metabolism, such as $NADH^+$, acetaldehyde and ethyl ester of fatty acid)

Contd....

Contd....

Other probable causes	Hyperlipidemia, gallstones (causing bile duct obstruction, the bile duct swells and lays pressure on capillaries of the pancreas leading to pancreatic inflammation)
Reason behind jaundice in acute pancreatitis	Swelled pancreas put pressure on bile duct resulting in obstructed flow of bile
Normal serum amylase	50–150 IU/L
Normal serum lipase	0–50 IU/L
Serum lipase is better marker than amylase	• Lipase is more specific for acute pancreatitis, as amylase is also produced by salivary glands • In acute pancreatitis, both rise at the same time (by 6 hours), but lipase remains elevated for longer duration as compared to amylase (10 days for lipase and only 10 days for amylase) • Raised amylase can also be seen in mumps, parotid glands damage • Due to macroamylasemia, there is high serum amylase without any pathological condition, because here, the amylase binds with proteins forming huge molecules which is not filtered by the kidneys, in some pathological conditions, high serum amylase is associated with high urine amylase also, which is not seen here, there is decreased urinary amylase

Age	40-year female, suffering from AIDS
Complains	Fever, diarrhea
On examination	Low diastolic blood pressure, high pulse, afebrile condition, hyperactive bowel sounds
	Investigations
pH	Low
Bicarbonates	Low
pCO_2	27 mm Hg
Sodium (N: 136–146 mmol/L)	138
Potassium (N: 3.5–5.3 mmol/L)	4.3
Total CO_2 (N: 23–27 mmol/L)	12
Chloride (N: 98–108 mmol/L)	116 (high)
Urea (N: 20–40 mg%)	52
Creatinine (N: 0.7–1.2 mg%)	1.8
Sugar (N: 70–100 mg%)	110
Diagnosis	Hyperchloremic metabolic acidosis due to bicarbonate loss by diarrhea
Anion gap	(138 + 4.3) – (116 + 4.3)
Compensatory response for the condition	Hyperventilation by high PCO_2, which will remove H^+ ions which will then correct chloride levels with increased retention of HCO_3^-
Other causes of acidosis	Duodenal fistula (loss of bicarbonates), glaucoma treatment drugs, such as carbonic anhydrase inhibitor drugs, renal disorders, such as less absorption of bicarbonates and hydrogen ion secretion

Age	68 years male
Complains	Breathlessness by very mild working, lying down position, swelling in legs
History	MI 2 years back, diabetic
On examination	Pedal edema, elevated jugular venous pressure, ascites, crepitations on auscultation
ECG	Features of CHD
Management on hospitalization	Digoxin started
Diagnosis	Congestive heart failure
Causes	MI 2 years back resulting in post-MI myocardium weakness and ischemia, vasculopathy due to diabetes, patients, such as these are more susceptible to silent attacks lading to decreased contractile cardiac functions, coronary arteries are also involved due to complication caused by diabetes

Contd....

Contd....

Cause of edema in CHF	There is increased hydrostatic pressure in the vessels because of decreased pumping of the heart resulting in fluid leak in the interstitial compartment
Cause of breathlessness	Congestion in lungs and poor pumping of heart with increased oxygen demand
Line of treatment	Need of strengthening contractility of myocardium, diuretics, restricted salt diet and associated complications are treated, such as diabetes and CAD
Role of digoxin	• Cardiac glycoside inhibiting Na^+-K^+ ATP-ase pump • There is increased entry of calcium in the myocardium due to increased intracellular sodium leading to stimulated contractility of myocardium • Ultimately there is good cardiac output thus decreasing hydrostatic pressure in the vascular compartment leading to decreased edema and correction of symptoms
Digoxin toxicity	Because of inhibited Na^+-K^+ ATP-ase pump, K^+ cannot enter the cells causing electrolyte disturbance
Blood investigation	Increased NT pro BNP, a peptide which is released from heart in response to failure of heart

OSCE—GOUT

1. **Scenario: Acute gout attack**
   Case: A 43-year-old man shows sudden pain/redness/swelling in the first metatarsophalangeal joint.
   Serum uric acid: 8.6 mg/dL (normal: 3.4–7.0 mg/dL)
   Synovial fluid analysis: Needle-shaped/negatively birefringent crystals under polarized light.
   Question: What is the interpretation?
   Interpretation: High serum uric acid/monosodium urate crystals in the synovial fluid indicates acute gout.
   Next steps: Treatment by NSAIDs/colchicine/lifestyle modifications/monitoring serum uric acid levels.
2. **Scenario: Chronic tophaceous gout**
   Case: A 68-year-old man with a history of recurrent gout comes with multiple nodular swellings on elbows.
   Serum uric acid: 9.3 mg/dL
   X-ray: rat-bite erosions.
   Question: What do these findings suggest?
   Interpretation: Chronic tophaceous gout is suggestive because of high uric acid levels/tophi/characteristic radiological result.
   Next steps: Start urate-lowering therapy such as allopurinol/anti-inflammatory medications for curing acute flares.
3. **Scenario: Hyperuricemia without symptoms**
   Case: A 43-year-old man comes for routine screening:
   Serum uric acid: 8.1 mg/dL
   No history of joint pain or swelling.
   Question: What is the management?
   Interpretation: Asymptomatic hyperuricemia. Treatment is not typically needed.
   Next steps: Lifestyle changes such as decreasing purine-rich food/no alcohol/proper hydration.
4. **Scenario: Uric acid nephrolithiasis**
   Case: A 37-year-old man presents with flank pain/hematuria.
   Serum uric acid: 9.1 mg/dL
   Urinalysis: pH 5.0; uric acid crystals.
   Imaging: Radiolucent stones seen in kidney.
   Question: What is the interpretation?
   Interpretation: Uric acid nephrolithiasis as indicated by acidic urine/hyperuricemia/radiolucent stones.
   Next steps: Alkalinize the urine by potassium citrate/more fluid intake/allopurinol.
5. **Scenario: Gout secondary to renal disease**
   Case: A 57-year-old man with chronic kidney disease complains of joint pain.
   Serum uric acid: 10.7 mg/dL
   Blood urea nitrogen: 45 mg/dL
   Creatinine: 3.1 mg/dL
   Question: How do you interpret?
   Interpretation: Hyperuricemia/gout secondary to low renal clearance of uric acid because of CKD.
   Next steps: Treat gout attacks/avoid medications that lead to impaired kidney function/use febuxostat and not allopurinol for long-term control.

6. **Scenario: Gout mimicking septic arthritis**
   Case: A 57-year-old man presents with monoarthritis in the knee.
   Synovial fluid analysis: high white blood cell count (20,000/mm^3); needle-shaped, negatively birefringent crystals seen
   Serum uric acid: 7.6 mg/dL
   Synovial fluid culture: No growth after 48 hours.
   Question: What is the interpretation?
   Interpretation: Gout is present. The absence of bacterial growth in synovial fluid culture confirms that there is no septic arthritis.
   Next steps: Treatment of gout using anti-inflammatory medications.
7. **Scenario: Drug-induced hyperuricemia**
   Case: A 65-year-old man with hypertension and chronic gout presents with worsening gout attacks. Medications include hydrochlorothiazide and aspirin.
   Serum uric acid: 9.8 mg/dL
   Question: What is the cause of his worsening symptoms?
   Interpretation: Hydrochlorothiazide and low-dose aspirin can cause hyperuricemia by reducing uric acid excretion.
   Next steps: Losartan that may lower uric acid levels) and evaluate the need for urate-lowering therapy.
8. **Scenario: Pseudo-gout**
   Case: A 70-year-old woman presents with acute knee pain and swelling.
   Serum uric acid: 5.5 mg/dL
   Synovial fluid analysis: Rhomboid-shaped, positively birefringent crystals under polarized light.
   Question: How should these findings be interpreted?
   Interpretation: The findings suggest calcium pyrophosphate deposition disease pseudo gout rather than gout, as indicated by the crystal morphology and birefringence.
   Next steps: Treat with NSAIDs or corticosteroids and manage any underlying conditions (e.g., hyperparathyroidism).
9. **Scenario: Acute gout in metabolic syndrome**
   Case: A 59-year-old man with obesity/hypertension/type 2 diabetes complains of acute ankle pain.
   Serum uric acid: 7.8 mg/dL
   Triglycerides: 258 mg/dL
   Fasting blood glucose: 169 mg/dL
   Question: How do you interpret this case?
   Interpretation: Hyperuricemia/acute gout is linked with metabolic syndrome, that is along with hypertriglyceridemia/obesity/insulin resistance.
   Next steps: Treatment of acute gout/lifestyle modifications/appropriate medications.
10. **Scenario: Allopurinol monitoring**
    Case: A patient with chronic gout has been taking allopurinol for 4 months.
    Serum uric acid: 5.1 mg/dL
    No recent gout attacks.
    Question: What do this interpret?
    Interpretation: Serum uric acid level is within the target range (<6 mg/dL) and there are no recent attacks, so the treatment is effective.
    Next steps: Continue allopurinol at the same dose and check out for any complications.

OSCE—ACID BASE DISORDERS

1. **Scenario: Respiratory acidosis (acute)**
   Case: A 62-year-old man having history of chronic obstructive pulmonary disease shows symptoms of shortness of breath and confusion.
   pH: 7.27 (normal: 7.35–7.45)
   $PaCO_2$: 61mmHg (normal: 35–45 mmHg)
   HCO_3^-: 29 mEq/L (normal: 22–26 mEq/L)
   PaO_2: 54 mmHg (normal: 75–100 mmHg)
   Question: What is the interpretation?
   Interpretation: The decreased pH, increased $PaCO_2$ exhibits respiratory acidosis. The bicarbonate is mildly high suggesting renal compensation, because the kidneys retain bicarbonate for balancing excess of CO_2. The PaO_2 is less so supports the logic of respiratory impairment.
   Diagnosis: Respiratory acidosis is probably secondary to COPD, that impairs elimination of carbon dioxide.
   Next steps: Ventilation by oxygen therapy/bronchodilators/noninvasive positive pressure ventilation like BiPAP).

2. **Scenario: Metabolic alkalosis (chronic)**
   Case: A 44-year-old woman with a history of more use of diuretics shows with weakness/dizziness.
   pH: 7.49 (normal: 7.35–7.45)
   $PaCO_2$: 45 mmHg (normal: 35–45 mmHg)
   HCO_3^-: 35 mEq/L (normal: 22–26 mEq/L)
   Serum chloride: 89 mEq/L (normal: 98–106 mEq/L)
   Question: What is the interpretation?
   Interpretation: The increased pH/high bicarbonate is indicative of metabolic alkalosis. The normal $PaCO_2$ is consistent with compensatory response, because lungs compensate by increasing retention of carbon dioxide. The less chloride concentration indicates alkalosis is because of volume depletion or high loss of chloride due to vomiting/use of diuretics.
   Diagnosis: Metabolic alkalosis is probably because of volume depletion by vomiting/diuretic therapy, resulting in loss of chloride along with retention of bicarbonate.
   Next steps: Correct main cause/replenish fluids/electrolytes such as chloride/discontinuing diuretics.
3. **Scenario: Mixed acid-base disorder (respiratory and metabolic acidosis)**
   Case: A 51-year-old man with complication of diabetic ketoacidosis shows with confusion/rapid breathing.
   pH: 7.11 (normal: 7.35–7.45)
   $PaCO_2$: 24 mmHg (normal: 35–45 mmHg)
   HCO_3^-: 13 mEq/L (normal: 22–26 mEq/L)
   Serum glucose: 358 mg/dL (normal: 70–110 mg/dL)
   Question: What is the interpretation?
   Interpretation: The low pH shows acidosis. The low bicarbonate shows metabolic acidosis, probably because of DKA that results in accumulation of all 3 ketone bodies, decreasing bicarbonate. The low $PaCO_2$ indicates compensation (respiratory)/metabolic acidosis (that is lungs blow off CO_2 to decrease acid concentration).
   Diagnosis: Mixed acid-base disorder that involves both metabolic acidosis because of DKA; respiratory alkalosis because of hyperventilation in response to the acidosis.
   Next steps: Treat DKA with insulin/fluids/monitor/correct acid-base balance.
4. **Scenario: Respiratory alkalosis (acute hyperventilation)**
   Case: A 27-year-old woman presents: dizziness/tingling in fingers following anxiety attack.
   pH: 7.51 (normal: 7.35–7.45)
   $PaCO_2$: 27 mmHg (normal: 35–45 mmHg)
   HCO_3^-: 21 mEq/L (normal: 22–26 mEq/L)
   Question: What is the interpretation?
   Interpretation: The high pH/low $PaCO_2$ shows respiratory alkalosis. The bicarbonate level is normal, indicating no significant metabolic compensation still took place. Hyperventilation that was the result of anxiety, results in more exhalation of CO_2, leading to respiratory alkalosis.
   Diagnosis: Acute respiratory alkalosis because of hyperventilation.
   Next steps: Breathing exercises/investigate for anxiety or main cause
5. **Scenario: Metabolic acidosis with anion gap**
   Case: A 53-year-old male with chronic renal failure has nausea and lethargy.
   pH: 7.21 (normal: 7.35–7.45)
   $PaCO_2$: 31 mmHg (normal: 35–45 mmHg)
   HCO_3^-: 17 mEq/L (normal: 22–26 mEq/L)
   Anion gap: 19 (normal: 8–16)
   Question: What is the interpretation?
   Interpretation: The decreased pH/decreased bicarbonate suggests metabolic acidosis. The high anion gap indicates the acidosis is because of accumulation of unmeasured anions which can be lactate/ketones/observed normally in renal impairment.
   Diagnosis: Metabolic acidosis and high anion gap because of uremic acidosis in the setting of CKD.
   Next steps: Hemodialysis for removing accumulated toxins. Monitor acid-base balance
6. **Scenario: Normal anion gap metabolic acidosis (hyperchloremic)**
   Case: A 31-year-old woman comes with muscle weakness/diarrhea.
   pH: 7.31 (normal: 7.35–7.45)
   $PaCO_2$: 39 mmHg (normal: 35–45 mmHg)
   HCO_3^-: 17 mEq/L (normal: 22–26 mEq/L)
   Serum chloride: 111 mEq/L (normal: 98–106 mEq/L)
   Question: What is the interpretation?
   Interpretation: The decreased pH/decreased bicarbonate suggests metabolic acidosis. The normal anion gap/high chloride indicates hyperchloremic metabolic acidosis, that is normally due to high loss of bicarbonate by diarrhea.
   Diagnosis: Diarrhea-induced metabolic acidosis because of loss of bicarbonate resulting in compensatory increase in chloride that is hyperchloremia
   Next steps: Fluid replacement/diarrhea management.

7. **Scenario: Respiratory acidosis (chronic)**
Case: A 72-year-old man with a history of obstructive sleep apnea complains of fatigue, morning headaches.
pH: 7.36 (normal: 7.35–7.45)
$PaCO_2$: 56 mmHg (normal: 35–45 mmHg)
HCO_3^-: 31 (normal: 22–26 mEq/L)
Question: What is the interpretation?
Interpretation: Respiratory acidosis. The high bicarbonate indicates renal compensation, that is kidneys retain bicarbonate for balancing increased CO_2.
Diagnosis: Chronic respiratory acidosis, possibly because of OSA that results in impaired ventilation and CO_2 retention.
Next steps: Improve ventilation/continuous positive airway pressure device for OSA treatment/monitoring of acid-base status.

OSCE—THYROID DISEASE

1. **Scenario: Hypothyroidism (primary)**
Case: A 37-year-old patient presents with fatigue/weight gain/cold intolerance.
Serum TSH: 13.0 µU/mL (normal: 0.4–4.0 µU/mL)
Free T4: 0.5 ng/dL (normal: 0.8–2.0 ng/dL)
Free T3: 1.3 pg/mL (normal: 2.0–4.4 pg/mL)
Question: What is the interpretation?
Interpretation: Primary hypothyroidism that is thyroid gland is not producing sufficient thyroid hormones.
Next steps: Initiate thyroid hormone replacement therapy/monitoring thyroid function tests.

2. **Scenario: Hyperthyroidism (Graves' disease)**
Case: A 41-year-old woman complains of loss in weight/palpitations/heat intolerance.
Serum TSH: <0.01 µU/mL (normal: 0.4–4.0 µU/mL)
Free T4: 3.6 ng/dL (normal: 0.8–2.0 ng/dL)
Free T3: 6.6 pg/mL (normal: 2.0–4.4 pg/mL)
TSH receptor antibodies: Positive
Question: What is the interpretation?
Interpretation: The suppressed TSH along with high Free T4 and Free T3/positive TSH receptor antibodies suggest Graves' disease, which is a autoimmune reason of hyperthyroidism.
Next steps: Antithyroid medications/radioactive iodine/thyroidectomy/Monitor thyroid function.

3. **Scenario: Subclinical hypothyroidism**
Case: A 51-year-old woman complains of fatigue and overt symptoms of hypothyroidism.
Serum TSH: 6.6 µU/mL (normal: 0.4–4.0 µU/mL)
Free T4: 1.1 ng/dL (normal: 0.8–2.0 ng/dL)
Free T3: 2.9 pg/mL (normal: 2.0–4.4 pg/mL)
Question: Interpret these findings?
Interpretation: Subclinical hypothyroidism, in which thyroid gland functions normally, however there is early sign of thyroid dysfunction.
Next steps: Patient is asymptomatic monitor thyroid functions/start treatment if symptoms become wors or TSH increase more.

4. **Scenario: Thyroiditis (Hashimoto's thyroiditis)**
Case: A 48-year-old man presents with goiter/constipation/gain in weight
Serum TSH: 9.9 µU/mL (normal: 0.4–4.0 µU/mL)
Free T4: 0.6 ng/dL (normal: 0.8–2.0 ng/dL)
Anti-TPO antibodies: high
Anti-Tg antibodies: high
Question: What is the interpretation?
Interpretation: Hashimoto's thyroiditis (autoimmune reason of hypothyroidism).
Next steps: Thyroid hormone replacement therapy.

5. **Scenario: Toxic multinodular goiter (Plummer's disease)**
Case: A 61-year-old man complains of tremors/palpitations/loss in weight
Serum TSH: <0.01 µU/mL (normal: 0.4–4.0 µU/mL)
Free T4: 3.1 ng/dL (normal: 0.8–2.0 ng/dL)
Free T3: 5.1 pg/mL (normal: 2.0–4.4 pg/mL)
Thyroid ultrasound: hypoechoic nodules

Question: What is the interpretation?
Interpretation: Toxic multinodular goiter (Plummer's disease), a reason behind hyperthyroidism.
Next steps: Antithyroid medications/radioactive iodine therapy/surgery. Monitoring of thyroid functions.

6. **Scenario: Primary hyperparathyroidism with hypercalcemia (thyroid related)**
Case: A 59-year-old woman complains of bone pain/kidney stones.
Serum TSH: 0.4 μU/mL (normal: 0.4–4.0 μU/mL)
Free T4: 1.3 ng/dL (normal: 0.8–2.0 ng/dL)
Free T3: 2.7 pg/mL (normal: 2.0–4.4 pg/mL)
Serum calcium: 11.0 mg/dL (normal: 8.5–10.2 mg/dL)
Parathyroid hormone: 99 pg/mL (normal: 10–65 pg/mL)
Question: What is the interpretation?
Interpretation: The low to normal TSH along with normal thyroid hormone concentration indicates euthyroid status. The high serum calcium plus PTH levels suggests primary hyperparathyroidism, that is not directly related to thyroid function however might present with symptoms which may overlap with thyroid disorders.
Next steps: Treat hyperparathyroidism/monitor calcium concentration.

7. **Scenario: Secondary hypothyroidism (pituitary dysfunction)**
Case: A 42-year-old woman complains of presenting with history of pituitary adenoma/weight gain.
Serum TSH: 0.01 μU/mL (normal: 0.4–4.0 μU/mL)
Free T4: 0.4 ng/dL (normal: 0.8–2.0 ng/dL)
Free T3: 1.1 pg/mL (normal: 2.0–4.4 pg/mL)
Prolactin: 79 ng/mL (normal: 3–20 ng/mL)
Question: What is the interpretation?
Interpretation: Secondary hypothyroidism because of pituitary dysfunction due to pituitary adenoma.
Next steps: MRI of pituitary gland/surgery/radiotherapy/hormone replacement therapy.

8. **Scenario: Thyroid storm (thyrotoxic crisis)**
Case: A 66-year-old woman with a history of hyperthyroidism complains of fever/tachycardia/altered mental status.
Serum TSH: <0.01 μU/mL (normal: 0.4–4.0 μU/mL)
Free T4: 6.6 ng/dL (normal: 0.8–2.0 ng/dL)
Free T3: 8.4 pg/mL (normal: 2.0–4.4 pg/mL)
Question: What is the interpretation?
Interpretation: The suppressed TSH/significant elevation of Free T4, Free T3 levels plus clinical signs are consistent with thyroid storm.
Next steps: Urgent treatment with antithyroid drugs/beta-blockers/supportive care.

9. **Scenario: Euthyroid sick syndrome**
Case: A 65-year-old woman with pneumonia shows with:
Serum TSH: 1.2 μU/mL (normal: 0.4–4.0 μU/mL)
Free T4: 0.5 ng/dL (normal: 0.8–2.0 ng/dL)
Free T3: 1.0 pg/mL (normal: 2.0–4.4 pg/mL).
Question: What is the interpretation?
Interpretation: Euthyroid sick syndrome which is nonthyroidal illness probably seen in cases of acute/chronic illness.
Next steps: No thyroid hormone replacement is necessary; focus on treating the underlying illness. Thyroid function may normalize once the illness resolves.

OSCE—EDEMA

1. **Scenario: Edema in heart failure**
Case: A 69-year-old male having history of congestive heart failure complains of swelling in lower extremities/shortness of breath/weight gain.
Serum albumin: 2.6 g/dL (normal: 3.5–5.0 g/dL)
Serum sodium: 134 mEq/L (normal: 136–145 mEq/L)
Serum creatinine: 1.4 mg/dL (normal: 0.6–1.2 mg/dL)
B-type natriuretic peptide: 810 pg/mL (normal: <100 pg/mL)
Question: What is the interpretation
Interpretation: The symptoms are due to congestive heart failure in which heart is not pumping properly resulting in fluid retention. Hypoalbuminemia decreases oncotic pressure/further aids in fluid accumulation in the tissues. High BNP confirm heart failure.

Diagnosis: Edema because of heart failure long with associated hypoalbuminemia.
Next steps: Diuretics for decreasing fluid overload/ACE inhibitors/beta-blockers/optimize fluid/electrolyte balance.

2. **Scenario: Edema in nephrotic syndrome**
   Case: A 42-year-old woman complains of swelling around her eyes/foamy urine.
   Serum albumin: 1.7 g/dL (normal: 3.5–5.0 g/dL)
   Urine protein: 4+ (normal: none)
   Serum cholesterol: 310 mg/dL (normal: <200 mg/dL)
   Serum creatinine: 0.8 mg/dL (normal: 0.6–1.2 mg/dL)
   Question: What is the interpretation?
   Interpretation: Edema/massive proteinuria/hypoalbuminemia/high serum cholesterol indicates nephrotic syndrome where kidneys lose protein, that reduces plasma oncotic pressure leading to fluid leakage in the tissues/edema.
   Diagnosis: Edema due to nephrotic syndrome.
   Next steps: Focus on the underlying renal disease/proteinuria/diuretics for fluid retention/immunosuppressive agents depending on the etiology.
3. **Scenario: Edema in liver cirrhosis**
   Case: A 59-year-old man with habit of alcohol consumption presents with abdominal distension/swelling of the leg.
   Serum albumin: 2.1 g/dL (normal: 3.5–5.0 g/dL)
   Serum bilirubin: 5 mg/dL (normal: 0.1–1.2 mg/dL)
   Prothrombin time: 19 seconds (normal: 10–13 seconds)
   Sodium: 131 mEq/L (normal: 136–145 mEq/L)
   Question: What is the interpretation?
   Interpretation: The symptoms are because of liver cirrhosis. The low albumin indicates reduced liver synthetic function resulting in fluid retention. High bilirubin/prolonged prothrombin time points to liver dysfunction. The low sodium is sign of hyponatremia because of fluid retention in cirrhosis.
   Diagnosis: Edema because of liver cirrhosis/portal hypertension.
   Next steps: Diuretics to manage edema/treat ascites. Monitor hepatic encephalopathy.
4. **Scenario: Edema in hypothyroidism**
   Case: A 48-year-old woman presents with edema/weight gain/fatigue. She has history of hypothyroidism.
   Serum TSH: 13 mIU/L (normal: 0.4–4.0 mIU/L)
   Free T4: 0.6 ng/dL (normal: 0.9–2.3 ng/dL)
   Serum sodium: 133 mEq/L (normal: 136–145 mEq/L)
   Question: What is the interpretation?
   Interpretation: The generalized edema is because of hypothyroidism. The high TSH/low free T4 suggests thyroid hormone levels are not sufficient, resulting in fluid retention plus decreased ability of clearing excess sodium. Hyponatremia can be seen in hypothyroidism.
   Diagnosis: Edema because of hypothyroidism.
   Next steps: Adjust thyroid hormone replacement therapy/fluid balance/sodium levels monitoring/diuretics
5. **Scenario: Edema in acute kidney injury (AKI)**
   Case: A 76-year-old man with a history of high blood pressure/diabetes shows with swelling in legs/difficulty breathing.
   Serum creatinine: 4.1 mg/dL (normal: 0.6–1.2 mg/dL)
   Serum urea: 67 mg/dL (normal: 10–20 mg/dL)
   Serum sodium: 137 mEq/L (normal: 136–145 mEq/L)
   Urine output: 205 mL/day
   Question: What is the interpretation?
   Interpretation: Acute kidney injury that leads to fluid retention because of kidneys' inability to excrete out the excess fluid. Oliguria is consistent with AKI.
   Diagnosis: Edema due to AKI.
   Next steps: Discontinue nephrotoxic drugs/optimize fluid status/supporting kidney functions/dialysis if situation worsens

OSCE—PANCREATITIS

1. **Scenario: Acute pancreatitis (typical case)**
   Case: A 48-year-old man presents with abdominal pain that radiates to the back/vomiting.
   Serum amylase: 810 U/L (normal: 30–110 U/L)
   Serum lipase: 1006 U/L (normal: 10–140 U/L)
   Liver function tests: Normal

Blood glucose: 126 mg/dL (normal: 70–110 mg/dL)
Question: What is the interpretation?
Interpretation: The high serum amylase/lipase levels suggest acute pancreatitis. The liver function tests are normal so there is no hepatic disorder. The blood glucose level is slightly high and this is common in acute pancreatitis because of stress-induced insulin resistance.
Next steps: Supportive care such as pain control/IV fluids/CT scan for finding cause of pancreatitis like gallstone/alcohol.

2. **Scenario: Chronic pancreatitis**
   Case: A 52-year-old man with a history of alcohol use abdominal pain/weight loss.
   Serum amylase: 156 U/L (normal: 30–110 U/L)
   Serum lipase: 189 U/L (normal: 10–140 U/L)
   Serum glucose: 1807 mg/dL (normal: 70–110 mg/dL)
   Fecal elastase: <40 µg/g (normal: 200–500 µg/g)
   Question: What is the interpretation?
   Interpretation: Chronic pancreatitis, although the enzymes can be less raised in comparison to acute pancreatitis. The high serum glucose indicates pancreatic endocrine function might be compromised, likely indicating developing diabetes mellitus as a side effect of chronic pancreatitis. The decreased fecal elastase level suggests exocrine pancreatic insufficiency, and this is common feature of chronic pancreatitis and leads to malabsorption.
   Next steps: Control pain/pancreatic enzyme replacement therapy for malabsorption/control blood glucose level/alcohol stoppage/abdominal ultrasound to assess pancreatic morphology.

3. **Scenario: Gallstone-induced pancreatitis**
   Case: A 39-year-old woman presents with epigastric pain/nausea after taking a fatty meal.
   Serum amylase: 606 U/L (normal: 30–110 U/L)
   Serum lipase: 708 U/L (normal: 10–140 U/L)
   Serum bilirubin: 2.6 mg/dL (normal: 0.1–1.2 mg/dL)
   ALT: 159 U/L (normal: 7–56 U/L)
   AST: 127 U/L (normal: 10–40 U/L)
   Question: What is the interpretation?
   Interpretation: The high amylase/lipase suggests acute pancreatitis. The high serum bilirubin/high ALT and AST, indicates that the pancreatitis is probably secondary to gall stones that is biliary pancreatitis that may be obstructing the common bile duct.
   Next steps: CT scan to assess gallstones/endoscopic retrograde cholangiopancreatography for removing them/cholecystectomy to prevent their recurrence.

4. **Scenario: Hypertriglyceridemia-induced pancreatitis**
   Case: A 41-year-old man complains of abdominal pain/vomiting. He presents with history of uncontrolled diabetes along with hyperlipidemia.
   Serum amylase: 510 U/L (normal: 30–110 U/L)
   Serum lipase: 752 U/L (normal: 10–140 U/L)
   Serum triglycerides: 910 mg/dL (normal: <150 mg/dL)
   Serum glucose: 253 mg/dL (normal: 70–110 mg/dL)
   Question: What is the interpretation?
   Interpretation: Pancreatitis is confirmed by the assays, high triglycerides are known risk factor for hypertriglyceridemia-induced pancreatitis. The high blood glucose level is because of stress/poor glycemic control.
   Next steps: Lowering of triglyceride levels/insulin therapy/plasmapheresis/managing blood glucose.

5. **Scenario: Pancreatitis in a child (cystic fibrosis)**
   Case: A 11-year-old boy with cystic fibrosis complains of abdominal pain/diarrhea.
   Serum amylase: 355 U/L (normal: 30–110 U/L)
   Serum lipase: 410 U/L (normal: 10–140 U/L)
   Sweat chloride test: 87 mEq/L (normal: <40 mEq/L)
   Question: What is the interpretation?
   Interpretation: Pancreatitis is common in children having cystic fibrosis because of pancreatic insufficiency. The sweat chloride test confirms diagnosis of cystic fibrosis.
   Next steps: Pancreatic enzyme replacement therapy/monitoring for pancreatic complications/respiratory/nutritional support.

6. **Scenario: Pancreatitis with hypercalcemia**
   Case: A 62-year-old man presents with severe epigastric pain/history of hypercalcemia/renal stones.
   Serum amylase: 710 U/L (normal: 30–110 U/L)
   Serum lipase: 910 U/L (normal: 10–140 U/L)
   Serum calcium: 15.0 mg/dL (normal: 8.5–10.2 mg/dL)
   Parathyroid hormone: 210 pg/mL (normal: 10–65 pg/mL)
   Question: What is the interpretation?

Interpretation: Pancreatitis is diagnosed and high calcium along with PTH levels indicates primary hyperparathyroidism, that may lead to pancreatitis because of hypercalcemia.
Next steps: Evaluate for parathyroid adenoma/hyperplasia. Treat hypercalcemia/parathyroid surgery may be needed.

7. **Scenario: Drug-induced pancreatitis**
   Case: A 47-year-old woman shows with abdominal pain after starting medicines for hyperlipidemia.
   Serum amylase: 510 U/L (normal: 30–110 U/L)
   Serum lipase: 620 U/L (normal: 10–140 U/L)
   Serum glucose: 140 mg/dL (normal: 70–110 mg/dL)
   Question: What could be the reason of pancreatitis?
   Interpretation: Pancreatitis is confirmed and one of the causes of this is medications such as statins/fibrates/diuretics. The high blood glucose is probably secondary to pancreatitis.
   Next steps: Discontinue the suspected medication/manage pancreatitis with supportive care.

CLINICAL MCQS

Gout

1. **A 76-year-old male presents with painful swelling in the big toe. Serum uric acid levels are high. What is the diagnosis?**
   a. Arthritis
   b. Osteoarthritis
   c. Gout
   d. Hyperthyroidism

   Answer: c. Gout
2. **In a patient with gout, which is typically high during an acute attack?**
   a. Blood urea nitrogen (BUN)
   b. Serum uric acid
   c. C-reactive protein (CRP)
   d. Aspartate transaminase (AST)

   Answer: b. Serum uric acid
3. **A patient with chronic gout shows hyperuricemia although he is taking treatment. Which investigation may aid to confirm presence of urate crystals in the joint?**
   a. Urine analysis
   b. Joint aspiration and crystal examination
   c. CT
   d. X ray

   Answer: b. Joint aspiration and crystal examination
4. **Which medication is used to low down uric acid levels in gout patient?**
   a. Allopurinol
   b. Methotrexate
   c. Prednisone
   d. Azithral

   Answer: a. Allopurinol

Thyroid Disease

5. **A 33-year-old female shows with fatigue, weight gain, cold intolerance. Low free T4: High TSH was reported. What is the diagnosis?**
   a. Secondary Hyperthyroidism
   b. Hypothyroidism
   c. Graves' disease
   d. Thyroiditis

   Answer: b. Hypothyroidism
6. **In a patient of hyperthyroidism, which lab findings is expected?**
   a. Low TSH/high free T4
   b. High TSH/low free T4
   c. Low TSH/low free T4
   d. Normal TSH, high free T4

   Answer: a. Low TSH/high free T4

7. **A patient with thyroid disorder has high TSH levels, low T3 and T4. Which is likely the reason?**
   a. Hyperthyroid crisis
   b. Primary hyperthyroid disease
   c. Secondary hypothyroidism
   d. Subclinical hyperthyroidism

   Answer: c. Secondary hypothyroidism

8. **A 66-year-old male patient complains of tachycardia, heat intolerance. Low TSH: high free T4. What is the diagnosis?**
   a. Graves' disease
   b. Hashimoto's thyroiditis
   c. Multinodular goiter
   d. Hypothyroidism

   Answer: a. Graves' disease

9. **Which test is used for monitoring treatment of hyperthyroidism in patients taking antithyroid therapy?**
   a. Free T4
   b. TSH
   c. Total T3, T4
   d. Thyroid antibodies

   Answer: b. TSH

Pancreatitis

10. **A 77-year-old male with habit of taking alcohol shows symptoms of abdominal pain, nausea, vomiting. Serum amylase, lipase are high. What is diagnosis?**
    a. Gallstone pancreatitis
    b. Chronic pancreatitis
    c. Acute pancreatitis
    d. Pancreatic malignancy

    Answer: c. Acute pancreatitis

11. **Which is the most specific enzyme to diagnose pancreatitis?**
    a. Serum amylase
    b. Serum lipase
    c. Alanine aminotransferase (ALT)
    d. Alkaline phosphatase (ALP)

    Answer: b. Serum lipase

12. **A patient suffering from acute pancreatitis shows serum lipase: 5 times than normal. Which is most probable diagnosis?**
    a. Hepatic disorder
    b. Renal disorder
    c. Pseudocyst formation
    d. Hypocalcemia

    Answer: c. Pseudocyst formation

13. **A 62-year-old female with abdominal pain/vomiting. High serum amylase. After 48 hours (2 days), the amylase level decreased but lipase remained high. What does this suggest?**
    a. Acute pancreatitis resolving
    b. Chronic pancreatitis
    c. A nonpancreatic source of amylase rise
    d. Pancreatic carcinoma

    Answer: a. Acute pancreatitis resolving

Acid-Base Disorders

14. **A patient presents with tachypnea, confusion, deep respirations. Arterial blood gas pH 7.32, $PaCO_2$ 30 mmHg, HCO_3 18 mEq/L. What can be the diagnosis?**
    a. Metabolic acidosis
    b. Metabolic acidosis
    c. Respiratory acidosis
    d. Metabolic alkalosis

    Answer: a. Metabolic acidosis

15. **A patient with chronic kidney disease shows symptoms of confusion, muscle weakness, serum bicarbonate level: 18 mEq/L. What is the reason behind these symptoms?**
    a. Acidosis
    b. Metabolic acidosis
    c. Respiratory acidosis
    d. Alkalosis

    Answer: b. Metabolic acidosis

16. **A 35-year-old female complains of vomiting and diarrhea for last 2 days and blood pH: 7.48, $PaCO_2$: 40 mmHg, HCO_3: 30 mEq/L. What acid-base disturbance can be present?**
    a. Acidosis
    b. Respiratory alkalosis
    c. Renal alkalosis
    d. Metabolic alkalosis

    Answer: d. Metabolic alkalosis

17. **A patient with diabetic ketoacidosis has an ABG report of pH of 7.1, bicarbonate: 10 mEq/L, high anion gap. Which acid-base disturbance can be present?**
    a. Metabolic acidosis
    b. Renal acidosis
    c. Respiratory acidosis
    d. Metabolic alkalosis

    Answer: a. Metabolic acidosis

Edema

18. **A patient shows symptoms of edema, serum albumin: 2.5 g/dL, very high cholesterol. Which is the diagnosis?**
    a. Nephrotic syndrome
    b. Nephrosclerosis
    c. Hepatitis
    d. Hyperthyroidism

    Answer: a. Nephrotic syndrome

19. **A 69-year-old male diagnosed with cirrhosis and has ascites symptoms along with lower limb swelling. Which biochemical assay is high?**
    a. Serum globulin
    b. Serum urea
    c. Serum ammonia
    d. Liver AST

    Answer: c. Serum ammonia

20. **A patient suffering from protein-losing enteropathy has edema. Serum protein electrophoresis: low albumins. What is the reason of edema?**
    a. Decreased albumin production
    b. Decreased albumin loss through the kidneys
    c. Decreased vascular permeability
    d. High sodium retention

    Answer: a. Decreased albumin production

VIVA VOCE

Gout

Q1. Discuss pathophysiology of gout.

Hyperuricemia → Monosodium urate crystal deposition in joints
Crystals trigger neutrophil activation → Inflammation
Common sites: 1st MTP joint/ankle/knee
Reasons of hyperuricemia: Overproduction as in ↑cell turnover, enzyme defects or underexcretion as in renal failure, diuretics

Q2. How do we diagnose gout?
Synovial fluid analysis:
Negatively birefringent needle-shaped crystals under polarized light
High WBCs/inflammatory joint fluid
Serum uric acid can be normal during acute attack
X-ray: Punched-out erosions with overhanging edges/rat-bite" lesions

Thyroid Disorders

Q3. Discuss causes of hyperthyroidism.
Graves' disease—Autoimmune (TSH receptor antibodies ↑T3/T4)
Toxic multinodular goiter
Toxic adenoma
Thyroiditis (subacute/postpartum) → Temporary hyperthyroidism

Q4. Differentiate primary vs. secondary hypothyroidism.
Primary hypothyroidism:
↑ TSH, ↓ T3/T4 like Hashimoto's thyroiditis
Secondary hypothyroidism: Pituitary/TSH deficiency—
↓ TSH, ↓ T3/T4 like pituitary adenoma/Sheehan's syndrome

Pancreatitis

Q5. Discuss diagnostic criteria for acute pancreatitis.
2 out of 3 criteria:
1. Epigastric pain radiating at back
2. Serum lipase/amylase >3x normal
3. CT scan exhibiting pancreatic inflammation

Q6. Discuss complications of chronic pancreatitis.
Pancreatic insufficiency → malabsorption, steatorrhea
Diabetes mellitus
Pancreatic pseudocyst
Increased risk of pancreatic cancer

Acid-base Disorders

Q7. Interpret an arterial blood gas (ABG).
Step 1: Look at pH → acidosis (<7.35)/alkalosis (>7.45)
Step 2: Check CO_2 (respiratory)/HCO_3 (metabolic)
pH ↓, CO_2 ↑ → Respiratory acidosis (COPD, hypoventilation)
pH ↓, HCO_3^- ↓ → Metabolic acidosis (diabetic ketoacidosis, lactic acidosis)
pH ↑, CO_2 ↓ → Respiratory alkalosis (hyperventilation, anxiety)
pH ↑, HCO_3^- ↑ → Metabolic alkalosis (vomiting, diuretics)

Q8. Explain anion gap and its utility.
Anion gap = $Na^+ - (Cl^- + HCO_3^-)$ (normal = 8–12 mEq/L)
Elevated anion gap metabolic acidosis: MUDPILES that is methanol, uremia, DKA, paraldehyde, isoniazid, lactic acidosis, ethylene glycol, salicylates
Normal anion gap metabolic acidosis: Diarrhea/renal tubular acidosis

Edema

Q9. Discuss causes of edema.
1. High capillary hydrostatic pressure → Heart failure/DVT
2. Low oncotic pressure → Nephrotic syndrome/liver failure/malnutrition
3. Lymphatic obstruction → Filariasis/malignancy
4. Raised capillary permeability → Sepsis/burns/angioedema

Q10. Differentiate transudative vs. exudative edema.
Transudate that is low protein/low LDH: CHF/Nephrotic syndrome/Cirrhosis
Exudate that is high protein/high LDH: Infection/Malignancy/Inflammation
Use Light's Criteria (for pleural effusion):
When pleural fluid/serum protein >0.5 → Exudate
When pleural fluid/serum LDH >0.6 → Exudate

SPOTTERS

Gout

Q1. Synovial fluid microscopy with needle-shaped crystals.

Spotter image: Polarized light microscopy exhibiting negatively birefringent/needle-shaped crystals
Interpret:
Gout/monosodium urate crystals
Negatively birefringent/yellow if parallel to light/blue if perpendicular
Observed in acute gouty arthritis

Q2. Gouty Tophus on ear helix.

Spotter image: Chalky white deposits on ear helix
Clinical significance:
Tophus/urate crystal deposit in chronic gout
Common locations: Ear/fingers/toes/olecranon bursa
Linked with long-standing hyperuricemia

Thyroid Disorders

Q3. Exophthalmos in Graves' disease.

Spotter image: Protruding eyes and lid retraction
Interpret:
Graves' disease/autoimmune hyperthyroidism
Caused by TSH receptor antibodies
Orbital fibroblast stimulation → Exophthalmos

Q4. Hashimoto's Thyroiditis Histology.

Spotter image: Lymphocytic infiltration with germinal centers and Hurthle cells
Interpret:
Hashimoto's thyroiditis/chronic lymphocytic thyroiditis
Autoimmune hypothyroidism
Linked with anti-TPO antibodies

Pancreatitis

Q5. Cullen's sign in acute pancreatitis.

Spotter image: Blue discoloration around umbilicus
Interpret:
Cullen's sign = Periumbilical hemorrhage
Indicates retroperitoneal bleeding in severe acute pancreatitis

Q6. Pancreatic pseudocyst on CT scan.

Spotter image: Well-defined fluid collection near the pancreas
Interpret:
Pancreatic pseudocyst/fluid-filled sac after pancreatitis
Lacks epithelial lining
Can result in infection or rupture

Acid-base Disorders

Q7. Arterial blood gas report exhibiting metabolic acidosis with elevated anion gap.

Spotter data:
pH = 7.25 (acidosis)
HCO_3^- = 15 mEq/L (low)
PCO_2 = 30 mmHg (compensatory ↓)
Anion gap = 20 (↑, Normal = 8–12)
Interpret:
Elevated anion gap metabolic acidosis
Reasons: Diabetic ketoacidosis/lactic acidosis/methanol poisoning

Q8. Kussmaul breathing in diabetic ketoacidosis (DKA).

Spotter image: Patient with deep, labored breathing
Interpret:
Kussmaul respiration = Compensatory hyperventilation
Observed in DKA/metabolic acidosis
Aids eliminate CO_2 to balance pH

Edema

Q9. Pitting edema in nephrotic syndrome.

Spotter image: Pressed skin on shin leaving a deep indentation
Interpret:
Pitting edema because of hypoalbuminemia
Common in nephrotic syndrome/heart failure/cirrhosis

Q10. Lymphedema (nonpitting edema).

Spotter image: Swollen lower limb with thickened skin (Stemmer's sign positive)
Interpret:
Nonpitting edema because of lymphatic obstruction
Reasons: Filariasis/malignancy/postsurgical
Does not respond to diuretics

REFLECTION

Describe the pathogenesis and clinical features of gout, thyroid disorders, pancreatitis, acid base disorders and edema. Describe the biochemical basis of the tests performed in these conditions.

32

CHAPTER

Biochemical Tests in Nephrotic Syndrome, Proteinuria, Renal Failure, Dyslipidemia and Myocardial Infarction

COMPETENCY

BC14.19: Explain the basis and rationale of biochemical tests done in the following conditions:
- Dyslipidemia
- Myocardial infarction
- Renal failure
- Proteinuria
- Nephrotic syndrome

LEARNING OBJECTIVES

After reading this chapter, the readers should be able to:
- Describe the pathogenesis and clinical features of nephrotic syndrome, proteinuria, renal failure, dyslipidemia and myocardial infarction.
- Describe the biochemical basis of the tests performed in these conditions.
- Understand the biochemical basis and rationale behind diagnostic tests used in various medical conditions.
- Explain how specific laboratory parameters are utilized in the diagnosis, monitoring, and management of different diseases.
- Interpret the results of biochemical tests in the context of specific clinical scenarios.
- Appreciate the role of biochemical investigations in understanding the pathophysiology of different medical conditions.

BLUE PRINT

Explanation of Biochemical Tests in Various Medical Conditions

Objective

By the end of the lecture, students should be able to:
1. Understand the biochemical basis and rationale behind diagnostic tests used in various medical conditions.
2. Explain how specific laboratory parameters are utilized in the diagnosis, monitoring, and management of different diseases.
3. Interpret the results of biochemical tests in the context of specific clinical scenarios.
4. Appreciate the role of biochemical investigations in understanding the pathophysiology of different medical conditions.

Duration: *60 minutes*

Materials Needed

1. Presentation slides illustrating the biochemical tests and their interpretation in different medical conditions.
2. Case studies or clinical vignettes representing each medical condition for interactive discussion.
3. Whiteboard or flipchart for drawing biochemical pathways and explaining concepts.
4. Handouts summarizing the biochemical tests and their significance in each medical condition.

Outline

I. **Introduction to biochemical testing in medicine** **(10 minutes)**
- Overview of the role of biochemical tests in the diagnosis and management of medical conditions.
- Importance of understanding the underlying biochemical mechanisms for interpretation of test results.

II. **Dyslipidemia** **(10 minutes)**
- Description of lipid profile tests including total cholesterol, LDL cholesterol, HDL cholesterol, and triglycerides.
- Significance of lipid profile in assessing cardiovascular risk and guiding lipid-lowering therapy.

III. **Myocardial infarction** **(10 minutes)**
- Discussion of cardiac biomarkers such as troponin, creatine kinase (CK), and CK-MB.
- Use of cardiac biomarkers in the diagnosis and risk stratification of myocardial infarction.

IV. **Renal failure and gout** **(10 minutes)**
- Explanation of renal function tests including serum creatinine, blood urea nitrogen (BUN), and uric acid.
- Relationship between renal function tests and the development of gout in renal failure.

V. **Proteinuria and nephrotic syndrome** **(10 minutes)**
- Overview of urinary protein tests and albuminuria measurement.
- Interpretation of proteinuria in the context of nephrotic syndrome and renal disease.

VI. **Conclusion and recap** **(5 minutes)**
- Summarize key points covered in the lecture regarding the biochemical tests used in various medical conditions.
- Emphasize the importance of interdisciplinary collaboration between clinicians and laboratory professionals in interpreting test results.

VII. **Question and Answer Session** **(5 minutes)**
- Encourage students to ask questions and seek clarification on any aspects of the lecture.
- Foster discussion on practical applications of biochemical tests in clinical practice.

Nephrotic syndrome	Increased permeability of glomerular basement membrane because of disorders of glomerulus		
Characteristics	• Proteinuria (due to increased permeability excretion of >3 g of protein in 24 hours) • Edema (due to decreased albumin in blood) • Hypoalbuminemia (excretion of albumin in urine) • Hyperlipidemia (hypoalbuminemia leads to excess lipoprotein synthesis by the liver)and (decreased lipoprotein lipase activity leads to less catabolism of lipoproteins) • Lipiduria (lipids may be filtered sometimes) • Hypercoagulability		
Causes	Glomerulonephritis that is the disease of glomerulus leads to increased permeability		
	Types of Glomerulonephritis		
Minimal change glomerulonephritis			
Diabetic nephropathy			
Infections	Beta hemolytic *Streptococcus*	Respiratory tract and gastro-intestinal tract infections	Hepatitis virus mainly B and C
Systemic inflammatory diseases	Rheumatoid arthritis	Systemic lupus erythematosus	
Drug toxicity	Nonsteroidal anti-inflammatory drugs (NSAIDs), like aspirin, ibuprofen		
Clinical manifestations	• Face swelling mainly in the morning • Swelling around ankles and feet may be present in heart patients • Fever, sore throat, diarrhea, dysuria (discomfort while urination), burning sensation, lethargy, weakness, less appetite, symptoms of associated complications like high blood pressure and diabetes mellitus (DM), anemia due to transferrin loss, low calcitriol due to decreased renal alpha 1 hydroxylase activity leading to vitamin D deficiency, malnutrition		

Rationale of Biochemical Tests Done

Serum proteins	Serum total proteins and albumin are decreased because of urinary excretion of these proteins
Urine proteins	Proteinuria is important manifestation

Contd...

Contd...

Urine examination	Red blood cell (RBCs), Hb are present, increased specific gravity due to proteinuria
Glomerular filtration rate (GFR)	Normal/less
Kidney function test (KFT)	Blood urea, creatinine, electrolytes, uric acid are estimated which may be normal/ increased
Lipid profile	Increased serum cholesterol and LDL-cholesterol
Electrophoresis of proteins	For evaluation of nature of protein excreted we do electrophoresis in serum and urine
Tests for other symptoms: LFT, tests for DM	
Tests to identify underlying diseases: Blood sugar in DM, urine, blood and throat swab culture for infections for identification of organisms and ultrasound of kidneys	
Management	• Glomerulonephritis respond well to steroids mainly in children • Treatment of underlying cause • Treatment of complications like edema is treated by salt restriction and diuretics

Proteinuria	Protein excretion in urine that is excretion of >150 mg per day of total proteins and >30 mg per day of albumin		
	Pathophysiology		
If the glomerular filtration membrane is damaged, the albumin and other plasma proteins escape this barrier and get excreted out in urine			
Structure of glomerular barrier, (3 layers)	Capillary endothelial layer having holes of 70–100 nm The basement membrane having proteins like laminin, entactin, type IV collagen, glycosaminoglycans (GAGs) like heparin and heparin sulfate The epithelial layer/podocyte layer, the foot processes of podocytes make filtration slits of 10–40 nm between them Glomerular membrane allows molecules up to the size of 8 nm to pass through it Though albumin is smaller than 8 nm, but it is prevented by the negatively charged heparin sulfate and sialic acid that repels albumin and most other plasma proteins which are also negatively charged at the pH of blood		
	Types of Proteinuria		
Three types	1. Glomerular proteinuria	2. Tubular proteinuria	3. Overflow proteinuria
Mechanism	Defect in glomerular filtration Albumin is mainly filtered and excreted early as it is small in size With more damage, large proteins also start excreting, RBC's may also pass which after getting mixed with urine get hemolyzed releasing Hb also It is pathological condition and excretion is >2 g/day	Due to excretion of small MW proteins secreted by tubules like beta 2 microglobulin and retinol binding protein. Tubular proteinuria can be isolated or associated with glomerular proteinuria	Due to excess circulating proteins
Causes	Nephrotic syndrome, glomerulonephritis and diabetic nephropathy, hypertensive nephropathy, stress, severe cold, high temperature, severe exercise	Renal tubular absorption defects like Fanconi's syndrome, amino acidurias, hypercalciuria	Multiple myeloma (increased synthesis of immunoglobulins) where small proteins like immunological light chains get excreted called Bence-Jones proteins detected by electrophoresis where dark thick band of gamma globulin is observed near the origin

Contd...

Contd...

Microalbuminuria	Albumin excretion ranging from 30–300 mg/day, earliest sign of diabetic kidney disease
Orthostatic proteinuria	Proteinuria during postural change like standing, benign, requires no treatment

Qualitative detection of proteinuria	**Quantitative estimation of proteinuria**
1. **Albustix method:**	**Sample:** 1. 24 hour urine sample is taken (first morning sample is discarded and then subsequently all samples during the day are collected, next day morning sample will be the last sample, refrigerated till examination, properly mixed aliquot is used) 2. Spot urine protein excretion/gram of creatinine in morning urine sample gives results comparable to 24 hour sample
Kit: It has a plastic strip, one end of which has an absorbent pad of cellulose, impregnate with bromophenol blue as indicator and a citrate buffer of pH 3.5	1. **Turbidimetric method:** Urinary proteins are precipitated with sulfosalicylic acid and sodium sulfate
Method: Strip is dipped in urine for 1 second and excess urine is removed, the color is compared with the test chart within 1 minute	**Principle:** Protein particles remain suspended in the solution and scatter the light that we pass through the solution, the transmitted light intensity is decreased I proportion to the suspended particles resent in the solution
Principle: At pH 3.5 the indicator is yellow but forms a blue color with increasing concentration of protein due to changing of indicator to divalent anion form	The concentration is calculated by comparing with the standard
Positive result shows albumin concentration of approximately 30 mg% or more	
2. Heat coagulation test	2. Immunoturbidimetric method for albuminuria where albumin gets precipitated by antibodies
3. Sulfosalicylic acid	3. Pyrogallol based methods for total protein estimation
4. Heller's nitric acid test	

Renal failure	Severe decline in the kidney functions leading to Azotemia that is accumulation of nitrogenous waste products like urea, creatinine, etc. in the blood, along with disturbance of extracellular fluid volume and acid base misbalance	
Uremia	Azotemia + clinical symptoms + multiorgan failure	
Types of renal failure	Acute	Chronic

Acute renal failure	Sudden decline in renal functions over days and weeks, generally associated with oliguria or Anuria
Mechanism	Decrease in glomerular filtration
Prerenal causes	• Decreased plasma volume → decreased renal blood flow → decreased GFR → retention of urea → increased blood urea • Diarrhea • Cholera • Vomiting • Intestinal obstruction • Burns • Shock • Severe hemorrhage • Accident • Trauma • Fluid depletion • Diabetic ketoacidosis
Renal causes	• Renal ischemia • Renal artery stenosis • Acute glomerulonephritis • Renal tubular necrosis

Contd...

Contd...

Post renal causes	• Decrease in GFR is due to obstruction to the flow of glomerular filtrate → increased intra-renal pressure and hydronephrosis (filtrate accumulates in kidneys) → increased pressure in renal capillaries and glomerulus → renal failure (when both the kidneys are affected) • Kidney, ureter and bladder stones • Kidney and bladder tumors • Enlargement of prostate • Urethral strictures
Clinical signs and symptoms	Polydipsia, nausea, vomiting, weakness, dizziness, postural hypotension, skin turgor is decreased, dry mucous membrane and tongue, pain in flanks, colicky pain
Laboratory investigations	• Blood urea, creatinine, electrolytes (hyperkalemia is very common) • To differentiate between prerenal and renal causes, urine sodium is done
Acute renal failure due to prerenal cause	Urinary sodium excretion is <10 mmol/L
Acute renal failure due to renal cause	Urinary sodium excretion is >20 mmol/L
For stones, renal artery stenosis	Radiological investigations
Aim of therapy	• To maintain volume of fluid • To correct hyperkalemia • To provide renal support by dialysis • To treat the underlying causes

Acute renal failure (ARF), when treated on time regains normal renal functions

Chronic renal failure	Chronic kidney disease (CKD) → loss of nephron activity → end stage renal disease (ESRD) → dialysis/ renal transplant	
CKD	Renal disorder of >3 months duration, along with reduced glomerular filtration rate	
Risk factors of CKD	• Old age • Family history of renal disorder • High blood pressure • DM • Past history of renal failure • Autoimmune disorders	
Five stages of CKD		
1.	CKD with renal damage	Normal GFR–90 mL/min/1.73 m^2
2.	CKD with mild decrease in GFR	60–89 mL/min/1.73 m^2
3.	CKD with moderate decrease in GFR	30–59 mL/min/1.73 m^2
4.	CKD with severe decrease in FR	15–29 mL/min/1.73 m^2
5.	Renal failure	<15 mL/min/1.73 m^2
Calculation of GFR	Equation which depends on plasma, creatinine, weight, height, etc.	
Cockroft Gault formula	• Creatinine clearance = (140–age) × body weight/72 × plasma creatinine (mg%) • For females the value obtained is multiplied by 0.85	
Causes of CRF	All kidney disorders, high blood pressure, DM	

Signs and symptoms of CRF:

- Edema with oliguria and Anuria
- **Electrolyte misbalance:** Hyperkalemia, hypernatremia, hyperphosphatemia, hypocalcemia
- Metabolic acidosis
- Erythropoietin deficiency leads to anemia
- Calcitriol deficiency results in osteomalacia
- Hypertriglyceridemia and decreased HDL cholesterol
- Protein–energy malnutrition (PEM)
- Heart failure or cardiomyopathy
- Hyper coagulation and increased atherosclerosis
- Bleeding tendency
- Less immunity

Hypocalcemia leads to secondary hyperparathyroidism

Contd...

Contd...

Laboratory investigations	• Blood urea, creatinine, GFR, electrolytes • Calcium, phosphate • Bicarbonate • Blood proteins and urine to evaluate proteinuria • Alkaline phosphatase (ALP) for bone disorder • Other investigations for DM, anemia, hyperlipidemia, coagulation abnormalities, etc.
Treatment approach	• Restrict protein diet (urea is formed from proteins and is excreted out by kidneys) • Treat anemia by giving iron and erythropoietin • Give calcitriol for bone disorders • Treat electrolyte disturbance • Maintain good control of DM and high blood pressure • Dialysis/renal transplant

Dyslipidemia	Abnormal alterations in the blood lipid levels, leading to increased risk of atherosclerosis causing myocardial infarction and stroke
Plasma lipids (present in lipoproteins except free fatty acid (FFA) which are present in loose bond with albumin)	Normal range
Total lipids	400–600 mg/dL
Total cholesterol (major lipid in LDL and HDL)	150–200 mg/dL
Total phospholipids	150–250 mg/dL
Triglycerides (major lipid in chylomicrons and VLDL)	50–150 mg/dL
Free fatty acids	10–20 mg/dL

Hyperlipoproteinemias: Genetic diseases associated with plasma lipid abnormalities

Type of hyperlipoproteinemia	Name of the disorder	Lipoprotein which is abnormal/ increased	Lipid abnormalities			
Type I	Familial chylomicronemia	Chylomicron	TG ↑↑↑↑	Chol ↑↑	LDL-C ↑	HDL-C ↓↓↓
Type II a	Familial hypercholesterolemia	LDL	TG N	Chol ↑↑↑	LDL-C ↑	HDL-C ↓
Type II b	Familial combined hyperlipidemia	LDL and VLDL	TG ↑↑	Chol ↑↑↑	LDL-C ↑↑	HDL-C ↓
Type III	Familial dysbetalipoproteinemia	IDL	TG ↑↑	Chol ↑↑	LDL-C ↓	HDL-C N
Type IV	Familial hyperlipidemia	VLDL	TG ↑↑	Chol N/↑	LDL-C ↓	HDL-C ↓↓
Type V	Familial hypertriglyceridemia	VLDL and chylomicrons	TG ↑↑↑↑	Chol ↑↑	LDL-C ↓	HDL-C ↓↓

Hypercholesterolemia	Increase of plasma total cholesterol level/non-HDL cholesterol level (total cholesterol—HDL cholesterol)

Normal lipid profile level in adults aged 20–40 years with lowest atherosclerotic cardiovascular disease risk (ACVD)

Total cholesterol	<200 mg%
Low-density lipoprotein cholesterol	<160 mg%
High-density lipoprotein cholesterol	>40 mg%
Triglycerides	<150 mg%

Causes of Hypercholesterolemia	
DM	Insulin deficiency → increased lipolysis → increased free fatty acids → increased oxidation of FFA → increased acetyl-CoA → increased cholesterol synthesis and other lipids → hypercholesterolemia
Hypothyroidism	Decreased thyroid hormones → decreased activation of 7 alpha hydroxylase enzyme → cholesterol does not convert to bile acids and salts which are to be excreted out in the bile → decreased thyroid hormones decrease this excretion → hypercholesterolemia
Obstructive jaundice	The obstruction to the flow of bile increases the blood cholesterol leading to hypercholesterolemia
Familial hypercholesterolemia	Defect of LDL receptor → decreased LDL uptake → decreased LDL catabolism → hypercholesterolemia

Hypertriglyceridemia	Increased serum triglycerides above 150 mg%
Blood TAG are present mainly in	Chylomicrons (Dietary TAG of exogenous origin)
	Very low-density lipoprotein (VLDL) (hepatic/endogenous origin)
Function of lipoprotein lipase enzyme	Lipoprotein lipase in peripheral tissue capillaries clear off the chylomicrons and VLDL and used for energy in muscle tissues or for storage in adipose tissues
Types and location of Apo B	Apo B 48 is present in chylomicrons and Apo B 100 is present in VLDL
Decreased lipase activity and defective Apo B formation	Results in hypertriglyceridemia
Common causes of hypertriglyceridemia	• High saturated lipid diet and high calorie intake (increase chylomicrons and TAG) • Obesity, DM (insulin resistance → increased lipolysis → Increased VLDL → hypertriglyceridemia • Intake of excess alcohol (excess acetyl-CoA promoting hyperlipidemia) • Hypothyroidism (promotes hypercholesterolemia by decreasing bile acid synthesis from cholesterol and also their excretion)

Genetic Causes of Hypertriglyceridemia	
1. Familial hypertriglyceridemia/type IV hyperlipoproteinemia:	Occurrence–1:500, polygenic (multiple gene defect), needs other associated conditions for its expression
2. Familial combined hypertriglyceridemia/type II B hyperlipoproteinemia:	Occurrence–1:1200, polygenic (multiple gene defect)
3. Familial dysbeta hypertriglyceridemia/type III hyperlipoproteinemia:	Occurrence–1:20,000, defective isoform APOE 3 present, needs other associated conditions for its expression

Classification of Hypertriglyceridemia	
Blood TG's level:	
Normal	>150 mg%
Borderline	150–199 mg%
High	200–499 mg%
Very high	>500 mg%
Chylomicronemia (serum samples are lipemic collected after 12 hours of fasting, when freezed at 4°C for some hours, chylomicrons float forming a creamy layer on top)	>1000 mg%
Patient exhibits yellow white xanthomatous patches on knees and elbows and retinal defects in eye	

Investigation of Dyslipidemia	
Lipid profile	Group of blood lipid tests for evaluating the risk of atherosclerosis
Risk factors for premature atherosclerosis	Hypercholesterolemia, hypertriglyceridemia, high LDL-cholesterol, low HDL-cholesterol and high lipoproteins, etc.
Foam cells	Cholesterol laden macrophages, and are the earliest cells to get deposited in the blood cells in atherosclerosis
Importance of HDL as a marker (good cholesterol)	Aids in removal of cholesterol from tissues to liver by reverse cholesterol transport
Importance of LDL as a marker (bad cholesterol)	Deposits cholesterol into the tissues making them more atherogenic
1. Serum total cholesterol (good indicator of dyslipidemia)	The serum has cholesterol, majorly as HDL and LDL and also minor as VLDL and chylomicrons
Normal level	150–200 mg% (lowest risk)
2. HDL-cholesterol/alpha lipoprotein/ good lipoprotein (high HDL is protective)	Removes cholesterol from peripheral tissues and with the help of LCAT enzyme and Apo A1 coenzyme lecithin cholesterol acyl transferase (LCAT)], esterify cholesterol and transfers it ultimately to the liver through LDL, VLDL, etc.
Reverse cholesterol transport	• HDL has LCAT and Apo A 1 • LCAT along with cofactor Apo A 1 esterify HDL-cholesterol • Cholesterol ester transfer protein (CTEP) transfers this esterified cholesterol to LDL and VLDL • Thus, there is decrease of free cholesterol in HDL • Thus, it takes up more cholesterol from the tissues through ABC 1 receptor, again esterify it and transfer to liver • Liver also takes up LDL and VLDL for catabolism
Normal level	>40 mg%
	• Drugs like progesterone and beta blockers used as treatment in high blood pressure decrease HDL-cholesterol • HDL-cholesterol can be increased by physical exercise and niacin
3. LDL-cholesterol (richest in cholesterol among all lipoproteins and important marker for evaluating CAD)	• It delivers 30% of the total cholesterol in the peripheral tissues so high LDL cholesterol means excess deposition of cholesterol in tissues and higher risk for atherosclerosis and coronary artery disease (CAD) • 30% LDL is thus taken up by the extrahepatic tissues and 70% goes to liver • When LDL-cholesterol is in excess, it will transfer more cholesterol to the peripheral tissues • Secondly, this transfer of cholesterol of LDL is through scavenger receptors and non-receptor-mediated endocytosis which are nonsaturable and nonregulated processes
Normal level	<160 mg%
Friedewald equation (since separation of LDL from serum needs ultracentrifugation for 18 hours so it is calculated and not estimated)	Total cholesterol = HDL-cholesterol + LDL-cholesterol + VLDL-cholesterol (mg%) LDL cholesterol = Total cholesterol–[HDL-C + VLDL-C] = Total cholesterol–[HDL-C + TG/5] since VLDL-C is taken to be 1/5th of serum TG level and is based on the logic that ratio of TG and cholesterol content of VLDL is 5:1 It should not be used in calculating LDL-C, if TG is >400 mg%/patient has type III hyperlipoproteinemia because in these conditions the composition of VLDL changes
LDL-C: HDL-C ratio	Good predictor of atherosclerosis
Normal	2–2.5
	High ratio, because of more LDL-cholesterol or less HDL-cholesterol, is a positive predictor for atherosclerosis
Triglycerides	• Derived from dietary lipids (exogenous/chylomicrons) and hepatic synthesis (endogenous/VLDL) • They increase in genetic disorders and metabolic disorders like DM and increased TG increase the risk of atherosclerotic cardiovascular disease
Normal value	Up to 150 mg%

Contd...

Apoproteins of Chylomicrons, VLDL and LDL

Chylomicrons:	Apo B 48
VLDL, IDL, LDL:	Apo B 100
	Apo B 48 and Apo B 100 are products of same gene
RNA editing:	B-48 is the part of apo B 100 formed due to mutation, changing a functional codon to stop codon

Risk Factors for Atherosclerosis, Coronary Artery Disease and Cerebral Stroke

Risk factor	Significance	Recommendations
A. Nonmodifiable		
1. Sex	Males are more prone Due to estrogen females in reproductive age are at low risk	In postmenopausal women, there is almost equal risk in both sex
2. Age	As the age increases the risk of CAD increases	–
B. Modifiable		
3. Sedentary lifestyle	Physical inactivity → obesity → DM, high blood pressure and atherosclerosis	Regular exercise results in decreased LDL-cholesterol and increased HDL- cholesterol
4. Obesity	Results in increased blood lipids and lead to CAD, high blood pressure and DM	Diet modification + regular exercise = Ideal weight
5. Smoking	Nicotine → vasoconstriction, lipolysis and hyperlipidemia → atherosclerosis	Stop smoking
6. Diet	High carbohydrate + high fat diet with saturated fatty acids → increased risk of atherosclerosis	Low fat diet with monounsaturated fatty acids and polyunsaturated fatty acids
7. Stress and anxiety	Catecholamine → vasoconstriction, lipid catabolism and increased VLDL leads to increased LDL	Avoid foods which are rich in cholesterol like meat, eggs
8. Hyperlipidemia	Risk factors mainly are excess cholesterol and triglyceride levels	Lifestyle modifications, with/without drugs
9. DM	Leads to dyslipidemia and increased risk of CAD	Good control of DM is the need
10. High blood pressure (above 140/90)	Mainly risk factor for CAD and cerebral stroke	Maintain normal BP of 120/80
11. Hyperhomocysteinemia	Increased homocysteine level in blood may lead to atherosclerosis	
12. Hypothyroidism	Leads to hypercholesterolemia	May be fatal
13. Lp(a), Apo(a)	Increased levels are dangerous	Diet modifications and drugs

Myocardial infarction (MI)	Acute cardiac emergency due to sudden stoppage of blood supply to a part of myocardium Sudden stoppage of blood supply (coronary artery block/its main branch) → ischemia → necrosis of that part of myocardium manifesting as chest pain radiating to jaw and left arm
Angina pectoris	Related disorder but here there is partial blockage of blood supply to the myocardium so there no complete ischemia, aggravates during increased activity as the blood supply does not increase in proportion to meet the extra demand, so chest pain is there because of myocardial ischemia
Typical sign of angina pectoris	The pain subsides when we stop the physical activity and take rest
Angina at rest	A pre myocardial infarction stage where the coronary artery blockage is almost complete giving very less blood supply and there is chest pain even at rest and not relieved by complete rest

Occurrence	• Common in left ventricle but can occur in atria or other parts of the myocardium • Common in middle, old age, and in females after menopause, although can occur in young boys and girls and rare in women before menopause
Causes	Atherosclerosis of coronary artery or its branches
Mechanism of plaque formation	• Fatty streak slowly increasing in size blocks partially or completely, the lumen of the artery, plaque is made of fats, foam cells, muscle cells covered by endothelium • Due to rupture of these plaques, circulation is blocked to the myocardium resulting in MI or angina
Unstable plaques	Old plaques not covered by endothelium which have a high tendency of getting ruptured, stable plaques rupture less
Risk factors	Old age, males, obese, sedentary life style, DM, high blood pressure, smoking, family history of CHD
Symptoms	• Chest pain/pressure behind the chest sternum which radiates to the jaw, left arm and upper abdomen • Tachycardia, anxiety, sinking sensation • Excess sweating, even in air condition environment • Breathlessness, fast irregular pulse, cardiac arrhythmias • Cardiogenic shock • The pain in DM is mild/absent because of neuropathy
Diagnosis	Diagnosed by the signs and symptoms along with ECG, and some biochemical investigations

Biochemical Investigations

CK isoenzymes II-CKMB/CK II	Isoenzyme of creatine phosphate kinase enzyme, not so much specific for heart CK III is 90% and CK II is 9%
Estimation	• CK-MB is estimated after precipitating CK III with CK III monoclonal antibody, supernatant mainly contains CK-MB • A specific enzymatic method is used for its estimation
Diagnosis	• In MI, total CK and CK-MB are increased • It is taken to be significant when rise in CK-MB is >6% of the total CK rise • It starts rising by 3–4 hours, peak is obtained in thirty hours and returns to normal by 3–4 days
Cardiac troponins	• Troponin T (TnT) and troponin I (TnI) • Both of them rise in MI • They are specific for heart
Diagnosis and LDH and SGOT	They rise by 3–4 hour, peak is got by 18–24 hours after onset, return to normal by 5–7 days

Treatment Approach
- Stabilize the shock
- Relieve pain and anxiety by giving analgesics and sedatives
- Nitroglycerine is given IV drip, that releases nitric oxide to do vasodilation
- Blood clots of arteries are dissolved by thrombolytic therapy by giving anticoagulants like heparin or streptokinase enzyme
- Streptokinase is given by a definite protocol of time, site and degree of blockage by plaque
- **Coronary artery intervention:** By coronary catheterization evaluation of coronary artery block is done and treated by angioplasty

Angioplasty

For restoration of blood supply/stopping re-blockage	A stent is placed in the lumen of the artery to clear the block
Stent	Metallic scaffold, coated with slow-releasing drugs to decrease thrombosis
Percutaneous transcoronary angioplasty	The technique of relieving the block through coronary artery
Blood thinning agents	75 mg aspirin increases the flow of blood

Treat dyslipidemia, high blood pressure and DM to decrease atherosclerosis

Follow up to increase vasodilation, decrease thrombosis and control the recurrence and other complications

Coronary Artery Bypass Graft
- This technique is used when stents are not benefitting the patient
- A small piece from a leg vein is taken and joined by surgery to bypass the block and the blood supply is restored

Age	5-year-old boy
Complains	Fever, chills, productive cough, swelling on face in the morning especially
On examination	Pitting edema on lower limbs
	Blood and Urine Report
Protein in urine	++
Urinary proteins	3,000 mg%
Total bilirubin	On higher side
ALT	Normal
AST	Normal
Total proteins	5 g/dL
Serum albumin	2.4 mg%
Blood urea	Normal
Serum creatinine	Normal
Lipid profile	Raised all parameters, low HDL
Diagnosis	Nephrotic syndrome (proteinuria, hypoalbuminemia, hypercholesterolemia)
Reason behind hypoalbuminemia	Loss of negative charges in the basement membrane and changed shape of podocytes result in albumin leakage resulting in excessive proteinuria
Reason behind increased lipid profile	Excess formation of apolipoproteins because of excess protein synthesis as compensatory increased process by the liver due to shortage of albumin in blood leads to increased lipid profile
Chances of any other complication in hypoalbuminemia	Calcium levels can be altered (calcium bound to albumin)
Line of treatment	Antibiotics, steroids, diuretics

Age	8-year-old girl
Complains	Face swelling especially around eyes, difficulty in passing urine
History	Throat infection but recovered
	Investigations
Hb	12.7 g/dL
Total Leukocyte count	9,900/cmm
DLC	P74 L24 E2M2
Urine sugar	–
Urine albumin	++ (210 mg) (normally >30 mg)
RBC's, casts	Present
Blood sugar	Normal
Blood urea	Normal
Serum creatinine	Normal
Serum proteins	Low
Serum albumin	2 g/dL
Total cholesterol	Normal
X-ray abdomen, chest	Normal

Contd...

Contd...

Diagnosis	Acute glomerulonephritis (difficulty in passing urine, hypoproteinemia causing edema, pus cells in urine showing signs of infection, proteinuria and RBC's in urine indicating damage of glomerulus)
Pathology of hypoproteinemia	Infection → Destroyed podocytes of basement membrane of glomerulus → loss of electrostatic charge on sialoproteins → proteins get filtered at the glomerulus
Criterion of proteinuria	Excreting proteins in urine of >150 mg per day and albumin of >30 mg per day

Age	30-year-old female
Complains	Feet swelling, recurrent urinary tract infection (UTI), oliguria
History	Diabetic, on treatment
On examination	Bilateral edema on ankles and feet, BP: 150/98 mm Hg
Investigations	
Hb	12 g/dL
TLC	7,500/cmm
Neutrophils	68%
Lymphocytes	35%
Monocytes	3%
Eosinophils	2%
Urine Report	
pH	5
SG	1.007 (decreased value shows doubtful urine concentration)
Volume	420 mL/day
Glucose	+++ (DM)
Proteins	++ (kidney damage increases filtration)
Red blood cells	12/HPF (glomerular/tubules damage)
WBC	10/HPF (UTI)
Epithelial cells	2-55/HPF
Casts	6/low power field
Blood Report	
Sugar	150 mg%
Creatinine	4 mg%
Urea	110 mg%
Calcium	7.8 mg% [N–9–11 mg%] (less calcitriol synthesis due to renal damage, resulting in less absorption of calcium)
Sodium	159 mEq/L (increased, because of retention of water as the kidneys fail to filter and absorb water, along with loss of dilution and concentration power of the kidneys)
Potassium	5 mEq/L (hyperkalemia, N–3.5-4.5 mEq/L) (excess H+ results in movement of K+ to the ECF from ICF)
Chloride	120 mEq/L
pH	7.20 (N- 7.36–7.44)–metabolic acidosis due to loss of kidney functions like reabsorption of the filtered bicarbonates, formation of new bicarbonates in the kidney tubules, excretion of hydrogen ions as ammonium ions
Bicarbonates	18 mEq/L (N–22–26 mEq/L)—metabolic acidosis
Diagnosis	Renal pathology (oliguria due to less capacity of filtration of the kidneys, pedal edema, increased serum creatinine, urea, hypertension, weakness, nausea indicating acute renal failure)
ARF	Abrupt low GFR over a very short period of time resulting in high presence of excretory products, fluid and electrolyte misbalance, oliguria and pedal edema

Age	55-year-old female
Complains	Nausea, vomiting, lethargy, loss of appetite
History	DM, hypertension, some kidney defect for which she got hospitalized earlier
On examination	High BP, anemia, RR–25/min
Hb	Low
TLC	7,555/cmm
Neutrophils	60
Lymphocytes	30
Monocytes	6
Eosinophils	2
Urine Report	
SG	1.020
Volume	780 mL/day
Glucose	++
Proteins	++
Red blood cells	3/HPF
Pus cells	3/HPF
Blood Report	
Sugar	168 mg%
Creatinine	3 mg%
Urea	70 mg%
Calcium	7.8 mg% (les calcitriol, resulting in less absorption of calcium)
Sodium	135 mEq/L
Potassium	4.8 mEq/L
Diagnosis	DM, hypertension, chronic renal failure (CRF)
Cause of CRF	DM complication of glomerulonephritis, low GFR resulting in low output of urine, leading to waste products accumulation, RFT's are imperfect and proteinuria is present
Reason behind anemia	Formation of erythropoietin in the kidneys is low because of kidney damage
Normal GFR	95–140 mL/min, determined by creatinine clearance
Stages of CKD (chronic kidney disease): 5	1. GFR >90 mL/min along with dysfunctions of kidney 2. GFR: 89-60 mL/min 3. GFR: 59-30 mL/min 4. GFR: 29-15 mL/min 5. GFR: 15 mL/min
Line of treatment	Dialysis, renal transplant, low protein and salts so as to decrease urea formation and water retention, vitamin D and erythropoietin for hypocalcemia and anemia, etc.
Chronic renal failure can lead to:	Metabolic bone disorder due to defective mineralization and vitamin D deficiency and increased osteoblastic action can lead to increased ALP

Age	55-year-old male, moderately obese
Routine Checkup	
History	DM
Report	
Fasting blood sugar	150 mg%
Postprandial blood sugar	190 mg%
Blood urea	35 mg%

Contd...

Contd...

Serum creatinine	1.5 mg%
SGOT	17 IU/L
SGPT	22 IU/L
ALP	155 IU/L
TC	298 mg% (N: <200 mg%)
TG	350 mg%
HDL-C	30 mg% (N: >35 mg%)
Diagnosis	Diabetes and hyperlipidemia (obese, type II DM, blood sugar fasting is >126 mg%, excess cholesterol and triglycerides, no renal and hepatic defect) shows risk for atherosclerosis
LDL-C?	LDL-C = TC–(HDL-C + VLDL-C)
	LDL-C = TC–(HDL-C + TG/5)
	= 298–(30 + 350/5) = ...mg% (N–<120 mg%)
Reason behind hyperlipidemia	Insulin deficiency → decreased glucose breakdown in peripheral tissues → decreased energy production → increased lipolysis to make up for less energy levels (increased glucagon) → increased oxidation of fatty acids → increased formation of acetyl-CoA → increased cholesterol synthesis and increased TG formation
Advice to the patient	Control diabetes by diet modification, regular exercise, reduce weight, stress-free lifestyle, complete follow up of DM, maintain lipid profile in normal range
Recommended diet:	Low calories, approximately 1500 cal/24 hours, low fatty diet, fats must be around 10% of total calories, MUFA:PUFA–1:3, excess fiber diet, protective elements like vitamins and minerals inclusion in the diet

Age	5-year-old boy
History	Father had cardiac arrest and died in early age
Complains	Subcutaneous xanthomas (white eruptions on skin)
	Investigations
Fasting blood glucose	90 mg%
TC	490 mg%
LDL-C	345 mg%
HDL-C	27 mg%
TG	126 mg%
Diagnosis	Familial hypercholesterolemia (type II a hyperlipoproteinemia)
Cause:	Defective LDL receptor (family history, high lipid profile)
Complications:	Atherosclerosis, CAD, MI, cerebrovascular stroke
Other investigations required?	Full checkup of heart, lipid lowering drugs, lifestyle modifications, stop smoking and alcohol use
Lipid lowering drugs:	Cholestyramine (increase conversion of cholesterol to bile acids and bile salts, up regulate receptors of LDL), clofibrate, HMG-CoA reductase inhibitors like statins (decrease formation of cholesterol) and sitosterol to bring down the level of TC below 200 mg% and LDL-C below 100 mg%

Age	55- year-old female
Complains	Nausea, epigastric pain
History	Diabetic ongoing oral antidiabetic drugs, had similar pain after exercise, parents expired after MI in the age of 55–60 years
On examination	Normal vitals
ECG	Mild ischemia

Contd...

Contd...

Enzymes profile

Total CK (N:0-200 IU/L): (Increased on 2 day but were in normal range)

- Day 1 was 130 IU/L
- Day 2 was 105 IU/L (6 AM)
- Day 2 was 156 IU/L (1 PM)
- Day 2 was 128 IU/L (11 PM)
- Day 3 was 104 IU/L (6 AM)

CK-MB (N: 7 IU/L): (Rise was above the normal range)

- Day 1 was 3.7 IU/L
- Day 2 was 3.0 IU/L (6 AM)
- Day 2 was 7.6 IU/L (1 PM)
- Day 2 was 4.2 IU/L (11 PM)
- Day 3 was 2.7 IU/L (6 AM)

Troponin I (N: <1.5 ng/mL):

- Day 1 was not detectable
- Day 2 was 1.3 IU/L (6 AM)
- Day 2 was 3.2 IU/L (1 PM)
- Day 2 was 2.2 IU/L (11 PM)
- Day 3 was not detectable (6 AM)

Diagnosis: Myocardial infarction (because of diabetic neuropathy, typical chest pain was not present, no sweating no radiating pain, but the family history showed indication of angina pectoris, but complications included DM, age of 5, postmenopausal female)

CK-MB as biochemical marker: ECG did not indicated myocardial injury then enzyme profile was done

We see that there was increase in CKMB which is specific for myocardium, it starts increasing by 3–4 hours, peak is obtained within 30 hours, and returns to normal by 3–4 days

Troponin I is very specific to myocardium, unlike CK which can also be correlated with skeletal muscle damage, CK-MB values showed signs of MI, all the more, Typically there was a rise in troponin I within 6-8 hours from the onset of the attack, reached peak by 36 hours, remain increased for longer period, almost 7 days, so it is important tool for patients coming late with the MI attack

Characteristic features of MI

- Coronary artery atherosclerosis
- Lipid deposits by foam cells in the endothelium of coronary artery leading to formation of fatty streaks
- Fatty streaks get coated by fibrous layers to form atherosclerotic plaques which get ruptured
- There is blocking of fine capillaries due to leakage of microthrombi in the blood resulting in MI
- Risk factors include a deranged lipid profile in form of high TC and TGs

Advise to patient after discharge: Low fat and carbohydrate diet, high fiber diet, daily workouts, weight maintenance, keep diabetes and hypertension in control, TC <200 mg%, TG <150 mg%, LDL-C <100 mg%, HDL-C >40 mg%, regular investigations and follow-ups, aspirin of 75 mg/day prevents aggregation of platelets along with formation of thrombus through cyclo-oxygenase enzyme by inhibiting formation of PG's and TX's

OSCE—MI

1. **Scenario: Acute myocardial infarction (AMI)—Elevated cardiac enzymes**
   Case: A 59-year-old male presents with severe chest pain, shortness of breath, and diaphoresis. He has a history of hypertension and smoking. His lab results show:
   Troponin I: 2.6 ng/mL (normal: <0.1 ng/mL)
   CK-MB: 36 U/L (normal: 0–25 U/L)
   Total CK: 455 U/L (normal: 30–170 U/L)
   LDH: 357 U/L (normal: 140–280 U/L)
   Question: What do this interpret?
   Interpretation: The high troponin I is an important marker for myocardial injury. Troponins are very specific for cardiac muscle injuries/remain raised for many days after infarction, that suggests acute myocardial infarction.
   High CK-MB/total CK also suggest myocardial injury, but they are less specific than troponins and increase earlier in AMI, peaking within one day.

LDH elevation, is also suggestive of tissue injury, but it is less specific for MI.
Diagnosis: Acute myocardial infarction, Non-ST elevation myocardial infarction based on the high level of cardiac markers.
Next Steps: Immediate management by aspirin/nitro-glycerine/oxygen/heparin. Reperfusion therapy/ECG for confirmation.

2. **Scenario: Myocardial infarction—Normal ECG, elevated troponin**
   Case: A 65-year-old female presents with chest discomfort/diaphoresis. Her ECG: no significant ST-segment changes.
   Troponin T: 1.6 ng/mL (normal: <0.01 ng/mL)
   CK-MB: 21 U/L (normal: 0-25 U/L)
   Total CK: 121 U/L (normal: 30-170 U/L)
   Question: What is the interpretation?
   Interpretation: ECG is normal, the markedly raised troponin T suggests myocardial injury. Troponin levels are sensitive plus specific for damage of the myocardium, this is suggestive of a non-ST elevation myocardial infarction.
   The CK-MB/total CK levels are mildly raised but are not as specific as troponin to diagnose myocardial infarction.
   Diagnosis: Non-ST elevation myocardial infarction
   Next Steps: Antiplatelet therapy/anticoagulation/angiography/revascularization. Monitor troponin levels that assess the extent of myocardial damage.

3. **Scenario: Myocardial infarction—Late presentation**
   Case: A 57-year-old male presents 48 hours after chest pain. Reports with mild exertional dyspnoea.
   Troponin I: 0.9 ng/mL (normal: <0.1 ng/mL)
   CK-MB: 21 U/L (normal: 0–25 U/L)
   Total CK: 137 U/L (normal: 30–170 U/L)
   LDH: 307 U/L (normal: 140–280 U/L)
   Question: How can the raised biomarkers be interpreted in this case what does this indicate regarding time of the infarction?
   Interpretation: The increased troponin I suggests ongoing myocardial damage, but the level is lower than in the acute phase. Troponin I remains high for up to seven days after myocardial infarction, and the slight decrease indicates the infarction occurred 48 hours before.
   The CK-MB/total CK are slightly high, and their levels tend to fall earlier than troponins and are less sensitive in diagnosing myocardial damage after the acute phase.
   LDH can remain high for a longer duration following myocardial infarction, and this also supports that myocardial injury has been in the recent past.
   Diagnosis: Acute myocardial infarction diagnosed within 48 hours of symptom onset.
   Next Steps: The patient is in the subacute phase, avoid further ischemic events can go for antiplatelet therapy/statins/lifestyle modifications. Cardiac rehabilitation plus more investigations for coronary artery disease can be taken up.

4. **Scenario: Myocardial infarction with renal impairment**
   Case: A 69-year-old diabetic male presents with chest pain/shortness of breath.
   Troponin T: 2.1 ng/mL (normal: <0.01 ng/mL)
   CK-MB: 49 U/L (normal: 0–25 U/L)
   Total CK: 619 U/L (normal: 30–170 U/L)
   BUN: 25 mg/dL (normal: 7–20 mg/dL)
   Creatinine: 1.6 mg/dL (normal: 0.6–1.3 mg/dL)
   Question: How does the renal impairment have impact on the interpretation of the troponin and CK levels?
   Interpretation: The high troponin T suggests myocardial injury. However, the high CK-MB/total CK levels can also be influenced by renal impairment. In patients with chronic kidney disease or renal dysfunction, CK levels remain high because of decreased clearance, and this can further complicate the interpretation of myocardial damage markers.
   BUN/creatinine concentrations suggest little renal impairment, that needs adjustments in the interpretation of some of the biomarkers.
   Diagnosis: Acute myocardial infarction along with associated renal impairment.
   Next Steps: Manage the myocardial infarction with reperfusion therapy/aspirin/statins/adjust drug dosages because of renal dysfunction. Monitor renal parameters.

5. **Scenario: Myocardial infarction—Troponin vs CK-MB**
   Case: A 72-year-old female presents with acute chest pain
   Troponin I: 3.1 ng/mL (normal: <0.1 ng/mL)
   CK-MB: 12 U/L (normal: 0-25 U/L)
   Total CK: 111 U/L (normal: 30-170 U/L)
   Question: What is the importance of high troponin I compared to CK-MB?
   Interpretation: The highly raised troponin I is a highly sensitive plus specific marker for myocardial injury, suggests acute myocardial infarction. Troponins remain high for a longer time than CK-MB, giving more proper reflection of myocardial injury over time.
   The CK-MB/total CK levels are less raised but are not as specific for myocardial injury in comparison to troponins. CK-MB concentration goes on peak earlier (within 1 day) and normalize soon, and troponins may remain high for up to 7 days following MI.

Diagnosis: Acute Myocardial Infarction based on the raised troponin I.
Next Steps: Antiplatelet therapy/anticoagulation/oxygen/PCI/thrombolytics.

OSCE—DYSLIPIDEMIA

1. **Scenario: Primary hypercholesterolemia**
   Case: A 48-year-old female presents with a history of familial hypercholesterolemia.
   Total cholesterol: 288 mg/dL (normal: <200 mg/dL)
   LDL cholesterol: 209 mg/dL (normal: <100 mg/dL)
   HDL cholesterol: 51 mg/dL (normal: >40 mg/dL)
   Triglycerides: 163 mg/dL (normal: <150 mg/dL)
   Question: What does this interpret?
   Interpretation: The raised total cholesterol/LDL cholesterol but normal triglyceride indicates primary hypercholesterolemia. This is because of familial hypercholesterolemia, that is frequently characterized by marked elevation of LDL leading to high risk of atherosclerotic cardiovascular disease.
   Diagnosis: Primary hypercholesterolemia because of familial hypercholesterolemia.
   Next Steps: Lifestyle modifications/Statin therapy/lipid-lowering agents for reducing LDL cholesterol plus decreasing cardiovascular risk.
2. **Scenario: Hypertriglyceridemia**
   Case: A 67-year-old male with poorly controlled diabetes mellitus presents with abdominal discomfort and xanthomas (fatty deposits under the skin). His lab results show:
   Total cholesterol: 323 mg/dL (normal: <200 mg/dL)
   LDL cholesterol: 133 mg/dL (normal: <100 mg/dL)
   HDL cholesterol: 401mg/dL (normal: >40 mg/dL)
   Triglycerides: 605 mg/dL (normal: <150 mg/dL)
   Question: What does the high triglyceride level indicate?
   Interpretation: Hypertriglyceridemia. This is very common in uncontrolled diabetes mellitus and can result in pancreatitis.
   Diagnosis: Hypertriglyceridemia, mostly secondary to uncontrolled diabetes mellitus.
   Next Steps: Blood glucose regulation, lifestyle modifications/omega-3 fatty acids for decreasing triglycerides. Statins for lowering LDL levels.
3. **Scenario: Combined hyperlipidemia**
   Case: A 52-year-old male with a history of hypertension/type 2 diabetes presents with fatigue
   Total cholesterol: 271 mg/dL (normal: <200 mg/dL)
   LDL cholesterol: 151 mg/dL (normal: <100 mg/dL)
   HDL cholesterol: 34 mg/dL (normal: >40 mg/dL)
   Triglycerides: 352 mg/dL (normal: <150 mg/dL)
   Question: What is the diagnosis?
   Interpretation: Pattern is consistent with combined hyperlipidemia, that is observed in cases of metabolic syndrome/type 2 diabetes.
   Diagnosis: Combined hyperlipidemia because of metabolic syndrome/type 2 diabetes.
   Next Steps: Manage diabetes/high blood pressure/diet/exercise/statins for LDL decrease/fibrates for triglycerides/niacin to increase HDL
4. **Scenario: Hypoalphalipoproteinemia (Low HDL)**
   Case: A 48-year-old female with a history of smoking/sedentary lifestyle
   Total cholesterol: 237 mg/dL (normal: <200 mg/dL)
   LDL cholesterol: 132 mg/dL (normal: <100 mg/dL)
   HDL cholesterol: 31 mg/dL (normal: >40 mg/dL)
   Triglycerides: 187 mg/dL (normal: <150 mg/dL)
   Question: What does this interpret?
   Interpretation: Patient is at high risk of atherosclerosis/cardiovascular disease.
   Diagnosis: Hypoalphalipoproteinemia with low good cholesterol.
   Next Steps: Smoking cessation/physical activity/weight management Statins to decrease LDL/fibrates to increase HDL
5. **Scenario: Secondary dyslipidemia (hypothyroidism)**
   Case: A 59-year-old female with a history of hypothyroidism presents with fatigue, weight gain, and elevated cholesterol levels. Her lab results show:
   Total cholesterol: 283 mg/dL (normal: <200 mg/dL)

LDL cholesterol: 194 mg/dL (normal: <100 mg/dL)
HDL cholesterol: 51 mg/dL (normal: >40 mg/dL)
Triglycerides: 182 mg/dL (normal: <150 mg/dL)
TSH: 11.0 μIU/mL (normal: 0.4–4.0 μIU/mL)
Question: How does hypothyroidism affect dyslipidemia?
Interpretation: The patient's high total cholesterol/LDL cholesterol is suggesting dyslipidemia, that is common feature in hypothyroidism. The high TSH shows that the thyroid dysfunction is contributing to the lipid metabolism abnormality. Hypothyroidism results in low LDL receptor activity plus low clearance of LDL from the blood.
Diagnosis: Secondary dyslipidemia because of hypothyroidism.
Next Steps: Thyroid hormone replacement therapy for correcting hypothyroidism/lipid levels should be corrected

6. **Scenario: Familial combined hyperlipidemia**
Case: A 38-year-old male with a family history of early heart disease shows with chest pain after vigorous exertion
Total cholesterol: 283 mg/dL (normal: <200 mg/dL)
LDL cholesterol: 172 mg/dL (normal: <100 mg/dL)
HDL cholesterol: 41 mg/dL (normal: >40 mg/dL)
Triglycerides: 303 mg/dL (normal: <150 mg/dL)
Question: What does this interpret?
Interpretation: Pattern of results is consistent with familial combined hyperlipidemia that is genetic disease which results in high LDL and high triglyceride levels, increasing the risk for CVD.
Diagnosis: Familial combined hyperlipidemia
Next Steps: As the patient has family history of early heart disease, immediate management with statins for LDL levels/fibrates for lowering triglyceride/diet/exercise is recommended.

OSCE—RENAL FAILUERE

1. **Scenario: Acute renal failure (prerenal)**
Case: A 69-year-old male with a history of congestive heart failure presents with decreased urine output and swelling in the lower extremities. His lab results show:
Serum creatinine: 2.6 mg/dL (normal: 0.6–1.2 mg/dL)
Blood urea nitrogen: 47 mg/dL (normal: 7–20 mg/dL)
Urine sodium: 10 mEq/L (normal: 20–40 mEq/L)
Urine osmolality: 510 mOsm/kg (normal: 300–900 mOsm/kg)
Fractional excretion of sodium: <1% (normal: <1%)
Question: What does this interpret?
Interpretation: Pattern suggest prerenal causes, means the renal failure is because of low renal perfusion due to heart failure
Diagnosis: Prerenal acute kidney injury because of congestive heart failure.
Next Steps: Improve cardiac output/fluid balance/diuretics/renal replacement therapy or dialysis

2. **Scenario: Chronic renal failure**
Case: A 58-year-old female with a history of hypertension and type 2 diabetes presents with fatigue, nausea, and increased urination. Her lab results are as follows:
Serum creatinine: 3.3 mg/dL (normal: 0.6–1.2 mg/dL)
Blood urea nitrogen 61 mg/dL (normal: 7–20 mg/dL)
Estimated glomerular filtration rate: 26 mL/min/1.73 m^2 (normal: >90 mL/min/1.73 m^2)
Urine albumin: 207 mg/dL (normal: <30 mg/dL)
Urine protein: 2+ (normal: none)
Question: What does this interpret?
Interpretation: Kidney damage might be related to diabetic nephropathy that is very common reason for CKD in diabetic patients.
Diagnosis: Chronic kidney disease due to diabetic nephropathy.
Next Steps: Manage blood glucose/blood pressure/lifestyle modification/Renal function monitoring

3. **Scenario: Acute renal failure (Intrinsic Renal)**
Case: A 42-year-old male with a history of taking nonsteroidal anti-inflammatory drugs for chronic pain shows with low urine output/swelling/history of recent fever.
Serum creatinine: 4.1 mg/dL (normal: 0.6–1.2 mg/dL)
Blood urea nitrogen: 51 mg/dL (normal: 7–20 mg/dL)
Urine protein: 3+ (normal: none)
Urine sodium: 24 mEq/L (normal: 20–40 mEq/L)

Urine osmolality: 300 mOsm/kg (normal: 300–900 mOsm/kg)
Fractional excretion of sodium: 2% (normal: <1%)
Question: What is the diagnosis?
Interpretation: The pattern is suggestive of intrinsic renal injury because of acute tubular necrosis that might be because of NSAIDs.
Diagnosis: Intrinsic acute kidney injury due to acute tubular necrosis induced by NSAID.
Next Steps: Advise to stop NSAID use/fluid balance/renal replacement therapy/no use of nephrotoxic agents

4. **Scenario: Postrenal failure**
   Case: A 77-year-old male with a history of benign prostatic hyperplasia complains of less urine output/abdominal pain/distended bladder.
   Serum creatinine: 2.1 mg/dL (normal: 0.6–1.2 mg/dL)
   Blood urea nitrogen: 41 mg/dL (normal: 7–20 mg/dL)
   Urine output: <100 mL/day
   Question: What does this suggest?
   Interpretation: Pattern is suggestive of acute kidney injury/postrenal obstruction mostly because of urinary retention/blockage due to prostatic hypertrophy.
   Diagnosis: Postrenal acute kidney injury because of urinary tract obstruction by benign prostatic hyperplasia
   Next Steps: A bladder ultrasound/catheterization procedure for reliving from urinary obstruction. Monitor renal damage

5. **Scenario: Renal Failure with hyperkalemia**
   Case: A 59-year-old male with a history of chronic hypertension and diabetes presents with weakness, nausea, and irregular heartbeats. His lab results show:
   Serum creatinine: 6.7 mg/dL (normal: 0.6–1.2 mg/dL)
   Blood urea nitrogen: 78 mg/dL (normal: 7–20 mg/dL)
   Serum potassium: 6.8 mEq/L (normal: 3.5–5.0 mEq/L)
   Serum calcium: 7.0 mg/dL (normal: 8.5–10.5 mg/dL)
   Question: What does it interpret?
   Interpretation: The raised serum creatinine/BUN/hyperkalemia points to acute kidney injury because of chronic kidney disease. Hyperkalemia is a usual complication of kidney failure because of impaired potassium excretion.
   Diagnosis: Acute kidney injury on the background of chronic kidney disease with hyperkalemia.
   Next Steps: Manage hyperkalemia control fluid/electrolyte balance.

Proteinuria

1. **Scenario: Proteinuria with hypertension**
   Case: A 58-year-old male with a history of hypertension presents with swelling in the legs and ankles. His lab results show:
   Urine protein: 4+ (normal: none)
   Serum albumin: 3.1 g/dL (normal: 3.5–5.0 g/dL)
   Serum creatinine: 1.1 mg/dL (normal: 0.6–1.2 mg/dL)
   Blood pressure: 160/100 mmHg
   Question: What is the interpretation?
   Interpretation: The presence of proteinuria/hypertension indicate that patient might be having hypertensive nephropathy, that might damage glomeruli, resulting in protein leakage in the urine. The serum albumin is mildly low, serum creatinine is normal, so no significant kidney dysfunction is there
   Diagnosis: Proteinuria because of hypertensive nephropathy.
   Next Steps: The patient should be managed with antihypertensive medications, such as ACE inhibitors or angiotensin II receptor blockers (ARBs), which can reduce proteinuria and slow the progression of kidney damage. Monitoring kidney function is important.

2. **Scenario: Proteinuria with diabetes mellitus**
   Case: A 69-year-old male with diabetes presents with generalized edema and frothy urine. His lab results are as follows:
   Urine protein: 2+ (normal: none)
   Serum albumin: 2.4 g/dL (normal: 3.5–5.0 g/dL)
   Serum glucose: 189 mg/dL (normal: 70–110 mg/dL)
   Serum creatinine: 1.4 mg/dL (normal: 0.6–1.2 mg/dL)
   Question: What is the interpretation?
   Interpretation: The results of lab assays suggest proteinuria is mainly due to diabetic nephropathy, that is a common complication of long-term diabetes. The mildly raised serum creatinine indicate that kidney function might decline soon.
   Diagnosis: Proteinuria because of diabetic nephropathy.
   Next Steps: Control blood glucose/reduce proteinuria/protect kidney functions.

3. **Scenario: Isolated Proteinuria in a Young Patient**
   Case: A 25-year-old male presents with incidental findings of proteinuria during a routine check-up. He has no symptoms and no significant medical history. His lab results show:
   Urine protein: 1+ (normal: none)
   Serum albumin: 4.3 g/dL (normal: 3.5–5.0 g/dL)
   Serum creatinine: 0.7 mg/dL (normal: 0.6–1.2 mg/dL)
   Question: What is the reason of proteinuria?
   Interpretation: Proteinuria is commonly seen in younger individuals, especially when urine is collected in a nonsupine position like standing).
   Diagnosis: Benign orthostatic proteinuria/transient proteinuria.
   Next Steps: The patient must be tested/advised for 24-hour urine collection/repeat urine tests after taking rest/in the supine position to confirm the diagnosis. If proteinuria persists the do further investigation like kidney function tests.
4. **Scenario: Proteinuria with acute kidney injury (AKI)**
   Case: A 49-year-old female with a history of systemic lupus erythematosus presents with worsening fatigue, leg swelling, and dark urine. Her lab results show:
   Urine protein: 3+ (normal: none)
   Serum albumin: 2.2 g/dL (normal: 3.5–5.0 g/dL)
   Serum creatinine: 2.1 mg/dL (normal: 0.6–1.2 mg/dL)
   Serum cholesterol: 257 mg/dL (normal: <200 mg/dL)
   Question: What is the diagnosis?
   Interpretation: The presence of massive proteinuria/hypoalbuminemia/acute kidney injury/history of systemic lupus erythematosus indicates lupus nephritis, a usual complication of SLE that results in glomerular damage/protein leakage.
   Diagnosis: Proteinuria by lupus nephritis.
   Next Steps: Corticosteroids/immunosuppressive agents for controlling underlying autoimmune disease. Renal function/urine protein levels should be maintained
5. **Scenario: Nephrotic syndrome with proteinuria**
   Case: A 38-year-old male presents with generalized edema and foamy urine. His lab results are as follows:
   Urine protein: 4+ (normal: none)
   Serum albumin: 2.3 g/dL (normal: 3.5–5.0 g/dL)
   Serum creatinine: 1.0 mg/dL (normal: 0.6–1.2 mg/dL)
   Serum cholesterol: 310 mg/dL (normal: <200 mg/dL)
   Question: What is the interpretation?
   Interpretation: The symptoms and results are characteristic features of nephrotic syndrome. The normal serum creatinine show that kidney function is normal.
   Diagnosis: Nephrotic syndrome that may be due to focal segmental glomerulosclerosis/minimal change disease.
   Next Steps: Treatment by corticosteroids/immunosuppressive agents, depending on the main cause. Diuretics for fluid retention/hyperlipidemia to be managed. A kidney biopsy may be considered.
6. **Scenario: Postrenal proteinuria**
   Case: A 59-year-old male presents with gross hematuria and mild proteinuria. He has a history of benign prostatic hyperplasia (BPH). His lab results show:
   Urine protein: 1+ (normal: none)
   Urine blood: 3+ (normal: none)
   Serum albumin: 4.1 g/dL (normal: 3.5–5.0 g/dL)
   Serum creatinine: 1.1 mg/dL (normal: 0.6–1.2 mg/dL)
   Question: What does presence of hematuria suggest?
   Interpretation: The presence of mild proteinuria/gross hematuria with benign prostatic hyperplasia indicates postrenal proteinuria, that is generally due to urinary tract obstruction/bladder dysfunction. Hematuria can be because of prostatic bleeding/urinary tract infection.
   Diagnosis: Postrenal proteinuria because of benign prostatic hyperplasia.
   Next Steps: A urinary tract ultrasound/CT scan for assessing obstructive reasons

OSCE—NEPHROTIC SYNDROME

1. **Scenario: Nephrotic syndrome with proteinuria**
   Case: A 38-year-old female presents with swelling of her legs and ankles. She has been noticing frothy urine for the past month. Her medical history is unremarkable, but she recently started a high-protein diet. Lab results:

Serum albumin: 2.3 g/dL (normal: 3.5–5.0 g/dL)
Urine protein: 4+ (normal: none)
Serum cholesterol: 295 mg/dL (normal: <200 mg/dL)
Serum creatinine: 1.1 mg/dL (normal: 0.6–1.2 mg/dL)
Question: What do the lab results suggest?
Interpretation: Nephrotic syndrome. The high serum cholesterol is consistent with nephrotic syndrome, that generally leads to lipid metabolism abnormalities, and finally hyperlipidemia.
Diagnosis: Nephrotic syndrome with proteinuria along with hyperlipidemia.
Next Steps: Identify the main cause that can be primary glomerulonephritis/secondary causes like diabetes, lupus etc. Corticosteroids/diuretics can be given for treating edema, proteinuria.

2. **Scenario: Nephrotic syndrome in a diabetic patient**
Case: A 62-year-old male with a history of diabetes mellitus presents with generalized edema and proteinuria. He has had poor blood sugar control in recent months. Lab results:
Serum albumin: 2.8 g/dL (normal: 3.5–5.0 g/dL)
Urine protein: 3+ (normal: none)
Serum glucose: 253 mg/dL (normal: 70–110 mg/dL)
Serum creatinine: 1.4 mg/dL (normal: 0.6–1.2 mg/dL)
Serum cholesterol: 238 mg/dL (normal: <200 mg/dL)
Question: What is the interpretation?
Interpretation: The patient's edema/proteinuria/decreased serum albumin/hyperlipidemia suggests nephrotic syndrome, mainly secondary to diabetic nephropathy. Diabetes can result in glomerular damage plus proteinuria, that is characteristic of nephrotic syndrome.
Diagnosis: Nephrotic syndrome secondary to diabetic nephropathy.
Next Steps: Blood sugar control, reduce proteinuria, use of diuretics for fluid retention. Monitor for progression to chronic kidney disease (CKD).

3. **Scenario: Nephrotic syndrome with hypertension**
Case: A 49-year-old male with a history of hypertension presents with lower extremity edema and weight gain. His blood pressure is elevated at 160/100 mmHg. Lab results:
Serum albumin: 1.9 g/dL (normal: 3.5–5.0 g/dL)
Urine protein: 4+ (normal: none)
Serum creatinine: 1.12 mg/dL (normal: 0.6–1.2 mg/dL)
Serum cholesterol: 328 mg/dL (normal: <200 mg/dL)
Urine sodium: 14 mEq/L (normal: 40–220 mEq/L)
Question: What is the interpretation?
Interpretation: Nephrotic syndrome. The urine sodium indicates that the kidneys are retaining sodium, probably because of renal dysfunction. This patient can suffer from primary glomerular disease, like focal segmental glomerulosclerosis which is complicated by high blood pressure.
Diagnosis: Nephrotic syndrome with hypertension, possibly due to focal segmental glomerulosclerosis.
Next Steps: Manage blood pressure with ACE inhibitors/ARBs, control fluid retention by diuretics/avoid hyperlipidemia. Biopsy for confirmation of underlying cause

4. **Scenario: Nephrotic syndrome in a child**
Case: A 86-year-old boy presents with swelling of his face/legs. His mother mentions that he has had frothy urine for the past few days. Lab results:
Serum albumin: 2.1 g/dL (normal: 3.5–5.0 g/dL)
Urine protein: 4+ (normal: none)
Serum cholesterol: 320 mg/dL (normal: <200 mg/dL)
Serum creatinine: 0.4 mg/dL (normal: 0.3–0.7 mg/dL)
Question: What is the interpretation?
Interpretation: The patient's symptoms are suggestive of nephrotic syndrome. In children, very common reason behind nephrotic syndrome is minimal change disease. The normal serum creatinine show that kidney function is normal.
Diagnosis: Nephrotic syndrome because of minimal change disease.
Next Steps: Corticosteroids/supportive care with diuretics/edema plus monitor for thromboembolic events.

5. **Scenario: Nephrotic Syndrome with Acute Kidney Injury (AKI)**
Case: A 59-year-old female with a history of lupus presents with new-onset swelling, weight gain, and fatigue. Her lab results:
Serum albumin: 2.0 g/dL (normal: 3.5–5.0 g/dL)
Urine protein: 4+ (normal: none)

Serum creatinine: 2.6 mg/dL (normal: 0.6–1.2 mg/dL)
Serum cholesterol: 267 mg/dL (normal: <200 mg/dL)
Urine output: 405 mL/day
Question: What is the interpretation?
Interpretation: Generalized edema/proteinuria/decreased albumin in serum/high serum cholesterol/acute kidney injury indicates nephrotic syndrome with acute kidney injury, probably secondary to lupus nephritis. Lupus nephritis is a common reason of nephrotic syndrome and can result in worsening of kidney function.
Diagnosis: Nephrotic syndrome with acute kidney injury because of lupus nephritis.
Next Steps: Control the main factor by immunosuppressive agents/optimize fluid/electrolyte balance, preventing thromboembolic events. Dialysis may be required

6. **Scenario: Nephrotic Syndrome with Hypercoagulability**
   Case: A 79-year-old male with known nephrotic syndrome presents with deep vein thrombosis (DVT). His lab results:
   Serum albumin: 2.2 g/dL (normal: 3.5–5.0 g/dL)
   Urine protein: 3+ (normal: none)
   Serum cholesterol: 296 mg/dL (normal: <200 mg/dL)
   Serum creatinine: 1.1 mg/dL (normal: 0.6–1.2 mg/dL)
   PT and aPTT: Normal
   D-dimer: High
   Question: What is the cause of the DVT?
   Interpretation: Nephrotic syndrome is linked with hypoalbuminemia/hyperlipidemia/proteinuria. Nephrotic syndrome is a very common reason behind hypercoagulability, resulting in high risk of venous thromboembolism/DVT. The high D-dimer indicates clot production that is consistent with the thromboembolic episodes.
   Diagnosis: Nephrotic syndrome with hypercoagulability resulting in DVT.
   Next Steps: Anticoagulation therapy for DVT treatment/reduce the risk of progressive thromboembolic episodes. Diuretics/corticosteroids for nephrotic syndrome management can be given.

CLINICAL MCQS

Nephrotic Syndrome

1. **A 49-year-old male shows generalized edema, hypoalbuminemia, proteinuria. What is the diagnosis?**
   a. Nephrotic syndrome
   b. Nephrosis
   c. Chronic glomerulonephritis
   d. Chronic kidney disorder
   Answer: a. Nephrotic syndrome
2. **In a patient of nephrotic syndrome, which biochemical observation is present?**
   a. High urine creatinine
   b. High serum cholesterol
   c. Raised blood urea nitrogen
   d. Less hemoglobin
   Answer: b. High serum cholesterol
3. **A 59-year-old patient of nephrotic syndrome has a 24-hour urine protein excretion: 4.6 g. What is the reason?**
   a. Minimal change disease
   b. Chronic pyelonephritis
   c. Acute kidney disease
   d. UTI
   Answer: a. Minimal change disease
4. **What is the reason of nephrotic syndrome in adults?**
   a. Diabetes mellitus
   b. Diabetes insipidus
   c. Focal segmental glomerulosclerosis
   d. Glomerulonephritis
   Answer: c. Focal segmental glomerulosclerosis

Proteinuria

5. A patient presents 2+ proteinuria after dipstick assay. What is the step to confirm diagnosis?
a. Kidney biopsy
b. Urine protein/creatinine ratio
c. 24-hour urine protein collection
d. Blood urea nitrogen

Answer: c. 24-hour urine protein collection

6. In a case of nephrotic syndrome, what is the range of 24-hour urine protein excretion?
a. <1 g/day
b. 1–2 g/day
c. 3–4 g/day
d. >5 g/day

Answer: d. >5 g/day

7. A 69-year-old male having diabetes shows persistent proteinuria. What investigation can confirm the degree of renal involvement?
a. Urine creatinine
b. Urine microalbumin
c. Serum sodium
d. 24-hour urine creatinine clearance

Answer: b. Urine microalbumin

Renal Failure

8. A 59-year-old patient shows high serum creatinine: 2.5 mg/dL, low glomerular filtration rate. What is diagnosis?
a. Chronic liver disease
b. Chronic kidney disease
c. Glomerulonephritis
d. Urinary tract infection

Answer: b. Chronic kidney disease

9. Which is the sensitive marker to detect early stages of kidney dysfunction?
a. Serum urea
b. Blood urea nitrogen
c. Estimated glomerular filtration rate
d. Urinary creatinine

Answer: c. Estimated glomerular filtration rate

10. A patient of renal failure shows BUN-to-creatinine ratio: 20:1. What is the reason?
a. Acute kidney disease
b. Prerenal kidney disease
c. Postrenal kidney disease
d. Chronic kidney disease

Answer: b. prerenal kidney disease

11. A 48-year-old male having history of high blood pressure, smoking shows serum creatinine: 3.0 mg/dL, high BUN. What is cause?
a. Acute kidney injury
b. Chronic kidney disease
c. Nephritis
d. Nephrotic syndrome

Answer: b. Chronic kidney disease

Dyslipidemia

12. A 49-year-old male with nephrotic syndrome presents with elevated cholesterol and triglycerides. Which of the following biochemical abnormalities is most likely?
a. Hyperalbuminemia
b. Hyperlipidemia

c. Hypernatremia
d. Hypercalcemia

Answer: b. Hyperlipidemia

13. In nephrotic syndrome, the high cholesterol, triglycerides are because of.
a. Increased hepatic lipoprotein synthesis
b. Increased clearance of lipoproteins
c. Decreased fat absorption
d. Proteinuria

Answer: a. Increased hepatic lipoprotein synthesis

14. A 65-year-old patient of dyslipidemia has high LDL, low HDL. Which is a likely cause of this result?
a. Nephrotic syndrome
b. Hypothyroidism
c. Diabetes mellitus
d. Chronic pancreatitis

Answer: a. Nephrotic syndrome

Myocardial Infarction

15. A patient with symptom of chest pain, high cardiac biomarkers. Which is the specific marker for MI?
a. Troponin I
b. Creatine kinase -3
c. Lactate dehydrogenase 1
d. Myoglobin

Answer: a. Troponin I

16. A 58-year-old male presents with suspected MI. Which marker is high during the first 6 hours of an MI?
a. Troponin I
b. CK-MB
c. Alanine aminotransferase
d. Serum amylase

Answer: b. CK-MB

17. In a patient of acute myocardial infarction, which is most probable marker to be high in the first 12 hours?
a. Troponin I
b. CK-MB
c. Serum lipase
d. Serum urea

Answer: b. CK-MB

18. A 60-year-old male shows with symptoms of acute chest pain. Serum troponin I: high. What is the reason behind this elevation?
a. Acute myocardial infarction
b. Chronic pancreatitis
c. Renal disorder
d. Pulmonary infection

Answer: a. Acute myocardial infarction

19. Which is a common finding in the first 24 hours after acute myocardial infarction?
a. High troponin I, CK-MB
b. High C-reactive protein
c. Low serum lipase
d. High serum cholesterol

Answer: a. High troponin I, CK-MB

20. A patient with a family history of myocardial infarction complains of high serum creatine kinase/troponin I. What is the interpretation of these results?
a. Ongoing myocardial injury
b. Renal disorder
c. Stable angina
d. Chronic pancreatitis

Answer: a. Ongoing myocardial injury

VIVA VOCE

Nephrotic Syndrome

Q1. Discuss the diagnostic criteria for nephrotic syndrome.
Significant proteinuria: >3.5 g/day
Hypoalbuminemia: <3.5 g/dL
Edema
Hyperlipidemia and lipiduria (fatty casts, oval fat bodies)

Q2. Discuss common factors causing nephrotic syndrome.
Primary/glomerular disorders: Minimal change disease/FSGS/Membranous nephropathy
Secondary: Diabetes/SLE/amyloidosis/infections (Hep B, HIV)/drugs

Proteinuria

Q3. Classify proteinuria.
Glomerular Proteinuria: Nephrotic syndrome/glomerulonephritis
Tubular Proteinuria: Tubulointerstitial diseases (Fanconi syndrome)
Overflow Proteinuria: Multiple myeloma (Bence-Jones protein)/Hemoglobinuria/Myoglobinuria
Postrenal Proteinuria: UTI/stones

Q4. What is microalbuminuria?
Excretion of Albumin: 30–300 mg/day
Early marker of diabetic nephropathy along with hypertension-related renal disease
Detected by urine albumin-to-creatinine ratio

Renal Failure

Q5. Discuss complications of chronic kidney disease.
Metabolic complications: Acidosis/hyperkalemia/hypocalcemia
Hematologic complications: Anemia (↓EPO)/platelet dysfunction
Cardiovascular complications: Hypertension/uremic pericarditis
Bone disorder: Renal osteodystrophy like osteitis fibrosa cystica/osteomalacia

Dyslipidemia

Q6. What are the major types of dyslipidemia and their causes?
Type I (hyperchylomicronemia): Deficiency of LPL or ApoC-II
Type IIa (familial hypercholesterolemia): Defective LDL receptors → ↑ LDL
Type IIb (combined hyperlipidemia): ↑ LDL & VLDL
Type III (dysbetalipoproteinemia): Defective ApoE
Type IV (hypertriglyceridemia): ↑ VLDL (common in diabetes)

Q7. What are the complications of dyslipidemia?
Atherosclerosis → MI/stroke
Pancreatitis if triglycerides > 1000 mg/dL
Xanthomas/Xanthelasma

Myocardial Infarction

Q8. What are the ECG changes in MI?
STEMI: ST elevation in ≥2 contiguous leads, reciprocal ST depression
NSTEMI: ST depression, T wave inversion, no ST elevation
Pathological Q waves: Suggests old MI

Q9. Discuss cardiac biomarkers of diagnosing MI?
Troponin I/T: Most specific, increases in 4–6 hours, peaks at 24 hours, last for 7–10 days
CK-MB: Increases in 3–6 hours, peaks at 24 hours, returns to normal in 48 hours
Myoglobin: Earliest marker/nonspecific

SPOTTERS

Nephrotic Syndrome

Q1. Urine microscopy showing oval fat bodies

Spotter image: Urine microscopy showing "Maltese cross" appearance under polarized light

Interpret:

Nephrotic syndrome because of lipiduria

Seen in minimal change disease/Membranous nephropathy/FSGS

Confirms massive protein loss and lipid presence

Q2. Electron microscopy of minimal change disease

Spotter Image: EM exhibiting podocyte foot process effacement

Interpret:

Observed in minimal change disease

Most common reason of nephrotic syndrome in children

Steroid-responsive

Proteinuria

Q3. 24-Hour urine protein report showing >3.5 g/day

Spotter Data: Urine protein = 4.2 g/day

Interpret:

Nephrotic range proteinuria (>3.5 g/day)

Requires serum albumin/lipid profile

Q4. Urine dipstick test showing proteinuria

Spotter Image: Urine dipstick test strip showing protein 3+

Clinical Relevance:

Nephrotic syndrome, glomerulonephritis, diabetic nephropathy

Requires confirmation with 24-hour urine protein or ACR

Renal Failure

Q5. Granular "muddy brown" casts in acute tubular necrosis

Spotter Image: Urine microscopy exhibiting granular casts

Interpret:

Acute Tubular Necrosis

Common causes: Ischemia/nephrotoxins

Differentiates intrinsic AKI from prerenal AKI

Q6. Shrunken kidneys after ultrasound

Spotter Image: Bilateral small/echogenic kidneys

Interpret:

Observed for Chronic Kidney Disease

Common causes: Diabetes/Hypertension/Chronic GN

Dyslipidemia

Q7. Achilles tendon xanthoma

Spotter Image: Yellow deposits on Achilles tendon

Interpret:

Familial Hypercholesterolemia (Type IIa Dyslipidemia)

Because of defective LDL receptors

Increased risk of premature atherosclerosis

Q8. Lipemic serum—milky

Spotter Image: Blood sample with milky/turbid plasma

Interpret:

Severe hypertriglyceridemia (>1000 mg/dL)

Risk: acute pancreatitis

Myocardial Infarction

Q9. ECG showing ST elevation in anterior leads
Spotter Image: ST elevation in V1-V6
Identify & Explain:
STEMI (Acute MI involving LAD artery)
Needs urgent reperfusion/PCI/thrombolysis

Q10. Show gross pathology of heart showing transmural infarct
Spotter Image: Cut section of the heart exhibiting pale infarcted area with hemorrhagic border
Interpret:
Myocardial infarction affecting full thickness of the wall
Observed in STEMI

REFLECTION

Describe the pathogenesis and clinical features of nephrotic syndrome, proteinuria, renal failure, dyslipidemia and myocardial infarction. Describe the biochemical basis of the tests performed in these conditions.

33

CHAPTER

Liver Function Test: An Overview

COMPETENCY

BC14.19: Explain the basis and rationale of biochemical tests done in the following conditions: Jaundice and liver diseases.

LEARNING OBJECTIVES

After reading this chapter, the readers should be able to:

- Describe the important functions of liver and explain the common diseases that affect the liver.
- Describe common clinical tests used to assess the functions of the kidney, liver, thyroid, and adrenal glands.
- Understand the principles behind these tests and their interpretation.
- Discuss the clinical significance of abnormal test results.

BLUE PRINT

Liver Function Tests

Objective

By the end of the lecture, students should be able to:

1. Describe common clinical tests used to assess the functions of the kidney, liver, thyroid, and adrenal glands.
2. Understand the principles behind these tests and their interpretation.
3. Discuss the clinical significance of abnormal test results.

Duration: ***60 minutes***

Materials Needed

1. Presentation slides covering common clinical tests for kidney, liver, thyroid, and adrenal function.
2. Handouts summarizing key points and tables listing diagnostic tests.
3. Whiteboard and markers for interactive explanations.
4. Clinical case studies or examples illustrating the interpretation of test results.

Outline

I. **Introduction to clinical tests for organ function** **(10 minutes)**
- Introduction to the importance of clinical tests in assessing organ function.
- Overview of the objectives and structure of the lecture.

II. **Tests for assessing kidney function** **(15 minutes)**
- Description of common renal function tests including serum creatinine, blood urea nitrogen (BUN), and glomerular filtration rate (GFR).
- Explanation of the principles behind each test and their interpretation.

III. **Tests for assessing liver function** **(15 minutes)**
- Discussion of liver function tests such as alanine aminotransferase (ALT), aspartate aminotransferase (AST), alkaline phosphatase (ALP), and bilirubin.
- Explanation of the clinical significance of abnormal liver function test results.

IV. **Tests for assessing thyroid function** **(10 minutes)**
- Presentation of thyroid function tests including thyroid-stimulating hormone (TSH), free thyroxine (FT4), and total triiodothyronine (T3) levels.
- Explanation of the interpretation of thyroid function test results in various thyroid disorders.

V. **Tests for assessing adrenal function** **(10 minutes)**
- Description of tests used to assess adrenal function such as cortisol levels, adrenocorticotropic hormone (ACTH) stimulation test, and aldosterone levels.
- Discussion of the clinical implications of abnormal adrenal function test results.

VI. **Clinical case studies and examples** **(10 minutes)**
- Present clinical case studies or examples illustrating the interpretation of test results for kidney, liver, thyroid, and adrenal function.
- Encourage students to analyze and discuss the cases in small groups.

VII. **Review and summary** **(5 minutes)**
- Review key points covered in the lecture.
- Summarize the common clinical tests for assessing organ function.

VIII. **Conclusion** **(5 minutes)**
- Conclude the lecture by emphasizing the importance of understanding clinical tests for organ function assessment.
- Encourage further study and exploration of the topic.

BLUE PRINT

Explanation of Biochemical Tests in Various Medical Conditions

Objective

By the end of the lecture, students should be able to:
1. Understand the biochemical basis and rationale behind diagnostic tests used in various medical conditions.
2. Explain how specific laboratory parameters are utilized in the diagnosis, monitoring, and management of different diseases.
3. Interpret the results of biochemical tests in the context of specific clinical scenarios.
4. Appreciate the role of biochemical investigations in understanding the pathophysiology of different medical conditions.

Duration: *90 minutes*

Materials Needed

1. Presentation slides illustrating the biochemical tests and their interpretation in different medical conditions.
2. Case studies or clinical vignettes representing each medical condition for interactive discussion.
3. Whiteboard or flipchart for drawing biochemical pathways and explaining concepts.
4. Handouts summarizing the biochemical tests and their significance in each medical condition.

Outline

I. **Introduction to biochemical testing in medicine** **(10 minutes)**
- Overview of the role of biochemical tests in the diagnosis and management of medical conditions.
- Importance of understanding the underlying biochemical mechanisms for interpretation of test results.

II. **Jaundice and liver diseases** **(10 minutes)**
- Description of liver function tests including bilirubin, AST, ALT, alkaline Phosphatase, and gamma-glutamyl transferase (GGT).
- Interpretation of liver function tests in diagnosing hepatobiliary disorders and assessing liver function.

III. **Conclusion and recap** **(5 minutes)**
- Summarize key points covered in the lecture regarding the biochemical tests used in various medical conditions.
- Emphasize the importance of interdisciplinary collaboration between clinicians and laboratory professionals in interpreting test results.

IV. **Question and answer session** **(5 minutes)**
- Encourage students to ask questions and seek clarification on any aspects of the lecture.
- Foster discussion on practical applications of biochemical tests in clinical practice.

Liver is the metabolic factory of our body

Synthetic functions of liver

Proteins	• Albumin • Alpha beta globulins • Clotting proteins • Transport proteins like transferrin • Storage proteins like ferritin
Lipids	• Cholesterol • Fatty acids • Phospholipids
Carbohydrates	• Regulation of blood glucose • Synthesize glucose from fats and proteins
Bile salts	Required for digestion and absorption of fats
Hormones	
Growth factors	
Enzymes	

Detoxification

Ammonia a toxic substance released from catabolism of proteins is detoxified by:	Urea cycle
Drugs and xenobiotics are converted to harmless substances	Xenobiotics metabolism

Excretory function

Excretion of bile acids	Excretion of cholesterol	Excretion of bilirubin

Metabolism of nutrients

Carbohydrates	Fats	Proteins	Heme

Storage function

Glycogen	Vitamins	Minerals

Enzymes activation

Enzymes related to digestion of food	Enzymes related to metabolism of nutrients

Viral hepatitis/hepatic jaundice	**Acute and infectious liver disease**
Causes	Five types of viruses are responsible A, B, C, D, E
	A, C, D, E are RNA viruses except hepatic virus B
Infection transmission route	
A and E	Feco-oral route
B, C and D	Through blood
Clinical manifestation	Hepatic jaundice
Biochemical disorder	Increased serum bilirubin and increased transaminase enzymes
Clinical course/outcomes	
Hepatitis A and E	Mild disorder leads to full recovery
Hepatitis C	Leads to chronic hepatitis
Hepatitis B	Progressing disease leads to hepatic carcinoma
Symptoms common to all	Loss of appetite, nausea, yellow discoloration of sclera, oral cavity and mucosa, fever, dark yellow color urine
Identification of viruses	Immunologically by surface proteins/specific antigens associated with various virus
Treatment of severe cases of hepatitis B and C	With interferon β
Hepatic jaundice	ALT (due to hepatic cells involvement) and AST (associated symptoms like fever) increase significantly (more than 30 IU/L), ALP is moderately increased (more than 13 KAU/dL), and conjugated hyperbilirubinemia occurs, apart from viral hepatitis other causes may be alcoholic liver cirrhosis, hepatic carcinoma and isoniazid which is antitubercular drug but hepatotoxic

Obstructive liver and biliary disorder	Obstruction to the flow of bilirubin and bile			
Biochemical derangements	Accumulation of conjugated bilirubin, bile salts, cholesterol, etc.			
Causes	Gallstones	Atresia in the common bile duct	Cancer of head of pancreas	Cancer of liver
Clinical manifestations	Clay color stools	Dark color urine	Itching due to bile salts	Cholesterol stones, bilirubin stones

Alcoholic liver disease

Cause	Chronic alcohol use
Stages	Fatty liver leading to alcoholic hepatitis and then leading to cirrhosis
Fatty liver	• End product of alcohol metabolism is acetyl-CoA • Acetyl-CoA Increases lipogenesis • Acetyl-CoA inhibits beta oxidation thus increasing fatty acids for excess triacylglycerol synthesis
Clinical manifestation	Enlarged and palpable liver
Biochemical derangement	• Moderate increase in serum bilirubin, AST, ALT and ALP • More increase in gamma glutamyl transpeptidase

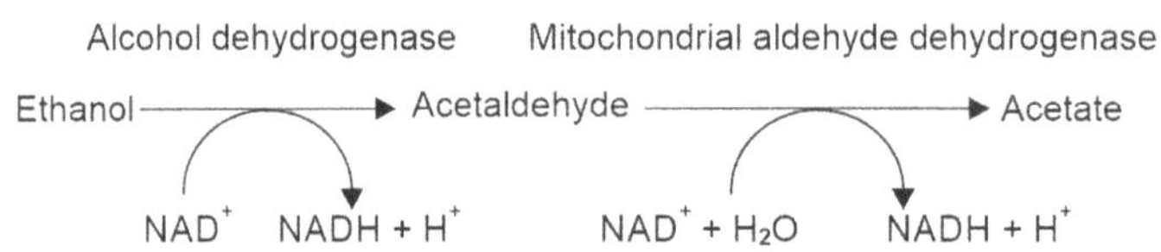

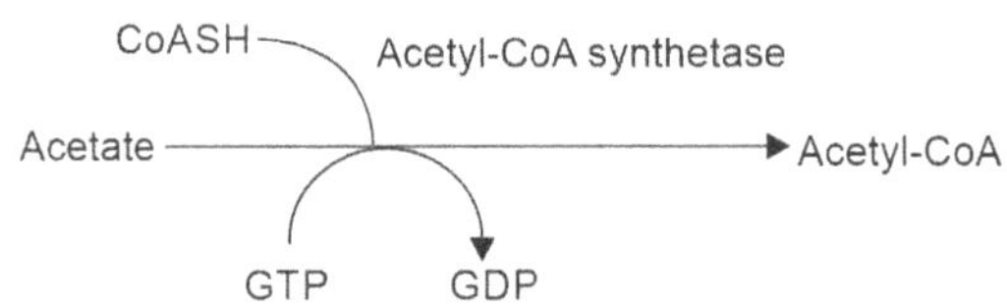

Nonalcoholic fatty liver disorder	Fatty liver without alcohol consumption
Causes	• Obesity • Diabetes mellitus • High blood pressure • Excess serum lipids
Characteristics	Generally without symptoms and abrupt onset

Liver cirrhosis	Irreversible chronic injury of liver parenchyma
	There is replacement of liver parenchyma by fibrous tissue resulting in deranged functions of liver
Causes	• Increased serum bilirubin (jaundice) • Decreased serum albumin (edema, ascites) • Defective formation of clotting factors (clotting diseases) • Ammonia intoxication (encephalopathy) • Alcohol intake • Hepatitis B, C • Chronic biliary obstruction • Hemochromatosis • Gaucher's disease • Wilson's disease • Nonalcoholic fatty liver

Contd....

Contd....

Clinical manifestations	Thin, emaciated appearance, distended abdomen, edema, hematemesis (fibrosis results in obstruction to the blood flow resulting in portal hypertension, which form dilated and thin veins which can rupture anytime or leak producing hemorrhage in the gut), disoriented, semiconscious, comatose, obstructive jaundice because of fibrosis of cells along with unconjugated hyperbilirubinemia as a result of loss of liver function of conjugation
Treatment	Prevent bleeding and clotting disorders, treat hypoalbuminemia, liver transplant

Liver function tests: All the tests done to assess the functions of liver

A. To assess the dysfunctioning of liver	B. To assess the damage of hepatocyte
1. Total and conjugated serum bilirubin	1. Aspartate transaminase (AST/SGOT) (mitochondrial matrix of liver cell)
2. Total protein, serum albumin, A:G ratio	2. Alanine transaminase (ALT/SGPT) (cytosol of liver cell)
3. Prothrombin time	3. Alkaline phosphatase (ALP)
4. Bile pigment in urine	4. Gamma glutamyl transferase (GGT)
5. Bile salt in urine	
6. Urobilinogen in urine	

Other special tests

Bromsulphthalein test	Flocculation/turbidity test	Computerized axial tomography (CAT-scan)	Ultrasonography (USG)	Magnetic resonance imaging (MRI)

To assess the type of cell (hepatocyte) damage

Aspartate transaminase (AST/SGOT)	**Alanine transaminase (ALT/SGPT)**
1. It is in mitochondrial matrix of liver cell	1. It is purely in cytosol of liver cell
2. **When AST increase > ALT increase:** It indicates infiltrative disorder that is plasma membrane damage + mitochondrial membrane damage	2. **When ALT increase > AST increase:** It indicates inflammatory/infective state of plasma membrane damage

To assess the excretory function of liver

Serum total bilirubin

Urine bile salts and bile pigments

To differentiate between hepatitis and obstructive jaundice

Serum conjugated bilirubin	Serum unconjugated bilirubin

To assess the hepatocellular damage

Aspartate transaminase (AST/SGOT)	Alanine transaminase (ALT/SGPT)

To check cholestasis

Alkaline phosphatase (ALP)

To assess the obstructive lesions

Gamma glutamyl transferase (gamma GT)

5′nucleotidase

Leucine amino peptidase

To assess the synthetic functions

Total protein	Serum albumin	Serum globulins	A/G ratio	Serum cholesterol

To assess detoxification function

Blood ammonia

Hippuric acid synthesis

To assess intermediary metabolic functions
Glucose/galactose tolerance test
Plasma amino acids
Prothrombin time

Normal range of LFT parameters	
Total bilirubin	0.2–1.0 mg/dL
Unconjugated/direct bilirubin	0.2–0.7 mg/dL
Conjugated/direct bilirubin	0.1–0.4 mg/dL
AST	5–30 U/L
ALT	5–40 U/L
ALP	30–120 IU/L
GGT	5–30 IU/L
Prothrombin time	11–15 seconds
Total protein	6–8 g/dL
Albumin	3.5–5.5 g/dL

Aspartate transaminase (AST/SGOT)	
Location: As its presence is in high concentration in all these places, increased AST is nonspecific for liver disorder	• Heart muscle (high concentration) • Skeletal muscle (high concentration) • Red blood cells (high concentration) • Kidney (high concentration)
AST is increased in following conditions	• Liver diseases (liver cell membrane damage results in release of AST in blood) – Cirrhosis – Cholestatic jaundice – Malignant infiltration of liver – Acute viral hepatitis – Toxic hepatitis • Myocardial infarction • Skeletal muscle disorders • Hemolysis • Trauma • Surgery • Shock • Hypoxia

Alanine transaminase (ALT/SGPT)	
Location: In comparison to AST increased plasma ALT is more specific to liver disorder	• Mainly in liver (purely cytosolic/high concentration) • Skeletal muscle (less concentration) • Heart (less concentration) • Kidney (less concentration)
ALT is increased in following conditions	• Shock • Hypoxia • Acute viral hepatitis • Toxic hepatitis • Cirrhosis • Congestive heart failure • Cholestatic jaundice • Surgery • Trauma

ALT and AST increase in liver damage but usually rise in ALT is more than AST.
In alcoholic diseases of liver rise in AST is more than rise in ALT which can also be normal sometimes.

Alkaline phosphatase (ALP)	Ectoenzyme containing zinc as metal ion and magnesium, manganese and cobalt act as co-activators of it					
Location	• Mucosa of small intestine • Proximal convoluted tubule (PCT) of kidney • Osteoblast of bone • Liver • Placenta					
Synthesis in liver cell induced by/increased in:	Biliary tract obstruction like stones	Hodgkin's lymphoma	CHD	Hyperthyroidism	Diabetes	Pancreatic cancer
	It is increased in cholestasis along with GGT and 5 nucleotidases					
Isoenzymes	Bone, placenta, intestine, liver					
Separation of isoenzymes	Electrophoresis, liver isoenzyme moves towards anode maximally					

Gamma glutamyl transferase/transpeptidase (γGT)	Microsomal enzyme
Significance	Differentiates liver disease from bone disease if ALP is increased, as its concentration is not elevated in bone disorders
Location	• PCT (quite high concentration) • Liver • Pancreas • Gastrointestinal tract (GIT)
Increased in:	Alcoholic liver disorder

Tests for assessing synthetic functions of liver

Albumin	Albumin is synthesized in liver
Prothrombin time	Except factor V the other clotting factors are made in the liver
Blood ammonia	When this level increases liver will not be able to detoxify it by conversion to urea

Urine investigations

Urinary bilirubin

In obstructive jaundice and hepatic jaundice, blood level of conjugated bilirubin is increased.
Conjugated bilirubin is water soluble so gets excreted in urine, while unconjugated bilirubin is not excreted out as it is insoluble in water

Fouchet's test	To detect the presence of bilirubin in urine
Positive Fouchet's test	Appearance of green color confirms the presence of conjugated bilirubin in urine and thus confirms obstructive jaundice/hepatic jaundice
Ictostix test	Reagent strip method to check for urine bilirubin
Principle	It has diazotized 2,4 dichloraniline theta combines with bilirubin to form azobilirubin
False positive test is given by	Chlorpromazine

Urinary bile salts

Hay's sulfur test	To detect the presence of bile salts in urine and confirming obstructive jaundice
Method	When we sprinkle sulfur powder on the surface of urine in a test tube, the sulfur powder sinks to the bottom if the bile salts are present in the urine
Principle of Hay's sulfur test	Bile salts decreases the surface tension so the sulfur powder sinks at the bottom of the test tube
Interpretation	Presence of bile salts in urine confirms obstructive jaundice

Contd....

Contd....

Urinary urobilinogen	
	Ehrlich's test
Normally:	UBG is formed in GIT from bilirubin and enters the enterohepatic circulation
In obstructive jaundice:	Bile does not reach the duodenum so UBG is not formed so a negative Erlich's test confirms obstructive jaundice
Urobilistix	Reagent strip method for detection of UBG in urine
Principle	It has para dimethyl aminobenzaldehyde that reacts with UBG
False positive test is given by	Para amino salicylic acid, some sulphonamides
Confirmation of hemolytic jaundice	Marked presence of UBG in urine and absence of bilirubin in urine

Serum bilirubin assessment: Total and conjugated		
Van den Bergh reaction	Main principle of serum bilirubin assessment	
Principle of van den Bergh test	Bilirubin + diazotized sulfanilic acid ⟶ Azobilirubin (purple)	
Two types of bilirubin	Direct bilirubin/conjugated bilirubin	Indirect bilirubin/unconjugated bilirubin
Two types of reactions are there in van den Bergh:	Direct reaction given by conjugated bilirubin	Indirect reaction given by unconjugated bilirubin
	To assess conjugated bilirubin	To assess unconjugated bilirubin
	Conjugated bilirubin is water soluble so gives van den Bergh reaction in aqueous medium itself	Unconjugated bilirubin is water insoluble so gives van den Bergh reaction only after addition of methyl alcohol
	It is positive in obstructive jaundice when the level of conjugated bilirubin increases	It is positive in hemolytic jaundice when the level of unconjugated bilirubin increases
For conjugated bilirubin:	The color is read before adding methyl alcohol in the reaction mixture	
For total bilirubin:	The color is read after adding methyl alcohol in the reaction mixture	
Unconjugated bilirubin:	Total bilirubin—conjugated bilirubin	
Biphasic van den Bergh reaction	There is immediate formation of purple color in the test which intensify after adding methyl alcohol	
Clinical Interpretation of biphasic reaction	Hepatic jaundice (serum has increased conjugated bilirubin as well as unconjugated bilirubin)	
Unconjugated hyperbilirubinemia causes	Hemolysis	Genetic disorders like Crigler–Najjar syndrome or Gilbert's syndrome
Conjugated hyperbilirubinemia causes	Liver defects	Biliary tree defects

Blood/urine/stool report in different types of jaundice			
Finding	Hemolytic jaundice/ prehepatic jaundice	Hepatic jaundice	Obstructive jaundice/post hepatic jaundice
Total bilirubin:	Increased	Increased	Increased
Conjugated/direct bilirubin:	↑	↑↑ (Edematous hepatic cell leads to intrahepatic cholestasis resulting in increased conjugated bilirubin)	↑↑↑ (Conjugated bilirubin is not able to excrete in bile so reabsorbs in the circulation)
In obstructive jaundice, it is the direct/conjugated bilirubin which gets effluxed in blood circulation due to obstruction in the passage of direct/conjugated bilirubin towards intestinal lumen			
Unconjugated/indirect bilirubin:	↑↑↑	↑↑ (Impaired hepatic functions results in increased unconjugated bilirubin)	↑

Contd....

Contd....

In hemolytic jaundice, unconjugated/indirect bilirubin is increased in plasma, as there is excess production of bilirubin and the capacity of the liver to conjugate and excrete this excess bilirubin is less (production exceeds conjugation), so the level of unconjugated bilirubin increases			
ALP	–	↑	↑ (Normally the cells lining the bile canaliculi secrete ALP in the bile but in obstruction, there is reabsorption of ALP into the blood)
γGT	–	–	↑
Stool color	Stercobilinogen gives dark color	Normal	Due to absence of stercoilin as obstruction prevents secretion of conjugated bilirubin into GIT so stercobilin is not formed—clay color/sticky due to obstruction preventing bile secretion which prevents emulsification and digestion of fats
Bilirubin	–	+/–	++
Bile salt in urine	–	+/–	++
UBG in urine	++ (because of increased UBG)	+	– (Bilirubin is not secreted into the intestine through the bile so UBG is not formed)

Blood ammonia	It is a byproduct of amino acid catabolism and a potential marker of hepatic encephalopathy
Role of liver	Detoxify ammonia by converting it to urea
Causes of hyperammonemia	Liver disorders and muscle wasting (muscles use ammonia to form glutamate, alanine, etc.)

Serum proteins

Albumin	Synthesized exclusively by liver			
Per day degradation	4%			
Half life	15–20 days			
Acute liver disease	Not a good marker because of its slow turn over			
Chronic liver disease/cirrhosis	Serum albumin <3 g/dL			
Causes of hypoalbuminemia	Nephrotic syndrome	Malnutrition	Chronic infections	Diabetic and hypertensive nephropathy

Globulins

Types	Alpha, beta and gamma
Synthesis	Alpha and beta globulins are made in hepatocytes while gamma globulins are made in plasma cells
Gamma globulins/antibodies	They are increased in chronic liver diseases like chronic hepatitis and cirrhosis as the liver cannot remove the antigens
What can happen in hemodilution/dehydration?	False variations in albumin/globulin levels
To rule out this false variation what can be done?	A:G ratio (it remains unchanged)

Prothrombin time	To measure factors II, V, VII, X
Half-life	• Factor VII has half-life of 6 hours • Fibrinogen has a half-life of 5 days
Role of liver	Except factor VIII, all clotting factors are made in liver
Role of vitamin K	Except factor V, vitamin K is required for synthesis of all factors
Poor liver function is indicated by:	Elevation of PT of >5 seconds in the presence of normal concentration of vitamin K

Contd....

Contd....

Conditions of poor liver function	Hepatitis	Cirrhosis
Liver biopsy	Last test to diagnose a particular liver disorder	
Indicated in:	Chronic liver diseases, where vague clinical findings are seen	
Procedure	Liver biopsy needle is inserted through the right hypochondrium into the liver, and the tissue is examined under the microscope for spotting any kind of lesion	

Age	62 years female alcoholic
Complains	Upper abdominal pain, weight loss
History	Blood vomiting, jaundice
On examination	Distended abdomen, muscle wasting, sclera jaundice, feet edema, ascites
Investigations	
PT	Increased
GGT (normal: 30 IU/L)	80 IU/L
SGOT (IU/L)	Raised
SGPT(IU/L)	Raised
Total proteins	Low
Serum albumin	Low
Urine sugar, proteins	Absent
Diagnosis	Alcoholic cirrhosis (history of consuming alcohol, jaundice, distended abdomen, edema of feet, hematemesis, hypoalbuminemia)
Reason behind edema of feet	Cirrhotic liver leads to less synthesis of albumin causing hypoproteinemia
Reason behind increased PT	Cirrhotic liver leads to less synthesis of clotting factors resulting in delayed clotting
Reason behind hematemesis	• Liver fibrosis leads to obstructed flow of blood resulting in portal hypertension • This results in dilation of veins at the arteriovenous junctions • There is possibility of leakage and rupture of veins resulting in gut hemorrhage resulting in hematemesis and bleeding from rectum in form of black stools of digested blood
Jaundice type in cirrhosis of liver	• Due to fibrosis of hepatic cells and canaliculi, it is mainly obstructive jaundice • In later stages, there is liver failure, it is like prehepatic with mainly unconjugated hyperbilirubinemia due to loss of conjugation function of liver
Reason behind encephalopathy	Cirrhotic liver cannot detoxify ammonia to urea, leading to ammonia intoxication
Other causes of cirrhosis besides alcoholism	NAFLD, hepatitis B and C, chronic biliary obstruction, Gaucher's disease
Complications of cirrhosis	• Hypoalbuminemia results in edema, ascites • Clotting abnormalities like hematemesis • Ammonia toxicity results in encephalopathy • Muscle wasting • Hepatic cancer

OSCE

1. **Scenario: Acute hepatitis—elevated liver enzymes**
   Case: A 39-year-old male presents with jaundice, lethargy and abdominal discomfort.
   Alanine aminotransferase: 204 U/L (normal: 7–56 U/L)
   Aspartate aminotransferase: 185 U/L (normal: 10–40 U/L)
   Alkaline phosphatase: 121 U/L (normal: 30–120 U/L)
   Bilirubin: 3.6 mg/dL (normal: 0.1–1.2 mg/dL)
   Albumin: 3.1 g/dL (normal: 3.4–5.4 g/dL)
   Question: What do this interpret?
   Interpretation: The raised ALT/AST are indicating to hepatocellular injury because ALT is mainly located in the liver and is more specific for liver damage. The moderate raise in ALP might indicate some degree of cholestasis/biliary obstruction, though the significant raise in ALT/AST is more suggestive of hepatitis.

The raised bilirubin shows jaundice, that is commonly seen in liver dysfunction. The low albumin points out that the liver's synthetic function is not appropriate oftenly seen in acute/chronic liver disease.

Diagnosis: Acute hepatitis might be because of viral infection like hepatitis A, B, or C/drug-induced liver injury/alcoholic hepatitis.

Next steps: Investigate more for viral hepatitis markers like anti-HAV, HBsAg, anti-HCV with history such as alcohol consumption/ medications to clarify underlying reason.

2. **Scenario: Chronic liver disease—elevated LFTs with decreased albumin**
   Case: A 59-year-old male with a history of chronic alcohol use presents for routine assays.
   ALT: 86 U/L (normal: 7–56 U/L)
   AST: 150 U/L (normal: 10–40 U/L)
   ALP: 155 U/L (normal: 30–120 U/L)
   Bilirubin: 2.1 mg/dL (normal: 0.1–1.2 mg/dL)
   Albumin: 2.7 g/dL (normal: 3.4–5.4 g/dL)
   Question: What is the interpretation?
   Interpretation: The raised ALT and AST, with AST higher than ALT, indicates chronic liver damage, might be related to alcohol consumption, as AST is higher than ALT in alcoholic liver disease. The high ALP indicate some degree of cholestasis/biliary obstruction, though the key problem appears to be hepatocellular damage.
   Bilirubin is mildly raised that support the presence of jaundice. The low albumin indicates impaired liver synthetic function, that is common in chronic liver disease.
   Diagnosis: Chronic alcoholic liver disease/cirrhosis, with evidence of impaired liver function.
   Next steps: Liver ultrasound/CT/biopsy to assess for cirrhosis, consider investigations for hepatitis B and C. Alcohol cessation and other supportive care.
3. **Scenario: Biliary obstruction—isolated ALP elevation**
   Case: A 69-year-old female with a history of gallstones presents with upper abdominal pain and nausea. Her lab results show:
   ALT: 49 U/L (normal: 7–56 U/L)
   AST: 51 U/L (normal: 10–40 U/L)
   ALP: 288 U/L (normal: 30–120 U/L)
   Bilirubin: 1.4 mg/dL (normal: 0.1–1.2 mg/dL)
   Albumin: 3.9 g/dL (normal: 3.4–5.4 g/dL)
   Question: What is your interpretation?
   Interpretation: The isolated rise of ALP and normal ALT, AST concentrations indicate cholestasis/biliary obstruction that is majorly associated with gallstones or biliary stricture or pancreatic malignancy. ALP is a marker for bile duct/bone tissue, and its rise in the context of normal hepatocellular enzymes (ALT/AST) suggests obstruction/cholestasis and not any primary liver injury.
   The mild rise in bilirubin supports the presence of cholestasis because its metabolism might become improper due to obstruction in bile duct. The normal albumin level points out that the liver's synthetic function is not significantly impaired up till now.
   Diagnosis: Biliary obstruction/cholestasis might be because of gallstones/bile duct obstruction.
   Next steps: Abdominal ultrasound/CT scan for assessing gallstones/biliary duct obstruction, endoscopic retrograde cholangiopancreatography.
4. **Scenario: Cirrhosis—elevated LFTs with ascites**
   Case: A 48-year-old female with a history of hepatitis B shows symptoms of weight gain, abdominal distension, and swelled legs.
   ALT: 42 U/L (normal: 7–56 U/L)
   AST: 95 U/L (normal: 10–40 U/L)
   ALP: 137 U/L (normal: 30–120 U/L)
   Bilirubin: 3.6 mg/dL (normal: 0.1–1.2 mg/dL)
   Albumin: 2.8 g/dL (normal: 3.4–5.4 g/dL)
   Prothrombin time: 19 seconds (normal: 11–13 seconds)
   Question: What do these results suggest?
   Interpretation: The mild increase in ALT/AST and moderate bilirubin rise indicates hepatocellular injury, majorly because of chronic hepatitis B. The mild rise of ALP indicates that obstruction is most probably not at the biliary level but rather because of liver damage.
   The low albumin and prolonged PT suggests impaired liver synthetic function, that is a feature of cirrhosis. Ascites that is accumulated fluid in the abdomen are strongly indicative of liver cirrhosis.
   Diagnosis: Cirrhosis, mostly because of hepatitis B infection (chronic).
   Next steps: Imaging for assessment of portal hypertension/liver architecture. Liver biopsy, manage cirrhosis complications.
5. **Scenario: Acute liver injury—elevated ALT/AST with no jaundice**
   Case: A 38-year-old female presents with right upper quadrant pain following an over-the-counter pain medication overdose.
   ALT: 303 U/L (normal: 7–56 U/L)
   AST: 285 U/L (normal: 10–40 U/L)
   ALP: 71 U/L (normal: 30–120 U/L)
   Bilirubin: 0. 6 mg/dL (normal: 0.1–1.2 mg/dL)

Albumin: 4.5 g/dL (normal: 3.4–5.4 g/dL)
Question: What does this interpret?
Interpretation: The significantly rise in ALT/AST suggest hepatocellular damage, probably because of toxic injury like acetaminophen overdose. The normal bilirubin plus normal albumin concentration indicates that liver's synthetic functions are proper.
Diagnosis: Acute liver injury because of drug-induced hepatotoxicity/likely acetaminophen toxicity.
Next steps: Urgent treat with N-acetylcysteine if acetaminophen toxicity is sure and monitor sliver functions for signs of acute liver failure. Frequently LFTs to be done.

CLINICAL MCQS

1. **A 49-year-old male complains of symptoms of jaundice/dark urine/pale stools. High total bilirubin, high conjugated bilirubin. Which is the cause?**
   a. Hepatitis C
   b. Gallstone obstruction
   c. Alcoholic liver disorder
   d. Anemia

   Answer: b. Gallstone obstruction
2. **A patient with acute viral hepatitis presents with high serum alanine aminotransferase, aspartate aminotransferase. Which findings you expect?**
   a. AST > ALT
   b. ALT > AST
   c. Normal AST/ALT
   d. Raised ALP but normal AST/ALT

   Answer: b. ALT > AST
3. **A 59-year-old female with a history of alcohol consumption has high AST, ALT, and gamma-glutamyl transferase. What is the diagnosis?**
   a. Hepatitis C
   b. Acute alcoholic hepatitis
   c. NAFLD
   d. Hepatitis B

   Answer: b. Acute alcoholic hepatitis
4. **Which is a sensitive marker to detect hepatocyte injury in patients of hepatitis?**
   a. Alkaline phosphatase
   b. Aspartate aminotransferase
   c. Alanine aminotransferase
   d. Bilirubin

   Answer: c. Alanine aminotransferase
5. **A 69-year-old male shows high liver enzymes serum alkaline phosphatase. Which is the cause of this pattern?**
   a. Hepatitis A
   b. Cirrhosis
   c. Cholestasis
   d. Hemolytic anemia

   Answer: c. Cholestasis
6. **A patient with chronic liver disease exhibits ALT: 50 IU/L, AST: 150 IU/L. What does this indicate?**
   a. Chronic liver injury
   b. Chronic liver injury with possible cirrhosis
   c. Hepatitis B
   d. Fatty liver

   Answer: b. Chronic liver injury with possible cirrhosis
7. **A patient with high AST, ALTALP levels is likely to have?**
   a. Toxic hepatitis
   b. Cholestatic liver disease
   c. Hemolytic anemia
   d. Chronic pancreatitis

   Answer: b. Cholestatic liver disease

8. A 48-year-old male with a history of nonalcoholic fatty liver disease presents with moderately high AST, ALT. Which tests would help evaluate the degree of hepatocyte damage?
a. Serum albumin
b. Prothrombin time
c. Serum bilirubin
d. Hepatitis B surface antigen

Answer: b. Prothrombin time

9. A patient with a history of liver cirrhosis shows high total bilirubin. Which is the cause?
a. Hepatic congestion
b. Impaired conjugation of bilirubin
c. Extreme red blood cell hydrolysis
d. Kidney failure

Answer: b. Impaired conjugation of bilirubin

10. Which is most increased in cases of cholestasis/obstructive jaundice?
a. ALT
b. AST, ALT
c. Conjugated bilirubin
d. Alkaline phosphatase

Answer: d. Alkaline phosphatase

VIVA VOCE

Q1. Explain main components of liver function tests.
1. *Hepatocellular injury markers*:
ALT/SGPT → Very specific for liver
AST/SGOT → Also located in muscle, heart
AST/ALT >2:1 indicates alcoholic liver disease
2. *Cholestasis markers*:
Alkaline phosphatase → Biliary obstruction/bone disease
Gamma-glutamyl transferase → Confirms liver source of ALP
3. *Synthetic function tests*:
Albumin → Less in chronic liver disease
Prothrombin time (PT/INR) → Prolonged in liver failure
4. *Excretory function*: Total & direct bilirubin → elevated in jaundice

Q2. What is the importance of albumin and prothrombin time in liver disorders?
Albumin → Low in chronic liver disease (cirrhosis) but normal in acute conditions
Prothrombin time (PT/INR) → Prolonged in acute liver failure (indicative of poor prognosis)
Reason? Liver makes albumin/clotting factors, therefore their deficiency shows synthetic failure

Q3. Differentiate unconjugated and conjugated hyperbilirubinemia.
Unconjugated/indirect bilirubin ↑
Reasons: Hemolysis/Gilbert's syndrome/Crigler–Najjar syndrome
Urine bilirubin negative due to unconjugated bilirubin being not water-soluble
Conjugated (direct) bilirubin ↑
Reasons: Hepatitis/biliary obstruction/Dubin–Johnson/Rotor syndrome
Urine bilirubin +

Q4. What is the importance of GGT in liver function tests?
GGT gets raised in:
Alcoholic liver disease—very specific
Biliary obstruction also with ALP
Drug-induced liver injury
Why is it significant?
Differentiates liver vs. bone ALP when ALP↑ but GGT is normal → Bone disease

SPOTTERS

Q1. AST/ALT ratio in alcoholic liver disease
Spotter data: Lab report: AST = 202, ALT = 81 (AST/ALT >2:1)
Interpret:
AST/ALT >2:1 indicates alcoholic liver disease
Reason: Alcohol damages mitochondria so AST is released more
Other findings: ↑ GGT, normal, mild raised bilirubin

Q2. Conjugated vs. Unconjugated hyperbilirubinemia
Spotter data: Total bilirubin = 5.1 mg/dL, Direct bilirubin = 4.1 mg/dL
Interpret:
Conjugated bilirubin predominant (direct >50%) → Obstructive or hepatocellular disease as in hepatitis/biliary obstruction
If indirect bilirubin high (>80%) → Hemolysis/Gilbert's syndrome

Q3. Isolated ALP elevation with normal GGT
Spotter data: ALP = 401 IU/L, GGT = Normal range
Clinical significance:
If ALP ↑ but GGT normal → Bone disease as in Paget's disease/osteomalacia
If both ALP & GGT ↑ → Cholestasis as in biliary obstruction

Q4. Prolonged prothrombin time (PT/INR) in liver disorder
Spotter data: PT = 19 sec (normal: 10–14 sec), INR = 2.5
Interpret:
Prolonged PT/INR = Liver synthetic failure as in acute liver failure or cirrhosis
Differentiate from vitamin K deficiency: If PT improves with vitamin K → Malabsorption as in cholestasis

Q5. Liver biopsy in Dubin–Johnson syndrome
Spotter image: Liver biopsy showing dark brown/black pigment in hepatocytes
Clinical significance:
Dubin–Johnson syndrome: Defect in bilirubin excretion/conjugated hyperbilirubinemia
Key result: Dark liver because of a melanin-like pigment in lysosomes
Rotor syndrome: Same but no pigmentation seen in liver

REFLECTION

Describe the important functions of the liver and explain the common diseases that affect the liver.

34

CHAPTER

Kidney Function Test: An Overview

COMPETENCY

BC14.19: Explain the basis and rationale of biochemical tests done in renal failure.

LEARNING OBJECTIVES

After reading this chapter, the readers should be able to:
- Describe the pathophysiology of kidney failure along with some clinical features.
- Learn the biochemical base of various tests that is performed in renal failure.

BLUE PRINT

Kidney Function Tests

Objective

By the end of this session, you should be able to:
1. Understand significance of kidney function tests
2. Understand different types of KFTs/clinical significance.
3. Interpret abnormal values in association of renal pathology.

Outline

I. **Introduction** **(10 minutes)**
- Discuss the role of kidneys in: Excretion, acid-base balance, fluid and electrolyte balance, endocrine functions, importance of assessing kidney function in diseases.

II. **Components of kidney function tests** **(30 minutes)**

A. **Serum markers** **(15 minutes)**

1. Serum creatinine
   Normal: 0.6–1.2 mg/dL
   Increased: renal dysfunction, dehydration, muscle breakdown
   Limitations: affected by muscle mass
2. Blood urea nitrogen
   Normal: 6–20 mg/dL
   Increased: renal dysfunction/high protein intake/GI bleeding
   Decreased: liver disease/ malnutrition
   BUN/Creatinine ratio: Differentiates prerenal (>20:1)/intrinsic renal (<10:1)/postrenal (10–20:1) failure
3. Cystatin C
   Early marker of kidney dysfunction, independent of muscle mass

B. **Urine tests** **(15 minutes)**

4. Urine albumin-to-creatinine Ratio (ACR)
   Used for early detection of diabetic nephropathy
   Normal: <30 mg/g
   Microalbuminuria: 30–300 mg/g
   Macroalbuminuria: >300 mg/g

5. Urine dipstick/microscopy
   Proteinuria → Indicates glomerular disease
   Hematuria → Indicates glomerular vs. postglomerular pathology
   Casts
   RBC casts → Glomerulonephritis
   WBC casts → Pyelonephritis/interstitial nephritis
   Granular casts → Acute tubular necrosis

III. **Advanced kidney function Tests** **(10 minutes)**

6. Glomerular filtration rate estimation
   eGFR (/CKD-EPI, MDRD equations
   Inulin clearance/gold standard but not practical
   Creatinine clearance/overestimates GFR
7. Fractional excretion of sodium
   Used in AKI differentiation
   <1% = Prerenal AKI
   >2% = Intrinsic renal AKI (ATN)

IV. **Clinical application and interpretation** **(15 minutes)**

- **Case-based discussion:** Provide cases with abnormal KFT values and discuss the differential diagnosis.
- **Example case:** A 60-year-old diabetic patient with eGFR of 50 ml/min and ACR 120 mg/g → Early CKD

V. **Summary and quick mnemonics** **(5 minutes)**

- Assessment **(10 minutes)**
- MCQs/short answer questions based on clinical scenarios.

Functions of kidney	Forming urine which is a waste product: 1. Filtration of 180 liters of plasma in 24 hours at the glomerulus 2. Glomerular filtrate has sugar, urea, creatinine, electrolytes 3. Finally, the tubules process the glomerular filtrate reabsorption of some substances, such as urea and secretion of some substances into the filtrate) where important compounds are retained and waste products are excreted, thus maintaining water, electrolyte, and acid base balance	Forming hormones, such as erythropoietin by interstitial cells, renin by Juxtaglomerular apparatus and calcitriol by proximal convoluted tubule	
What is the need for doing KFT	To find out the damage done in the renal system in many clinical situations	To find the progress of damage done in the renal system	To set the dose of potentially toxic drugs

Kidney function tests (KFT)

They assess the different functions of kidney

Types

Glomerular function tests	Glomerular filtration capacity testing			Glomerular filtration barrier integrity testing		
	Clearance test	Plasma urea	Plasma creatinine	Proteinuria	Urine protein electrophoresis	Hematuria
Tubular function tests	Reabsorption test		Concentration test/Na+ excretion test		Renal tubular acidosis test	

Glomerular filtration capacity testing

Clearance test: Measure of glomerular filtration rate, and depends on the renal metabolism of the substance

Substance that is only filtered	Clearance is equal to GFR	Inulin, cystatin (low MW protein)
Substance that is filtered plus reabsorbed	Clearance is less than GFR	Urea
Substance that is filtered plus secreted	Clearance is more than GFR	Creatinine

Contd...

Contd...

Relation between GFR and plasma creatinine	Creatinine is a good indicator of GFR and more sensitive than urea, it gives a fair estimate of GFR at low plasma creatinine levels
Significant increase in plasma creatinine	50% less GFR

Glomerular Filtration Barrier Integrity Testing

Glomerular damage/glomerular injury leads to decreased GFR

Proteinuria	Urine protein electrophoresis		Hematuria
Excretion of total proteins in one day is more than 150 mg	Less glomerular damage (selective proteinuria)	Severe glomerular damage	Red blood cells are otherwise not allowed by a perfect intact glomerulus, but due to severe injury of glomerulus, RBC's start leaking
Excretion of albumin in one day is more than 30 mg	Low MW proteins, such as albumin, alpha-1 antitrypsin, transferrin appear in urine	Albumins, immunoglobulins	
Microalbuminuria that is between 30–300 mg/day shows earliest evidence of kidney damage as in high blood pressure and diabetes mellitus			

Tubular Functions

Reabsorption test: Good indicators of this test are the following which are reabsorbed in proximal convoluted tubule	Glucose (glycosuria can also be in normal blood glucose level)
	Phosphorus (low blood level indicate tubular damage)
	Uric acid (low blood level indicate tubular damage)
	Bicarbonates (low blood level indicate tubular damage)
	Potassium (low blood level indicate tubular damage)
	Beta 2 microglobulin (detected by electrophoresis)

Renal Concentration Ability/H_2O Deprivation Test

Normal osmolality of a random urine sample	850–900 mOsmol/kg	
Water deprivation test	Restriction of fluid intake for 18 hours, osmolality measured in first morning sample of urine	
Low ADH activity	**Less response to ADH**	**Normal**
Disorders of hypothalamus or pituitary gland: Osmolality is below 300 mOsmol/kg	Nephrogenic diabetes insipidus osmolality is below 300 m osmol/kg	osmolality exceeds 850 mOsmol/kg
Interpretation	After 12–18 hours of fluid restriction if the urine osmolality is more than 600 mOsm/kg, it means that renal concentration ability is normal	

Assessment of Renal Concentration Ability

Concentration of urine can be measured by: • Urinary osmolality • Specific gravity	 • Less common but more accurate • More common but less accurate
Normal urinary osmolality depends on the state of hydration	Normal range is 50–1400 mOsm/kg
Normal specific gravity of urine measured by urinometer	1.010

Assessment of Renal Dilution Capacity

Method	After 12 hour night fast, patient is given 1 liter of water to drink in half hour, and then 4 urine samples are collected in 4 hours
Interpretation	Specific gravity of 1.003 or below in any of these urine samples denotes that tubules are properly functioning

Contd...

Contd...

Sodium Excretion Test	
To assess	Renal tubular capacity to conserve/excrete Na as per the body need
Method	• For a week, the patient is given 5 g of salt per day (100 mmols) • Test his urinary excretion of sodium in next 3 days • It should ideally be around 85 mmols per day or 3.3 g per day
Interpretation	• About 85% of sodium is excreted in urine, and remaining is excreted by skin/feces • Then the patient is given salt free diet (10 mmol/0.4 g salt) for some days, and again measure the urinary excretion of sodium • It should be decreased to around 10 mmol per day
Clinical interpretation	Kidneys cannot conserve sodium in CRF (chronic renal failure), uncontrolled diabetes mellitus and Addison's disease

Ammonium Chloride Test		
To assess	H^+ secretion capacity of the kidney tubule	
Requirement of the test	If the urinary pH is more than 5.5	
Method	Ammonium chloride is given to the patient according to the body weight (100 mg per kg body weight) Eight samples for 8 hours are collected and pH measured in urine	
Interpretation	Normal	Renal tubular acidosis
	At least one of the samples should have a pH of 5.5 or less	pH does not fall below 6.5 in any of the sample

Blood Urea Assessment	
Introduction	Main nitrogenous waste of protein catabolism
Composition	About 75% non-protein nitrogen that is excreted out
Route of excretion	About 90% by kidneys, and 10% from gastrointestinal tract and skin
Characteristics	Freely filtered by glomeruli, so whenever filtration is affected due to any disorder of glomeruli, there is accumulation of urea in plasma and we can measure the plasma urea level which gives a fair idea of renal functions
Methods	
1. **DAM-TSC/ Fearon method:** (Chemical method)	Urea + diacetyl monoxime (DAM) + Fe^{+++} → pink-colored complex measured at 540 nm TSC is thiosemicarbazide, used to intensify the color Initially, diazine is yellow which is intensified to pink by TSC
2. **Berthelot's method:** (Enzymatic method)	$\text{Urea} + 2H_2O \xrightarrow{\text{Urease}} 2NH_4^+ + CO_3^{--}$ $NH_4^+ + \text{2-oxoglutarate} \xrightarrow[\text{NADH} \rightarrow \text{NAD}^+]{\text{Glutamate dehydrogenase}} \text{Glutamate} + H_2O$ Rate of disappearance of NADH is measured at 340 nm We can quantify the released NH_4 + by: • Color change associated with pH indicator • Glutamine synthetase • Pyruvate kinase • Pyruvate oxidase

Serum Urea vs BUN

- 60 g of urea has 28 g of nitrogen
- Conversion factor for changing value of urea to BUN is: 0.46

To change BUN to blood urea the conversion factor is 2.14

Assessment of Serum Creatinine

Methods: Kinetic Jaffe method— non- specific, interference by acetone, acetoacetate, glucose, vitamin C, pyruvate

Creatinine + picric acid $\xrightarrow{\text{Alkaline medium}}$ red orange-colored alkaline picrate that is read at 490 nm

Coupled enzymatic method

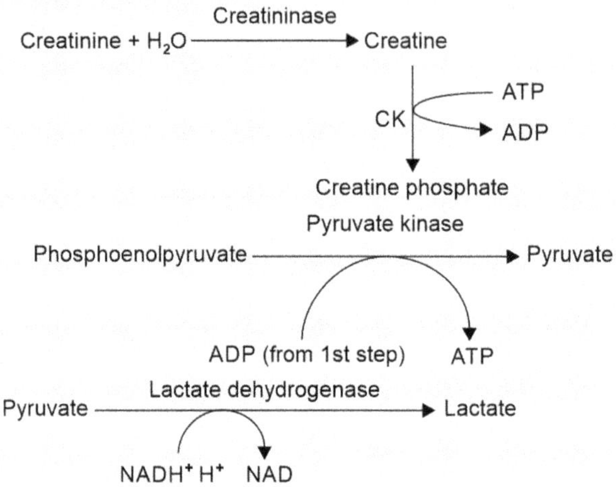

Assessment of Uric Acid

Phosphotungstic acid/Caraway method	Uric acid + Phosphotungstic acid $\xrightarrow{\text{Alkaline medium}}$ tungsten blue of which the absorbance is measured at 650 nm
Uricase/enzymatic method	Uric acid $\xrightarrow{\text{Uricase}}$ Allantoin + H_2O_2 H_2O_2 $\xrightarrow{\text{Peroxidase}}$ H_2O + [O] [O] + chromogen ⟶ pink-colored complex

Clearance	Plasma volume which is completely cleaned off an substance by the kidneys in unit time			
Endogenous substances used for clearance study	Creatinine	Urea (clearance is less than GFR as 40–60% filtered urea is reabsorbed)		
Exogenous substances used for clearance study	Inulin	Iohexol	51 Cr-EDTA	99m Tc-diethylenetriamine pentaacetic acid
To assess renal blood flow	Para-aminohippuric acid (totally filtered by glomeruli and secreted by tubules so clearance value is more than GFR)			

Creatinine Clearance

Introduction	• Creatinine–endogenous excretory substance formed from creatine at a constant rate • It is freely filtered from the glomeruli and minimum reabsorption takes place in proximal convoluted tubule, very useful to assess GFR
Formula	Creatinine clearance = UV/P mL/minute U = creatinine concentration in urine (mg%) V = volume of urine excreted in one minute (mL) P = plasma concentration of creatinine (mg%)

Calculation

24 hour urine is taken and urine volume per minute is calculated	Urine volume per minute = total volume of urine in 24 hours (mL)/24 × 60

Contd...

Contd...

Correction Factor		
Both creatine and creatinine depends on body mass, so there is a need of a correction factor	The correction factor is 1.73/A Where A is body surface area of the patient Thus the final formula becomes: Creatinine clearance = UV/P × 1.73/A	
Normal creatinine clearance	**Males:** 100–125 mL/minute	**Females:** 90–115 mL/minute
After taking correction factor for body surface area	Creatinine clearance in males and females come to be 100 mL/minute	
Importance of creatinine clearance	• Estimate GFR • Assess the glomerular filtration ability	
Urea Clearance		
Introduction	• It is not taken into consideration for study of clearance due to following reasons: • Urea clearance is less than GFR (60% of filtered urea is reabsorbed by PCT) • Urea in blood as well as its excretion by the kidneys (clearance) depends/varies with content of proteins taken in diet so accurate assessment of glomerular function is not possible	
Types of urea clearance	Maximum urea clearance When the rate of output of urine is more than 2 mL per minute	Standard urea clearance When the rate of output of urine is less than 2 mL per minute
Formulas	UV/P	U V/P
Normal values	75 mL/minute	54 mL/minute

OSCE

1. **Scenario: Acute kidney injury (AKI)—elevated serum creatinine and BUN**
   Case: A 69-year-old male presents with oliguria (reduced urine output), fatigue, and swelling in the legs. His lab results show:
   Serum creatinine: 3.6 mg/dL (normal: 0.7–1.3 mg/dL)
   Blood urea nitrogen: 47 mg/dL (normal: 7–20 mg/dL)
   Urine output: 251 mL in the last 24 hours
   Question: How do you interpret this?
   Interpretation: The raised serum creatinine/BUN suggest acute kidney injury, as creatinine and BUN are important markers of kidney filtration. High serum creatinine shows impaired glomerular filtration rate.
   Oliguria supports the diagnosis of AKI. The high BUN is consistent with azotemia.
   Diagnosis: AKI, because of prerenal, intrinsic, or postrenal reasons.
   Next Steps: Urine analysis/ultrasound for obstructive reasons/evaluation of hydration status. Dialysis.
2. **Scenario: Chronic kidney disease (CKD)—gradual increase in creatinine**
   Case: A 59-year-old female with a history of hypertension/diabetes:
   Serum creatinine: 2.1 mg/dL (normal: 0.7–1.3 mg/dL)
   Blood urea nitrogen: 29 mg/dL (normal: 7–20 mg/dL)
   Urine albumin-to-creatinine ratio: 355 mg/g (normal: <30 mg/g)
   Estimated GFR: 46 mL/min/1.73 m^2 (normal: >90 mL/min/1.73 m^2)
   Question: What do these lab results indicate?
   Interpretation: The raised serum creatinine/BUN/reduced eGFR suggest chronic kidney disease. The low GFR is suggests impaired renal functions and point to stage 3 CKD that is GFR between 30-59 mL/min/1.73 m^2.
   The high urine ACR point towards proteinuria, that is a sign of glomerular damage and is quite common in diabetic nephropathy as well as hypertensive nephropathy.
   Diagnosis: CKD by diabetic nephropathy/hypertensive nephropathy.
   Next Steps: Monitor serum creatinine, eGFR and urine protein concentration. Control blood glucose/blood pressure, prevent proteinuria.

3. **Scenario: Postrenal acute kidney injury—elevated creatinine and BUN**
   Case: A 77-year-old male presents with difficulty in urination/lower abdomen pain, history of prostate enlargement.
   Serum creatinine: 5.0 mg/dL (normal: 0.7–1.3 mg/dL)
   Blood urea nitrogen: 56 mg/dL (normal: 7–20 mg/dL)
   Urine output: 51 mL in 24 hours
   Urine sodium: 11 mEq/L (normal: 20–40 mEq/L)
   Question: How do you interpret this case?
   Interpretation: The raised serum creatinine/BUN suggest acute kidney injury (postrenal type). Postrenal AKI happens because of some blockage in the urinary tract, leading to low urine output that is oliguria and high waste products such as creatinine/BUN in the blood.
   The low urine sodium indicates prerenal reasons of AKI.
   Diagnosis: Postrenal AKI, because of urinary tract obstruction from benign prostatic hyperplasia/bladder outlet obstruction.
   Next Steps: Abdominal ultrasound/CT scan for assessing hydronephrosis/urinary tract obstruction. Treatment: Relieve the obstruction by catheterization and surgery and restore normal renal function.
4. **Scenario: Dehydration—prerenal acute kidney injury**
   Case: A 48-year-old male presents with dizziness, dehydration, low urine output after a day of extreme exercise in very hot conditions.
   Serum creatinine: 1.9 mg/dL (normal: 0.7–1.3 mg/dL)
   Blood urea nitrogen: 32 mg/dL (normal: 7–20 mg/dL)
   Urine output: 99 mL in the last 24 hours
   Urine sodium: 4 mEq/L (normal: 20–40 mEq/L)
   Question: What do you interpret?
   Interpretation: The raised serum creatinine/BUN indicate towards acute kidney injury. The decreased urine sodium is suggestive of prerenal AKI, that is typical in dehydration condition, where the kidneys have to conserve sodium for to maintaining fluid balance.
   The low urine output (100 mL) also suggests oliguria, which is commonly seen in prerenal causes of AKI due to reduced renal perfusion.
   Diagnosis: Prerenal AKI secondary to dehydration because of loss of fluids during exercise in hot conditions.
   Next Steps: Rehydration with IV fluids/monitor renal functions/repeat creatinine/BUN levels
5. **Scenario: Diabetic nephropathy—proteinuria and elevated serum creatinine**
   Case: A 59-year-old patient male having history of diabetes presents with:
   Serum creatinine: 1.6 mg/dL (normal: 0.7–1.3 mg/dL)
   Blood urea nitrogen: 26 mg/dL (normal: 7–20 mg/dL)
   Urine albumin-to-creatinine ratio: 255 mg/g (normal: <30 mg/g)
   Estimated GFR: 49 mL/min/1.73 m^2 (normal: >90 mL/min/1.73 m^2)
   Question: What is the interpretation?
   Interpretation: The raised serum creatinine/BUN but decreased eGFR suggest CKD, mostly because of diabetic nephropathy. The albumin-to-creatinine ratio of shows marked proteinuria, and this is main feature of diabetic nephropathy/reflecting glomerular damage.
   Diagnosis: Diabetic nephropathy/stage 3 chronic kidney disease
   Next Steps: Proper glycemic control, manage blood pressure monitor renal function tests - serum creatinine, eGFR, ACR), Refer nephrologist.

CLINICAL MCQS

1. **A 69-year-old male with family history of diabetes, high blood pressure has high serum creatinine of 2.5 mg/dL low glomerular filtration rate. What is the diagnosis?**
   a. Acute kidney damage
   b. Chronic kidney disease
   c. Nephrosclerosis
   d. Nephropathy
   Answer: b. Chronic kidney disease
2. **A 39-year-old female complains of edema, decreased urine output, high serum creatinine: 3.6 mg/dL. Which is the test to confirm the stage of kidney failure?**
   a. Serum potassium
   b. Urinary 24-hour protein

c. Serum uric acid
d. Estimated glomerular filtration rate

Answer: d. Estimated glomerular filtration rate

3. **A 56-year-old patient with high blood pressure and serum creatinine: 1.9 mg/dL, BUN: 29 mg/dL. What is interpretation?**
a. Acute renal failure
b. Prerenal azotemia
c. Chronic kidney disease
d. Urinary tract disease

Answer: c. Chronic kidney disease

4. **A 29-year-old male complains of hematuria, decreased urine output. Serum creatinine: 4.2 mg/dL. Which is the best next step in this evaluation?**
a. Creatinine clearance
b. Renal ultrasound
c. 24-hour urine protein collection
d. Urea clearance

Answer: b. Renal ultrasound

5. **Which is a main indicator of acute kidney injury in patients with high serum creatinine?**
a. Decreased Blood Urea Nitrogen
b. Reduced GFR
c. Raised hemoglobin
d. High urine specific gravity

Answer: b. Reduced GFR

6. **A patient with CKD shows eGFR: 35 mL/min/1.73m^2. How can this GFR value classified?**
a. Stage 1
b. Stage 2
c. Stage 3
d. Stage 4

Answer: c. Stage 3

7. **A 69-year-old known diabetic patient complains of proteinuria and high serum creatinine. What is best assay for assessing for diabetic nephropathy?**
a. 24-hour urine protein
b. Urine microscopy
c. Biopsy of kidney
d. Serum globulin

Answer: a. 24-hour urine protein

8. **A 49-year-old male having upper respiratory tract infection suffers from acute renal failure. BUN: 45 mg/dL, serum creatinine: 4.8 mg/dL. What would be the cause?**
a. Postrenal obstruction
b. Nephrotic syndrome
c. Acute tubular necrosis
d. Chronic glomerulonephritis

Answer: c. Acute tubular necrosis

9. **Which is the accurate test for the diagnoses of renal tubular dysfunction in case of unexplained electrolyte disorder?**
a. Creatinine clearance
b. Urine osmolality
c. Urinary sodium
d. Fractional excretion of sodium

Answer: d. Fractional excretion of sodium

10. **A 49-year-old male with a history of consuming alcohol use shows with BUN of 30 mg/dL, serum creatinine of 1.5 mg/dL. Which can be cause?**
a. Chronic liver disease
b. Glomerulonephritis
c. Prerenal azotemia
d. Nephrotic syndrome

Answer: c. Prerenal azotemia

VIVA VOCE

Q1. Discuss key kidney function tests, and their importance.

Serum tests: Creatinine, BUN, Cystatin C
Urine tests: Urine albumin, ACR, Urine microscopy, Creatinine clearance
GFR estimation: eGFR (CKD-EPI, MDRD), Inulin clearance (gold standard)
Significance: Aids to assess kidney function/diagnosing CKD, AK/monitoring of disease progression

Q2. Discuss about BUN/Creatinine ratio.

Normal: 10:1 to 20:1
>20:1 → Prerenal AKI as in dehydration/heart failure
<10:1 → Intrinsic renal failure as in ATN/glomerulonephritis
10:1 to 20:1 → Postrenal obstruction as in stones/BPH

Q3. What is the importance of urine albumin-to-creatinine ratio?

Normal: <30 mg/g
Microalbuminuria: 30-300 mg/g → Early marker of CKD for diabetes/hypertension
Macroalbuminuria: >300 mg/g → Advanced renal disease
Significance: ACR confirms about early kidney damage before GFR reduces

Q4. Explain limitations of serum creatinine as marker of kidney function.

Delayed rise → Not an early marker of AKI
Affected by muscle mass that is low in elderly and high in athletes
Inaccurate for pregnant women/malnutrition/liver disease
Does not differentiate acute vs. chronic renal disease
Better alternative: Cystatin C that is unaffected by muscle mass

SPOTTERS

Q1. Show urine microscopy with RBC casts.

Spotter image: Microscopic slide of RBC casts

Identify and Explain:

RBC casts indicating glomerulonephritis

Observed in IgA nephropathy/poststreptococcal GN/lupus nephritis

Q2. Show blood urea nitrogen/creatinine ratio chart.

Spotter data: Table exhibiting different BUN/creatinine ratios

Interpret:

>20:1 → Prerenal AKI s in dehydration/heart failure

10:1–20:1 → Postrenal AKI as in obstruction/ stone/ BPH

a<10:1 → Intrinsic renal disease as in ATN/glomerulonephritis

Q3. Urine Dipstick + for Proteinuria.

Spotter: Urine dipstick test strip with proteinuria of +3

Clinical significance:

Indicates nephrotic syndrome (if >3.5g/day)

Common reason: Minimal Change Disease/FSGS/Membranous nephropathy

Requires confirmation with 24-hour urine protein estimation/ACR

Q4. eGFR Calculation Using CKD-EPI Formula.

Spotter data: Serum creatinine value/age of patient/gender/race

Interpret:

eGFR <60 mL/min/1.73m^2 → CKD

CKD staging:

Stage 1: eGFR >90 along with kidney damage

Stage 2: eGFR 60–89

Stage 3: eGFR 30–59

Stage 4: eGFR 15–29

Stage 5: eGFR <15 (ESRD)

Q5. Granular "Muddy Brown" Casts in Acute Tubular Necrosis (ATN).

Spotter image: Microscopy showing granular casts

Identify and explain:

Observed for Acute Tubular Necrosis

Common reasons: Ischemia as in shock /a nephrotoxins in aminoglycosides/ contrast dye/ myoglobin in rhabdomyolysis

Differentiates intrinsic AKI from prerenal AKI

REFLECTION

Learn the biochemical base of various tests that is performed in renal failure and describe the pathophysiology of kidney failure along with some clinical features.

35

CHAPTER

Pancreatic and Gastric Function Tests

COMPETENCY

BC14.19: Explain the basis and rationale of biochemical tests done in pancreatitis.

LEARNING OBJECTIVES

After reading this chapter, the readers should be able to:
- Describe pathophysiology along with clinical aspects of pancreatitis and biochemical basis of tests that is done for diag nosis of pancreatitis.
- Describe the gastric function tests along with clinical interpretations.

BLUE PRINT

Pancreatic and Gastric Function Tests

Objective

By the end of the lesson, students should be able to:
1. Understand physiological basis of pancreatic/gastric function tests.
2. Identify clinical significance of tests.
3. Interpret test results.

Outline (45–60 minutes)

I. **Introduction** **(10 minutes)**
   - Discuss role of pancreas/stomach in digestion.
   - Explain why functional assessment is significant in relation to gastrointestinal diseases.

II. **Pancreatic function tests** **(20 minutes)**
   - **Direct tests:** (Stimulate pancreas and measure secretions)
     - *Secretin-stimulated test*:
       - *Principle*: Secretin stimulates pancreas to release bicarbonate-rich fluid.
       - *Clinical significance*: Chronic pancreatitis/cystic fibrosis.
     - *Lundh meal test*:
       - *Principle*: Test meal stimulates pancreatic enzyme secretion.
       - *Clinical significance*: Exocrine pancreatic insufficiency.
   - **Indirect tests:** To measure enzyme activity in blood/stool/urine)
     - *Fecal elastase-1 test*:
       - *Principle*: Measures elastase in stool.
       - *Clinical significance*: Chronic pancreatitis, cystic fibrosis.
     - *Serum amylase and lipase*:
       - *Principle*: Released into circulation during pancreatic inflammation.
       - *Clinical significance*: Acute pancreatitis.
     - *Urinary D-xylose test*:
       - *Principle*: Measures carbohydrate absorption.
       - *Clinical significance*: Malabsorption syndromes.

III. **Gastric function tests** **(20 minutes)**
- **Tests for gastric acid secretion**
  - *Basal acid output and maximal acid output*:
    - *Principle*: Measures gastric acid secretion before and after stimulation like pentagastrin.
    - *Clinical significance*: Zollinger-Ellison syndrome (↑ MAO)/Achlorhydria (↓ BAO).
  - *Gastrin levels*:
    - *Principle*: High in Zollinger-Ellison syndrome.
    - *Clinical significance*: Gastrinoma diagnosis.
- **Tests for gastric mucosal integrity**
  - *Urea breath test*:
    - *Principle*: Detection of *H. pylori*
    - *Clinical significance*: Peptic ulcer
  - *Fasting serum gastrin*:
    - *Principle*: High in gastric acid hypersecretion states.
    - *Clinical significance*: Gastrinoma, atrophic gastritis.

IV. **Summary and clinical correlation** **(5–10 minutes)**
- Comparison of direct vs. indirect tests.
- Case scenarios.
- Important takeaways.

V. **Assessment and discussion**
- Short MCQs or viva questions.
- Clinical case presentation.

Pancreatic function test	
Exocrine function of pancreas	Secretion of pancreatic fluid with pH 8–8.3
Composition of pancreatic fluid	Bicarbonate, enzymes, such as trypsin, amylase, lipase, etc.
Function of pancreatic juice	Digestion and absorption of carbohydrates, proteins and lipids
One day volume of pancreatic juice	3 liters
Pancreatic diseases	
1. **In children:** Morphogenesis diseases	• Annular pancreas • Pancreas divisum • Pancreatic hypoplasia • Pancreatic agenesis
Inherited syndrome	Cystic fibrosis
Acquired pancreatitis	• Idiopathic • Traumatic • Drugs
2. **In adults:** Causes of acute pancreatitis	• Gallstones • Alcohol • Infections, such as mumps • Tumors of pancreas • Drugs, such as Azathioprine, estrogen, steroids • After surgery
Causes of chronic pancreatitis	• Alcohol • Nutritional • Trauma • Idiopathic • Hypercalcemia

Pancreatic function tests: Two types

Invasive	**Non invasive**
–	Tubeless
–	Comfortable
–	Lack sensitivity and specificity
–	Until half acinar cells are destroyed and there are 90% symptoms developed, this can give false tests

Invasive tests

Gold standard test	Secretin-cholecystokinin/secretin ceruletide tests
Collection of sample	• Secretin IV injection is given followed by Ceruletide injection or C terminal cholecystokinin octapeptide sequence of intact hormone—CCK • Assessment of bicarbonate and enzymes is done in the collected pancreatic juice
Lundh meal	Previously this meal having 6% fat, 15% carbohydrates and 74% fiber was given which provided stimulus for secretion of pancreatic juice

Non-invasive test

1. Fecal elastase test	Assess the reduction in the level of fecal enzyme elastase as a marker of pancreatic insufficiency
2. 13C-mixed chain triglyceride breath test	• Oral administration of labeled 13C fatty acid containing mixed TG is done • Breath is tested for labeled 13 CO_2 • If lipase enzyme is normal in intestine then adequate amount of 13C will be exhaled in the breath, otherwise, it will be absent in pancreatic insufficiency

Gastric function tests

Tests for *Helicobacter pylori* (*H. pylori*) infection:

H. pylori	Spiral shape bacterium, localize in the gastric antrum
Mechanism of action of *H. pylori*	Produces enzyme urease that breaks down urea to bicarbonate and ammonia, which are needed for surviving this organism in the stomach
Urea breath test for *H. pylori*	Non-invasive test for detecting *H. pylori* infection
Method	• Patient is asked to take urea 13C labeled as capsule • If the patient has the infection, this urea is converted to bicarbonate and ammonia • This bicarbonate has 13C and after getting absorbed from stomach to blood, gets broken down to 13CO_2 which is exhaled out
Mass spectrometry	• Detects 13CO_2 in breath sample collected 45–60 minutes after taking the labeled urea • In absence of the infection, there is no urease in the intestinal lumen then the labeled urea is absorbed intact in the blood and is excreted as such in the urine
1. Serological test for *H. pylori* infection	*H. pylori* specific antibodies IgG and IgA can be detected
2. PCR	Detection of nuclear sequence specific of *H. pylori* detects it in feces and saliva

Test for gastric acid secretion and gastrinomas

Earlier patients with gastric/duodenal ulcers were tested for basal and maximal acid output in the gastric juice analysis

But now there are non-invasive tests, such as:	• Plasma gastrin measurement • Endoscopy • CT scan • MRI
Gastrin	Secreted by G cell of antral mucosa, and G cell of proximal duodenum and delta cell of the pancreatic cell
Function of gastrin	Stimulates gastric acid secretion, intrinsic factor, pepsinogen, pancreatic bicarbonate and enzymes
Gastric acid output estimation	Standard alkali is used of 0.1 N NaOH
Normal basal acid output (BAO)	1–2.5 mmol of acid/hour
Normal maximum acid output (MAO)	20–40 mmol/hour

Clinical interpretation

Zollinger-Ellison syndrome consist of:	• Multiple peptic ulcer • Gastric hyper secretion • Non-beta islet cell tumor of pancreas secreting gastrin

OSCE

1. **Scenario: Acute pancreatitis—elevated amylase and lipase**
   Case: A 41-year-old male presents with sudden onset of severe upper abdominal pain radiating to the back, nausea, and vomiting. His lab results show:
   Serum amylase: 803 U/L (normal: 30–120 U/L)
   Serum lipase: 1220 U/L (normal: 10–140 U/L)
   Liver function tests (LFTs): Normal
   Ultrasound: No gallstones or biliary obstruction
   Question: What does this interpret?
   Interpretation: The significant raise of serum amylase/lipase indicates acute pancreatitis, because the enzymes are produced by the pancreas and released into the blood during inflammation of the pancreas.
   Amylase is often elevated early in acute pancreatitis, while lipase tends to remain elevated longer and is more specific to pancreatic injury.
   Diagnosis: Acute pancreatitis, cause being alcohol consumption/pancreatic duct obstruction
   Next steps: Evaluate the causes like alcohol use, triglyceride levels, CT scan for pancreatic complications.
2. **Scenario: Chronic pancreatitis—normal amylase, elevated fecal fat**
   Case: A 58-year-old male with a history of alcohol abuse presents with weight loss, steatorrhea, and chronic upper abdominal pain. His lab results show:
   Serum amylase: 121 U/L (normal: 30–120 U/L)
   Serum lipase: 165 U/L (normal: 10–140 U/L)
   Fecal fat test: 12 g/24 hours (normal: <7 g/24 hours)
   Liver function tests (LFTs): Normal
   Question: What is the interpretation?
   Interpretation: Normal serum amylase/lipase is present, but presence of raised fecal fat predicts malabsorption, mainly due to chronic pancreatitis where pancreas is damaged, and production of digestive enzymes like lipase is the result and this leads to steatorrhea.
   Diagnosis: Chronic pancreatitis, may be because of alcohol abuse that results in exocrine pancreatic insufficiency
   Next steps: CT scan/MR for assessing extent of pancreatic damage, along with pancreatic enzyme replacement therapy
3. **Scenario: Gastric acid secretion—elevated gastrin and low pH**
   Case: A 33-year-old male presents with chronic heartburn, epigastric pain, and occasional nausea. His lab results show:
   Serum gastrin: 820 pg/mL (normal: 50–200 pg/mL)
   Gastric pH: 1.4 (normal: 1.5–3.5)
   Helicobacter pylori (H. pylori) stool antigen: Negative
   Question: How do we interpret the diagnosis?
   Interpretation: The raised serum gastrin/low gastric pH is indicating gastritis/Zollinger-Ellison syndrome. Gastrin is produced in excess from gastrinoma, leading to excess formation of acid/low gastric pH.
   The negative *H. pylori* stool antigen suggests that *H. pylori* infection is not the cause of the elevated gastrin levels.
   Diagnosis: Likely Zollinger-Ellison syndrome (ZES), a condition characterized by gastrin-secreting tumors (gastrinomas) causing increased gastric acid secretion and peptic ulcers.
   Next steps: Further imaging (e.g., CT, MRI, somatostatin receptor scintigraphy) to identify the gastrinoma. Initiate proton pump inhibitors (PPIs) for acid suppression and consider surgical management of the Tumor.
4. **Scenario: Peptic ulcer disease—low gastric pH, normal gastrin**
   Case: A 44-year-old female presents with intermittent epigastric pain and occasional bloating. Her lab results show:
   Serum gastrin: 154 pg/mL (normal: 50–200 pg/mL)
   Gastric pH: 2.1 (normal: 1.5–3.5)
   H. pylori stool antigen: Positive
   Question: What does this interpret?
   Interpretation: The normal serum gastrin/low gastric pH and positive *H. pylori* stool antigen indicates reason of this peptic ulcer *H. pylori* infection.
   H. pylori is a very common reason behind peptic ulcers. The low gastric pH is expected because of raised acid secretion. In the absence of elevated gastrin, Zollinger-Ellison syndrome is unlikely to take place.
   Diagnosis: Peptic ulcer disease caused by *H. pylori* infection.
   Next steps: Eradication therapy for *H. pylori* (combination of antibiotics and proton pump inhibitors). Repeat testing after treatment to confirm eradication.
5. **Scenario: Pancreatic exocrine insufficiency—low amylase, elevated fecal fat**
   Case: A 61-year-old female with a history of chronic pancreatitis presents with weight loss, bloating, and indigestion.
   Serum amylase: 52 U/L (normal: 30–120 U/L)
   Serum lipase: 72 U/L (normal: 10–140 U/L)

Fecal fat test: 16 g/24 hours (normal: <7 g/24 hours)
Question: What does this interpret?
Interpretation: The decreased serum amylase/lipase is indicative of pancreatic exocrine insufficiency, a state where pancreas is not producing digestive enzymes. Reason can be chronic pancreatic damage leading to malabsorption symptoms.
The raised fecal fat is suggestive of fat malabsorption, that is a highlight for exocrine pancreatic insufficiency.
Diagnosis: Exocrine pancreatic insufficiency secondary to chronic pancreatitis.
Next steps: Pancreatic enzyme replacement therapy.

6. **Scenario: Gastric acid secretion—increased gastrin with low pH and ulcer formation**
   Case: A 51-year-old male presents with recurrent epigastric pain, nausea, vomiting. duodenal ulcers.
   Serum gastrin: 610 pg/mL (normal: 50–200 pg/mL)
   Gastric pH: 1.4 (normal: 1.5–3.5)
   Helicobacter pylori test: Negative
   Question: What is the interpretation?
   Interpretation: The raised serum gastrin suggests Zollinger-Ellison syndrome. Syndrome is caused by a gastrin-secreting Tumor that leads to excess secretion of gastric acid which forms peptic ulcer. The negative *H. pylori* test aids rule out infection as the reason of the ulcers.
   Diagnosis: Zollinger-Ellison syndrome characterized by hyperacid formation along with duodenal ulcers.
   Next steps: Further imaging for finding the gastrinoma/treatment with proton pump inhibitors/surgical resection of tumor.

CLINICAL MCQS

Pancreatic Function Tests

1. **A 49-year-old male shows symptoms of weight loss, steatorrhea, abdominal pain. Serum amylase, lipase levels: normal, secretin stimulation: decreased bicarbonate. What is the diagnosis?**
   a. Pancreatitis
   b. Chronic pancreatitis
   c. Pancreatic Tumor
   d. Celiac disorder
   Answer: b. Chronic pancreatitis
2. **A 53-year-old female comes with epigastric pain, nausea. Serum amylase is elevated, lipase levels are raised. What is the reason?**
   a. Acute pancreatitis
   b. Pancreatic malignancy
   c. Chronic pancreatitis
   d. Cirrhosis
   Answer: a. Acute pancreatitis
3. **Which is the sensitive test for evaluating exocrine pancreatic function in a patient with suspected pancreatic insufficiency?**
   a. Serum lipase
   b. Serum amylase
   c. Fecal elastase
   d. Secretin stimulation assay
   Answer: c. Fecal elastase
4. **A 68-year-old male with chronic alcohol use presents with abdominal pain, nausea, and vomiting. His serum lipase is elevated. Which specific test confirms damage of pancreas?**
   a. Serum glucose
   b. Urinary creatinine
   c. Serum lipase
   d. C-reactive protein
   Answer: c. Serum lipase
5. **A 47-year-old male presents with frequent epigastric pain. Secretin stimulation test: low bicarbonate secretion. What is the cause?**
   a. Pancreatic insufficiency
   b. Chronic pancreatitis
   c. Gastroesophageal reflux disease
   d. Hepatitis A
   Answer: a. Pancreatic insufficiency

Gastric Function Tests

6. **A 47-year-old female shows dyspepsia and takes up gastric acid secretion test. Increased basal acid output, normal maximal acid output. What is the diagnosis?**
   a. Peptic ulcer
   b. Malabsorption syndrome
   c. Chronic gastritis
   d. Dyspepsia

   Answer: c. Chronic gastritis

7. **A patient shows symptom of frequent ulcers, diarrhea, weight loss. Gastric acid secretion test: high BAO and MAO levels. Which is the most likely diagnosis?**
   a. Zollinger-Ellison syndrome
   b. *H. pylori* infection
   c. Peptic ulcer
   d. Metabolic acidosis

   Answer: a. Zollinger-Ellison syndrome

8. **A 39-year-old male shows weight loss, abdominal pain, frequent diarrhea. A secretin stimulation test shows high serum gastrin level. What is diagnosis?**
   a. Peptic ulcer disease
   b. Zollinger-Ellison syndrome
   c. Gastric carcinoma
   d. GERD

   Answer: b. Zollinger-Ellison syndrome

9. **Which assay is useful to diagnose Helicobacter pylori infection in peptic ulcer disease?**
   a. Gastric acid secretion test
   b. Urea breath test
   c. Serum amylase
   d. Serum pepsin

   Answer: b. Urea breath test

10. **A 68-year-old male with chronic dyspepsia takes up gastric acid secretion test. High basal acid output, normal maximal acid output. What is the diagnosis?**
    a. Zollinger-Ellison syndrome
    b. Helicobacter pylori infection
    c. Functional dyspepsia
    d. Gastric carcinoma

    Answer: c. Functional dyspepsia

VIVA VOCE

Q1. Why do we prefer serum lipase over amylase for diagnoses of acute pancreatitis?
Lipase is more specific to the pancreas, and remains high for longer time than amylase, and is less affected by non-pancreatic reasons.

Q2. Which PFT is more reliable for detection of chronic pancreatitis?
Fecal elastase-1 test, it reflects exocrine pancreatic insufficiency and remains unaffected by pancreatic enzyme replacement treatment.

Q3. Give principle of the secretin-stimulated PFT?
Secretin stimulates pancreas to release bicarbonate-rich fluid, that can be measured in duodenal aspirates. Less bicarbonate levels indicate chronic pancreatitis/cystic fibrosis.

Q4. Differentiate between Zollinger-Ellison syndrome and normal gastric acid hypersecretion?
The process of differentiating is by measurement of fasting serum gastrin levels/perform a secretin stimulation test—in Zollinger-Ellison syndrome, gastrin paradoxically increases after administering secretin.

Q5. What is the clinical importance of the urea breath test?
Detection of Helicobacter pylori infection by measurement of labeled CO_2 in exhaled breath after ingestion of C-13 or C-14-labeled urea, suggesting active infection in states such as peptic ulcer disease.

SPOTTERS

Q1. Show a clinical scenario where patient presents with epigastric pain/raised serum lipase/amylase.
Spot diagnosis: Acute pancreatitis

Q2. Show a report of stool test with low fecal elastase-1 in a case of chronic diarrhea/weight loss.
Spot diagnosis: Exocrine pancreatic insufficiency as in chronic pancreatitis/cystic fibrosis

Q3. Show a report of case with frequent peptic ulcers: fasting serum gastrin level >1000 pg/mL.
Spot diagnosis: Zollinger-Ellison syndrome/gastrinoma

Q4. Urea breath test + for patient with epigastric pain.
Spot diagnosis: *Helicobacter pylori* infection as in peptic ulcer/gastritis

Q5. Show that Basal acid output is absent in a patient with pernicious anemia.
Spot diagnosis: Achlorhydrias observed for atrophic gastritis/pernicious anemia

REFLECTION

Describe pathophysiology along with clinical aspects of pancreatitis and biochemical basis of tests that is done for diag nosis of pancreatitis. Describe the gastric function tests along with clinical interpretations.

CHAPTER 36

Enzymes as Disease Markers

COMPETENCY

BC14.19: Explain the basis and rationale of biochemical tests done in the following conditions:
- Diabetes mellitus
- Obesity, dyslipidemia, fatty liver, myocardial infarction, renal failure, gout, proteinuria, nephrotic syndrome, edema, jaundice, liver diseases, pancreatitis, disorders of acid- base balance.

LEARNING OBJECTIVES

After reading this chapter, the readers should be able to:
- Describe the principles of all the enzymes required for diagnosis of diseases.
- Interpret laboratory results of enzyme activities.
- Describe the clinical utility of various enzymes as markers of pathological conditions.
- Understand the significance of enzyme assays in clinical diagnosis and management.

BLUE PRINT

Understanding Enzyme Activity in Clinical Diagnosis

Objective

By the end of the lecture, students should be able to:
1. Interpret laboratory results of enzyme activities.
2. Describe the clinical utility of various enzymes as markers of pathological conditions.
3. Understand the significance of enzyme assays in clinical diagnosis and management.

Duration: *90 minutes*

Materials Needed

1. PowerPoint presentation or visual aids
2. Whiteboard and markers
3. Handouts with key points and diagrams
4. Examples of enzyme activity profiles in clinical scenarios (optional)

Outline

I. **Introduction to enzyme activity interpretation** **(10 minutes)**
- Brief overview of the lecture's objectives and agenda.
- Explanation of the importance of enzyme activity interpretation in clinical diagnosis.

II. **Basics of enzyme activity measurement** **(20 minutes)**
- Overview of the methods used to measure enzyme activity in laboratory settings.
- Discussion on the principles of enzyme assays and factors influencing assay results.

III. **Interpretation of laboratory results** **(30 minutes)**
- Explanation of how enzyme activity levels are interpreted in clinical practice.
- Description of reference ranges and cutoff values for normal and abnormal enzyme activity.
- Discussion on the significance of changes in enzyme activity levels in different pathological conditions.

IV. **Clinical utility of various enzymes** **(20 minutes)**
- Description of specific enzymes commonly used as markers of pathological conditions, such as:
- Creatine kinase (CK) for muscle injury.
- Alanine aminotransferase (ALT) and aspartate aminotransferase (AST) for liver damage.
- Amylase and lipase for pancreatic diseases.
- Explanation of how changes in enzyme levels correlate with specific diseases and clinical presentations.

V. **Case studies and examples** **(10 minutes)**
- Presentation of case studies or examples illustrating the interpretation of enzyme activity results in clinical scenarios.
- Discussion on the implications of enzyme activity findings for diagnosis and patient management.

VI. **Conclusion and recap** **(10 minutes)**
- Summary of key points covered in the lecture.
- Emphasis on the clinical relevance of interpreting enzyme activity results.
- Encouragement for further exploration of enzyme assays in clinical practice.

SPOTS/CLINICAL CASES

CASE 1: MYOCARDIAL INFARCTION

Age, gender	55 years, female
Complains	Pain in left side of chest, radiating in arm
Family history	Mother died of heart attack
Blood Report	
Total CPK (normal: 40–170 U/L)	215 U/L
CPK (MB) (normal: 3–10 U/L)	16 U/L
AST (0–35 IU/L)	87 IU/L
Cardiac troponin I	↑
High sensitive cardiac troponin T	↑
What is the clinical condition in the patient?	Myocardial infarction (MI)
Reasons:	1. Typical clinical history 2. Increased cardiac profile markers 3. CPK-MB is 7.5% of total CPK wherein normally it should be <5%

The rising time, the peaks and the duration of cardiac enzymes in serum:

Enzyme marker	Normal range	Start increasing	Peak	Till (maximum)
CPK	40–170 U/L	3–6 hours	24–36 hours	4 days
AST	0–35 IU/L	8–12 hours	24 hours	6 days
LDH	55–140 IU/L	12–24 hours	48–72 hours	14 days
Troponins	Not detected	3–12 hours	18–24 hours	10 days

CASE 2: ACUTE PANCREATITIS

Age, gender, characteristic feature	68 years, male, chronic alcoholic
Complains	Pain in epigastric region in abdomen radiating in back
On examination	Fever, diminished bowel sounds, distended abdomen
Family history	–
Blood Report	
Serum amylase (normal: 80–180 Somogyi units/mL)	500 Somogyi units/mL
Serum lipase (normal: 5–45 U/L) (more specific)	120 U/L

Contd...

Contd...

Blood glucose (R)	200 mg/dL
What is the clinical condition of the patient?	Acute pancreatitis
Reasons	1. Very common causes of acute pancreatitis is gallbladder stones and chronic consumption of alcohol 2. Epigastric pain radiating back 3. Elevation of serum amylase and lipase
Imaging abdomen	Confirms acute pancreatitis

CASE 3: PROSTATE CANCER

Age, gender	57 years, male
Complains	Frequent passing of urine, urinary incontinence
Family history	–
On examination	Prostate firm, enlarged
Blood Report	
Prostate specific antigen (normal: <4 ng/mL)	55 ng/mL
What is the diagnosis?	Prostate cancer
Reasons	1. Enlargement of the prostate gland (either because of benign prostatic hyperplasia/prostate cancer) 2. Increased prostate-specific antigen (PSA)
Biopsy	Confirms prostate cancer

CASE 4: HEMOLYTIC JAUNDICE

Age, gender	15 years, female child
Complains	Lethargy, recurrent pain in lower limbs, weakness, says that urine is normal color and feces is dark colored
On examination	Anemic, yellow discoloration of sclera and mucous membrane, tender abdomen, mild hepatomegaly
Family history	–
Blood Report	
Total bilirubin	14 mg/dL (0.3–1 mg/dL)↑
Conjugated bilirubin	0.4 mg/dL (0.1–0.3 mg/dL) N
Unconjugated bilirubin	10 mg/dL (0.2–0.7 mg/dL)↑
AST	20 IU/L (0–35 IU/L) N
ALT	34 IU/L (0–35 IU/L) N
ALP	50 IU/L (30–120 IU/L) N
Urine Report	
Bile pigments	–
Bile salts	–
Urobilinogen	+++
Stool	
Stercobilinogen	+++
What is the clinical condition in the patient?	Prehepatic hemolytic jaundice

Contd...

Contd...

Justification	• Increased plasma unconjugated bilirubin but normal conjugated bilirubin (no obstruction in the excretion of conjugated bilirubin via bile, so obstructive jaundice is definitely not there) • Liver enzymes are normal so no hepatic jaundice • Visible pallor, pain in lower limbs indicate sickle cell disease as a reason for hemolytic jaundice
Electrophoresis	HbS band is observed
Other probable reasons of hemolytic jaundice	G6PD deficiency, malarial parasite

CASE 5: HEPATIC JAUNDICE

Age, gender	25 years, male
Complains	Fever, headache, nausea, loss of appetite, weakness, says that urine is yellow color and normal feces color
On examination	Mild hepatomegaly
Family history	–
	Blood Report
Total bilirubin	9 mg/dL (0.3–1 mg/dL) ↑
Conjugated bilirubin	2.4 mg/dL (0.1–0.3 mg/dL) ↑
Unconjugated bilirubin	5.0 mg/dL (0.2–0.7 mg/dL) ↑
AST	1,200 IU/L (0–35 IU/L) ↑
ALT	1,000 IU/L (0–35 IU/L) ↑
ALP	155 IU/L (30–120 IU/L) ↑
	Urine Report
Bile pigments	+
Bile salts	+
Urobilinogen	++
	Stool
Stercobilinogen	++
What is the clinical condition in the patient?	Hepatic jaundice
Reasons of justification	• Fever suggests infection • Conjugation of bilirubin is affected as there may be deficiency of enzyme required for conjugation called glucoronyl transferase • Obstruction of bile flow due to edematous cells of liver, blocking the liver sinusoids resulting in increased conjugated bilirubin also • Increased liver enzymes—AST, ALT, ALP support our diagnosis
Other common probable reasons of hepatic jaundice:	Viral infection, drugs toxicity

CASE 6: OBSTRUCTIVE JAUNDICE

Age, gender	55 years, female
Complains	Severe pain abdomen (upper right), says that urine is yellow color and clay colored feces for past few days
On examination	Sclera—yellow discoloration, skin scratch marks seen
Family history	–

Contd...

Contd...

Blood Report	
Total bilirubin	9 mg/dL (0.3–1 mg/dL) ↑
Conjugated bilirubin	8.0 mg/dL (0.1–0.3 mg/dL) ↑
Unconjugated bilirubin	2.0 mg/dL (0.2–0.7 mg/dL) ↑
AST	30 IU/L (0–35 IU/L) N
ALT	35 IU/L (0–35 IU/L) N
ALP	355 IU/L (30–120 IU/L) ↑
Urine Report	
Bile pigments	++
Bile salts	++
Urobilinogen	–
Stool	
Stercobilinogen	–
What is the clinical condition in the patient?	Obstructive jaundice
Reasons of justification:	• Increased conjugated bilirubin because of obstruction in flow of bile resulting in regurgitation of conjugated bilirubin in the plasma • Dark color of the urine is because of excretion of water-soluble conjugated bilirubin • Since there is obstruction to the flow of bile, there is no bilirubin in the intestinal lumen so urobilinogen and stercobilinogen are not formed in the intestinal lumen showed as no UBG in urine and clay colored stool in the report • The liver cells are normal so AST and ALT are normal • ALP is increased in obstructive jaundice
Other causes of obstructive jaundice:	Biliary tract stones, duct stricture, cancer of the head of pancreas
Investigation tests recommended in urine:	• Bilirubin—Fouchet's test • Bile salts—Hay's sulfur test • Urobilinogen—Ehrlich's test

OSCE

1. **Scenario: Myocardial infarction—elevated cardiac enzymes (CK-MB, troponin)**
   Case: A 51-year-old male presents with pain in chest /sweating/shortness of breath.
   Creatine kinase (CK): 304 U/L (normal: 22–198 U/L)
   CK-MB: 75 U/L (normal: <25 U/L)
   Troponin I: 3.6 ng/mL (normal: <0.01 ng/mL)
   Liver function tests (LFTs): Normal
   Question: What is the interpretation?
   Interpretation: The raised CK-MB/Troponin I levels are suggestive of myocardial infarction.
   CK-MB: Cardiac-specific isoenzyme of creatine kinase, its elevation is linked with myocardial damage.
   Troponin I: Sensitive/specific marker for MI.
   Diagnosis: Myocardial infarction. The significant rise of Troponin I indicates progressive myocardial damage /confirms diagnosis of acute Myocardial infarction.
   Next Steps: Reperfusion therapy /manage complications
2. **Scenario: Acute hepatitis - Elevated ALT and AST**
   Case: A 31-year-old female presents with jaundice, dark urine
   Alanine aminotransferase: 1201 U/L (normal: 7–56 U/L)
   Aspartate aminotransferase: 1005 U/L (normal: 10–40 U/L)
   Total bilirubin: 6 mg/dL (normal: 0.1–1.2 mg/dL)

Alkaline phosphatase: 122 U/L (normal: 44–147 U/L)
Question: What does this interpret?
Interpretation: The rise of ALT/AST/bilirubin plus jaundice, are indicating towards acute liver injury, because of acute viral hepatitis.
ALT is more specific towards liver cell injury, and its rise is observed in liver diseases like hepatitis.
AST is less specific and may be increased in many states like muscle injury/liver disease. The ALT:AST ratio in acute viral hepatitis is more than 1.
Diagnosis: Acute viral hepatitis.
Next Steps: Identify the type of hepatitis/supportive care/monitor complications.

3. **Scenario: Pancreatitis—elevated lipase and amylase**
Case: A 47-year-old male presents with severe epigastric pain that is radiating to his back, nausea, and vomiting.
Serum amylase: 510 U/L (normal: 30–120 U/L)
Serum lipase: 1006 U/L (normal: 10–140 U/L)
Liver function tests (LFTs): Normal
Complete blood count (CBC): Mild leukocytosis seen
Question: What does this interpret?
Interpretation: The significant rise of serum amylase along with lipase is indicative of acute pancreatitis.
Both the enzymes are produced by pancreas, and their concentrations increase markedly in acute pancreatitis because of pancreatic cell injury along with enzyme release.
Lipase is more specific for pancreatic injury and remain increased for more time in comparison to amylase, making it a more reliable marker for the state of pancreatitis.
Diagnosis: Acute pancreatitis, because of gallstones or alcohol use
Next Steps: Supportive treatment like fluid resuscitation/ultrasound/CT scan for further finding underlying reason.

4. **Scenario: Rhabdomyolysis—elevated CK and myoglobin**
Case: A 34-year-old male presents with muscle pain, weakness, and dark urine after physical exercise.
Creatine kinase (CK): 5070 U/L (normal: 22–198 U/L)
Myoglobin: 1506 ng/mL (normal: <100 ng/mL)
Serum creatinine: 3.0 mg/dL (normal: 0.6–1.2 mg/dL)
Question: What does this interpret?
Interpretation: The marked increase of CK/myoglobin/creatinine, are suggestive of rhabdomyolysis, involving breakdown of muscles and release of muscle proteins into the circulation
CK: Enzyme present in muscles, and its concentration increase in muscle injury, like rhabdomyolysis.
Myoglobin: Released from damaged muscle tissue leading to renal function abnormality
Diagnosis: Rhabdomyolysis, because of aggressive physical activity/muscle trauma.
Next Steps: Fluid resuscitation to avoid more kidney damage/check out for renal failure.

5. **Scenario: Bone disease—elevated alkaline phosphatase (ALP)**
Case: A 61-year-old female presents with bone pain/fractures.
Alkaline phosphatase: 351 U/L (normal: 44–147 U/L)
Calcium: 9.1 mg/dL (normal: 8.5–10.5 mg/dL)
Phosphate: 3.1 mg/dL (normal: 2.5–4.5 mg/dL)
Vitamin D: Decreased
Question: What does this interpret?
Interpretation: The raised ALP but normal calcium/phosphate concentrations is pointing towards bone disease, like osteomalacia/Paget's disease.
Alkaline phosphatase: Enzyme associated with formation of bone and in increased bone turnover conditions like osteomalacia/bone metastasis, its concentration increases in blood.
The decreased level of vitamin D level is suggesting the same state of osteomalacia, a state where impaired bone mineralization is present because of Vitamin D deficiency.
Diagnosis: osteomalacia because of deficient Vitamin D.
Next Steps: Vitamin D supplements to be given determine bone density, manage underlying causes like malabsorption/dietary deficiency.

6. **Scenario: Acute cholestasis—elevated ALP and GGT**
Case: A 41-year-old female presents with jaundice, pruritus, and dark urine.
Alkaline phosphatase: 302 U/L (normal: 44–147 U/L)
Gamma-glutamyl transferase: 183 U/L (normal: 9–48 U/L)
Total bilirubin: 3.1 mg/dL (normal: 0.1–1.2 mg/dL)
Liver function tests: Mild rise of ALT and AST
Question: What does this interpret?

Interpretation: The conditions suggest cholestasis, that is obstruction/impairment of bile flow.
ALP/GGT are markers for cholestatic liver diseases, and their rise is indicating obstruction/bile duct injury, that might be due to primary biliary cirrhosis/biliary obstruction/cholelithiasis.
Diagnosis: Cholestasis, because of biliary obstruction/liver disease.
Next Steps: ultrasound/MRI for assessing gallstones/bile duct obstruction.

CLINICAL MCQS

1. **A 58-year-old male presents with chest pain, shortness of breath. Serum creatine kinase troponin levels are high. Which is the diagnosis?**
   a. Myocardial infarction
   b. Chronic pancreatitis
   c. Kidney failure
   d. Hepatitis

   Answer: a. Myocardial infarction
2. **A 49-year-old female shows report of jaundice and presents with abdominal pain. Serum alkaline phosphatase is significantly high, serum bilirubin is high. What is the diagnosis?**
   a. Acute liver failure
   b. Cholestasis
   c. Hepatitis A
   d. Acute pancreatitis

   Answer: b. Cholestasis
3. **A 66-year-old male with a habit of consuming alcohol presents with high serum alanine aminotransferase, AST levels. What is the cause of these high concentration of enzymes?**
   a. Hepatitis A
   b. Acute alcoholic hepatitis
   c. NAFLD
   d. Acute liver disease

   Answer: b. Acute alcoholic hepatitis
4. **A 53-year-old male with abdominal pain, nausea, vomiting has high serum amylase, lipase levels. What is the diagnosis?**
   a. Acute pancreatitis
   b. Peptic ulcer
   c. GIT disorder
   d. Cirrhosis

   Answer: a. Acute pancreatitis
5. **A 37-year-old female presents with fatigue, weight loss, and a high serum CK-MB. Which is the most likely reason?**
   a. Myocardial infarction
   b. Skeletal muscle injury
   c. Renal disorder
   d. Tissue disorder

   Answer: b. Skeletal muscle injury
6. **A 71-year-old male presents with high serum lactate dehydrogenase after past trauma. Which is the cause?**
   a. Liver disorder
   b. MI
   c. Hemolysis or tissue injury
   d. Renal disorder

   Answer: c. Hemolysis or tissue injury
7. **A 61-year-old female with a family history of diabetes, hypertension/shows increased serum troponin I and CK-MB after getting chest pain. What is the diagnosis?**
   a. Acute myocardial infarction
   b. Pulmonary infection
   c. Angina
   d. Heart failure

   Answer: a. Acute myocardial infarction

8. **A 48-year-old male presents with jaundice, and high reporting of serum alanine aminotransferase. Liver biopsy shows liver cell necrosis. What is cause?**
   a. Acute viral hepatitis
   b. Chronic hepatitis A
   c. NAFLD
   d. Cirrhosis

   Answer: a. Acute viral hepatitis

9. **A 52-year-old male presents with high serum C-reactive protein, serum alkaline phosphatase. Which is the diagnosis?**
   a. Chronic pancreatitis
   b. Cholestatic liver disease
   c. Rickets
   d. Arthritis

   Answer: b. Cholestatic liver disease

10. **A 37-year-old female shows symptoms of abdominal pain, high serum amylase, lipase. Which investigation confirms diagnosis of acute pancreatitis?**
    a. Serum glucose
    b. Serum ALP
    c. Serum triglycerides
    d. Serum HDL

    Answer: c. Serum triglycerides

VIVA VOCE

Q1. What is the importance of measuring serum amylase/lipase levels?
Serum amylase and lipase are key markers for acute pancreatitis. Lipase is more specific in comparison to amylase and also remains high for longer time than amylase.

Q2. Name enzyme of marker for myocardial infarction, and justify.
Troponins (cTnI, cTnT)—gold standard. CK-MB was initially used. CK-MB increases within 3-6 hours, peak is at 12-24 hours, and returns to normal in 48-72 hours.

Q3. Why is ALP measured in liver/bone diseases?
ALP is raised in cholestasis that is biliary obstruction/Paget's disease/rickets/osteomalacia. In liver disorders gamma-glutamyl transferase aids to differentiate hepatobiliary causes from bone disorders.

Q4. What enzyme is high in hemolytic anemia/why?
Lactate dehydrogenase because of RBC destruction, resulting in release of intracellular LDH into blood.

Q5. How is acid phosphatase clinically important?
ACP—marker for prostate cancer, along with prostate-specific antigen. ACP is significant in forensic investigations/rape cases because of its presence in seminal fluid.

SPOTTERS

Q1. Show a blood report with high CK-MB/troponin levels.
Spot Diagnosis: Myocardial infarction

Q2. Show a clinical scenario of a patient of jaundice who has highly elevated ALP/GGT and normal AST/ALT.
Spot Diagnosis: Obstructive /cholestatic jaundice

Q3. A child image of bone deformities and his report with increased serum ALP levels.
Spot Diagnosis: Rickets

Q4. Clinical scenario of a patient with a history of alcohol abuse has high serum amylase/lipase.
Spot Diagnosis: Acute pancreatitis

Q5. A case of hemolysis with high LDH/low haptoglobin.
Spot Diagnosis: Hemolytic anemia

REFLECTION

Interpret laboratory results of enzyme activities and describe the clinical utility of various enzymes as markers of pathological conditions, also describe the principles of all the enzymes required for diagnosis of diseases.

37

CHAPTER

Interpretation of Laboratory Result: Amino Acid Metabolism

COMPETENCY

BC14.19: Explain the basis and rationale of biochemical tests done in various conditions (amino acid metabolism).

LEARNING OBJECTIVES

After reading this chapter, the readers should be able to:
- Describe the clinical interpretation related to tests done in amino acid metabolism.

BLUE PRINT

Interpretation of Tests Done in Amino Acid Metabolism

Objective

By the end of the lesson, students should be able to:
1. Understand normal amino acid metabolism/significance.
2. Interpret abnormal lab results associated with amino acid metabolism.
3. Identify metabolic disorders based on lab findings.
4. Correlation of biochemical abnormalities with clinical symptoms and manifestations.

Outline

I. **Introduction** **(10 minutes)**
- Brief introduction of amino acid metabolism.
- Significance of amino acids in protein synthesis and energy production.
- Functions of metabolic pathways like urea cycle/transamination/deamination.
- Importance of lab tests for diagnoses of metabolic disorders.

II. **Key lab investigations in amino acid metabolism** **(15 minutes)**
- *Plasma amino acid profile*: For identifying abnormal amino acid levels.
- *Urine amino acid analysis*: For detecting metabolic disorders.
- *Blood ammonia levels*: Foe evaluating urea cycle disorders.
- *Organic acid analysis (urine plus plasma)*: For diagnoses of metabolic acidosis-related diseases.
- *Enzyme activity tests*: For confirming particular enzyme deficiencies.

III. **Interpretation of lab results—case-based discussion** **(30 minutes)**
- **Case 1:** Phenylketonuria (PKU)
  - *Lab findings*: High phenylalanine, decreased tyrosine, ferric chloride tests positive.
  - *Interpretation*: Deficiency of enzyme—phenylalanine hydroxylase.
  - *Clinical features*: Like developmental delay/musty odor/light skin/eczema.
- **Case 2:** Maple syrup urine disease (MSUD)
  - *Lab findings*: High valine, leucine, isoleucine/ketonuria/urine with a "maple syrup" odor.
  - *Interpretation*: Deficient enzyme branched-chain ketoacid dehydrogenase.
  - *Clinical features*: inadequate feeding/seizures/lethargy/metabolic acidosis.

- **Case 3:** Homocystinuria
  - *Lab findings*: High homocysteine in blood and urine, decreased cystathionine synthase.
  - *Interpretation*: Deficient cystathionine beta-synthase.
  - *Clinical features*: Marfanoid habitus/lens dislocation/deep vein thrombosis.
- **Case 4:** Tyrosinemia Type I
  - *Lab findings*: High tyrosine, succinylacetone positive in urine, liver dysfunctioning.
  - *Interpretation*: Deficient fumarylacetoacetate hydrolase.
  - *Clinical features*: Liver failure/kidney dysfunction/cabbage-like odor.
- **Case 5:** Urea cycle disorder—ornithine transcarbamylase deficiency
  - *Lab findings*: Hyperammonemia/respiratory alkalosis/normal anion gap.
  - *Interpretation*: Urea cycle enzyme defect resulting in ammonia accumulation.
  - *Clinical features*: Vomiting/encephalopathy/lethargy.

IV. **Summary and recap** **(10 minutes)**
- Key lab tests, significance in amino acid metabolism.
- Interpretation of abnormal results in metabolic disorders.
- Significance of early detection in newborn screening programs.
- Importance of dietary/enzyme replacement therapies in management.

V. **Assessment** **(10 minutes)**
- *Spotters*: Identify lab findings in amino acid metabolism diseases.
- *Short answer questions*: Discuss lab abnormalities in particular metabolic conditions.
- *Case scenario discussion*: To give lab reports, diagnose/explain metabolic disorder.

Materials Required

1. PowerPoint slides of case images/lab reports.
2. Sample lab reports.
3. Flowcharts—metabolic pathways.

SPOTS/CLINICAL CASES

CASE 1: DISORDER OF UREA CYCLE

Age, gender	3-year-old, boy
Complains	Vomiting, aversion for protein diet
On examination	Tiredness, mentally retarded
	Blood report
Ammonia	High
	Urine report
Orotic acid	Positive
What is the diagnosis? Characteristics?	• Urea cycle disorder • Deficiency of ornithine transcarbamoylase (OTC) enzyme • X linked disease where males are affected more in comparison to heterozygous females • Increased orotic acid is seen because carbamoyl phosphate is not utilized in urea cycle due to deficiency of enzyme—OTC, so it diffuses to cytosol and gets diverted to form pyrimidine nucleotides • Excess ammonia in blood and delayed consultation with the doctor is the reason behind mental retardation

CASE 2: MAPLE SYRUP URINE DISORDER

Age, gender	4-month-old, female
Complains	Lack of appetite, fits, urine smells like burnt sugar
History	Normal at birth but over a period of 5 days condition got serious

Contd....

Contd....

	Urine report
Dinitrophenylhydrazine test	Yellow white precipitate
Ferric chloride test	Bluish gray color
What is the diagnosis?	Maple syrup urine disease
Reasons	Branched chain aciduria/maple syrup urine disorder/oxoaciduria–autosomal recessive disease
Enzyme deficient	Branched chain alpha keto acid dehydrogenase complex/decarboxylase (2 enzyme of catabolism of branched chain amino acids)
Gene mutation	• Gene coding enzyme E1, E2 or E3 of the enzyme complex, and this extent is responsible for the degree of disease severity • Neurological disorders are observed after 4 days of birth, manifested as mental disturbances, apnea, seizures and even death
Advised mother	Branched chain amino acid free diet particularly leucine is given

CASE 3: CLASSICAL/TYPICAL HOMOCYSTINURIA

Age, gender	3-year-old, boy
Complains	Skeletal deformation, defect in vision
On examination	Genu valgum, osteoporosis, anomaly of vertebra, cardiovascular system not normal, myopia, ectopia lentis (lens dislocation)
What is the diagnosis?	Homocystinuria
Reasons	Defective amino acid metabolism—methionine
Subclasses of the disease	Type I (typical or classical): Deficiency of enzyme cystathionine beta synthase, B6 dependent enzyme
	Type II: Deficiency of N5, N10-methylenetetrahydrofolate reductase
	Type III: Deficiency of homocysteine methyltransferase
	Type IV: Deficiency of vitamin B_{12} along with methylmalonic acidemia
Typical homocystinuria	Autosomal recessive
	Symptoms
Eye	Subluxation of lens, secondary glaucoma, optic atrophy, retinal detachment
Central nervous system (CNS)	Cerebellar ataxia, nystagmus, aphasia, hypotonia, weakness of muscles, mental retardation
Vascular	Atherosclerosis
Skeletal	Arachnodactyly, osteoporosis, scoliosis
Treatment	Dietary restriction of proteins and methionine, B6 stimulates the activity of the enzyme cystathionine beta synthase, B_{12}, methyltetrahydrofolate and betaine supplementation

CASE 4: ALKAPTONURIA

Age, gender	13-year-old, female
Complains	Backache, knee pain, urine turns black after exposure to atmospheric oxygen
What is the diagnosis?	Typically alkaptonuria
Reasons	Autosomal recessive
Enzyme deficient	Homogentisic acid oxidase
Metabolism disorder	Tyrosine and phenylalanine catabolism (metabolism of homogentisic acid stops)
Reason behind black color urine	Homogentisic acid is colorless, excretes in urine, undergoes auto oxidation and forms quinone, which then polymerize to form black alkapton bodies giving black color to urine
	Homogentisic acid deposits in cartilages of knees, hips, shoulders leading to arthritis
Reason behind backache	Homogentisic acid deposits in intervertebral disc
Ochronosis	These alkapton bodies deposits in the tissues like ear pinnae and above mentioned tissues

CASE 5: PHENYLKETONURIA

Age, gender	8-months-old child
Complains	Fits
History	Normal delivery, no use of forceps
On examination	Delayed milestones gray color hair, mousy odor in skin, hair and urine, tiredness, improper neurological development
What is the diagnosis?	Phenylketonuria
Screening test	Ferric chloride test in urine gives leafy green color as a positive test for phenyl acetate
Confirmatory test	Guthrie test in the patient blood
	Reasons
Enzymes deficient	Phenylalanine hydroxylase Dihydrobiopterin reductase Dihydrobiopterin synthase
Reason behind impaired neurological development	Alternate pathways open leading to formation of phenyl ketones
Reason behind mousy odor of skin, sweat and urine	Formation of alternate unwanted products like phenyl acetate
Reason behind gray hair	1. Melanin synthesis does not take place because tyrosine is required for melanin synthesis, and here phenylalanine is not converted to tyrosine due to deficiency of some enzymes 2. Tyrosinase enzyme which is required for melanin formation is inhibited competitively by phenyl alanine
Advised mother	Restrict diet having phenylalanine and supplement tyrosine in the diet

CASE 6: ALBINISM

Age, gender	18-year-old, male
Complains	Vision defect, photophobia, white skin and hair, nystagmus
What is the diagnosis?	Albinism (autosomal recessive)
Enzyme deficient	Tyrosinase
Gene mutation of	Enzyme–tyrosinase (required for melanin formation)
Melanin	Pigment required for black pigmentation of skin and hair

OSCE

1. **Scenario: Phenylketonuria (PKU)—elevated phenylalanine**
   Case: A 2-month-old infant presents with developmental delay, seizures, musty smell.
   Phenylalanine: 36 mg/dL (normal: 1–2 mg/dL)
   Tyrosine: 0.4 mg/dL (normal: 2–4 mg/dL)
   Glucose: 96 mg/dL (normal: 70–100 mg/dL)
   Question: What does this interpret?
   Interpretation: The high phenylalanine but decreased tyrosine is suggestive of phenylketonuria
   PKU: Metabolic disease due to deficiency of phenylalanine hydroxylase, resulting in accumulation of phenylalanine, that is neurotoxic.
   There is also reduction in conversion of phenylalanine to form tyrosine.
   Diagnosis: Phenylketonuria.
   Next steps: Restrict phenylalanine in diet/monitor blood phenylalanine concentration. Avoid irreversible brain damage.
2. **Scenario: Maple syrup urine disease (MSUD)—elevated branched-chain amino acids**
   Case: A newborn present with poor feeding/maple syrup smell in the urine.
   Leucine: 310 μmol/L (normal: 80–200 μmol/L)
   Isoleucine: 96 μmol/L (normal: 30–70 μmol/L)

Valine: 151 μmol/L (normal: 60–150 μmol/L)
Blood glucose: 53 mg/dL (normal: 70–100 mg/dL)
Question: What does this indicate?
Interpretation: The raised branched-chain amino acids indicate maple syrup urine disease
MSUD: deficiency disorder of enzyme branched-chain α-keto acid dehydrogenase that is required for hydrolysis of branched chain amino acids. On accumulating in the blood, they cause neurotoxicity and other symptoms mentioned above.
Diagnosis: Maple syrup urine disease (MSUD).
Next steps: Restrict branched-chain amino acids in diet/intravenous glucose for avoiding metabolic crises.

3. **Scenario: Homocystinuria—elevated homocysteine and methionine**
   Case: A 6-year-old boy presents with symptoms of developmental delay/dislocated lenses/long limbs.
   Homocysteine: 32 μmol/L (normal: 5–15 μmol/L)
   Methionine: 156 μmol/L (normal: 30–60 μmol/L)
   Vitamin B12: Normal
   Folate: Normal
   Question: What does this interpret?
   Interpretation: Suggestive of homocystinuria, a disease related to metabolism of methionine
   Common reason of Homocystinuria is deficient enzyme—cystathionine β-synthase needed to convert homocysteine to form cystathionine. Homocysteine accumulation causes vascular/ocular/skeletal deformities like lens dislocation and long limbs
   Secondary finding: High methionine.
   Diagnosis: Homocystinuria, because of deficient enzyme—cystathionine β-synthase.
   Next steps: Vitamin B6 supplementation, restrict methionine/folic acid to aid to lower homocysteine concentration.
4. **Scenario: Alkaptonuria—elevated homogentisic acid**
   Case: A 41-year-old man presents with dark urine and joint pain. Blood tests show:
   Homogentisic acid: 21 mg/dL (normal: <0.1 mg/dL)
   Urinary creatinine: 182 mg/dL (normal: 70–120 mg/dL)
   Question: What does this suggest?
   Interpretation: The high homogentisic acid in urine suggests alkaptonuria, due to deficient enzyme homogentisate 1,2-dioxygenase.
   Accumulation of homogentisic acid, leads to dark urine and Ochronosis, plus dark sclera/ear cartilage.
   All these complications can lead to arthritis with time.
   Diagnosis: Alkaptonuria due to raised homogentisic acid.
   Next steps: Symptomatic treatment for joint pain/vitamin C supplementation to reduce homogentisic acid.
5. **Scenario: Tyrosinemia—elevated tyrosine and methionine**
   Case: A 3-week-old infant presents with failure to thrive, enlargement of liver
   Tyrosine: 603 μmol/L (normal: 40–90 μmol/L)
   Methionine: 122 μmol/L (normal: 30–60 μmol/L)
   Alanine aminotransferase: 253 U/L (normal: 7–56 U/L)
   Total bilirubin: 11 mg/dL (normal: 0.1–1.2 mg/dL)
   Question: What does this indicate?
   Interpretation: The raised tyrosine/methionine/liver enzymes/bilirubin indicates tyrosinemia.
   Tyrosinemia: Due to deficient enzyme fumarylacetoacetate hydrolase, that is required for breaking down tyrosine. Accumulation of toxic metabolites is the result and finally leads to liver dysfunction/renal tubular damage/neurological symptoms.
   Diagnosis: Tyrosinemia type 1, due to defective fumarylacetoacetate hydrolase.
   Next steps: Production of toxic metabolites should be prevented, low-tyrosine and phenylalanine diet. Early diagnosis will prevent liver failure.

CLINICAL MCQS

1. **A 3-day-old infant shows symptoms of vomiting/fatigue/irritability. High plasma phenylalanine levels were seen. What is the diagnosis?**
   a. MSUD
   b. Phenylketonuria
   c. Tyrosinosis
   d. Tyrosinemia

   Answer: b. Phenylketonuria

2. **A 31-year-old male complains of developmental delay, psychiatric symptoms, lens dislocation. High Plasma homocysteine, High methionine levels are seen, cysteine levels are decreased. Which conditions is present?**
   a. PKU
   b. Tyrosinemia II
   c. Homocystinuria
   d. MSUD

   Answer: c. Homocystinuria
3. **A 4-year-old child having presents with poor feeding, vomiting, irritability, leucine levels are elevated. What is the diagnosis?**
   a. Tyrosinosis
   b. Maple syrup urine disease
   c. Homocystinuria
   d. PKU

   Answer: b. Maple syrup urine disease
4. **A 28-year-old male with a history of muscle weakness, pain after exercise, high plasma ammonia, branched-chain amino acids. What is the most likely diagnosis?**
   a. Urea cycle disorder
   b. Phenylketonuria
   c. Maple syrup urine disease
   d. Homocystinuria

   Answer: c. Maple syrup urine disease
5. **A newborn screening test exhibits high phenylalanine levels, no apparent symptoms at birth. What is the management?**
   a. Start a low-protein diet immediately
   b. Confirm diagnosis with a urinary amino acid analysis
   c. Reassure the parents, as the infant is asymptomatic
   d. Confirm diagnosis with a plasma phenylalanine test after 1 week

   Answer: b. Confirm diagnosis with a urinary amino acid analysis
6. **A 46-year-old male presents with a history of osteoarthritis, dark urine on exposure to air. Which findings support alkaptonuria?**
   a. Elevated urinary homocysteine
   b. Elevated plasma tyrosine
   c. Dark-colored urine after oxidation
   d. Raised serum ammonia

   Answer: c. Dark-colored urine after oxidation
7. **A 4-year-old child presents with developmental delay, musty odor in urine. Normal Plasma phenylalanine levels seen. Which is diagnosis?**
   a. Tyrosinosis
   b. Tyrosinemia II
   c. Trimethylaminuria
   d. MSUD

   Answer: c. Trimethylaminuria
8. **A 11-month-old infant presents with vomiting, hyperreflexia. Plasma phenylalanine, tyrosine levels high. What is the most likely cause of this state?**
   a. Cystinuria
   b. Tyrosinemia
   c. PKU
   d. Alkaptonuria

   Answer: b. Tyrosinemia
9. **A 48-year-old male presents with cognitive decline, high plasma ammonia levels. Urinary orotic acid is high. Which underlying disorder is present?**
   a. Deficient OTC
   b. PKU
   c. Urea cycle disorder
   d. Homocystine in urine

   Answer: a. Deficient OTC

10. A 6-month-old child with symptoms of vomiting, irritability, and abnormal gait high plasma levels of methionine. What condition may be present?

a. Homocystinuria
b. MSUD
c. PKU
d. Tyrosinemia I

Answer: a. Homocystinuria

VIVA VOCE

Q1. What is the importance of high phenylalanine level in a newborn screening test?
Follow-up: What condition does this suggest/name underlying metabolic defect?

Q2. Interpret a urine sample with presence of ketone bodies/high tyrosine/high phenylalanine in a patient showing with developmental delay.
Follow-up: What disorder is this/further tests to confirm diagnosis?

Q3. What does high blood ammonia level, plus normal blood urea nitrogen level indicate?
Follow-up: How to link with urea cycle disorders?

Q4. Interpret a urine sample with high methionine in a patient with failure to thrive.
Follow-up: What condition is indicated/diagnosis/treated?

Q5. What is the importance of raised urinary excretion of branched-chain amino acids?
Follow-up: What condition is this/potential complications?

SPOTTERS

Q1. Show sample of urine with maple syrup smell/high branched-chain valine, leucine, isoleucine. What is the interpretation/ underlying cause?

Maple syrup urine disease; Deficiency of enzyme—branched-chain ketoacid dehydrogenase.

Q2. Show a report of blood test with high phenylalanine but normal tyrosine levels in a newborn. What does this interpret?

Phenylketonuria (PKU); Deficient phenylalanine hydroxylase.

Q3. Show urine report with high homocysteine levels. What is the interpretation?

Homocystinuria; Deficient cystathionine beta-synthase.

Q4. Urine sample showing high levels of tyrosine, with a history of jaundice and liver dysfunction. What is the likely diagnosis, and what enzyme deficiency is involved?

Tyrosinemia type I; Deficiency in fumarylacetoacetate hydrolase.

Q5. Show a report of blood ammonia levels high/urine is negative for ketones in a case of encephalopathy/failure to thrive. What is the interpretation?

Urea cycle disorder; Deficient in one of the urea cycle enzymes like carbamoyl-phosphate synthetase 1.

REFLECTION

Interpret laboratory results of analytes associated with amino acid metabolism; describe the clinical interpretation related to tests done in amino acid metabolism.

38

CHAPTER

Interpretation of Laboratory Result: Protein Metabolism

COMPETENCY

BC14.19: Explain the basis and rationale of biochemical tests done in various conditions (Protein metabolism).

LEARNING OBJECTIVES

After reading this chapter, the readers should be able to:
- Describe the clinical interpretation related to tests done in protein metabolism.
- Understand the laboratory tests used to assess protein metabolism.
- Interpret laboratory results related to protein metabolism analytes.
- Discuss the clinical significance of abnormal findings in protein metabolism tests.

BLUE PRINT

Interpreting Laboratory Results in Protein Metabolism

Objective

By the end of the lecture, students should be able to:
1. Understand the laboratory tests used to assess protein metabolism.
2. Interpret laboratory results related to protein metabolism analytes.
3. Discuss the clinical significance of abnormal findings in protein metabolism tests.

Duration: *90 minutes*

Materials Needed

1. PowerPoint presentation or visual aids
2. Whiteboard and markers
3. Handouts with key laboratory reference ranges and interpretation guidelines
4. Examples of laboratory reports for demonstration

Outline

I. **Introduction to laboratory tests in protein metabolism** **(10 minutes)**
   - Overview of the lecture's objectives and agenda.
   - Importance of laboratory tests in assessing protein metabolism.

II. **Laboratory analytes associated with protein metabolism** **(30 minutes)**
   - Description of common laboratory tests related to protein metabolism, including:
     - Total protein and albumin levels
     - Serum protein electrophoresis
     - Urinary protein analysis
     - Nitrogen balance studies
   - Explanation of the principles and methodologies behind each test.

III. **Interpretation of laboratory results** **(30 minutes)**
- Step-by-step guide to interpreting laboratory results in protein metabolism tests.
- Discussion on normal reference ranges and significance of abnormal findings.
- Illustration of interpretation guidelines using case examples.

IV. **Clinical significance and case studies** **(15 minutes)**
- Present clinical case studies related to abnormal protein metabolism test results.
- Facilitate a discussion on the clinical implications and management strategies for abnormal findings.

V. **Future directions and research** **(5 minutes)**
- Brief overview of emerging trends and advancements in laboratory testing for protein metabolism.
- Encouragement for students to explore research opportunities and advancements in this field.

VI. **Conclusion and recap** **(5 minutes)**
- Summary of key points covered in the lecture.
- Emphasis on the importance of accurate interpretation of laboratory results in clinical practice.
- Encouragement for students to continue learning and staying updated on developments in laboratory diagnostics.

SPOTS/CLINICAL CASES

CASE 1: KWASHIORKOR

Age, gender	4-year-old, male
Complains	Weakness, swelling on the body, lethargy
On examination	Pitting pedal edema, muscular atrophy, abdomen is distended, hepatomegaly
	Blood report
Total protein	4.8 g/dL (N: 6.5–8 g/dL)
Albumin	1.7 g/dL (N: 4–6 g/dL)
Random sugar	105 mg% (N: 90–140 mg%)
Total cholesterol	97 mg% (N: <200 mg%)
What is the diagnosis?	Kwashiorkor
Reasons	Disorder caused due to proper calorie intake but less protein intake in the diet
Characteristics	• Moon face • Bilateral extremity swelling • Protruded abdomen • Atrophy of muscles • Observed mostly in children till 5 years
Main cause	Staple diet of maize, rice cassava
Reason behind pedal edema	Fluid misbalance between hydrostatic and oncotic pressure across the walls of capillaries Albumin maintains the oncotic pressure and keeps the fluid within the vasculature, here the albumin levels are below than normal

CASE 2: MARASMUS

Age, gender	1-year-old, male
Complains	Lethargy, eyes shrunken, weight loss
On examination	Rib cage was prominent
	Blood report
Total protein	6.3 g/dL (N: 6.5–8 g/dL)
Albumin	3.2 g/dL (N: 4–6 g/dL)
Random sugar	70 mg% (N: 90–140 mg%)
Minerals	Deficient

Contd...

Contd...

What is the diagnosis?	Marasmus
Reasons	Malnutrition disorder caused due to improper carbohydrate as well as protein intake in the diet
	Comparison between two
Kwashiorkor	**Marasmus**
Disorder caused due to proper calorie intake but less protein intake in the diet	Malnutrition disorder caused due to improper carbohydrate as well as protein intake in the diet
More prevalent in children between age of 6 months to 3 years	Common in children under the of 1 year
Subcutaneous fat observed	Subcutaneous fat not observed
Edema present	Edema absent
Enlarged fatty liver	Fatty liver absent
No prominent ribs	Prominent ribs
Lethargy	Alert but irritable
Muscle wasting not seen/mild	Severe muscle wasting
Appetite poor	Voracious feeding
Treatment—requires proper proteins in the diet	Treatment—requires carbohydrates, proteins and fats in the diet

CASE 3: NEPHROTIC SYNDROME

Age, gender	5-year-old, male
On admission	Puffiness on face, mainly in the morning, weakness, poor appetite
	Blood report
Total protein	5 g/dL (N: 6.5–8 g/dL)
Albumin	2.7 g/dL (N: 4–6 g/dL)
Globulin	2.6 g/dL (N: 1.5–3.5 g/dL)
Total cholesterol	480 mg% (N: <20 mg%)
Blood urea	100 mg% (N: 10–40 mg%)
Serum creatinine	1.9 mg% (N: <1 mg%)
Urinary total protein 24 hour sample	4.7 g (N: <150 mg%)
What is the diagnosis?	Nephrotic syndrome
Reasons	Nephrotic syndrome is a group of disorders characterized by loss of proteins in the urine
Reason of puffiness on face	Loss of albumin from plasma leading to fluid exudation from intravascular space
Two types	Primary and secondary
Primary childhood nephrotic syndrome characteristics	Focal segmental glomerulonephritis Membranoproliferative glomerulonephritis
Secondary childhood nephrotic syndrome characteristics	Associated with other disorders, such as diabetes, IgA vasculitic, hepatitis, lupus, malaria, HIV, streptococcal infection
	Diagnostic criterion for nephrotic syndrome
Proteinuria >3 g/Dl	
Hypoalbuminemia	
Hypercholesterolemia	
Edema	
Hypertension	

CASE 4: ALCOHOLIC LIVER DISORDER

Age, gender	50-year-old, male, chronic alcoholic
Complains	Weight loss, weakness, nausea, vomiting, pain in right upper quadrant
On examination	Ascites, hepatomegaly, yellow discoloration of eyes, clubbing of fingers, palmar erythema
	Blood report
Total protein	5.6 g/dL (N: 6.5–8 g/dL)
Albumin	2.7 g/dL (N: 4–6 g/dL)
Total bilirubin	1.9 mg%
Conjugated bilirubin	0.9 mg%
Unconjugated bilirubin	1.0 mg%
AST	412 IU/L
ALT	206 IU/L
AST: ALT ratio	2:1
GGT	375 IU/L
PT	Increased
What is the diagnosis?	Alcoholic cirrhosis
Reasons	Fibrosis of liver, reduced mass of liver, disrupted LFT's
Cause of edema, ascites	Albumin synthesis is reduced, causing edema and ascites
Cause of increased PT	Disrupted LFT's leads to impaired posttranslational modifications of clotting factors
Cause of increased GGT	Proliferation of endoplasmic reticulum
De-Ritis index/AST:ALT ratio: Normal is 1:1 as AST, ALT concentration in the plasma is almost same (30–40 IU/L)	2:1 indicates alcoholic liver disease ALT is present in cytoplasm of hepatocytes alone AST is present in hepatocyte cytoplasm as well as mitochondria
Isoenzymes of AST	Cytosolic—cAST Mitochondrial—mAST (more prevalent)

CASE 5: MULTIPLE MYELOMA

Age, gender	59-year-old, male, employed in leather industry
Complains	Pain in bones, weakness, numbness of lower limbs
History	Relapsing infection of lungs
On examination	Anemia
	Blood report
Total protein	7.6 g/dL (N: 6.5–8 g/dL)
Albumin	3.1 g/dL (N: 4–6 g/dL)
Globulin	4.7 g/dL
Serum urea	59 mg%
Serum creatinine	1.7 mg%
ALP	57 IU/L
Serum total calcium	11.8 mg%
Hb	7.2 g/dl
Serum uric acid	7.9 mg%
X-ray skull	Punched out lesion
Protein electrophoresis	M band seen

Contd...

Contd...

Urine	Bence-Jones protein present
What is the diagnosis?	Multiple myeloma (malignant proliferation of plasma cell derived from one clone)
Reasons	Susceptibility of infections are common (due to diffuse hypogammaglobulinemia)
Reason behind punched out lesion in skull	Osteoclastic activating factors lead to osteolytic lesions
Reason for anemia	Expanding tumor cell displaces normal marrow and decreased production of erythropoietin by the kidney

OSCE

1. **Scenario: Protein-energy malnutrition (PEM)—low serum albumin and total protein**
   Case: A 4-year-old child presents with symptoms of slow growth/edema/wasting of muscles.
   Serum albumin: 2.1 g/dL (normal: 3.5–5.0 g/dL)
   Total protein: 4.4 g/dL (normal: 6.0–8.0 g/dL)
   Blood glucose: 82 mg/dL (normal: 70–100 mg/dL)
   Question: What does this interpret in the child?
   Interpretation: The low serum albumin along with total protein suggest protein-energy malnutrition that is mainly observed in states such as kwashiorkor/marasmus.
   In kwashiorkor, the main problem is protein deficiency despite of adequate calorie intake, resulting in hypoalbuminemia/edema, and wasting muscles.
   Marasmus specifically includes both calories as well as protein deficiency but is rarely show significant edema.
   Diagnosis: Protein-energy malnutrition more probability of kwashiorkor as there are symptoms of edema/less albumin.
   Next Steps: Urgent intervention by protein supplementation/caloric intake /micronutrient correction. Hospitalization for proper supportive therapy.
2. **Scenario: Liver disease—elevated serum aminotransferases and decreased albumin**
   Case: A 52-year-old man presented with history of consuming alcohol is suffering from jaundice/ascites/peripheral edema.
   Serum albumin: 2.4 g/dL (normal: 3.5–5.0 g/dL)
   Serum AST: 126 U/L (normal: 5–40 U/L)
   Serum ALT: 147U/L (normal: 7–56 U/L)
   Total protein: 5.3 g/dL (normal: 6.0–8.0 g/dL)
   Question: What do the high AST and ALT, and decreased albumin indicate?
   Interpretation: The high AST/ALT and low albumin suggest liver dysfunctioning mainly because of chronic liver disease like alcoholic cirrhosis.
   AST and ALT are the enzymes that are released from damaged hepatocytes (concentrations become elevated in hepatic damage).
   The low albumin level is suggestive of improper liver protein synthesis, a highlight for cirrhosis.
   Diagnosis: Chronic liver disease mainly alcoholic cirrhosis with improper liver functions.
   Next Steps: The patient must go for liver function tests, get his ascitic fluid analyzed for liver imaging. Treatment can be avoiding alcohol plus nutritional support, and treating ascites.
3. **Scenario: Nephrotic syndrome—increased urinary protein excretion**
   Case: A 7-year-old child shows symptoms of generalized edema/frothy urine. Urine tests was done:
   Urine protein: 510 mg/dL (normal: <30 mg/dL)
   Urine creatinine: 2.1 g/dL (normal: 0.1–0.2 g/dL)
   Serum albumin: 2.1 g/dL (normal: 3.5–5.0 g/dL)
   Serum cholesterol: 355 mg/dL (normal: 140–200 mg/dL)
   Question: What does this interpret?
   Interpretation: The elevated urinary protein less serum albumin/high serum cholesterol is consistent with disorder of nephrotic syndrome, a state where there can be proteinuria/hypoalbuminemia/hyperlipidemia.
   In nephrotic syndrome, the kidneys excrete protein, mainly albumin, resulting in edema. The liver compensates these conditions through increasing cholesterol formation which ends up in hyperlipidemia.
   Diagnosis: Nephrotic syndrome.
   Next Steps: Further evaluate for underlying cause, that can be minimal change disease or focal segmental glomerulosclerosis/membrane nephropathy. Treatment: Focus on corticosteroids/diuretics/lipid-lowering drugs

4. **Scenario: Acute inflammation—increased C-reactive protein (CRP) and fibrinogen**
Case: A 41-year-old woman having history of rheumatoid arthritis shows symptoms of fever, lethargy swelling in joints
C-Reactive Protein: 51 mg/L (normal: <10 mg/L)
Fibrinogen: 452 mg/dL (normal: 200–400 mg/dL)
Serum albumin: 3.1 g/dL (normal: 3.5–5.0 g/dL)
Question: What does this suggest?
Interpretation: The high CRP/fibrinogen and decreased albumin is indicative of acute inflammatory response, that can be presented in rheumatoid arthritis.
CRP/fibrinogen: Acute-phase reactants which elevate in response to any kind of inflammation. The low serum albumin: Negative acute-phase protein, lowering down in inflammation.
Diagnosis: Acute inflammation because of rheumatoid arthritis flare-up.
Next Steps : Regularly keep monitoring inflammatory markers, treat rheumatoid arthritis.

5. **Scenario: Liver failure—low serum albumin and high ammonia**
Case: A 61-year-old patient having cirrhosis shows confusion/jaundice.
Serum albumin: 1.7 g/dL (normal: 3.5–5.0 g/dL)
Serum ammonia: 101 μmol/L (normal: 15–45 μmol/L)
Total bilirubin: 8.1 mg/dL (normal: 0.1–1.2 mg/dL)
Question: What does this interpret?
Interpretation: The decreased albumin/high ammonia suggests liver dysfunctioning mainly because of cirrhosis/liver failure. The liver is not synthesizing albumin, resulting in hypoalbuminemia plus edema. The high ammonia is because the liver is not able to detoxify it and accumulation, of ammonia is causing hepatic encephalopathy/confusion.
Diagnosis: Cirrhosis along with hepatic encephalopathy.
Next Steps: Manage hepatic encephalopathy with lactulose/restrict protein intake manage ascites. Liver transplantation when required.

CLINICAL MCQS

1. **A 56-year-old man shows fatigue/edema/frothy urine. Serum albumin: 2.1 g/dL (reference: 3.5–5.0 g/dL), 24-hour urinary protein excretion: 4.6 g/day (reference: <150 mg/day). What is the diagnosis?**
   a. Chronic kidney damage
   b. Acute liver disease
   c. Nephrotic syndrome
   d. Kwashiorkor

   Answer: c. Nephrotic syndrome

2. **A 46-year-old woman shows with symptoms of muscle weakness. Plasma ammonia: 90 μmol/L (reference: 10–50 μmol/L), serum urea: 10 mg/dL (reference: 15–40 mg/dL). Which condition is linked with these findings?**
   a. Urea cycle disorder
   b. Hepatic cell encephalopathy
   c. Renal failure
   d. Hyperammonemia

   Answer: a. Urea cycle disorder

3. **A 5-year-old child presents with developmental delay, "musty" odor. High plasma phenylalanine, low tyrosine levels. What is diagnosis?**
   a. Tyrosinemia
   b. Maple syrup disease
   c. Phenylketonuria
   d. Homocystinuria

   Answer: c. Phenylketonuria

4. **A patient with chronic liver disease exhibits: serum albumin: 2.9 g/dL (reference: 3.5–5.0 g/dL), total protein: 5.1 g/dL (reference: 6.0–8.0 g/dL), prothrombin time: 21 seconds (reference: 11–13 seconds), Which lab parameter exhibits synthetic liver function?**
   a. Serum albumin
   b. Total protein
   c. Prothrombin time
   d. ACP

   Answer: c. Prothrombin time

5. **A newborn has high citrulline concentration plus high ammonia. What enzyme deficiency is present?**
   a. Arginosuccinate lyase
   b. OTC
   c. Arginosuccinate synthetase
   d. Carbamoyl phosphate synthetase II

   Answer: c. Arginosuccinate synthetase

6. **A 58-year-old chronic alcoholic person shows confusion/tremors/high serum ammonia/normal serum creatinine level. What treatment is required for decreasing serum ammonia?**
   a. Fluids intravenously
   b. Lactulose
   c. High-protein intake advised
   d. Hemodialysis

   Answer: c. Lactulose

7. **A 28-year-old boy presents with bilateral lens dislocation, thrombosis, homocysteine levels are high. What vitamin deficiency is present?**
   a. Vitamin B5
   b. Vitamin B6
   c. Folic acid
   d. All mentioned above

   Answer: d. All mentioned above

8. **A 34-year-old man presents with hyperpigmented skin/joint pain/homogentisic acid positive in urine. What is the diagnosis?**
   a. Alkaptonuria
   b. MSUD
   c. Phenylketonuria
   d. Tyrosinosis

   Answer: a. Alkaptonuria

9. **A patient shows serum total protein level: 4.5 g/dL (reference: 6.0–8.0 g/dL) with normal globulin. Which condition is present?**
   a. Acute inflammation
   b. Multiple myeloma
   c. Hypoalbuminemia
   d. Hyperglobulinemia

   Answer: c. Hypoalbuminemia

10. **A patient with burns has high serum urea, low serum albumin. What is the reason of hyperuremia?**
    a. Urea cycle disease
    b. Increased protein catabolism
    c. Alkaptonuria
    d. Renal disease

    Answer: b. Increased protein catabolism

VIVA VOCE

Q1. What does high serum albumin level indicate/what is underlying causes?
Follow-up: How to interpret a decreased serum albumin level in a patient?

Q2. What are the important findings in a 24-hour urine collection for protein/how they diagnose nephrotic syndrome?
Follow-up: What is the importance of proteinuria in relation to kidney damage?

Q3. What does abnormal ratio of albumin to globulin in a serum protein electrophoresis indicate?
Follow-up: Interpret monoclonal gammopathy in serum protein electrophoresis?

Q4. Interpret high blood urea nitrogen/creatinine ratio on basis of kidney function?
Follow-up: What is reason behind raised BUN without a raise in creatinine?

Q5. What does a decreased total protein assay suggest/give important cause of hypoproteinemia?
Follow-up: Interpret a low total protein level and a normal albumin-to-globulin ratio?

SPOTTERS

Q1. Show serum protein electrophoresis exhibiting monoclonal spike (M-spike). What is the condition/which further tests can be done?
Multiple Myeloma/other plasma cell dyscrasias; Serum free light chains/bone marrow biopsy.

Q2. Show urine dipstick exhibiting positive result for protein that is 3+. What is the result indicative of/give causes of proteinuria?
Proteinuria, that suggests nephrotic syndrome/glomerulonephritis/kidney damage.

Q3. Show serum albumin level highly low (<2.5 g/dL) and a normal globulin level. What does this interpret?
Hypoalbuminemia, that may suggest liver disease/nephrotic syndrome/malnutrition.

Q4. Show serum BUN highly increased but creatinine is normal. What does this interpret and give causes?
Prerenal azotemia; because of dehydration/heart failure/ high protein consumption.

Q5. Show 24-hour urine collection exhibiting >3.5 g of protein. What condition is indicated/next step for management?
Nephrotic syndrome; Checking for reasons like diabetic nephropathy/minimal change disease/membranous nephropathy.

REFLECTION

Interpret laboratory results of analytes associated with protein metabolism also describe the clinical interpretation of tests done in protein metabolism.

39

CHAPTER

Interpretation of Laboratory Result: Lipid Metabolism

COMPETENCY

BC14.19: Explain the basis and rationale of biochemical tests done in various conditions (lipid metabolism).

LEARNING OBJECTIVES

After reading this chapter, the readers should be able to:

- Interpret laboratory results of analytes associated with lipid metabolism.
- Understand the significance of lipid-related parameters in health and disease.
- Apply knowledge of lipid metabolism to clinical scenarios.
- Discuss on certain lab reports related to lipid profile.
- Can do tests done to find out dyslipidemia and its type and the rationale behind it.

BLUE PRINT

Understanding Laboratory Results in Lipid Metabolism

Objective

By the end of the lecture, students should be able to:

1. Interpret laboratory results of analytes associated with lipid metabolism.
2. Understand the significance of lipid-related parameters in health and disease.
3. Apply knowledge of lipid metabolism to clinical scenarios.

Duration: *90 minutes*

Materials Needed

1. PowerPoint presentation or visual aids
2. Whiteboard and markers
3. Handouts with key lipid-related laboratory parameters and their interpretation
4. Clinical case studies related to lipid metabolism

Outline

I. **Introduction to lipid-related laboratory parameters** **(10 minutes)**
   - Overview of the lecture's objectives and agenda.
   - Explanation of the importance of lipid-related laboratory tests in clinical practice.

II. **Common lipid profile tests** **(20 minutes)**
   - Description of common lipid profile tests, including:
     - Total cholesterol
     - LDL cholesterol
     - HDL cholesterol

  - Triglycerides
  - Lipoprotein(a) [Lp(a)]
- Explanation of reference ranges and interpretation of results for each parameter.

III. **Additional lipid-related tests** **(20 minutes)**
- Discussion on additional lipid-related tests, including:
  - Apolipoproteins (apoB, apoA1)
  - Lipoprotein particle size and density
  - Lipid ratios (e.g., LDL/HDL ratio)
- Interpretation of results and clinical significance of these tests.

IV. **Clinical correlation and case studies** **(30 minutes)**
- Present clinical case studies related to lipid metabolism disorders.
- Facilitate a discussion on how to interpret laboratory results in the context of specific clinical scenarios.

V. **Quality control and assurance** **(5 minutes)**
- Brief overview of quality control measures for lipid-related laboratory tests.
- Importance of accurate and reliable lipid testing for patient care.

VI. **Conclusion and recap** **(5 minutes)**
- Summary of key points covered in the lecture.
- Emphasis on the importance of interpreting lipid-related laboratory results in clinical practice.
- Encouragement for further study and research in lipid metabolism and laboratory medicine.

SPOTS/CLINICAL CASES

Lipid profile in healthy adults

TC	Desired	<200 mg%
	Border	200–239 mg%
	High	>240 mg%
HDL-C	40–75 mg%	
LDL-C	Normal	<100 mg%
	Near to normal	100–129 mg%
	Borderline	130–159 mg%
	High	160–189 mg%
	Extremely high	>190 mg%
TG	60–150 mg%	
VLDL	<40 mg%	
FFA	200–800 micromole/liter	
Lipoprotein (a)	0–30 mg%	

Friedewald equation: Method for LDL-C estimation by calculation

LDL-C	[TC]–[HDL cholesterol]–[TAG/5]
	Where TAG/5 is VLDL cholesterol because TAG is approximately 5 times to that of cholesterol in VLDL
When not to apply this formula?	Sample having TAG is >400 mg%
	Chylomicron in the non-fasting sample can vary TAG
	Type III hyperlipoproteinemia (VLDL composition is not normal, so cannot apply TAG/5)

LAB REPORT 1

Age	46 years
Complain	Yellow nodules around the eye for last 4 months
Lipid profile	
TC	396 mg%
TG	150 mg%
HDL-C	30 mg%
LDL-C	325 mg%
VLDL	30 mg%
Interpret your report	
Diagnosis	Familial hypercholesterolemia—Type II a hyperlipoproteinemia
Heterozygous type	Manifests only in adults, prevalence—1:500
Homozygous type	Manifests only in children, prevalence—1:1 million
Causes	LDL clearance is defective, due to LDL receptor mutation/mutation of Apo B 100 of LDL
Characteristics	Tendon xanthomas
	Xanthelasma
	Vascular defect

LAB REPORT 2

Age	40 years
Complain	Acute pancreatitis
Lipid profile	
TC	190 mg%
TG	355 mg%
HDL-C	34 mg%
LDL-C	98 mg%
VLDL	76 mg%
Interpret your report	
Diagnosis	Isolated hypertriglyceridemia presenting with acute pancreatitis:
	Either type I familial hypertriglyceridemia/Type V hyperlipoproteinemia
Type I hyperlipidemia	Deficiency of enzyme—lipoprotein lipase resulting in increased VLDL and chylomicron
Type V hyperlipidemia	Deficiency of Apo C resulting in increased VLDL and chylomicron

LAB REPORT 3

Age	40 years
History	Cardiac disease
Lipid profile	
TC	340 mg%
TG	355 mg%
HDL-C	39 mg%
LDL-C	240 mg%
VLDL	72 mg%

Contd....

Contd....

Interpret your report	
Diagnosis	Type II b hyperlipoproteinemia (Familial combined hyperlipidemia)
Cause	1. More secretion of VLDL from liver resulting in high TG also
	2. Improper clearance of LDL from the plasma
Characteristics	High TC
	High LDL-C
	High TG

LAB REPORT 4

Age	45 years, healthy male, routine test
History	Nil
Lipid profile	
TC	250 mg%
TG	255 mg%
HDL-C	43 mg%
LDL-C	140 mg%
VLDL	52 mg%
Lipoprotein electrophoresis	Broad beta band
Interpret your report	
Diagnosis	Type III hyperlipoproteinemia/Familial dysbetalipoproteinemia
Characteristics	Generally asymptomatic till the development of vascular disorder
	Palmer/Tuberous xanthoma formation may be there

LAB REPORT 5

Age	55 years
History	Diabetic
Lipid profile	
TC	185 mg%
TG	355 mg%
HDL-C	43 mg%
LDL-C	79 mg%
VLDL	72 mg%
Interpret your report	
Diagnosis	Type IV hyperlipoproteinemia
Cause	More secretion of VLDL from liver because of idiopathic reason resulting in high TG also
Characteristics	Asymptomatic/vascular features may be there

OSCE

1. **Scenario: Hyperlipidemia—elevated total cholesterol and LDL**
   Case: A 55-year-old male lipid profile reveals:
   Total cholesterol: 2807 mg/dL (normal: <200 mg/dL)
   Low-density lipoprotein (LDL): 1901 mg/dL (normal: <100 mg/dL)

High-density lipoprotein (HDL): 34 mg/dL (normal: >40 mg/dL)
Triglycerides: 200 mg/dL (normal: <150 mg/dL)
Question: What do the elevated total cholesterol and LDL, along with low HDL, suggest in this patient?
Interpretation: The elevated total cholesterol high LDL and low HDL are suggestive of dyslipidemia, specifically hyperlipidemia. High LDL is a key risk factor towards atherosclerosis plus cardiovascular diseases as it increases cholesterol in the walls of the arteries.
Low HDL reduces the body's ability to remove excess cholesterol from the bloodstream.
Elevated triglycerides contribute even more towards risk of CVD.
Diagnosis: Hyperlipidemia with a dyslipidemic profile (high LDL, low HDL, high triglycerides).
Next steps: The patient must be assessed for risk factors like high blood pressure/diabetes/cardiovascular diseases. Lifestyle modification by diet and exercise/statin therapy might be indicated looking at the overall cardiovascular risk.

2. **Scenario: Familial hypercholesterolemia—marked elevation of LDL**
Case: A 30-year-old female with a family history of heart disease and presents with the following lipid profile:
Total cholesterol: 331 mg/dL (normal: <200 mg/dL)
LDL: 261 mg/dL (normal: <100 mg/dL)
HDL: 44 mg/dL (normal: >40 mg/dL)
Triglycerides: 140 mg/dL (normal: <150 mg/dL)
Question: What does the marked raise of LDL suggest?
Interpretation: The marked raise of LDL with a normal HDL plus little raised triglycerides is indicative of familial hypercholesterolemia.
FH: Inherited state when there is a deficiency/malfunction of the LDL receptor, resulting in markedly raised LDL cholesterol concentration.
Individuals with FH have a significantly increased risk of early atherosclerotic cardiovascular disease (ASCVD) due to the persistent high LDL levels.
Diagnosis: Familial hypercholesterolemia (FH).
Next steps: Genetic testing for LDL receptor mutations/early initiation of lipid-lowering therapy like statins/lifestyle modifications/low-cholesterol diet.

3. **Scenario: Hypertriglyceridemia—elevated triglycerides**
Case: A 50-year-old man with type 2 diabetes plus obesity presents with:
Total cholesterol: 246 mg/dL (normal: <200 mg/dL)
LDL: 122 mg/dL (normal: <100 mg/dL)
HDL: 34 mg/dL (normal: >40 mg/dL)
Triglycerides: 404 mg/dL (normal: <150 mg/dL)
Question: What does this interpret?
Interpretation: The elevated triglyceride level in the context of low HDL and normal LDL suggests hypertriglyceridemia, which is associated with insulin resistance, type 2 diabetes, obesity.
Hypertriglyceridemia rises risk of pancreatitis/atherosclerosis.
Elevated triglycerides are marker of poor metabolic regulation in diabetes.
Diagnosis: Hypertriglyceridemia, associated with insulin resistance/obesity.
Next steps: The patient must focus on improving the glycemic control by lifestyle modifications/medications for decreasing TG's. Statins may be advised when a high risk of cardiovascular disease is present.

4. **Scenario: Secondary hyperlipidemia due to hypothyroidism—elevated cholesterol and LDL**
Case: A 62-year-old woman with complains of weight gain, fatigue, and dry skin is found to have:
Total cholesterol: 297 mg/dL (normal: <200 mg/dL)
LDL: 205 mg/dL (normal: <100 mg/dL)
HDL: 43 mg/dL (normal: >40 mg/dL)
Triglycerides: 188 mg/dL (normal: <150 mg/dL)
Thyroid function tests:
TSH: 16.0 mU/L (normal: 0.4–4.0 mU/L)
Free T4: 0.5 ng/dL (normal: 0.7–1.8 ng/dL)
Question: What does this interpret?
Interpretation: The elevated total cholesterol, LDL, and triglycerides, along with low HDL, in the context of elevated TSH and low Free T4 suggest secondary hyperlipidemia because of hypothyroidism.
Hypothyroidism is well known to lead to increased cholesterol formation and decreased clearance of lipoproteins, resulting in elevated LDL plus total cholesterol.
Diagnosis: Hypothyroidism with secondary hyperlipidemia.
Next steps: Initiate thyroid hormone replacement (levothyroxine) for normalizing thyroid functions. The lipid profile will improve with treatment of the thyroid disorder. Statin therapy might be considered if cardiovascular risk remains more.

5. **Scenario: Fatty liver disease—elevated liver enzymes and lipid profile changes**
Case: A 39-year-old male with a history of alcohol consumption and obesity presents with:
Total cholesterol: 239 mg/dL (normal: <200 mg/dL)
LDL: 155 mg/dL (normal: <100 mg/dL)
HDL: 37 mg/dL (normal: >40 mg/dL)
Triglycerides: 259 mg/dL (normal: <150 mg/dL)
Liver function tests:
AST: 71 U/L (normal: 5–40 U/L)
ALT: 81 U/L (normal: 7–56 U/L)
Question: What do this interpret?
Interpretation: The elevated liver enzymes plus hyperlipidemia are indicative of non-alcoholic fatty liver disease/alcoholic liver disease.
Both these states can result in elevated liver enzymes and are linked with dyslipidemia, specifically hypertriglyceridemia and raised LDL.
NAFLD is very common in overweight and obese and along with insulin resistance, while alcoholic fatty liver disease is associated with alcohol consumption.
Diagnosis: Likely non-alcoholic fatty liver disease/alcoholic fatty liver disease.
Next steps: Perform more liver imaging/consider liver biopsy. Focus on weight management alcohol avoidance managing lipid levels with statins/fibrates.

VIVA VOCE

Q1. What are the reference ranges for lipid profile parameters?
Next question/Follow-up: How these values are different in high cardiovascular risk patients?

Q2. What is the importance of a high LDL/HDL ratio, and how it is associated with atherosclerosis?
Next question/Follow-up: Why is HDL taken as protective against CVD?

Q3. How to interpret a lipid profile exhibiting isolated hypertriglyceridemia?
Next question/Follow-up: What are the usual reasons/complications of severe hypertriglyceridemia?

Q4. What does a raised lipoprotein(a) level suggest in a lipid profile?
Next question/Follow-up: Why is lipoprotein(a) taken to be independent risk factor for CVD?

Q5. Differentiate between primary/secondary reasons behind dyslipidemia on basis of lab results.
Next question/Follow-up: Which endocrine disorders cause secondary dyslipidemia?

SPOTTERS

Q1. Show a report of lipid profile with elevated LDL/decreased HDL/elevated total cholesterol. What is the interpretation/give major risk linked with it?

Dyslipidemia; High risk of atherosclerosis plus cardiovascular disease.

Q2. Show a report of lipid profile exhibiting very high triglyceride levels that is >1000 mg/dL. What is the probable diagnosis/major complication?

Severe hypertriglyceridemia; Complication of acute pancreatitis.

Q3. Show a graph with inverse relationship between HDL/cardiovascular risk. What is the importance of HDL in lipid metabolism/cardiovascular health?

HDL is protective against atherosclerosis by mechanism of reverse cholesterol transport.

Q4. Show electrophoresis/ultracentrifugation pattern exhibiting high chylomicrons. What is the condition/enzyme deficiency involved?

Familial chylomicronemia syndrome; deficient Lipoprotein lipase.

Q5. Show lipid profile of a patient exhibiting nephrotic syndrome with elevated LDL and high triglycerides. Why does nephrotic syndrome lead to this lipid abnormality?

Loss of albumin increases hepatic lipoprotein formation resulting in secondary dyslipidemia.

REFLECTION

Discussion on certain lab reports related to lipid profile also describe test done to find out dyslipidemia and its type and the rationale behind it. Describe the clinical interpretation of the tests done in lipid metabolism.

40 CHAPTER

Interpretation of Laboratory Result: Purine Nucleotide Metabolism

COMPETENCY

BC14.19: Explain the basis and rationale of biochemical tests done in various conditions (purine nucleotide metabolism).

LEARNING OBJECTIVES

After reading this chapter, the readers should be able to:
- Understand the laboratory tests used in the diagnosis of gout and Lesch–Nyhan syndrome.
- Interpret the results of these tests in the context of the biochemical abnormalities associated with each condition.
- Discuss the clinical implications of abnormal laboratory findings in patients with gout and Lesch–Nyhan syndrome.

BLUE PRINT

Interpretation of Laboratory Results of Purine Nucleotide Metabolism

Objective

By the end of the lecture, students should be able to:
1. Understand the laboratory tests used in the diagnosis of gout and Lesch–Nyhan syndrome.
2. Interpret the results of these tests in the context of the biochemical abnormalities associated with each condition.
3. Discuss the clinical implications of abnormal laboratory findings in patients with gout and Lesch–Nyhan syndrome.

Duration: ***60 minutes***

Materials Needed

1. Presentation slides outlining laboratory tests and results for gout and Lesch–Nyhan syndrome.
2. Handouts summarizing key points and case studies.
3. Whiteboard and markers.

Outline

I. **Introduction to gout and Lesch–Nyhan syndrome** **(5 minutes)**
- Introduction to the biochemical basis and clinical manifestations of gout and Lesch–Nyhan syndrome.
- Overview of the objectives and structure of the lecture.

II. **Laboratory tests for gout** **(20 minutes)**
- Description of laboratory tests used in the diagnosis of gout, including serum uric acid levels, synovial fluid analysis, and imaging studies.
- Interpretation of abnormal laboratory findings and their significance in the diagnosis and management of gout.
- Discussion of differential diagnoses and potential confounding factors.

III. **Laboratory tests for Lesch–Nyhan syndrome** **(20 minutes)**
- Overview of laboratory tests used in the diagnosis of Lesch–Nyhan syndrome, including urine uric acid levels, hypoxanthine-guanine phosphoribosyltransferase (HGPRT) enzyme activity assay, and genetic testing.

- Interpretation of abnormal laboratory results and their implications for the diagnosis and management of Lesch-Nyhan syndrome.
- Discussion of genetic counseling and family screening considerations.

IV. **Case studies and examples** **(10 minutes)**
- Presentation of case studies or examples illustrating laboratory findings in patients with gout and Lesch-Nyhan syndrome.
- Facilitation of discussion on the interpretation of laboratory results and their clinical significance.

V. **Clinical management and follow-up** **(5 minutes)**
- Overview of treatment options and management strategies for patients with gout and Lesch-Nyhan syndrome.
- Discussion of the role of laboratory monitoring in disease management and follow-up care.

VI. **Recap and application** **(5 minutes)**
- Summary of key points covered in the lecture.
- Application of knowledge through case-based questions or scenarios.

VII. **Conclusion** **(5 minutes)**
- Concluding remarks on the importance of laboratory testing in the diagnosis and management of gout and Lesch-Nyhan syndrome.
- Encouragement for further study and research in the field of metabolic disorders.

CASE 1: GOUT

Age	47 years, consumed alcohol with nonvegetarian diet on previous day
Complains	Pain in right wrist and left metatarsophalangeal joint
	Blood report
Total protein	7.1 g/dL
Albumin	3.8 g/dL
Blood urea	39 mg%
Serum creatinine	1 mg%
Serum uric acid	8.9 mg%
Diagnosis	Acute attack of Gout
Gout	Acute/chronic arthritis because of deposition of monosodium urate crystals in joints and soft tissues
	Disease along with hyperuricemia because of metabolic defect in production of uric acid or impaired renal excretion affecting mainly elder males and postmenopausal females
Effect of alcohol	1. There is excess formation of adenosine monophosphate which is a precursor of uric acid, due to degradation of adenine nucleotide as a result of metabolism of ethanol to acetyl CoA 2. There is increased lactate level of blood due to alcohol metabolism which inhibits excretion of uric acid
Gold standard of diagnosis	Synovial fluid—observing monosodium urate crystals
Monosodium urate crystals	Negatively birefringent crystals
	When plane polarized light falls on these crystals, they show a characteristic color
When the axis of monosodium urate crystals is parallel to the polarizer	They appear yellow
When the axis of monosodium urate crystals is perpendicular instead of parallel again	They appear blue

CASE 2: LESCH–NYHAN SYNDROME

Age	3 years
Complains	Involuntary movements of upper limb, habit of biting lips and fingers, orange discoloration of diaper
	Blood report
Serum uric acid	9.1 mg%
Diagnosis	Lesch–Nyhan syndrome
Lesch–Nyhan syndrome	X-linked recessive disorder of purine metabolism, affecting only male children
Cause	Deficient enzyme—hypoxanthine guanine phosphoribosyl transferase (HGPRT)
Hypoxanthine guanine phosphoribosyl-transferase (HGPRT)	Enzyme of salvage pathway of purine nucleotide metabolism Excessive hypoxanthine is diverted for degradation and uric acid synthesis
Characteristics	• Spasticity • Choreoathetosis • Increase uric acid • Self-mutilation • Aggressive nature • Normal at birth, but in 6–8 months, show signs of progressive generalized spastic paresis and bilateral athetosis

OSCE

1. **Scenario: Gout—elevated uric acid**
   Case: A 58-year-old male presents with symptoms of acute pain/swelling in big toe, along with a history of heavy alcohol consumption. Serum uric acid: 9.6 mg/dL (normal: 3.5–7.2 mg/dL).
   Laboratory results:
   Serum uric acid: 9.6 mg/dL (high)
   Creatinine: 1.1 mg/dL (normal)
   Hemoglobin: 13 g/dL (normal)
   Question: What does this interpret?
   Interpretation: The elevated serum uric acid level is suggestive of gout, a state caused by the deposition of uric acid crystals in the joints, leading to inflammation/pain.
   Gout results from overproduction/underexcretion of uric acid, which is a product of purine metabolism.
   Alcohol usage in excess is a well-known risk factor for gout because it elevates purine turnover along with lowering uric acid excretion.
   Diagnosis: Gout, likely because of hyperuricemia.
   Next steps: Treatment must target on acute management with NSAIDs/colchicine/long-term management with allopurinol for reducing uric acid levels.
2. **Scenario: Lesch–Nyhan syndrome—hyperuricemia and neurological symptoms**
   Case: A 2-year-old child presents with symptoms of self-mutilating behavior that is biting of fingers and lips/developmental delay/gout-like symptoms. Uric acid: 13 mg/dL (normal: 3.5–7.2 mg/dL).
   Laboratory results:
   Serum uric acid: 13 mg/dL (high)
   Creatinine: 0.7 mg/dL (normal)
   Liver enzymes: Normal
   Question: What does this interpret?
   Interpretation: The elevated uric acid level of 13 mg/dL plus neurological symptoms are indicative of Lesch–Nyhan syndrome that is a genetic disorder caused by a deficiency of enzyme hypoxanthine-guanine phosphoribosyltransferase that is important in purine salvage.
   This deficiency may lead to increased purine degradation, resulting in elevated uric acid concentration.
   Neurological symptoms are characteristic of this condition/linked with dopamine dysfunction.
   Diagnosis: Lesch–Nyhan syndrome, a disease of purine metabolism.
   Next steps: The management must focus on the symptoms and control neurological problems and also allopurinol to control the uric acid levels.

3. **Scenario: Purine nucleotide metabolism in cancer—increased purine synthesis**
   Case: A 49-year-old woman with a recently diagnosed leukemia has elevated concentration of purine metabolites in her blood. Uric acid level: 11.1 mg/dL (normal: 3.5–7.2 mg/dL).
   Laboratory results:
   Serum uric acid: 11.1 mg/dL (high)
   Lactate dehydrogenase (LDH): 1210 U/L (elevated)
   White blood cell count: 16000/mm^3 (elevated)
   Question: What does this result interpret?
   Interpretation: The elevated uric acid in this leukemia patient is indicative of Tumor lysis syndrome that happens when very large amounts of purine nucleotides are released from the lysed cancer cells.
   The hydrolysis of purine nucleotides from rapidly multiplying cancer cells stimulates the formation of uric acid, leading to state of hyperuricemia.
   Lactate dehydrogenase is raised because of tissue breakdown plus leukocytosis is seen in leukemia.
   Diagnosis: Tumor lysis syndrome in the context of leukemia.
   Next steps: The patient must be managed with proper hydration/medications like allopurinol for avoiding acute renal failure because of uric acid crystal precipitation.
4. **Scenario: Hyperuricemia in chronic kidney disease**
   Case: A 65-year-old male with chronic kidney disease presents with the following symptoms: fatigue, joint pain, and swelling. uric acid: 9 mg/dL (normal: 3.5-7.2 mg/dL).
   Laboratory results:
   Serum uric acid: 9 mg/dL (high)
   Creatinine: 3.57 mg/dL (elevated)
   Glomerular filtration rate (GFR): 31 mL/min (decreased)
   Question: What does this indicate?
   Interpretation: The raised uric acid along with CKD is indicative of reduced renal excretion of uric acid due to defective renal function.
   In CKD, the kidneys are not able to excrete enough uric acid, leading to hyperuricemia.
   Hyperuricemia in CKD can result in gout plus kidney stones.
   Diagnosis: Hyperuricemia due to CKD.
   Next steps: The patient must be managed with urate-lowering treatment like allopurinol plus therapy of underlying kidney disorder. Careful follow up and proper monitoring of renal functions is important for preventing any further side effects.
5. **Scenario: De Novo purine synthesis—elevated purine derivatives**
   Case: A 5-year-old child with symptoms like failure to thrive, delayed development, along with signs of hyperactivity undergoes: Urine test exhibits high uric acid along with high xanthine levels.
   Laboratory results:
   Urinary uric acid: 22 mg/day (elevated)
   Urinary xanthine: 16 mg/day (elevated)
   Question: What does this interpret?
   Interpretation: The elevated urinary uric acid along with xanthine concentration suggest disorder in purine nucleotide metabolism, mostly xanthinuria, a rare inherited state because of deficiency enzyme xanthine dehydrogenase.
   This enzyme converts xanthine to form uric acid in the purine degradation metabolism. When this enzyme gets deficient, xanthine accumulates, starts excreting in the urine, and uric acid levels remain elevated.
   Diagnosis: Xanthinuria, a disease of purine metabolism.
   Next steps: The patient may need increased fluid intake for avoiding xanthine stones in the kidneys. Monitoring of urinary purine metabolites is significant.

CLINICAL MCQS

1. **A 49-year-old man presents with severe pain in big toe, uric acid level: 9.2 mg/dL (reference: 3.5–7.2 mg/dL). Synovial fluid analysis: needle-shaped crystals that are negatively birefringent in polarized light. What is the diagnosis?**
   a. Gout
   b. Pseudogout
   c. Rheumatoid arthritis
   d. Arthritis

   Answer: a. Gout

2. **A 7-month-old boy has frequent infections, low T, B lymphocytes, high deoxyadenosine triphosphate. Which enzyme deficiency is present?**
   a. Adenosine deaminase
   b. Hypoxanthine-guanine phosphoribosyltransferase
   c. Purine nucleoside phosphorylase
   d. Xanthine oxidase

   Answer: a. Adenosine deaminase
3. **A 36-year-old man presents with symptoms of kidney stones, uric acid is high in serum/urine pH: 5.0. What dietary recommendation will prevent formation of more stones?**
   a. More purine-rich food intake
   b. Alkalinize the urine with potassium citrate
   c. Restrict calcium
   d. Reduce consumption of fluids

   Answer: b. Alkalinize the urine with potassium citrate
4. **A patient with gout is taking treatment of allopurinol. Two weeks later, uric acid concentration is less and development of a maculopapular rash is seen. What is the mechanism here?**
   a. Inhibition of enzyme xanthine oxidase
   b. Stimulation of HGPRT
   c. Activation of purine nucleoside phosphorylase
   d. Stimulation of uric acid absorption

   Answer: a. Inhibition of enzyme xanthine oxidase
5. **A 11-year-old boy has habit of self-mutilating/gout/developmental delay/hyperuricemia, low HGPRT action. What is the likely diagnosis?**
   a. Lesch-Nyhan syndrome
   b. Arthritis
   c. Adenosine deaminase stimulation
   d. Purine nucleoside phosphorylase activation

   Answer: a. Lesch-Nyhan syndrome
6. **A patient with gout is prescribed with drug febuxostat, but serum uric acid levels are still high/urinary uric acid concentration is normal. What is the most likely underlying cause of their gout?**
   a. Over formation of uric acid
   b. Under excretion of uric acid
   c. Xanthinuria
   d. Enzyme activation in purine salvage

   Answer: b. Under excretion of uric acid
7. **A 29-year-old woman presents with a recurrent kidney stone, xanthine plus hypoxanthine are positive in urine, testing confirms xanthine oxidase deficiency. Which dietary modification is required?**
   a. Increase purine-rich food products
   b. Decrease purines in diet
   c. Increase vitamin C in diet
   d. Restrict protein consumption

   Answer: b. Decrease purines in diet
8. **A 9-year-old boy has gouty arthritis, neurological abnormalities, absent HGPRT enzyme activity. Which is a consequence/effect of this enzyme deficiency?**
   a. High purine synthesis
   b. Increased uric acid formation
   c. Decreased accumulation of adenosine
   d. Improper pyrimidine synthesis

   Answer: b. Increased uric acid formation
9. **A 6-year-old child presents with recurrent infections plus neurological dysfunction, low immunoglobulin and hypouricemia. What enzyme deficiency is most likely?**
   a. Purine nucleoside phosphorylase
   b. Adenosine deaminase
   c. HGPRT
   d. Xanthine oxidase

   Answer: a. Purine nucleoside phosphorylase

10. **A 53-year-old man with a history of gout shows symptoms of acute renal failure, significantly high serum uric acid, potassium, recently started chemotherapy for leukemia. What is the diagnosis?**
    a. Tumor lysis syndrome
    b. CKD
    c. Uric acid nephropathy
    d. Nephrolithiasis

    Answer: a. Tumor lysis syndrome

VIVA VOCE

Q1. What is the key cause of gout, and which joints get most affected?
Next question/Follow-up: Why is the first metatarsophalangeal joint the most affected site of gout?

Q2. What are the typical microscopic findings in synovial fluid assay of a gouty patient?
Next question/Follow-up: How does urate crystals different from calcium pyrophosphate crystals under polarized light?

Q3. What is the function of xanthine oxidase in gout, and how does allopurinol work?
Next question/Follow-up: Why should allopurinol not be initiates during an acute gout attack?

Q4. Discuss tophi, and where are they usually found in chronic gout?
Next question/Follow-up: Why does chronic gout result in destruction of joint?

Q5. What are the factors for developing gout, and what is the effect of diet in this scenario?
Next question/Follow-up: Why does alcohol consumption increase the risk of developing gout attacks?

Q6. What is the genetic concept of Lesch–Nyhan syndrome, and name enzyme that is deficient?
Next question/Follow-up: How does the deficiency of this enzyme result in hyperuricemia?

Q7. What are the characteristic features of Lesch–Nyhan Syndrome?
Next question/Follow-up: Why patients having Lesch–Nyhan syndrome show self-mutilation?

Q8. How is Lesch–Nyhan syndrome diagnosed?
Next question/Follow-up: Which biochemical markers are raised in this condition?

Q9. Why does Lesch–Nyhan syndrome result in neurological symptoms despite it is metabolic disorder?
Next question/Follow-up: What significance does purine metabolism has in brain function?

Q10. What are the therapy options for Lesch–Nyhan Syndrome, and how will they manage symptoms?
Next question/Follow-up: Why does allopurinol aids in controlling hyperuricemia but not the neurological symptoms?

SPOTTERS

Q1. Show an image of needle-shaped negatively birefringent crystals in polarized light. Identify the condition displayed/substance seen in this microscopy.

Gout; monosodium urate crystals.

Q2. Show a photo of a swollen/red/first metatarsophalangeal joint (Podagra). What is the interpretation/why is this joint usually affected?

Gout; affected because of low temperature/slow blood flow.

Q3. Show an X-ray exhibiting punched-out erosions along with overhanging edges. Identify this condition/characteristic radiological finding.

Chronic gout; Rat-bite erosions.

Q4. Show picture of a patient with tophi on the ear/elbow/fingers. What are these/their significance?

Tophi because of chronic gout, they represent monosodium urate crystal accumulation.

Q5. Show serum uric acid level chart having high elevated values. What condition is this/and what factors are causing it?

Hyperuricemia observed in gout, due to high purine consumption/kidney disease/enzyme defects.

Q6. Image of a child showing self-mutilation injuries on lips/fingers. What is syndrome and what are the biochemical defects that are causing it?

Lesch–Nyhan syndrome; Enzyme—HGPRT deficiency.

Q7. Show photo of orange sand-like crystals in a diaper (they are uric acid crystals). What is the condition/why it occurs?

Lesch–Nyhan syndrome; Because of excessive uric acid excretion.

Q8. Show a pedigree chart exhibiting X-linked recessive inheritance pattern. What metabolic disorder follows this inheritance, and what is the reason?

Lesch–Nyhan syndrome; deficient HGPRT enzyme.

Q9. Show MRI scan with basal ganglia abnormalities. What disorder can lead to these changes, and how does it link to neurological symptoms?

Lesch–Nyhan syndrome; Dysfunctional purine metabolism affecting basal ganglia, resulting in movement disorders.

Q10. Show chemical pathway diagram of purine metabolism focusing HGPRT enzyme. What disorder results from the deficient focused enzyme, and what are important features?

Lesch–Nyhan syndrome; Hyperuricemia, neurological dysfunction/self-mutilation.

REFLECTION

Discuss the laboratory results of analytes associated with gout and Lesch-Nyhan syndrome also describe the clinical interpretation of the tests done in purine nucleotide metabolism.

41

CHAPTER

Clinical Manifestations of Deficiencies Associated with Vitamins and Minerals

COMPETENCY

BC14.19: Explain the basis and rationale of biochemical tests done in various conditions (vitamins and minerals).

LEARNING OBJECTIVES

After reading this chapter, the readers should be able to:

- Describe the clinical manifestation of deficiencies associated with vitamins and minerals.
- Understand the biochemical roles of vitamins in the body.
- Explain the manifestations of vitamin deficiencies.
- Discuss the importance of adequate vitamin intake for maintaining health.
- Understand the importance of mineral metabolism for overall health.
- Identify and describe common disorders associated with mineral metabolism.
- Discuss the etiology, clinical manifestations, diagnosis, and management of these disorders.

BLUE PRINT

Biochemical Role of Vitamins and Manifestations of Deficiency

Objective

By the end of the lecture, students should be able to:

1. Understand the biochemical roles of vitamins in the body.
2. Explain the manifestations of vitamin deficiencies.
3. Discuss the importance of adequate vitamin intake for maintaining health.

Duration: ***60 minutes***

Materials Needed

1. Presentation slides outlining the biochemical roles of vitamins and manifestations of deficiency.
2. Handouts summarizing key points and case studies.
3. Whiteboard and markers.

Outline

I. **Introduction to vitamins** **(5 minutes)**
- Introduction to the importance of vitamins in maintaining health and well-being.
- Overview of the objectives and structure of the lecture.

II. **Water-soluble vitamins** **(25 minutes)**
- Description of water-soluble vitamins (e.g., vitamin C and B-complex vitamins).
- Explanation of their biochemical roles in metabolism, including enzyme cofactors and antioxidants.
- Discussion of the manifestations of deficiency for each water-soluble vitamin.

III. **Fat-soluble vitamins** **(25 minutes)**
- Overview of fat-soluble vitamins (e.g., vitamin A, D, E, and K).
- Explanation of their roles in various physiological processes, such as vision, bone health, and blood clotting.
- Discussion of the clinical manifestations of deficiency for each fat-soluble vitamin.

IV. **Case studies and examples** **(5 minutes)**
- Presentation of case studies or examples illustrating the biochemical roles of vitamins and manifestations of deficiency.
- Facilitation of discussion on the importance of recognizing and addressing vitamin deficiencies.

V. **Clinical implications and dietary recommendations** **(5 minutes)**
- Discussion of the clinical implications of vitamin deficiencies and their impact on health.
- Overview of dietary recommendations and supplementation strategies for preventing vitamin deficiencies.

VI. **Recap and application** **(5 minutes)**
- Summary of key points covered in the lecture.
- Application of knowledge through case-based questions or scenarios.

VII. **Conclusion** **(5 minutes)**
- Concluding remarks on the significance of understanding the biochemical roles of vitamins and recognizing deficiencies.
- Encouragement for further study and research in the field of nutrition and metabolic health.

BLUE PRINT

Mineral Metabolism

Objective

By the end of the lecture, students should be able to:
1. Understand the importance of mineral metabolism for overall health.
2. Identify and describe common disorders associated with mineral metabolism.
3. Discuss the etiology, clinical manifestations, diagnosis, and management of these disorders.

Duration: *60 minutes*

Materials Needed

1. Presentation slides outlining disorders associated with mineral metabolism.
2. Handouts summarizing key points and tables listing mineral metabolism disorders.
3. Clinical case studies or examples illustrating each disorder.
4. Whiteboard and markers for interactive explanations.

Outline

I. **Introduction to mineral metabolism disorders** **(10 minutes)**
- Introduction to the significance of mineral metabolism for physiological processes.
- Overview of the objectives and structure of the lecture.

II. **Disorders of calcium metabolism** **(15 minutes)**
- Description of disorders such as hypercalcemia, hypocalcemia, osteoporosis, and hyperparathyroidism.
- Explanation of etiology, clinical manifestations, diagnostic criteria, and management strategies for each disorder.

III. **Disorders of phosphorus metabolism** **(15 minutes)**
- Discussion of disorders including hyperphosphatemia, hypophosphatemia, and disorders of phosphate excretion.
- Presentation of clinical case studies or examples to illustrate key concepts.

IV. **Disorders of potassium metabolism** **(10 minutes)**
- Description of disorders such as hyperkalemia and hypokalemia.
- Explanation of underlying mechanisms, clinical manifestations, and treatment options.

V. **Other mineral metabolism disorders** **(10 minutes)**
- Overview of disorders associated with magnesium, sodium, iron, and other minerals.
- Discussion of etiology, clinical features, and management strategies.

VI. **Case studies and interactive discussion** **(10 minutes)**
- Presentation of clinical case studies or scenarios for interactive discussion.
- Encourage students to apply their knowledge to analyze and solve clinical problems related to mineral metabolism disorders.

VII. **Review and summary** **(5 minutes)**
- Review key points covered in the lecture.
- Summarize the main disorders associated with mineral metabolism and their clinical implications.

VIII. **Conclusion** **(5 minutes)**

- Conclude the lecture by emphasizing the importance of understanding mineral metabolism disorders for clinical practice.
- Encourage further exploration of the topic and its relevance in healthcare.

WATER-SOLUBLE VITAMINS

Vitamin C (Ascorbic Acid)

Scurvy

Age	45-years male
History	Bleeding gums, petechial hemorrhages on skin, diet deficient of fruits and vegetables
On examination	Swelled and bleeding gums
Blood vitamin C	0.13 mg% (Normal: 0.20–2.00 mg%)
Diagnosis	Scurvy (due to deficiency of vitamin C)
Reason of bleeding gums	Proline, Lysine forms Hydroxyproline, Hydroxylysine required for collagen stabilization in presence of enzymes—Prolyl hydroxylase, lysyl hydroxylase
	Vitamin C acts as a coenzyme in this reaction required for forming collagen important for forming wall of blood vessels
	If vitamin C is deficient, then unstable collagen leads to weak blood vessel wall and fragility resulting in bleeding gums and ecchymosis on skin
Rich source of vitamin C:	Amla, guava, lime

Vitamin B_1

Wernicke-Korsakoff Syndrome

Age	55-years male
Complains	Poor appetite, weakness of muscles, forgetfulness, hand tremors, nystagmus
History	Alcoholic
On examination	Unsteady gate, tremors, mental confusion
Diagnosis	Thiamine deficiency causing Wernicke-Korsakoff syndrome
Causes	Observed in chronic alcoholics with poor diet intake and impaired nutrient absorption from GIT
Estimation in plasma	RBC transketolase activity is assessed for assessing the deficiency of B1
Treatment	Vitamin B1 supplementation
Symptoms in mild cases	Loss of appetite, lethargy, irritation, peripheral neuropathy
Symptoms in moderately severe cases	• Clinical triad of global confusion, ophthalmoplegia, ataxia • Amnestic state and patient presents improper recent memory, confabulation (false belief that what he believes, in filling recent memory gap, is true)
	There is a permanent damage at medial thalamic nuclei and mammillary bodies of brain
Severe deficiency of vitamin B1	Beriberi

Wet Beriberi

Age	6-years-old child
Complains	Lethargy, poor appetite, irritable, pitting pedal edema
History	Eats mainly polished rice (B1 is present on outer aleurone layer of cereals, which is removed by polishing)
Diagnosis	Beriberi
Dry beriberi	Neuromuscular abnormalities, muscular atrophy, emaciation
Wet beriberi	Neuromuscular abnormalities, muscular atrophy, emaciation and pedal edema

Ariboflavinosis (Vitamin B_2 Deficiency)

Age	15-year-old boy
Complains	Repeated ulcers at mouth corner, swelling and pain in tongue
History	Strict vegetarian
On examination	Dry lips, ulcers at mouth corner, red and swelled tongue, circumcorneal vascularization
Diagnosis	B_2 deficiency
RDA of vitamin B_2	1.5 mg%
Sources of vitamin B_2	Egg, milk, milk products, fish, liver, yeast, cereals
Main symptoms of vitamin B_2 deficiency	• Glossitis • Angular stomatitis • Dry and scaly lips • Bulbar conjunctiva proliferation • Circumcorneal vascularization

Vitamin B_3 Deficiency—Pellagra

Age	38-year-old male
Complains	Dry scaly lesions around the neck
History	Frequent diarrhea
On examination	Characteristic lesions around the neck and on dorsum of hand
Diagnosis	B_3 deficiency—Pellagra
Main symptoms of vitamin B_3 deficiency: 3D's	• Diarrhea • Dementia • Dermatitis • Casal necklace deformity (lesions on neck) • Gloved hand deformity (dry scaly lesions on hand)

Vitamin B_6 Deficiency (Pyridoxine)

Age	38-year-old male
Complains	Tingling, numbness in peripheries, dry and scaly scalp
History	Suffering from pulmonary tuberculosis and taking antitubercular treatment
Diagnosis	• B_6 deficiency • Antitubercular drug isoniazid is associated with deficiency of vitamin B_6
Functions of pyridoxine phosphate: (Coenzyme form)	• Transamination • Decarboxylation • Glycogen synthase activity for glycogen synthesis • Glycogen phosphorylase activity for glycogenolysis • ALA synthase for heme synthesis • Cystathionine beta synthase, cystathionase for metabolism of sulfur containing amino acids • Patients excrete Xanthurenic acid in the urine, which is made by kynurenine in alternate pathway of tryptophan metabolism, when the normal route is impaired because of lack of activity of kynureninase enzyme

Biotin Deficiency (Vitamin B_7)

Age	25-year-old male
Complains	Hair loss, red scaly rashes around mouth, nose and eyes, tingling sensation on extremities
History	Takes raw eggs
Diagnosis	Biotin deficiency
Sources of biotin	Cereals, rice, spinach, egg yolk

Contd....

Contd....

Symptoms	• Periorificial dermatitis • Alopecia • Lesions on skin as like zinc deficiency
Functions of biotin:	Required by carboxylase enzymes for CO_2 fixation reactions
1. Gluconeogenesis	Pyruvate carboxylase
2. Protein metabolism	• Beta-methylcrotonyl-CoA carboxylase • Propionyl-CoA carboxylase
3. Synthesis of fatty acids	Acetyl-CoA carboxylase
Treatment	Oral biotin 5 mg/day
Function of biotinidase enzyme	Releases biotin from dietary protein
Deficiency of biotinidase	Autosomal recessive disease where deficiency of biotin is due to no release of biotin from dietary protein

Vitamin B_{12} Deficiency

Age	26-year-old female, strict vegetarian
Complains	Weakness, tiredness
On examination	Looks pale
Peripheral smear	Megaloblastic anemia
Diagnosis	Megaloblastic anemia is due to deficiency of vitamin B_{12}
Cause	Vitamin B_{12} is obtained from foods of animal origin, such as meat, fish
Functions of vitamin B_{12}	Contains mineral cobalt, needed by enzymes methylmalonyl-CoA mutase in 2′-deoxyadenosylcobalamin form and methionine synthase in methyl cobalamine form

FAT-SOLUBLE VITAMINS

Vitamin A Deficiency

Age	5-year-old child
History	Less vision after sunset, repeated URI
On examination	Follicular hyperkeratosis on back of arm, dry eyes, white patches on sclera
Diagnosis	Vitamin A deficiency
Characteristics	• Patients are prone to repeated infections as vitamin A does the down regulation of keratin synthesis • Deficiency of vitamin A causes excess keratinization of skin and mucous membrane
In skin	Shows as follicular hyperkeratosis
In mucous membrane	• Show as keratinization of respiratory, gastrointestinal and genitourinary tracts which favor colonization of microorganisms and infections • There is increased mortality in case of vitamin A deficiency due to diarrhea, dysentery, malaria, respiratory disorders, etc.
Sources of vitamin A	Yellow and green vegetables, mango, banana, carrot, tomato, pumpkin

Vitamin D Deficiency

Osteomalacia

Age	60-year-old postmenopausal woman
Complain	Backache
On examination	Kyphosis
X-ray	Porous matrix, loss of osteoid matrix
History	2 recent fractures in foot

Contd....

Contd....

Diagnosis	• Osteomalacia • Vitamin D deficiency results in hypocalcemia and hypophosphatemia • There is improper mineralization of bone matrix protein, leading to bowing of weight-bearing extremities and easy skeletal fractures • Proximal myopathy may be seen
Particular findings inosteomalacia	• Pseudofractures • Looser zones in scapula, pelvis, femoral neck

Rickets

Age	8-year-old child
Complain	Deformity of bones, widening of wrist
On examination	Prominent chest
Diagnosis	Rickets
	Vitamin D deficiency—Rickets
Characteristics	• There is improper mineralization of bone resulting in soft and pliable bones • Normal osteoid matrix and cartilages • Before the fusing of epiphyseal plate, the deficiency of vitamin D causes widening of growth plate in long bones (causing bowed legs) and costochondral junction (causing rachitic rosary)
Treatment	Vitamin D is give in therapeutic doses and physiotherapy is advised

Vitamin D Toxicity

Age	8-year-old child
History	Vomiting, headache, bulging fontanelle, vitamin D injections were given over a period of >12 months
X-ray	Metastatic calcification of calf muscle and renal tract stones
Diagnosis	Vitamin D toxicity
Upper tolerable limit of vitamin D toxicity in adults	4000 IU/day
Upper tolerable limit of vitamin D toxicity in children	• 2000 IU/day • There is demineralization of bones here also as in rickets but it is because of excess reabsorption of calcium from the bone • There is high blood level of calcitriol and calcium

MINERALS AND CLINICAL MANIFESTATIONS OF THEIR PLASMA LEVELS ABNORMALITIES

Iron Deficiency Anemia

Age	12-year-old child
Complain	Loss of appetite, early fatigue, lethargic, frequent headache
On examination	Flat nails with pallor, shrunken eyes, brittle nails
Peripheral smear	Hypochromic microcytic picture
	Blood report
Hb	7 g/dL (Normal: 12–14 g/dL)
Serum iron	43 ng/dL (Normal: 50–150 g/L)
Serum ferritin	25 mg/dL (Normal: 50–200 mg/dL)
Diagnosis	Iron deficiency anemia
	Deficiency of iron results in impaired heme synthesis

Contd....

Contd....

Causes	• Dietary deficiency of iron and high content of phytates in the diet which form insoluble complexes with iron and impairs absorption of iron • Worm infestation • Bleeding piles
Cause of early fatigue	The RBC's are not able to supply enough O_2 to the tissues
Sources of iron	Pulses, meat, black gram, Jaggery
Other investigations required	Total iron binding capacity, transferrin saturation

Hypocalcemia

Age	30-year-old male
Complains	Nocturnal muscle cramps
On examination	On cheek stroking, there was facial twitching, spasm in fingers when taking blood pressure
Diagnosis	Hypocalcemia
Chvostek sign	On cheek stroking, there appears facial twitching
Trousseau's sign	Adduction of thumb and flexion of metacarpophalangeal joints and extension of interphalangeal joints and flexion of wrist on inflating the blood pressure 20 mm Hg above the systolic pressure for 3 minutes
Normal ionized calcium level	4.9 mg%
In hypocalcemia	<4.7 mg%

Fluorosis

Age	10-year-old boy
Complains	Short stature, bowing of legs, mottling teeth with rough ridge, his co-villagers also showed similar features
Diagnosis	• Fluorosis • Excess intake of fluorine in drinking water of >5 ppm
RDA	1–2 mg (0.5–0.9 ppm)
Other sources of fluorine	Sea food, cheese
Functions of fluorine	• Makes strong bones and teeth • Keeps the teeth resistant to dental caries/cavities • Keeps the bones resistant to osteoporosis • Deficiency causes dental caries and osteoporosis
Characteristics of dental fluorosis	• Mottled/spotting teeth • Discoloration of teeth with pitting • In severe cases, skeletal fluorosis occur (intake of >20 ppm), making deformed bones

Wilson's Disease

Age	20-year-old male
Admission	Presents with bizarre behavior, crying phases
On examination	Hand tremors, limb movements were not coordinated, dysarthria, dysphagia, eyes showed golden brown ring around corneal rim
	Blood report
Serum ceruloplasmin	10 mg% (Normal: 18–35 mg%)
Biopsy—copper content in liver	310 mg/g of tissue (Normal: 20–50 mg/g)
Urinary copper (24 hour)	290 mg (Normal: 20–50 mg)

Contd....

Contd....

Diagnosis	• Wilson's disease • Autosomal recessive • Mutation of ATP 7B gene that encodes membranous copper transporting ATPase • There is a defect in biliary secretion of copper leading to accumulation of copper in liver and liver toxicity
Reason behind low ceruloplasmin in serum	• There is lack of incorporation of copper into apoceruloplasmin • Free copper in plasma goes on increasing and then starts depositing in brain and eye causing neurological as well as psychiatric diseases and Kayser-Fleischer rings around the cornea develops
	Treatment
1. Zinc	• Zinc blocks intestinal absorption of copper • Zinc forms metallothionine that can bind with copper in non-toxic form and decreases its toxicity
2. Trientine	It is a copper chelator

Iodine Deficiency

Age	30-year-old woman
Complains	Neck swelling for last few months which is increasing now
History	Recent weight gain, lethargy, oligomenorrhea
Diagnosis	Goitrous hypothyroidism
Cause	Deficiency of dietary iodine
Functions of iodine	Synthesis of thyroid hormones T3 and T4
In deficiency of iodine	There is enlargement of thyroid gland because of its follicle proliferation for compensating thyroid hormone production so it presents as multi nodular goiter (MNG)
Treatment	Supplementation of iodine

Acrodermatitis Enteropathica (Zinc deficiency)

Age	4-year-old child
Complains	Stunted growth, irritable, diarrhea, loss of taste, alopecia, erythematosus rashes on face, perineum and extremities
On examination	Lesions on the face and perineum are typically symmetrical
Diagnosis	• Deficiency of zinc called acrodermatitis enteropathica • Autosomal recessive • Defect in absorption of zinc
Treatment	Oral zinc supplementation: 60 mg two times a day
Zinc toxicity	Exposure to welding fumes, characterized by fever, respiratory distress, excess salivation, headache, sweating

OSCE

1. **Scenario: Vitamin A deficiency—night blindness**
   Case: A 28-year-old female shows symptoms of difficulty seeing in low light along with dry eyes. She is a vegetarian strictly and does not take any vitamin supplements. Serum vitamin A: 20 µg/dL (normal: 20–80 µg/dL).
   Laboratory results:
   Serum vitamin A: 20 µg/dL (low)
   Hemoglobin: 13 g/dL (normal)
   LFT: Normal

Question: What does this value of vitamin A indicate?
Interpretation: The low vitamin A level with symptoms of night blindness along with dryness of eyes is indicative of deficiency of fat-soluble vitamin A which is required for vision, specifically rhodopsin formation in the retina.
The deficiency of this vitamin results in night blindness/xerophthalmia/keratomalacia that is corneal damage).
Diagnosis: Deficiency of Vitamin A
Next steps: He must be given oral vitamin A supplements/dietary intake of beta-carotene that is present in orange and green vegetables.

2. **Scenario: Vitamin D deficiency—rickets**
Case: A 5-year-old child shows with symptoms of pain in bones along with delayed growth, bowed legs, soft skull. The mother says that he takes very little sun exposure and also do not drink milk.
Laboratory results:
Serum calcium: 8.4 mg/dL (low-normal)
Serum phosphate: 2.1 mg/dL (low)
Serum 25-hydroxyvitamin D: 09 ng/mL (low, normal: 20–50 ng/mL)
Question: What does this result interpret?
Interpretation: The low serum vitamin D along with hypocalcemia and bowed legs, soft skull, are consistent with disease called rickets, a state which is due to vitamin D deficiency.
Vitamin D is important for the normal absorption of minerals—calcium and phosphate from the intestines. Deficiency of this vitamin results in improper bone mineralization, leading to rickets in children and osteomalacia in adults.
Diagnosis: Vitamin D deficiency resulting in rickets.
Next steps: The patient must get vitamin D supplementation/dietary intake of calcium and vitamin D along with increasing sun exposure.

3. **Scenario: Vitamin C deficiency—scurvy**
Case: A 45-year-old man presents with bleeding gums, easy bruising, and joint pain. He tells that his history is consuming poor diet/no fresh fruits/vegetables.
Laboratory results:
Serum vitamin C: 0.2 mg/dL (low, normal: 0.6–2 mg/dL)
Platelet count: 222,000/mm^3 (normal)
Hemoglobin: 14 g/dL (normal)
Question: What does this result interpret?
Interpretation: The low vitamin C level/clinical symptoms of bleeding gums, easy bruising, and joint pain are indicative of scurvy, a state due to vitamin C deficiency.
Vitamin C is important for the synthesis of collagen, that is crucial structural protein for connective tissues. Deficiency can lead to scurvy, that is characterized by bleeding gums/delayed wound healing/joint pain.
Diagnosis: Scurvy because of vitamin C deficiency.
Next steps: He must be treated with oral vitamin C supplements/dietary intake of citrus fruits/green leafy vegetables.

4. **Scenario: Vitamin B_{12} deficiency—pernicious anemia**
Case: A 64-year-old female presents with symptoms of fatigue/pallor/neuropathy. She is strict vegetarian. Hemoglobin: 9 g/dL (normal: 12–15 g/dL), Serum vitamin B_{12}: 120 pg/mL (normal: 200–900 pg/mL).
Laboratory results:
Serum vitamin B_{12}: 120 pg/mL (low)
Mean corpuscular volume (MCV): 111 fL (elevated)
Serum homocysteine: 19 µmol/L (elevated)
Question: What does this result interpret?
Interpretation: The low vitamin B_{12} concentration/macrocytic anemia/high homocysteine is indicative of vitamin B_{12} deficiency. The neuropathy/fatigue direct toward pernicious anemia that is a type of B_{12} deficiency anemia due to autoimmune destruction of intrinsic factor/parietal cells of stomach, resulting in impaired absorption of the vitamin B_{12}.
Diagnosis: Vitamin B_{12} deficiency along with pernicious anemia.
Next steps: She must be treated with intramuscular vitamin B_{12} injections/dietary adjustments to take more B_{12}-rich foods like dairy products/eggs/fortified cereals etc.

5. **Scenario: Iron deficiency anemia—microcytic hypochromic anemia**
Case: A 38-year-old female presents with symptoms of fatigue/pale skin/shortness of breath after work. She says there is history of heavy menstrual periods some days back.
Laboratory results:
Serum ferritin: 11 ng/mL (low, normal: 20–300 ng/mL)
Serum iron: 31 µg/dL (low, normal: 50–150 µg/dL)
Mean corpuscular volume (MCV): 71 fL (low, normal: 80–100 fL)
Question: What do these results interpret?

Interpretation: The low serum ferritin/low serum iron and microcytic hypochromic anemia that is due to low MCV is indicative of iron deficiency anemia.
This condition is very common reason of microcytic anemia and can also be due to chronic blood loss like in or during heavy menstrual periods/insufficient dietary consumption of iron.
Diagnosis: Iron deficiency anemia.
Next steps: She must be treated with oral iron supplements like ferrous sulfate/consume more iron-rich foods.

6. **Scenario: Folate deficiency—megaloblastic anemia**
Case: A 41-year-old male presents with symptoms of fatigue/pallor/sore tongue. He was continuously taking alcohol in the past and have poor dietary habits.
Laboratory results:
Serum folate: 2 ng/mL (low, normal: 5–25 ng/mL)
Serum vitamin B_{12}: 410 pg/mL (normal)
Mean corpuscular volume (MCV): 120 fL (high)
Question: What does this result interpret?
Interpretation: The low serum folate level/macrocytic anemia that is suggested by high MCV plus clinical symptoms suggest folic acid deficiency.
Folate is important for formation of DNA and this is the reason that results in megaloblastic anemia.
Alcohol use disorder can result in folate deficiency because of malabsorption/poor dietary intake.
Diagnosis: Folate deficiency.
Next steps: The patient must get oral folic acid supplements/dietary intake of folate-rich foods like leafy greens/legumes.

CLINICAL MCQS

1. **A 35-year-old woman shows symptoms of night blindness, dry, scaly skin. Which vitamin deficiency is present?**
a. Vitamin A
b. Vitamin D
c. Vitamin B
d. Vitamin C
Answer: a. Vitamin A

2. **A 52-year-old man presents with easy fractures, weak muscle low serum calcium, low serum 25-hydroxyvitamin D. What condition is present?**
a. Rickets
b. Osteomalacia
c. Pellagra
d. Osteoporosis
Answer: b. Osteomalacia

3. **A 61-year-old woman presents with symptoms of glossitis, cheilitis, macrocytic anemia, high homocysteine concentration. Which vitamin deficiency is present?**
a. Folate
b. Vitamin B_{12}
c. Vitamin B_3
d. Pantothenic acid
Answer: a. Folate

4. **A 6-year-old boy presents with bowlegs, wide epiphyseal plates. What is the deficiency?**
a. Calcium
b. Vitamin D
c. Sodium
d. Phosphorus
Answer: b. Vitamin D

5. **A 41-year-old man presents with 3 D symptoms of dermatitis, diarrhea, and dementia. What vitamin deficiency is present?**
a. Vitamin C
b. Vitamin B_3
c. Vitamin B_5
d. Vitamin B_{12}
Answer: b. Vitamin B_3 (Niacin)

6. **A patient presents with bleeding gums, poor wound healing. Which vitamin deficiency is present?**
   a. Vitamin C
   b. Vitamin B
   c. Vitamin A
   d. Niacin

   Answer: a. Vitamin C

7. **A newborn is having bleeding from the umbilical stump, intracranial hemorrhage. What vitamin deficiency is present?**
   a. Vitamin K
   b. Vitamin D
   c. Vitamin E
   d. Vitamin B_{12}

   Answer: a. Vitamin K

8. **A 46-year-old man presents with peripheral neuropathy, hemolytic anemia. Which vitamin deficiency is most likely?**
   a. Vitamin E
   b. Vitamin C
   c. Vitamin B
   d. Folic acid

   Answer: a. Vitamin E

9. **A 39-year-old woman presents with brittle nails/microcytic hypochromic anemia. Which mineral deficiency is present?**
   a. Iron
   b. Selenium
   c. Copper
   d. Calcium

   Answer: a. Iron

10. **A 5-year-old child presents with delayed wound healing, perioral dermatitis. Which mineral deficiency is present?**
    a. Zinc
    b. Calcium
    c. Copper
    d. Iron

    Answer: a. Zinc

11. **A patient presents with peripheral neuropathy, elevated homocysteine levels. Which vitamin deficiency is present?**
    a. Vitamin B_6
    b. Vitamin B_5
    c. Folic acid
    d. Vitamin A

    Answer: a. Vitamin B_6

12. **A 3-year-old child shows irritability/poor appetite/delayed psychomotor development/decreased level of serum copper. Which condition is present?**
    a. Menkes disease
    b. Wilson's disease
    c. Anemia
    d. Iron deficiency anemia

    Answer: a. Menkes disease

13. **A vegetarian individual shows symptom of fatigue/glossitis/megaloblastic anemia/methylmalonic acid concentration is very high. Which vitamin deficiency is present?**
    a. Vitamin B_{12}
    b. Pantothenic acid
    c. Vitamin B_5
    d. Vitamin C

    Answer: a. Vitamin B_{12}

14. **A patient suffering from Crohn's disease shows symptoms of muscle cramps/hypocalcemia/low level of magnesium in serum. What is the deficiency?**
    a. Magnesium
    b. Iron

c. Vitamin C
d. Sodium

Answer: a. Magnesium

15. **A 51-year-old woman shows symptom of goiter/hypothyroidism. Which mineral deficiency is present?**
a. Iodine
b. Calcium
c. Zinc
d. Copper

Answer: a. Iodine

16. **A patient with habit of taking alcohol presents with confusion, ataxia, ophthalmoplegia. What vitamin deficiency is present?**
a. Vitamin B_1
b. Pyridoxine
c. Vitamin B_3
d. Cobalamin

Answer: a. Vitamin B_1

17. **A premature infant shows symptoms of hemolytic anemia, retinopathy. What vitamin deficiency is present?**
a. Vitamin E
b. Vitamin B_5
c. Vitamin D
d. Vitamin C

Answer: a. Vitamin E

18. **A patient shows pale skin, fatigue, and pica, decreased hemoglobin, hematocrit with decreased ferritin levels. What deficiency is present?**
a. Iron
b. Vitamin B_6
c. Folic acid
d. Calcium

Answer: a. Iron

19. **A child complains of poor growth, skeletal abnormalities, enamel hypoplasia. Which mineral deficiency is present?**
a. Calcium
b. Phosphorus
c. Copper
d. Sodium

Answer: a. Calcium

20. **A 66-year-old man shows symptoms of muscle weakness, cardiac arrhythmias, decreased serum potassium, magnesium. Which mineral deficiency is most likely contributing to these findings?**
a. Magnesium
b. Potassium
c. Copper
d. Calcium

Answer: a. Magnesium

VIVA VOCE

Q1. What are the clinical signs of deficiency of Vitamin K, and why the neonates are at higher risk?
Next question/Follow-up: What is the effect of Vitamin K deficiency on coagulation tests (PT/INR)?

Q2. What is the function of Pyridoxine/which symptom arise from the deficiency of B6?
Next question/Follow-up: Why is Vitamin B6 deficiency very common in patients who are on isoniazid therapy?

Q3. What are the final effects of deficient Biotin, and in which conditions they are usually seen?
Next question/Follow-up: Why does excessive raw egg consumption results in Biotin deficiency?

Q4. Explain megaloblastic anemia, and which vitamin deficiencies can cause it?
Next question/Follow-up: Why does folic acid deficiency develop faster than Vitamin B_{12} deficiency?

Q5. What are the dermatological/neurological manifestations of riboflavin deficiency?
Next question/Follow-up: How can deficiency of riboflavin be diagnosed clinically?

Q6. What are the clinical features of deficiency of calcium, and how will it affect neuromuscular function?
Next question/Follow-up: What do you understand by Chvostek's sign, and why it occurs in hypocalcemia?

Q7. How does deficient magnesium affect cardiovascular/nervous system?
Next question/Follow-up: Why does hypomagnesemia lead to Hypokalemia?

Q8. What are the hematological and systemic complications of deficient copper?
Next question/Follow-up: How copper deficiency results in anemia/neutropenia?

Q9. What is the importance of selenium, and what are the deficiency consequences?
Next question/Follow-up: How selenium deficiency contributes towards Keshan disease?

Q10. What are the symptoms of Hypokalemia and why is it fatal?
Next question/Follow-up: How Hypokalemia affect ECG results?

SPOTTERS

Q1. Image of Bitot's spots on conjunctiva. Identify the condition and the vitamin deficiency which is responsible.

Bitot's spots because of deficient Vitamin A.

Q2. Picture of a child with bow legs (Rickets). What is the condition, and which vitamin deficiency is responsible?

Rickets because of Vitamin D deficiency.

Q3. Image of bleeding gums/perifollicular hemorrhages. Identify the condition and the vitamin deficiency responsible.

Scurvy due to Vitamin C deficiency.

Q4. Picture of a patient with hyperpigmented/scaly skin rash specially on sun-exposed areas (Pellagra). What is the deficiency, and which vitamin is responsible?

Pellagra because of deficient Niacin.

Q5. Picture of an anemic patient with peripheral neuropathy along with glossitis. Which vitamin deficiencies could be responsible for these findings?

Vitamin B_{12}/Folate (B9) deficient.

Q6. ECG exhibiting prolonged QT interval. Identify the electrolyte imbalance and also mineral deficiency involved.

Hypocalcemia because of deficient calcium.

Q7. Photo of a patient with goiter. Which mineral deficiency is linked with this condition?

Deficient iodine.

Q8. Picture of a patient with koilonychia/spoon-shaped nails. What is the probable mineral deficiency responsible for this condition?

Iron deficiency/Iron deficiency anemia.

Q9. Picture of a child with muscle weakness/delayed growth/Kwashiorkor-like features. Which mineral deficiency can be associated to this presentation?

Deficiency of Zinc.

Q10. Picture of a person with Keshan disease/cardiomyopathy/muscle weakness). Which mineral deficiency is associated here?

Deficient Selenium.

REFLECTION

Visit to the department of skin and identify skin changes due to deficiency of Vitamin B complex, vitamin C and zinc deficiency and cutaneous changes in vitamin A deficiency also identify the clinical features of the vitamins deficiencies and make a diagnosis.

42

CHAPTER

Energy Content of Food Items and Glycemic Index

COMPETENCY

BC14.23: Calculate energy content of different food items and identify the food items with high and low glycemic index and explain the importance of these in the diet.

LEARNING OBJECTIVES

After reading this chapter, the readers should be able to:

- Calculate energy content of different food Items, identify food items with high and low glycaemic index and explain the importance of these in the diet.

BLUE PRINT

Energy Content of Various Food Items

Objective

By the end of the lecture, students should be able to:

1. Calculate the energy content of different food items using macronutrient composition.
2. Identify food items with high and low glycemic index (GI).
3. Explain the importance of glycemic index in the diet and its implications for health.

Duration: *60 minutes*

Materials Needed

1. Nutrient composition tables or databases for various food items.
2. Worksheets or handouts with sample data for energy content and glycemic index calculations.
3. Whiteboard or presentation slides for visual aids.

Outline

I. **Introduction to energy content of food items** **(15 minutes)**
- Explanation of the concept of energy content in food.
- Overview of macronutrients contributing to energy: Carbohydrates, proteins, and fats.
- Discussion of the energy yield per gram for each macronutrient (carbohydrates: 4 kcal/g, proteins: 4 kcal/g, fats: 9 kcal/g).
- Introduction to the formula for calculating energy content: Energy (kcal) = Carbohydrates (g) × 4 + Proteins (g) × 4 + Fats (g) × 9.

II. **Calculation of energy content** **(20 minutes)**
- Step-by-step demonstration of calculating the energy content of different food items using sample data.
- Practical exercises for students to calculate the energy content of various food items based on their macronutrient composition.
- Discussion of factors influencing the energy content of foods, such as processing and cooking methods.

III. **Introduction to glycemic index (GI)** **(10 minutes)**
- Definition of glycemic index and its significance in nutrition.
- Explanation of how GI ranks carbohydrates based on their effect on blood glucose levels compared to a reference food (usually glucose or white bread).
- Overview of GI classification: Low GI (<55), medium GI (55–69), high GI (≥70).
- Importance of GI in managing blood sugar levels, weight control, and overall health.

IV. **Calculation of glycemic index** **(15 minutes)**
- Explanation of methods for determining glycemic index, including laboratory testing and clinical trials.
- Practical demonstration of calculating glycemic index using sample data and reference values.
- Examples of food items with high and low glycemic index and their implications for dietary choices.

V. **Conclusion and recap** **(5 minutes)**
- Summary of key points covered in the calculation of energy content and glycemic index of food items.
- Emphasis on the importance of understanding energy content and glycemic index in making informed dietary decisions.

VI. **Question and answer session** **(10 minutes)**
- Encourage students to ask questions and seek clarification on the concepts and calculations discussed.
- Discuss practical applications of energy content and glycemic index in meal planning and dietary management.

INTRODUCTION

Food gives the essential nutrients and proper energy that human body requires for proper functioning.

Two fundamental concepts are there when we consider the nutritional value of food and they are:

Energy Content

Glycemic Index

It is crucial to understand these concepts in order to promote optimal health, to manage conditions such as diabetes, and also to maintain optimal performance in routine daily activities long with physical exercises. This competency explores the energy content of food, how it can be measured, its significance in the body, and the glycemic index (GI) that measures how various carbohydrate-containing foods can affect blood glucose levels.

Energy Content of Food

The energy content of food refers to the amount of energy which can be derived from a specific quantity of food. It can be measured in kilocalories (kcal) or kilojoules (kJ).

Proximate Principles

Carbohydrates, proteins and fats are called as proximate principles of the diet.

Food Energy Determination

Lavoisier proved that the production of energy by the food inside our body is same as it is produced outside our body by combustion in aerobic condition in presence of oxygen. Oxidation is same as combustion in presence of oxygen. Thus, energy formed by combustion is measured easily by Bomb Calorimeter. Although there are some factors to be kept in mind like there are some foods that are not fully digested and absorbed and are even metabolized incompletely like proteins and many residual intermediates like keto acids and urea are excreted out. So, these factors must be taken care of while deciding the energy value of foods.

Flow of Food Energy in Body

- **GE**: Gross energy is the total energy present in the food taken or consumed.
- **FE**: Fecal energy is part of energy lost in undigested food excreted in feces.
- **GE**: Gaseous energy is energy lost in form of gases like methane, hydrogen, short chain volatile acids.
- **UE**: Of the remaining digested food and absorbed, some part may not be completely metabolized like proteins and this gets excreted out in the urine as urinary energy.
- Diet-induced thermogenesis/specific dynamic action of food: Of the remaining food metabolized and the energy produced from it, the METABOLIC ENERGY, some portion is lost from the surface of the body, and some portion is utilized by processes of energy generation itself.
- In the end, after all these above losses of energy, of the remaining metabolic energy, 2/3 is captured as ATP.

Energy is given by the three primary macronutrients:

1. Carbohydrates
2. Proteins
3. Fats

Every macronutrient mentioned above contributes differently to the total caloric content of food.

Calorific Value of Different Foods

Carbohydrates and Energy Content

Carbohydrates are the primary source of energy for human beings. After digestion, carbohydrates are hydrolyzed and break into simpler sugars like monosaccharide glucose that the body can use for energy purpose.

The energy yield from carbohydrates is approximately: 4 kcal per gram of carbohydrate.

Dietary carbohydrates include sugars, starches, and fiber. Simple sugars, like glucose and sucrose, are rapidly digested and give rapid energy. Starches, found in foods like bread and potatoes, take longer time for digestion and give more sustained energy. Fiber, that is not digestible, plays an important role in digestive health.

Proteins and Energy Content

Proteins are crucial for building as well as in repairing the tissues. They also serve as a very important source of energy when the stores of carbohydrate are depleted. Proteins are hydrolyzed to form amino acids, which are used by the body to perform various functions.

The energy yield from proteins is: 4 kcal per gram of protein.

However, proteins are not the body's preferred source of energy and are typically important more for their role in building of muscles and performing enzymatic functions rather than being used as a primary fuel source.

Fats and Energy Content

Fats are the most energy-dense macronutrients and are the body's most preferred long-term energy storage form. Lipids are hydrolyzed to form fatty acids and glycerol that can be used by the body for energy purpose, especially during periods of rest or prolonged activity.

The energy yield from fats is: 9 kcal per gram of fat.

Fats are significant not only for energy but also for insulation, protection of organs, and absorption of fat-soluble vitamins like A, D, E, and K.

Alcohol and Energy Content

Although it is not a macronutrient that is required to perform body functions, but it provides energy for our body.

The energy yield from alcohol is: 7 kcal per gram of alcohol.

However, alcohol gives empty calories, as it does not provide any essential nutrients like vitamins or minerals, and it can even interfere with various metabolisms and health when it is consumed in excess.

Steps for Calculation of Food Energy

- Note the amount of carbohydrate, protein and fat in a given food
- Calculate energy formed by each component:
  - Energy from carbohydrate (Kcal) = 4× amount of carbohydrate in grams
  - Energy from protein (Kcal) = 4× amount of protein in grams
  - Energy from fat (Kcal) = 9× amount of fat in grams
- Add the Kcal to get total Kcal given by the food

Log Activity

Calculate the energy given by a chapati made of 25 grams of dry whole wheat flour. Carbohydrate content is 72%, protein content is 12% and fat is 1.6% in the flour:

Carbohydrates in 25 g chapati = 72/4 = 18 g

Proteins in 25 g chapati = 12/4 = 3 g

Fats in 25 g chapati = 1.6/4 = 0.4 g

Energy Produced

Carbohydrates = 18 × 4 = 72 Kcal
Proteins = 3 × 4 = 12 Kcal
Fats = 0.4 × 9 = 3.6 Kcal
Total energy given by one wheat chapati of 25 g = 72 + 12 + 3.6 = 87.6 Kcal

Energy Requirements

Energy requirement vary a lot and is based on factors like age, gender, body composition, and physical activity levels.

On an average, adults need approximately: 2,000–2,500 kcal/day for women and 2,500–3,000 kcal/day for men

Athletes or people leading life with higher physical activity levels need more energy to support muscle function, recovery, and maintaining overall health.

Glycemic Index (GI)

The glycemic index (GI) is a ranking system which measures how rapidly carbohydrate-containing foods increase blood glucose levels. Foods are ranked on a scale from 0–100, with glucose (a simple monosaccharide) having a GI value of 100. GI is used to assess the effect of various foods on blood sugar level, and understanding GI is very significant in managing states such as diabetes, where blood sugar balance and regulation is critical.

GI is a comparative value with glucose therefore GTT is done with the food and glucose. The relative increase in blood glucose following ingestion of food having 50 grams of carbohydrates is compared with the ingestion of 50 grams of pure glucose.

GI in % = area under the curve of test meal/area under the curve of glucose.

Low, Medium, and High GI Foods

Low GI foods that are having GI value of 55 or less cause a slow and more gradual increase in blood glucose levels. Examples include whole grains, legumes, fruits, and non-starchy vegetables.

Medium GI foods that are having GI value between 56 and 69 cause a moderate increase in blood glucose levels. Examples include foods like whole wheat bread, sweet potatoes, and brown rice.

High GI foods that are having GI value of 70 or above lead to a rapid and significant rise in blood glucose levels. Examples include white bread, sugary cereals, and certain processed snacks.

Factors Affecting GI

Various factors have an impact on the GI of a food:

1. **Carbohydrate type:** Simple sugars generally have a higher GI in comparison to the complex carbohydrates such as starch.
2. **Food processing:** Highly processed foods (e.g., white bread) have a high GI in comparison to less processed foods (e.g., whole grain bread).
3. **Fiber content:** Foods rich in fiber tend to have a low GI because fiber slows down digestion as well as the absorption of carbohydrates.
4. **Fat and protein content:** Foods that have fat and protein tend to have a low GI as fat and protein slow down the absorption of glucose.
5. **Ripeness of fruit:** Ripe fruits typically have a high GI as their starch content has converted to sugar.
6. **Cooking methods:** The way the food is cooked can also affect its GI. For example, pasta has a low GI when it is firm compared to when it is overcooked.

Importance of GI in Diet and Health

The GI of food plays a very important role in managing blood glucose levels, and this is particularly significant for diabetic patients. Foods having a low GI aid in maintaining stable blood sugar levels and preventing insulin spikes, which can result in insulin resistance with time. Additionally, a low-GI diet has been associated with less risk of chronic diseases, including cardiovascular diseases and life style disorder of obesity.

1. **Diabetes management:** A low-GI diet helps individuals with both, type 1 and type II diabetes in managing their blood glucose levels in a more effective manner.
2. **Weight management:** Low-GI foods tend to promote satiety, reduce hunger and helps in weight management.
3. **Chronic disease prevention:** Researchers suggest that diets rich in low-GI foods can aid prevent cardiovascular diseases, type 2 diabetes, and some type of cancers.

Relationship between Energy Content and Glycemic Index

Both energy content as well as glycemic index affects and influence how food affects the body. While the energy content refers to how much energy a food provides, the glycemic index refers to how that particular food impacts blood sugar and levels of insulin. Together, they give a clearer picture of a food's effect on the body.

Combining Energy and GI in Healthy Eating

Balanced Meals

A balanced meal must not only consider the energy content of foods but also their GI. For instance, consuming a high-energy food with a high GI can lead to quick increase in blood sugar, leading to energy crashes. To avoid this state, it's significant to combine high-energy foods with low-GI foods, like pairing a slice of whole-grain bread having low GI with an egg or avocado that is a source of fat and protein.

Sustained Energy

Foods having a low GI release energy slowly over time, helping to maintain energy levels for the whole day without causing significant blood glucose fluctuations.

Practical Applications of GI in Diet Plans

For individuals who look forward to optimize their diet for health purpose or performance purpose or avoiding medical conditions like diabetes they have to consider both energy content and glycemic index in their diet plan. They can use food combinations like:

Pre-Workout

Foods with a moderate GI are 100 % ideal for fueling exercise, as they give a steady release of energy. For example, whole grain pasta or oatmeal is often recommended before any physical activity.

Post-Workout

After exercise, consuming high-GI foods like fruits (e.g., banana) combined with proteins (e.g., Greek yogurt) can aid replenish glycogen stores rapidly while also helping in muscle recovery.

CONCLUSION

Understanding the two basic fundamentals, energy content and glycemic index of foods, it is significant for making informed dietary choices which can support long-term health and well-being of an individual. While energy content gives the body with the fuel it requires to perform daily activities, the glycemic index helps to manage blood glucose levels along with prevention of insulin resistance, and lowering the risk of various chronic diseases. By combining foods with appropriate energy content as well as glycemic index, one can maintain steady energy levels, optimize performance, and improve overall health. Proper awareness of these two factors can result in healthier eating habits and an excellent balanced approach to nutrition.

OSCE

1. **Scenario: Understanding glycemic index**
   Case: A nutritionist has to advise patient having diabetes for food choices. The patient ask questions regarding how immediately foods can increase blood glucose concentration along with glycemic index of various foods. Explanation was given to the patient that food which have high GI will result in quick raise in blood sugar, and there will be a gradual rise in the blood sugar when foods with a low GI are consumed.
   Foods and glycemic index values:
   White bread: GI = 75
   Oatmeal: GI = 55
   Apple: GI = 35
   Question: How can the glycemic index of these foods have an impact patient's blood glucose regulation?
   Interpretation: Foods with a more glycemic index will be quickly digested/absorbed, leading to quick spike in blood glucose levels. However, low GI foods are digested lowly, resulting in a gradual rise in blood glucose.

Recommendation: The patient must eat low-GI foods, like oatmeal/apples, to help regulate the stable blood glucose levels and also prevent quick spikes, that are specifically significant for the management of diabetes.

2. **Scenario: Glycemic index and meal planning**
Case: A diabetic patient needs planning meal which can aid to control their blood sugar levels. The patient is taking up these food items and their glycemic index.
Foods they can choose:
Baked potato (GI = 85)
Sweet potato (GI = 54)
Brown rice (GI = 50)
Whole-wheat bread (GI = 70)
Question: What is correct combination of foods as far as the individual glycemic indexes are concerned?
Interpretation: To minimize fluctuating levels of blood glucose fluctuations, the patient must take up foods with low glycemic index. *Options*:
Sweet potato (GI – 54) and brown rice (GI = 50) are the best combinations because they both have moderate to low GIs and would result in slow elevation in blood sugar.
Whole-wheat bread and baked potato have higher GIs and should be consumed in moderation.
Recommendation: The patient must focus on sweet potato and brown rice for regulation of blood sugar levels.

3. **Scenario: Calculating energy content of a food item**
Case: A dietician has to calculate total energy content of a food item for planning a diet. The patient is consuming 100 grams of a food containing these macronutrients:
Carbohydrates: 30 g
Proteins: 10 g
Fats: 5 g
Question: How to calculate total energy content of this food?
Interpretation: For calculating energy content of food, we need to use the caloric values of every macronutrient:
Carbohydrates: 4 kcal per gram
Proteins: 4 kcal per gram
Fats: 9 kcal per gram
Calculation:
Energy from carbohydrates = 30 g × 4 kcal/g = 120 kcal
Energy from proteins = 10 g × 4 kcal/g = 40 kcal
Energy from fats = 5 g × 9 kcal/g = 45 kcal
Total energy content = 120 kcal + 40 kcal + 45 kcal = 205 kcal
Answer: The energy content of the food item: 205 kcal/100 g.

4. **Scenario: Glycemic index and weight management**
Case: The patient is considering consuming those foods that have low GI in order to control appetite and prevent obesity.
Foods to consider:
Low-GI food: Brown rice (GI = 50)
High-GI food: White bread (GI = 75)
Question: How can glycemic index of these foods relate to management of weight management, and points to focus on for the patient?
Interpretation: Since the low-GI food are digested slowly, resulting in slow and gradual increase in blood glucose levels, the patient must focus on this low GI food. This leads to better controlled insulin release, that might aid in regulation of appetite along with prevention of more hunger.
High-GI foods, like white bread, leads to rapid spikes in blood glucose, and also rapid drop in the level, that might result in more hunger that leads to overeating.
Recommendation: The patient must focus on low-GI foods to aid in weight management by helping to control appetite and prevent quick fluctuations in blood sugar.

5. **Scenario: Calculation of energy from macronutrients in a meal**
Case: A meal consists of:
Carbohydrates: 45 g
Proteins: 20 g
Fats: 12 g
The patient needs energy content of this meal.
Question: How would you calculate the total energy content of the meal?
Interpretation: The energy content is calculated by multiplying the grams of each macronutrient by their individual caloric values:
Carbohydrates: 4 kcal per gram
Proteins: 4 kcal per gram
Fats: 9 kcal per gram

Calculation:
Energy from carbohydrates = 45 g × 4 kcal/g = 180 kcal
Energy from proteins = 20 g × 4 kcal/g = 80 kcal
Energy from fats = 12 g × 9 kcal/g = 108 kcal
Total energy content = 180 kcal + 80 kcal + 108 kcal = 368 kcal
Answer: The total energy content of the food items is: 368 kcal.

CLINICAL MCQS

1. **A food product has 10 grams: carbohydrates, 5 grams: protein, and 2 grams: fat. Calculate total energy content? (Carbohydrates, proteins = 4 kcal/g, Fat = 9 kcal/g)**
   a. 74 kcal
   b. 69 kcal
   c. 61 kcal
   d. 56 kcal

   Answer: a. 74 kcal
2. **An individual consumes about 50 grams: carbohydrates, 10 grams: protein, and 20 grams: fat. What is total energy contents?**
   a. 490 kcal
   b. 431 kcal
   c. 372 kcal
   d. 523 kcal

   Answer: a. 490 kcal
3. **Which macronutrients contains highest energy content/gram?**
   a. Carbohydrates
   b. Protein
   c. Fat
   d. Green vegetables

   Answer: c. Fat
4. **An item having glycemic index: 85 is classified as:**
   a. Low to high GI
   b. Medium to low GI
   c. High GI
   d. Very low GI

   Answer: c. High GI
5. **Why is the glycemic index significant in clinical nutrition?**
   a. It aids to determine the fat content of food.
   b. It measures the impact of carbohydrates on blood glucose levels.
   c. It focus on protein content of meals.
   d. It gives the mineral content of food.

   Answer: b. It measures the impact of carbohydrates on blood glucose levels.
6. **A diabetic person is consuming food meal with low glycemic index. Which of the foods is most appropriate?**
   a. White bread
   b. Brown rice
   c. Sugary cereal
   d. Fried oats

   Answer: b. Brown rice
7. **A meal with a glycemic load: 20 is considered: (Glycemic load = GI × carbohydrate content (g)/100)**
   a. Low to high GL
   b. Medium GL
   c. High GL
   d. Very high GL

   Answer: b. Medium GL

8. **Which of the statements is correct regarding glycemic index?**
   a. Less GI foods cause rapid spikes in blood sugar.
   b. High GI foods are best to maintain stable glucose levels.
   c. Less GI foods provide sustained energy release.
   d. GI is relevant for protein-rich food items.

   Answer: c. Less GI foods provide sustained energy release.

9. **A person takes 100 grams of a foods having GI: 70 and 30 grams: carbohydrates. What is the glycemic load?**
   a. 21
   b. 32
   c. 52
   d. 71

   Answer: a. 21
   Explanation: GL = (GI × carbohydrate content)/100 = (70 × 30)/100 = 21.

10. **Why is less glycemic index food recommended for patients having diabetes mellitus?**
   a. They increase insulin resistance.
   b. They prevent rapid spikes in postprandial blood glucose.
   c. They reduce rate of protein metabolism.
   d. They result in increased basal metabolic rate.

   Answer: b. They prevent rapid spikes in postprandial blood glucose.

VIVA VOCE

Q1. What is the energy content of 4 important macronutrients?
Carbohydrates: 4 kcal/g
Proteins: 4 kcal/g
Fats: 9 kcal/g
Alcohol: 7 kcal/g

Q2. What is the way to measure energy content of food?
By bomb calorimeter, that determines heat released when the food gets burned.

Q3. What is the Respiratory Quotient/how does relates to energy metabolism?
RQ = CO_2 produced/O_2 consumed
Carbohydrates: RQ = 1.0
Proteins: RQ = 0.8
Fats: RQ = 0.7
Utilized for assessing substrate utilization in al metabolisms.

Q4. What is Basal Metabolic Rate/give factors influencing BMR
BMR: energy needed for vital body functions at rest.
Factors affecting: Age, gender, body composition, hormones specially thyroxine and temperature.

Q5. Give the formula to calculate total energy expenditure?
TEE = BMR + Physical Activity Energy Expenditure + Thermic Effect of Food

Q6. Define Glycemic Index?
Measure of how quickly a carbohydrate-containing food increases blood glucose levels in comparison to glucose (GI = 100).

Q7. How are foods classified based on glycemic index?
Low GI: ≤55 like lentils, oats
Medium GI: 56–69 like brown rice, sweet potato
High GI: ≥70 like white bread, glucose

Q8. What factors affect GI of food?
Type of carbohydrate that is simple vs. complex
Presence of fiber, fat/protein
Cooking methods like boiling vs. frying
Processing like whole grain vs. refined

Q9. What is Glycemic Load/how does is it different from GI?
GI × Carbohydrate content per serving/100
GI measures quality, and GL considers both quality and quantity of carbohydrates.

Q10. Why is the glycemic index significant in clinical practice?
Aids in diabetes management that is lower GI foods voids glucose spikes.
Weight management that is low GI foods promote satiety.
Decreases risk of CVD/metabolic syndrome.

SPOTTERS

Q1. Plate having white bread, white rice, and glucose solution. What category is this/how it can affect blood glucose?

Glycemic index: High GI foods (≥70). They result in quick increase in blood glucose levels.

Q2. Comparison chart showing apple (GI 36) vs. white bread (GI 75). Which food is better for a patient of diabetes?

Apple is better in comparison to white bread because it has a low GI, resulting in slow/more stable glucose response.

Q3. Graph that shows blood glucose levels over time after having white bread vs. oats. Which food has a higher glycemic index and what is the reason?

White bread has a high GI as it results in sharp glucose spike, and oats results in gradual rise.

Q4. A meal with brown rice, vegetables, and grilled chicken. Is this meal ok for patient of diabetes in terms of GI?

Yes, as brown rice has a low GI in comparison to white rice, and protein/fiber helps slow glucose absorption.

Q5. Label showing calories/gram of macronutrients: Carbs = 4 kcal/g, Proteins = 4 kcal/g, Fats = 9 kcal/g. Which macronutrient gives the highest energy?

Fats (9 kcal/g) give highest energy/gram.

Q6. Image of a nutrition label exhibiting total energy content of 250 kcal/serving. How is this calculated?

By summing up calories from all 3 macronutrients in the food item.

Q7. Graph comparing energy expenditure at rest, lighter activity, and vigorous activity. What is the main source of energy at rest vs. activity?

Rest: Fat oxidation
Activity: Carbohydrates

Q8. Table showing the energy content of different foods like almonds = 579 kcal/100g, banana = 88 kcal/100g. Why do nuts have a higher energy content than fruits?

Nuts are high in fats, that give more energy/gram in comparison to carbohydrates.

REFLECTION

43

CHAPTER

Baseline Diagnostic Prognostic and Discharge Investigations of Clinical Biochemistry

COMPETENCY

BC14.24: Observe and interpret and discuss the baseline diagnostic prognostic and discharge investigations of clinical biochemistry.

LEARNING OBJECTIVES

After reading this chapter, the readers should be able to:

- Understand the baseline diagnostic prognostic and discharge investigations of clinical biochemistry.

BLUE PRINT

To Observe and Interpret Baseline Diagnostic, Prognostic and Discharge Investigations of Clinical Biochemistry

Duration: *60 minutes*

Objectives

By the end of this lesson, learners should be able to:

1. Define baseline, diagnostic, prognostic, and discharge investigations.
2. Differentiate between these investigations.
3. Identify investigations in every category along with examples.
4. Apply in patient management/diagnosis.

Outline

I. **Introduction** **(10 minutes)**
- Importance of investigations in clinical practice.
- Overview of different categories:
  - Baseline investigations—early patient assessment.
  - Diagnostic investigations—confirm a disease.
  - Prognostic investigations—for predicting disease course and outcomes.
  - Discharge investigations—ensuring proper health of patient before discharging.

II. **Baseline investigations** **(10 minutes)**
- *Definition*: Routine tests done on admission to assess the patient's general health status.
- *Examples*:
  - Complete blood count for detection of anemia/infections
  - Renal function tests for baseline kidney status.
  - Liver function tests for baseline liver status.
  - Random blood sugar for detecting undiagnosed diabetes.
  - Electrocardiogram for baseline cardiac status.
- *Clinical importance*: Guide management.

III. **Diagnostic investigations** **(10–15 minutes)**
- Tests performed to confirm or rule out a suspected diagnosis.
- *Infectious diseases*: Blood cultures, PCR for TB, COVID-19 RT-PCR.

- *Cardiovascular*: Troponin I/T for MI, echocardiography.
- *Respiratory*: Chest X-ray/Pulmonary function tests
- *Neurology*: CT/MRI-stroke, EEG-epilepsy.
- *Case-based discussion*: Given a clinical scenario like fever, chest pain, students suggest appropriate diagnostic tests.

IV. **Prognostic investigations** **(10 minutes)**
- *Definition*: Tests that predict disease progression and long-term outcomes.
    - D-dimer/BNP—heart failure.
    - HbA1c—diabetes for long-term control.
    - Tumor markers like CEA/AFP—cancer prognosis.
    - CD4 count—HIV for disease progression.
- *Clinical importance*: Aids in monitoring, advising treatment intensity/counselling patients.

V. **Discharge investigations** **(10 minutes)**
- *Definition*: Tests performed before discharging a patient for ensuring stability for home care.
    - Hb levels in post-surgery patients.
    - Electrolytes and RFT in dehydrated patients.
    - Chest X-ray for post-pneumonia treatment.
    - INR/PT for anticoagulation therapy patients.
- *Significance*: Avids re-admission, ensures safe transition from hospital to home care.

Assessment and Review **(10 minutes)**

Quick Quiz

Conclusion and Take-Home Message **(5 minutes)**

BASELINE DIAGNOSTIC INVESTIGATIONS

Diagnostic Investigations

In today's world of clinical practice, diagnostic investigations are extremely fundamental in order to detect as well as identify various diseases, understanding the nature of these disorders, and starting appropriate treatments and therapies.

These investigations are testing and examining different biological fluids, tissues, and enzymatic biomarkers which can reflect the underlying pathological conditions and states.

Blood Glucose

Blood glucose levels are measured for identifying states and conditions like diabetes mellitus and hypoglycemia. There are some routine investigations like fasting blood glucose, postprandial glucose, and HbA1c. This aids in diagnosing diabetes and also in assessing its regulation and control. An HbA1c level of more than 6.5% typically has an indication towards diabetes, while if the values fall between 5.7% and 6.4%, this can suggest pre-diabetic states. Blood glucose investigation is mandatory to monitor the response to treatment as well as therapies along with preventing side effects and complications such as diabetic retinopathy and nephropathy.

Liver Function Tests (LFTs)

Liver function tests are a group of blood investigations required for assessing the liver's health and condition by measuring enzymes, proteins, and other substances that are processed by the liver.

There are some primary markers that include:
- ALT (Alanine Aminotransferase) and AST (Aspartate Aminotransferase), that are enzymes released when the hepatocytes get damaged.
- ALP (Alkaline Phosphatase), that may be higher side and elevated in conditions like obstruction of the bile duct or liver tumors.
- Bilirubin levels aid in detecting conditions like jaundice, liver disease, or bile duct obstructions and blockages.
- Elevated liver enzymes may indicate towards hepatitis, cirrhosis, liver damage, or biliary obstructions.

Kidney Function Tests (KFTs)

Kidney function is assessed by investigations like serum creatinine, BUN (blood urea nitrogen), and the calculated GFR (glomerular filtration rate). These investigations become crucial in order to diagnose as well as monitor conditions such as acute kidney injury (AKI) or chronic kidney disease (CKD).

The investigations of creatinine levels are a direct marker of renal functions, and increased levels of this parameter indicate reduced renal clearance.

BUN levels elevate when kidney functions declines.

GFR is required for estimating filtration ability of the kidney along with classifying the stages of kidney disease.

Complete Blood Count (CBC)

The CBC measures various components of the blood, like red blood cells (RBCs), white blood cells (WBCs), platelets, hemoglobin, and hematocrit. Abnormal results might indicate a different and wide range of states and conditions, like anemia, infections, leukemia, and bleeding disorders.

Hemoglobin levels aid in diagnosing anemia, while WBC counts can reveal any infection, inflammation, or immune response.

Platelet counts are significant to assess clotting functions.

Electrolyte Panel

Electrolytes like sodium, potassium, chloride, and bicarbonate are extremely vital to maintain fluid balance, nerve functions, along with muscle contractions. Abnormal levels may indicate states of dehydration, kidney dysfunctioning, heart abnormalities, or hormonal imbalances and disorders. For example low levels of potassium (hypokalemia) can result in muscle weakness and arrhythmias, while elevated levels of potassium (hyperkalemia) can lead to many life-threatening heart rhythms.

Lipid Profile

The lipid profile measurement includes measurements of total cholesterol, LDL (low-density lipoprotein), HDL (high-density lipoprotein), and triglycerides. High and elevated LDL cholesterol and triglycerides are important major risk factors of CVD that is cardiovascular diseases, along with atherosclerosis, stroke, and coronary artery disease. A well regulated lipid profile helps in assessing the different risks of heart diseases and also guides therapeutic interventions, like lifestyle modifications and statin therapies.

Prognostic Investigations

Prognostic investigations give an insight into the very likely course and outcomes of disorders. These investigations are made use of in order to predict the progression, severity, and complications that are associated with specific states. Prognostic investigations also are significant in decision-making for planning treatment strategies, identifying patients who might be benefited from early interventions.

Tumor Markers

Tumor markers are the substances that are found in the blood, urine, or tissues that might indicate the presence of malignancy. They are not always specific to cancer, but they can be helpful in assessing the prognosis, track disease progression, and also monitor the effectiveness of the treatment.

PSA (prostate-specific antigen): Elevated PSA levels in men can indicate prostate cancer or benign prostatic hyperplasia.

CA-125: This marker is increased in condition like ovarian cancer and can aid in monitoring treatment response.

CEA (carcino-embryonic antigen): Elevated levels of CEA might indicate colorectal cancer, pancreatic cancer, or other malignancies.

C-Reactive Protein (CRP)

CRP is an acute-phase reactant formed by the liver in response to inflammation. It is a key marker to monitor the activity of inflammatory disorders such as rheumatoid arthritis, inflammatory bowel disease (IBD), and systemic lupus erythematosus (SLE). High CRP levels may suggest ongoing inflammation and are helpful for assessing the risk of cardiovascular events and complications in different conditions.

B-Type Natriuretic Peptide (BNP)

BNP is a peptide released by the ventricles of the heart in response to stress, like in heart failure. Elevated level of BNP indicates the severity of heart failure along with helping in predicting the prognosis. BNP levels are key for distinguishing between cardiac and non-cardiac reasons of shortness of breath and to assess the patient's risk of hospitalization or death because of heart failure.

Procalcitonin (PCT)

Procalcitonin is a precursor of the hormone calcitonin. It is produced in response to bacterial infections, specifically sepsis. It is highly sensitive and specific for bacterial infections, aids in distinguishing them from viral infections. High levels of PCT indicate a severe bacterial infection, and monitoring levels can also guide the duration of antibiotic therapy.

HbA1c

For diabetic patients, HbA1c investigation is very critical prognostic tool. It can measure the average blood glucose level over the previous two to three months. An elevated HbA1c is associated with an increased risk of diabetes and its related complications, like neuropathy, retinopathy, and cardiovascular disease. If we keep HbA1c within target ranges then this will help in reducing long-term complications.

Arterial Blood Gases (ABGs)

ABGs give information on a patient's acid-base regulation, oxygenation status, and levels of carbon dioxide. This is specifically valuable for assessing respiratory and metabolic states like COPD, asthma, diabetic ketoacidosis, or respiratory failure. ABG abnormalities might predict complications and also guide interventions like oxygen therapy/mechanical ventilation.

Discharging Investigations

Before we discharge a patient from the hospital, various investigations are done for ensuring the patient has stabilized and is also fit for discharge. These investigations are a key and are important to confirm that the patient is now no longer at risk for getting any complications and that they are also ready for outpatient care.

Renal Function Tests (for patients with kidney conditions)

For patients who recovered from kidney-related issues, it is very vital to assess renal functions before their discharge. Serum creatinine, BUN, and GFR are re-evaluated before their discharge to confirm that renal functions have improved and are stable. If these tests show worsening renal functions, further treatment or prolonged hospitalization might be required and necessary.

Cardiac Biomarkers

In patients who have recovered from a myocardial infarction (MI) or other cardiac events, cardiac biomarkers like troponin I/T and CK-MB are tested for assessing whether the heart muscles have been sufficiently repaired properly. Normalization of troponin ranges suggests that the further risk of heart damage is less, making discharge safer.

Coagulation Profile

Patients who have undergone surgery or are on anticoagulation therapies are investigated for their coagulation condition and status before their discharge. A prothrombin time (PT), international normalized ratio (INR), and activated partial thromboplastin time (a PTT) are a key for ensuring that bleeding risks are minimized or not. Proper anticoagulation levels aids in preventing clotting disorders, like deep vein thrombosis (DVT) or pulmonary embolism (PE).

Liver and Renal Function Tests

Patients with liver and kidney disorders like cirrhosis, hepatitis, or those patients who were on nephrotoxic drugs, require regular monitoring of liver and kidney function markers. Improved and stable functions on discharge reduce the risk of long-term damages along with facilitating the transition to outpatient care.

Complete Blood Count (CBC)

A CBC is done before discharge for ensuring that the patient's hemoglobin and white blood cell count is within the normal limits. A hemoglobin level within normal range is important for post-surgical recovery, and a normal WBC count indicate towards no ongoing infection. This investigation also helps to detect potential bleeding or clotting disorders.

Blood Glucose Monitoring (for Diabetic Patients)

For diabetic patients, blood glucose levels are closely monitored before their discharge. We ensure that the glucose levels are under control and this is important for preventing any post-discharge side effects and like complications, like diabetic ketoacidosis and hypoglycemic episodes.

CONCLUSION

Diagnostic, prognostic, and discharging investigations in clinical biochemistry are key and necessary tools in patient management. Diagnostic tests aids in identifying diseases, while prognostic tests predict outcomes and also guide treatment strategies. Discharging investigations confirm recovery along with assessing readiness for outpatient care. By ensuring accurate and timely biochemical testing, physicians can enhance patient outcomes, reduce hospital readmissions, and also optimize healthcare resources. These investigations when performed appropriately, play a key and pivotal role in modern medical practice and also contribute significantly to personalized patient care and treatment.

OSCE

1. **Scenario: Baseline diagnostic investigation**
   Case: A 47-year-old patient presents with symptoms of fatigue, muscle weakness, and weight loss. The doctor advises baseline lab tests for assessing his full health status as:
   Complete blood count (CBC): Mild anemia (Hb: 10 g/dL)
   Serum electrolytes: Sodium: 137 mEq/L, Potassium: 3.4 mEq/L
   Liver function tests (LFTs): ALT: 21 U/L, AST: 19 U/L, ALP: 91 U/L
   Renal function tests (RFTs): Creatinine: 0.9 mg/dL, Urea: 18 mg/dL
   Question: Based on the baseline results, what are the possible interpretations, and what additional tests would be recommended for further investigation?
   Interpretation:
   The mild anemia indicates potential nutritional deficiency/chronic disease/blood loss.
   Serum electrolytes are normal, suggestive of there are no urgent concerns as far as electrolyte imbalance is concern.
   The Liver Function Tests are in normal limits, indicating no significant liver damage.
   Renal function tests are normal, with no signs and symptoms of renal dysfunction.
   Recommendation for further testing:
   Explore the reason for anemia, further testing such as Iron studies, Vitamin B12, Folate levels might be indicated.
   As patient suffer from fatigue/muscle weakness, an assessment of Thyroid function tests (TSH, T3, T4) must be done.
   HbA1c can be checked for ruling out diabetes.
2. **Scenario: Diagnostic investigation for cardiac symptoms**
   Case: A 56-year-old patient male presents with chest pain along with breath shortness. The doctor suspects of cardiac event. Diagnostic investigations are advised:
   Troponin I: 0.15 ng/mL (Normal range: 0–0.01 ng/mL)
   Creatine Kinase-MB (CK-MB): 50 U/L (Normal range: 0–24 U/L)
   ECG: ST-segment elevation in leads II, III, and aVF
   Question: What does these diagnostic results indicate, and what is the next move for management?
   Interpretation:
   High troponin I levels (0.15 ng/mL, above the normal range) suggest myocardial injury or myocardial infarction (MI).
   High CK-MB (50 U/L) also supports this diagnosis, as CK-MB is a specific marker for cardiac muscle damage.
   The ECG findings of ST-segment elevation in leads II, III, and aVF are peculiar of an acute inferior myocardial infarction.
   Next step in management:
   Immediate treatment in a coronary care unit.
   The patient must get antiplatelet therapy like aspirin/anticoagulants/thrombolytics or proceed to percutaneous coronary intervention if required.
   Repeat Troponin measurements over next 6–12 hours for assessing progress of the myocardial injury.
3. **Scenario: Prognostic investigations in liver disease**
   Case: A patient with cirrhosis presents for routine checkup. The prognostic assessment was done as:
   Serum bilirubin: Total: 3.2 mg/dL (Normal range: 0.2–1.2 mg/dL)
   Albumin: 2.5 g/dL (Normal range: 3.5–5 g/dL)
   Prothrombin time (PT): 17 seconds (Normal range: 11–13 seconds)
   AFP (Alpha-fetoprotein): 50 ng/mL (Normal range: <10 ng/mL)
   Question: What results indicate regarding prognosis of the patient, and what next steps must be taken?
   Interpretation:
   High bilirubin (3.2 mg/dL) suggests impaired liver function and indicates that liver is not properly clearing waste products.
   Low albumin (2.5 g/dL) is indicative of liver synthetic dysfunctioning and is a poor prognostic sign in state of cirrhosis.

The prolonged prothrombin time (PT) (17 seconds) also exhibits liver dysfunction as well as inability to form clotting factors in effective way.
High AFP (50 ng/mL) is suggestive of hepatocellular carcinoma, mainly in the setting of cirrhosis.
Prognosis and next steps:
The patient has advanced liver disorder with possible compensated cirrhosis and must be monitored for development of HCC.
Ultrasound of the liver/CT scan must be done for assessment of liver nodules.
Refer to a liver transplant center to evaluate a liver transplant might be important based on severity of liver failure.

4. **Scenario: Discharging investigation in kidney disease**
Case: A patient with chronic kidney disease has to be discharged following an episode of acute kidney injury). Before discharge lab results:
Serum creatinine: 1.4 mg/dL (Normal range: 0.6–1.2 mg/dL)
Blood urea nitrogen (BUN): 26 mg/dL (Normal range: 7–20 mg/dL)
Urine output: 1.3 L/day (Normal: 1–2 L/day)
Urinalysis: Mild proteinuria (1+)
Question: What is the clinical significance and how to proceed with the discharge plan?
Interpretation:
High serum creatinine/BUN is suggestive of renal dysfunction, though the values are not very high at this stage.
Normal urine output indicates normal functions of kidneys and also at a relatively stable level.
Mild proteinuria suggests some level of kidney damage/glomerular dysfunction.
Discharge planning:
The patient must be discharged with close follow-up for monitoring renal function along with proteinuria states.
The doctor must assess for etiology of kidney disorder along with consideration of more investigations like urinary protein-to-creatinine ratio/renal ultrasound.
Medications for controlling blood pressure like ACE inhibitors/ARBs, can be continued/adjusted as required.
Patient should be educated regarding proper hydration, dietary modifications, and the significance of frequent follow-up to avoid further deterioration of the renal system.

5. **Scenario: Baseline investigations in preoperative assessment**
Case: A 61-year-old patient is scheduled for elective surgery. Baseline tests were done:
CBC: Normal
Serum electrolytes: Sodium: 140 mEq/L, Potassium: 4.2 mEq/L
Liver function tests: Normal
Renal function tests: Serum Creatinine: 1.1 mg/dL
ECG: Normal sinus rhythm
Question: What do these results suggest, and what would you recommend before surgery?
Interpretation:
All baseline lab results are within normal ranges, that suggest that the patient is in good health as far as metabolic/organ function are concerned.
Normal CBC, electrolytes, LFTs, and renal function indicate no significant underlying systemic concerns.
Normal ECG reflects immediate concerns are not needed regarding heart's electrical activity.
Recommendation:
Proceed with surgery as the baseline investigations exhibits no major concerns and complications.
Preoperative clearance must be taken by anesthesiology department for confirming fitness of patient.
Ensure that the patient's medications are reviewed, mainly for patients affecting bleeding time.
The patient must be informed properly regarding postoperative recovery procedure and some needed lifestyle management after surgery.

CLINICAL MCQS

1. **A 51-year-old man shows symptom: Pain in chest. Troponin I: high. What is the main diagnostic significance?**
   a. Acute kidney damage
   b. Myocardial infarction
   c. Pulmonary embolism
   d. Liver dysfunction

   Answer: b. Myocardial infarction

2. **A patient having chronic kidney disease presents with baseline serum creatinine: 2.0 mg/dL. During hospitalization, it rises to 4.0 mg/dL. What does this suggest?**
   a. Acute on chronic kidney injury
   b. Normal variation in kidney function
   c. Liver dysfunctioning
   d. Rhabdomyolysis

   Answer: a. Acute on chronic kidney injury

3. **A 61-year-old woman presents with jaundice. High alanine aminotransferase, aspartate aminotransferase with a normal alkaline phosphatase. What is the most likely reason?**
   a. Acute viral hepatitis
   b. Obstructive jaundice
   c. Hepatitis
   d. Metastatic liver disorder

   Answer: a. Acute viral hepatitis

4. **A patient is admitted in hospital with sepsis. Baseline investigations: Lactate level: 5 mmol/L. What is the clinical interpretation?**
   a. Hypoglycemic condition
   b. Lactic acidosis indicating tissue hypoperfusion
   c. Liver disorder
   d. Electrolyte disturbance

   Answer: b. Lactic acidosis indicating tissue hypoperfusion

5. **A 46-year-old man with a history of diabetes shows symptom of confusion. His baseline glucose: 35 mg/dL. What is the urgent clinical interpretation?**
   a. Hyperglycemic state
   b. Hypoglycemia causing neuroglycopenia
   c. Metabolic/diabetic ketoacidosis
   d. Hyperosmolar hyperglycemic condition

   Answer: b. Hypoglycemia causing neuroglycopenia

6. **A 37-year-old woman with suspected thyroid dysfunction has a TSH level: 0.05 mIU/L, elevated free T3 and T4. What is the clinical interpretation?**
   a. Primary hypothyroidism
   b. Secondary hypothyroidism
   c. Primary hyporthyroidism
   d. Euthyroid sick syndrome

   Answer: c. Primary hypothyroidism

7. **A 66-year-old man with liver cirrhosis was evaluated for prognosis. Serum albumin: 2.5 g/dL, INR: 2.0, bilirubin: 5 mg/dL. Which prognostic score is appropriate?**
   a. MELD score
   b. APACHE II score
   c. CHA2DS2-VASc score
   d. Ranson's criteria

   Answer: a. MELD score

8. **A patient shows symptoms of shortness of breath, edema. Baseline investigations: BNP (B-type natriuretic peptide): 900 pg/mL. What is the clinical interpretation?**
   a. Acute kidney damage
   b. Congestive heart failure
   c. Chronic liver disorder
   d. Pulmonary embolism

   Answer: b. Congestive heart failure

9. **A 71-year-old man with a history of prostate cancer comes for discharge investigations. PSA: Elevated in comparison to baseline. What does this indicate?**
   a. Normal aging
   b. Progression or recurrence of prostate cancer
   c. Chronic prostatitis
   d. UTI

   Answer: b. Progression or recurrence of prostate cancer

10. A patient with chronic obstructive pulmonary disease comes with ABG at discharge as: pH = 7.36, $PaCO_2$ = 55 mmHg, HCO_3^- = 30 mmol/L. What is the clinical interpretation?

a. Respiratory acidosis
b. Compensated respiratory acidosis
c. Metabolic alkalosis
d. Diabetic acidosis

Answer: b. Compensated respiratory acidosis

VIVA VOCE

Q1. What is the difference between diagnostic and prognostic investigations?

....

....

....

Q2. Give two examples of baseline and discharge investigations.

....

....

....

Q3. Why is HbA1c a prognostic test?

....

....

....

SPOTTERS

Baseline Investigations

Q1. A complete blood count: Hb = 12 g/dL, WBC = 7,000/mm^3, platelets = 250,000/mm^3. What category this test belongs to, and what is the reason of its performance?

Baseline investigation: It is at the time of admission for assessing the overall health/detecting anemia/infection,/bleeding tendencies.

Q2. Serum creatinine = 1.2 mg/dL, blood urea nitrogen = 14 mg/dL. Which category it belongs/why is it significant?

Baseline investigation: Aids for evaluating renal function prior to start of any nephrotoxic drugs/procedures.

Diagnostic Investigations

Q3. Chest X-ray exhibiting bilateral infiltrates in case with fever/cough. What is category/what is the likely diagnosis?

Diagnostic investigation: Suggestive of pneumonia, performed for confirmation of the disease.

Q4. Troponin I report exhibiting raised levels in a case having chest pain. What category is this belonging to?

Diagnostic investigation: Confirming acute myocardial infarction

Prognostic Investigations

Q5. HbA1c: 8.6% for diabetic patient. What category is this test falling into, and what does it suggest?

Prognostic investigation: For assessing long-term glucose control in diabetics.

Q6. Brain natriuretic peptide: 801 pg/mL in a heart failure case. What category/why significant?

Prognostic investigation: Raised BNP suggest worsening of condition of heart failure.

Discharge Investigations

Q7. INR = 2.5 in a patient on warfarin therapy prior discharge. What category is this/why is it required?

Discharge investigation: For ensuring therapeutic anticoagulation prior sending the patient to home.

Q8. Serum sodium = 137 mEq/L, potassium = 4.1 mEq/L in a patient recovering from dehydration. What category, and why is it important?

Discharge investigation: For confirming electrolyte stability prior to the discharge.

REFLECTION

Case Scenario: Present a case of a patient and ask the students to properly choose appropriate investigations.

44

CHAPTER

Point-of-Care Testing/ Bedside Testing

COMPETENCIES

BC14.3: Describe the physical properties chemical constituents of normal urine and abnormal constituents of urine and perform urine analysis to determine normal and abnormal constituents including DIPSTICKS method demonstrations.
BC14.7: Perform estimation of glucose by manual or semiautomated analyzer method and demonstrate GLUCOMETER usage and interpretation of results with clinical scenarios.

LEARNING OBJECTIVES

After reading this chapter, the readers should be able to:
- Describe the points of care testing or bedside testing.

BLUE PRINT

Care Testing/Bedside Testing

Duration: *60 minutes*

Objectives

By the end of this lesson, learners should be able to:
1. Define point-of-care testing/its significance.
2. Identify POCT devices/clinical applications.
3. Describe advantages/limitations
4. Explain quality control measures/regulatory considerations
5. Demonstrate uses of POCT devices.

Outline

I. **Introduction** **(5–10 minutes)**
II. **Common POCT devices and their applications** **(10 minutes)**
III. **Advantages and limitations of POCT** **(10 minutes)**
IV. **Quality control and regulatory aspects** **(10 minutes)**
- Importance of calibration/validation of devices
- Adhering to CLIA
- Operator training/proper documentations

V. **Demonstration & hands-on practice** **(15–20 minutes)**

Assessment and Review **(5–10 minutes)**

Quick Quiz

Case scenario discussion: Given a clinical scenario, ask students to decide whether POCT is useful and justify their choice.

Conclusion and take-home message **(5 minutes)**
- POCT is revolutionizing patient care with quick diagnostics.

SPOTTERS

POCT (point-of-care testing)	It is called bedside testing as it refers to clinical laboratory testing done at the bedside of the patient
	There are 2 types of settings where it can be employed:
1. Primary care testing	Home, workplace, clinic, paramedical support vehicle, etc.
2. Secondary care testing	OT, ICU, OPD, emergency wards, etc.
Advantages	• The results are immediately obtained • Turnaround time is decreased as there is minimal time wastage for collection, transportation, reporting, etc. • It is comfortable for the patient as it decreases the stay in the hospital • Sometimes, time is a critical factor for the patients, physicians can start the treatment at their earliest by POCT
POCT system	Some important requirements of this system are: • Simple and flexible menu • Portable instruments, with high data storage facilities • Noninvasive methods should be included • Sample processing should not be present, sample to be used as such • Minimum maintenance, cost effective, reagents should be stable at room temperature
	POCT assays
1. Instrument based	Home blood glucose monitoring system, noninvasive pulse oximetry
2. Noninstrument based	• Enzyme assays, immunoassays, chemical reaction base assays • Sample requirement is minimum • Blood, serum, plasma, CSF, urine, amniotic fluid, saliva can be taken
3. Qualitative	Pregnancy home kit, urinary dip stick for glucose, troponin T test for MI
4. Semi-quantitative	Urinary dipsticks
5. In vivo	Portable X-rays
6. In vitro	Blood glucose, urinary dipsticks
7. Ex vivo	Blood gas analysis
	Urine Dipsticks Test
Principle	• Dry chemistry-based test strip is present • The strip reacts with the sample of urine • There is a color change observed, that we can read visually • The strips can be of 2 types—paper and plastic • Paper strips are specific for 1 test • Plastic strips, having multiple pads each impregnated with specific reagents, can do multiple tests simultaneously • Qualitative strips give a + or–results • Semi-quantitative strips give results as 1+, 2+, 3+ or 4+ giving an approximate concentration of the parameter
1. Glucose estimation by urinary dipstick test	Based on glucose oxidase method
2. Ketone bodies estimation by urinary dipstick method	Sodium nitroprusside + acetoacetic acid in alkaline medium by ammonia forms purple color complex
3. Bilirubin estimation by urinary dipstick method	Diazotization reaction: Bilirubin + diazonium salt (2,4 dichloraniline) in acid medium to form a pink color azo dye
4. Urobilinogen estimation by urinary dipstick method	Based on Ehrlich's reaction where UBG + diethylaminobenzaldehyde in acid medium to form a pink color complex

Contd....

Contd....

5. Proteins	• The pads of strips have tetrabromophenol blue in acid buffer to maintain the pH • When the proteins are absent, at a pH of 5, indicator appear yellow, and then with the increasing concentration of protein, the color changes to different shades of green and then finally blue • The color of the indicators change due to transfer of protons from the indicator to the protein
6. Detection of nitrites in urine infections caused by nitrite forming organisms, such as *E. coli*	–
7. pH	• Needs fresh voided midstream sample • Measures pH in the range of 5–9 • Uses 2 indicators • For pH range 4–6–methyl red (color changes from red to yellow) • For pH range 6–9–bromothymol blue (color changes from yellow to green and dark blue)
8. Specific gravity	• Strip has poly methyl vinyl ether Maleic anhydride in basic medium • It ionizes and form protons in proportion to the number of cations present in the sample • The more the cations, more are the protons liberated, and that we can detect by bromothymol blue • Color varies from dark blue (specific gravity—1.000) to yellow (specific gravity—1.030)
9. Blood	Red color is got
10. Intact RBC's	Microscopically
11. Hb	• Pseudoperoxidase reaction • There is peroxidase activity associated with heme proteins, such as Hb and Mb, thus heme of both of them catalyze the oxidation of tetramethylbenzidine to form a colored oxidized chromogen • Two color charts are given for free Hb and Mb detection • Negative result is shown by tallow color, and green blue color shows strong positive result • Results are given as traces, 1+, 2+, etc.

	Blood glucose estimation by glucometer
Sample	Freshly taken arterial capillary blood got from finger tip
Strip contains	Enzyme-based assay technique—glucose oxidase method
Result	Reflectance photometry: Displays on a recalibrated device
Calibration/quality assurance	There is a bar code, precaution should be taken to use the strip of recommended bar code within the expiry date
Advantages	This method can estimate 10 mg% to 500 mg% blood sugar and the sample required is 0.5–1.0 µL, results are available by 10 seconds

OSCE

1. **Scenario: POCT: Blood glucose monitoring**
   Case: A 57-year-old diabetic patient complains of dizziness, weakness, POCT was ordered for blood glucose monitoring. Result: blood glucose level: 325 mg/dL.
   Question: What is the clinical interpretation what actions can be taken up?
   Interpretation: A blood glucose level of 325 mg/dL is significantly high and elevated, suggestive of hyperglycemia, this might be a result of poorly controlled diabetes/an acute episode such as diabetic ketoacidosis/hyperosmolar hyperglycemic state.
   Immediate actions:
   The patient must be assessed for symptoms of DKA like fruity breath, confusion, dehydration/HHS like altered mental status, extreme thirst.
   Insulin therapy may be needed depending on severity, along with hydration, electrolyte balance management.
   The physician can go for further confirmatory tests such as urine ketones, arterial blood gases, serum electrolytes for a more comprehensive assessment and evaluation.

2. **Scenario: POCT: Rapid antigen detection**
   Case: A 36-year-old patient comes with symptoms of fever, sore throat, cough. The doctor suspects streptococcal pharyngitis and advise a rapid antigen test for group A streptococcus.
   Question: What is the clinical significance of this result, how would it influence the treatment further?
   Interpretation: A positive rapid antigen test result for Group A Streptococcus confirms the presence of bacteria, that is indicative of streptococcal throat infection.
   Treatment:
   The patient must be started on antibiotics, either penicillin/amoxicillin, for treatment of the infection along with preventing side effects and complications like rheumatic fever.
   If the test was negative, a throat culture can be done for confirming the diagnosis, empirical treatment can be considered which is based on the clinical presentation.

3. **Scenario: POCT for pregnancy testing**
   Case: A 29-year-old woman comes with symptoms of missed periods, nausea. She wants to know if she is pregnant. The doctor advises for urine pregnancy test (POCT), which is positive.
   Question: What does this positive test indicate, what further steps can be taken up?
   Interpretation: A positive urine pregnancy test indicates presence of human chorionic gonadotropin, that gets typically elevated in early pregnancy.
   Next steps:
   A blood test for hCG can be ordered for accurate estimation of the pregnancy hormone concentration.
   The patient can be advised an ultrasound for confirming viability of pregnancy and assessing gestational age.
   The doctor can discuss different option, give guidance for prenatal care/potential risk factors on the basis of patient's health.

4. **Scenario: POCT: Coagulation testing**
   Case: A 71-year-old patient having history of atrial fibrillation is going for elective surgery. The doctor advises for bedside prothrombin time international normalized ratio test for assessing patient's anticoagulation status before operation. Result is INR 3.5.
   Question: What does the high INR suggest, and what steps can be taken before the operation?
   Interpretation: An INR of 3.5 is high and indicates that the patient's blood is more prone to bleeding than usual, likely because of over-anticoagulation from warfarin/another anticoagulant.
   Next steps:
   The patient's anticoagulant therapy must be stopped/decreased for some days before the surgery, depending on the kind of anticoagulant and the urgency of the procedure.
   A vitamin K injection might be advised for reversing the effects of warfarin if the INR is very elevated.
   The doctor must monitor INR and observe bleeding risk before going for surgery.

5. **Scenario: POCT: Arterial blood gas**
   Case: A 66-year-old patient having chronic obstructive pulmonary disease has symptoms of shortness of breath. The doctor advises bedside arterial blood gas test to evaluate for oxygenation/acid-base status. The results were:
   pH: 7.32 (Low)
   $PaCO_2$: 55 mm Hg (High)
   PaO_2: 60 mm Hg (Low)
   HCO_3^-: 28 mEq/L (Normal)
   Question: What does ABG suggest, and what interventions are important?
   Interpretation:
   The low pH, high $PaCO_2$ is indicating respiratory acidosis, likely because of CO_2 retention by COPD exacerbation.
   The low PaO_2 indicates hypoxemia/low oxygen levels in the blood, that is consistent with COPD/acute respiratory failure.
   The normal HCO_3^- indicates the kidneys have not yet compensated for the acidotic condition.
   Interventions:
   The patient must receive supplemental oxygen and closely monitored for respiratory failure state
   If required non-invasive positive pressure ventilation like BiPAP might be started for aiding in CO_2 removal and improving the oxygenation.
   Bronchodilators and steroids can be administered for managing COPD exacerbation.

6. **Scenario: POCT: Electrolyte imbalance**
   Case: A 47-year-old patient in the emergency department presents with confusion, muscle weakness, arrhythmias. The doctor advises a POCT for electrolytes:
   Serum sodium: 124 mEq/L (low)
   Serum potassium: 6.3 mEq/L (high)
   Serum calcium: 9.0 mg/dL (normal)
   Question: What does these electrolyte imbalances suggest, and what quick actions are needed?
   Interpretation:
   Low sodium suggest hyponatremia, that may be due to syndrome of inappropriate antidiuretic hormone/renal failure.

High potassium indicates hyperkalemia, that is a dangerous electrolyte disorder observed in renal failure/adrenal insufficiency/use of ACE inhibitors.

Immediate actions:

Correction of both electrolyte imbalances.

Hyperkalemia to be managed immediately with calcium gluconate/sodium bicarbonate/insulin and glucose to shift the potassium into the cells.

Hyponatremia to be corrected slowly because rapid correction can result in central pontine myelinolysis.

Investigate the key reason like kidney function tests/adrenal function tests.

7. **Scenario: POCT: Cholesterol screening**

Case: A 42-year-old male with a family history of heart disorder undergoes a POCT to do cholesterol screening:

Total cholesterol: 243 mg/dL (high)

HDL cholesterol: 32 mg/dL (low)

LDL cholesterol: 161 mg/dL (high)

Triglycerides: 180 mg/dL (normal)

Question: What does this indicate, and what steps should be next?

Interpretation:

Elevated total cholesterol/elevated high LDL cholesterol suggest high risk for atherosclerosis/CVD.

The low HDL cholesterol increases the risk of CVD because HDL is good cholesterol and is protective.

Next steps:

The patient can be advised lifestyle modifications like dietary changes, more physical activity, and stop smoking.

If required statin therapy to decrease LDL cholesterol and decrease cardiovascular risk.

Monitoring/risk stratification, assess blood pressure/diabetes status.

CLINICAL MCQS

1. **What defines point-of-care testing?**
   a. Laboratory testing performed only in central labs
   b. Diagnostic testing performed at or near the site of patient care
   c. Research testing for research reasons
   d. Tests needing complex lab infrastructure

   Answer: b. Diagnostic testing performed at or near the site of patient care

2. **A patient having diabetes mellitus does monitoring of blood glucose by glucometer. Which kind of testing does this represent?**
   a. Point-of-care testing
   b. Diagnostic
   c. Screening
   d. Reference

   Answer: a. Point-of-care testing

3. **What is application of POCT against traditional lab test?**
   a. Higher analytical sensitivity
   b. Reduced cost of consumables
   c. Faster turnaround time for results
   d. Lower training requirements for users

   Answer: c. Faster turnaround time for results

4. **Which is a common quality control measure in POCT?**
   a. Daily calibration of devices using control solutions
   b. Use of manual testing methods
   c. Sending samples to central laboratories for confirmation
   d. Eliminating external quality assurance programs

   Answer: a. Daily calibration of devices using control solutions

5. **A patient shows with symptoms of acute chest pain. A POCT device is taken up for measuring troponin levels at the bedside. What is the advantage?**
   a. Higher specificity for myocardial infarction
   b. Rapid diagnosis for immediate decision-making

c. Elimination of pre-analytical errors
d. Ability to measure all cardiac markers simultaneously

Answer: b. Rapid diagnosis for immediate decision-making

6. **Which is a limitation of POCT in comparison to the traditional lab testing?**
a. POCT is less time-efficient.
b. POCT results are less reliable in all settings.
c. POCT has a higher likelihood of operator-dependent errors.
d. POCT requires more infrastructure than centralized labs.

Answer: c. POCT has a higher likelihood of operator-dependent errors.

7. **Bedside testing of ABG by using portable analyzer is frequently made use in critical care settings. What is a main advantage?**
a. Lower cost compared to lab-based ABG analysis
b. Faster identification of acid-base imbalances
c. Higher precision than centralized testing
d. Reduced need for clinical interpretation

Answer: b. Faster identification of acid-base imbalances

8. **Which bedside test is useful for quick assessment of coagulation status in patient going for surgery?**
a. Activated partial thromboplastin time (aPTT)
b. Prothrombin time (PT)
c. Thromboelastography (TEG)
d. Platelet count

Answer: c. Thromboelastography (TEG)

9. **What is main error linked with glucose meters used in POCT?**
a. Inadequate sample volume
b. Device malfunction
c. Calibration drift
d. Incorrect software configuration

Answer: a. Inadequate sample volume

10. **A lab introduces a POCT device to estimate hemoglobin What is a critical competency for technician to learn?**
a. Proficiency in troubleshooting complex instruments
b. Ability to interpret results in the clinical context
c. Advanced knowledge of laboratory biochemistry
d. Training in chromatography techniques

Answer: b. Ability to interpret results in the clinical context

VIVA VOCE

Q1. Explain about point-of-care testing?
POCT: Medical diagnostic testing done at/near the patient's location, giving quick results for urgent/immediate clinical diagnosis and decision-making.

Q2. What are the advantages of POCT?
Quick turnaround time, immediate clinical decisions, decreased sample transportation requirements, improved interpretations and patient outcomes.

Q3. Name common POCT devices?
Glucometer for blood glucose testing for diabetes management, blood gas analyzers in emergency medicine and ICU, pregnancy test kits, rapid antigen tests like COVID-19 and influenza/portable coagulation analyzers for INR monitoring, cardiac markers like troponin for diagnosis of acute coronary syndrome.

Q4. What are the main challenges in POCT?
Accuracy/reliability issues/require regular calibration/quality control/more costly investigation and potential for user-related errors.

Q5. How is quality control maintained in POCT?
By regular calibration, using control samples, strictly adhering to standardized protocols, operator skill and training, and external quality assurance.

REFLECTION

Appendix

REFERENCE VALUES OF BIOCHEMICAL PARAMETERS

Laboratory parameter	Reference range	Unit
	Diabetes test	
	Blood sugar	
Fasting	70–100	mg%
Post prandial	70–140	mg%
Random	70–130	mg%
	Oral GTT	
Fasting	>92	mg%
One hour	>180	mg%
Two hours	>153	mg%
	HbA1c	
Nondiabetic	<6	%
Excellent control	6–7	%
Good control	7–8	%
Fair control	8–9	%
Poor control	>9	%
	RFT	
Urea	10–45	mg%
Creatinine	0.4–1.2	mg%
	Electrolytes	
Sodium	135–145	mmol/L
Potassium	3.5–5.1	mmol/L
Chloride	97–112	mmol/L
Uric acid	3.5–7.2	mg%
Blood urea nitrogen	6–21	mg%
	LFT	
SGOT	10–45	IU/L
SGPT	10–45	IU/L
Total bilirubin	0.2–1	mg%
Direct bilirubin	0–0.25	mg%
Indirect bilirubin	0–0.75	mg%
ALP	Till 85	IU/L
Total protein	6.6–8.3	g/dL

Contd...

Contd...

Albumin	3.5–5	g/dL
Globulin	2.3–3.5	g/dL
A:G ratio	1.2–1.5	–
	Lipid profile	
Total Cholesterol	120–150	mg%
TG	0–170	mg%
HDL	30–70	mg%
LDL	0–150	mg%
VLDL	0–35	mg%
	Cardiac profile	
CPK Total	46–171	IU/L
CPK-MB	0–25	IU/L
LDH	200–400	IU/L
TROP-T	+/–	–
	Minerals	
Calcium	8–10	mg/dL
Phosphorus	2.5–5.0	mg/dL
Magnesium	1.5–2.6	mg/dL
	PFT	
Amylase	Till 85	IU/L
Lipase	Till 85	IU/L
	Iron profile	
Serum iron (males)	60–160	microg/dL
Serum iron (females)	35–145	microg/dL
Serum iron (new born)	150–220	microg/dL
Ferritin	15–150	ng/mL
Total iron binding capacity	250–400	microg/dL
	Thyroid tests	
T3	0.8–2	ng/mL
T4	4.6–11	mcg/dL
TSH	0.4–4.2	microIU/mL
fT3	2–4	pg/mL
fT4	0.93–1.7	ng/dL
	Tumor markers	
CEA	0–5	ng/mL
PSA	0–4	ng/mL
Cancer antigen 125	0–135	IU/mL
AFP	<8.5	ng/mL
B12 (adults)	200–835	pg/mL
B12 (infants)	160–1300	pg/mL
Vitamin D deficiency	<10	ng/mL
Vitamin D toxicity	>100	ng/mL
Procalcitonin (low risk)	<0.5	ng/mL

Contd...

Contd...

Procalcitonin (high risk)	>2	ng/mL
Parathormone	10–15	pg/mL
CRP	0–10	mg/L
CSF Parameters		
Sugar	50–80	mg/dL
Protein	15–45	mg/dL
Pleural fluid sugar	70–130	mg/dL
Pleural fluid protein	2.5–3.5	g/dL
Urine 24 hour protein	0–150	mg/24 h
Protein creatinine ratio	<0.2	–
Miscellaneous		
LH (males)	3–15	mU/mL
LH (females, follicular)	3–22	mU/mL
FSH (males)	5–15	mU/mL
FSH (females, follicular)	5–20	mU/mL
Prolactin (males)	4.04–15.2	ng/mL
Prolactin (females)	4.79–23.3	ng/mL
Anti mullerian hormone	1–6	ng/mL
Estradiol	21–251	pg/mL
COVID-19 protocol tests: (ROCHE)		
CRP	0–10	mg/L
Serum Ferritin	30–400	ng/L
IL-6	<7	pg/mL
LDH	200–400	U/L
Procalcitonin	<0.5–>2.0 (low risk, high risk)	ng/mL
D dimer	<500	ng/mL

COVID-19 PROGRESSION

Increased WBC, increased neutrophils, decreased lymphocytes, decreased platelets due to bacterial infections, less immunological response and disseminated coagulopathy; blood gases may show abnormality; there may be increased LDH, ALT, AST, total bilirubin, creatinine, urea, troponin (cardiac), D dimer, PT, prolactin, CRP, ferritin, cytokines due to lung injury, liver failure, kidney failure, cardiac failure, blood clotting activation, severe viral infection, inflammation and cytokine storm syndrome; there may be decreased albumin due to improper liver functions.

Index

EU GSPR Authorised Reprsentative
Logos Europe, 9 rue Nicolas Poussin
1700, La Rochelle, France
Phone: +33 (0) 6 67 93 73 78
E-mail: contact@logoseurope.eu

www.ingramcontent.com/pod-product-compliance
Ingram Content Group UK Ltd.
Pitfield, Milton Keynes, MK11 3LW, UK
UKHW051924100926
8556IPUK00021B/1358
9789356960749

U

V

W

X

Z